MW00352539

ULTIMATE GUIDE TO
WEIGHT-FREE EXERCISES

GENERAL DISCLAIMER
The contents of this book are intended to provide useful information to the general public. All materials, including text and images, are for informational purposes only and are not a substitute for medical diagnosis, advice, or treatment for specific medical conditions. All readers should seek expert medical care and consult their own physicians before commencing any regimen for any general or specific health issues. The author and publishers do not recommend or endorse specific treatments, procedures, advice, or other information found in this book and specifically disclaim all responsibility for any and all liability, loss, or risk, personal or otherwise, which is incurred as a consequence, directly or indirectly, of the use or application of any of the material in this publication.

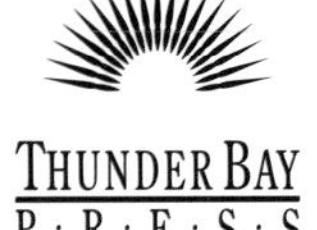

Thunder Bay Press
An imprint of Printers Row Publishing Group
9717 Pacific Heights Blvd, San Diego, CA 92121
www.thunderbaybooks.com • mail@thunderbaybooks.com

All notations of errors or omissions should be addressed to Thunder Bay Press, Editorial Department, at the above address. Author and illustration inquiries should be addressed to Moseley Road Inc., smoore@moseleyroad.com.

Thunder Bay Press
Publisher: Peter Norton
Associate Publisher: Ana Parker
Senior Development Editor: April Graham Farr
Acquisitions Editor: Kathryn C. Dalby
Production Team: Beno Chan, Mimi Oey, Rusty von Dyl

Produced by Moseley Road Inc., www.moseleyroad.com
President: Sean Moore
Art Director: Lisa Purcell
Production Director: Adam Moore
Editor: Finn Moore
Photography: Naila Ruechel. www.nailaruechel.com

Library of Congress Control Number: 2021941108
ISBN: 978-1-64517-914-6

Printed in China

26 25 24 23 22 1 2 3 4 5

ULTIMATE GUIDE TO
WEIGHT-FREE EXERCISES

WITH DETAILED INSTRUCTIONS AND ANATOMICAL ILLUSTRATIONS FOR 154 WEIGHT-FREE EXERCISES

Hollis Liebman, Sophie Cornish-Keefe,
Nancy J. Hajeski, Alex Geissbuhler

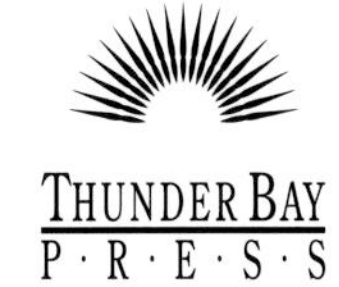

THUNDER BAY
P·R·E·S·S

San Diego, California

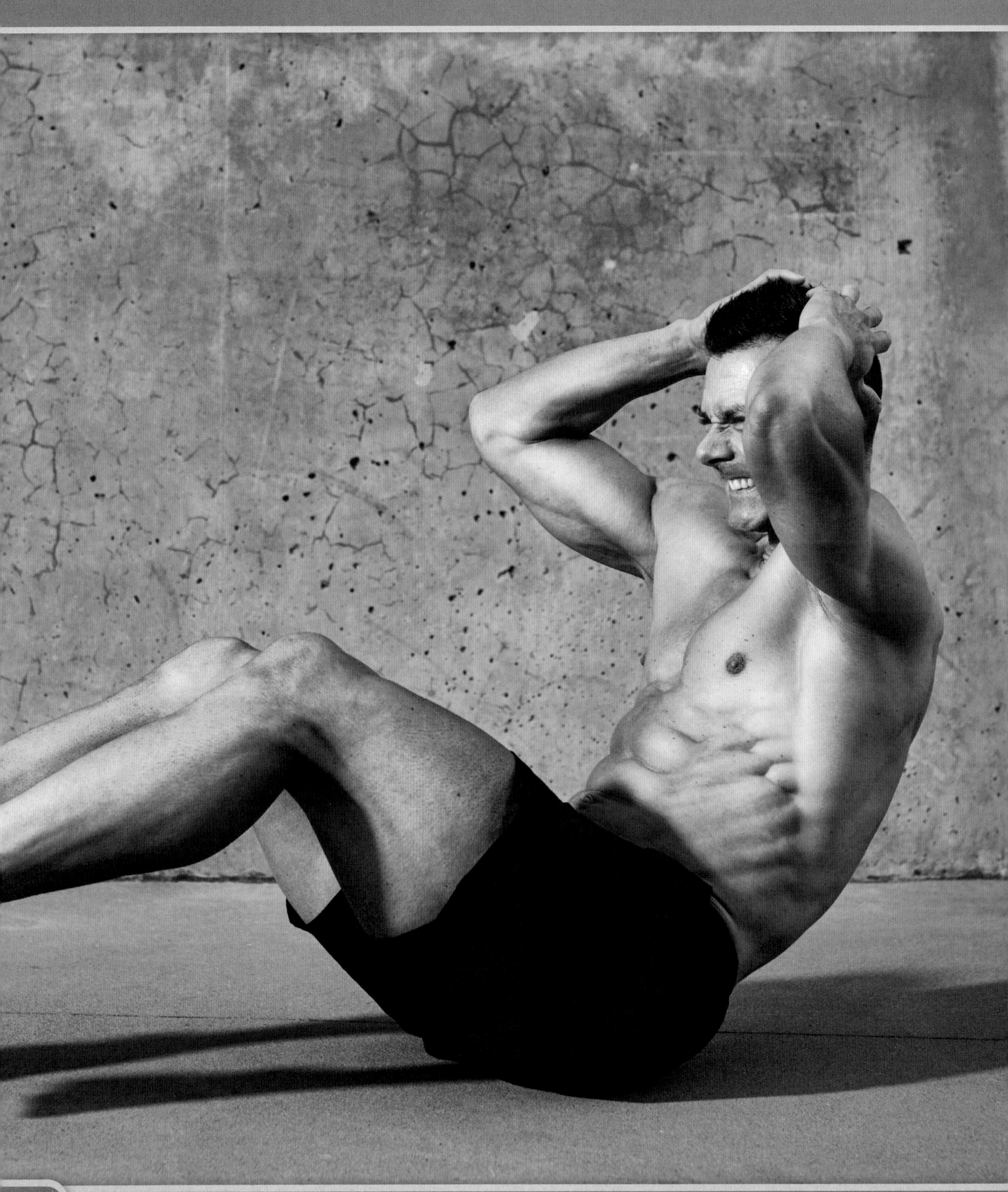

CONTENTS

Who Is Weight-Free For?

Gyms—you either love them or hate them! There are plenty of people out there who need their fix at the gym, and who are motivated by the camaraderie and shared sense of purpose engendered by gyms, but there are far more who are put off by the price of gym membership, the distance to travel to get to the gym, the complexity or limited access to equipment, or who simply don't like the idea of exercising in public—this book is for those people. It is also for all of us who have been spending way more time at home, so being able to work out from home has never been more vital. And for those who travel for work, or for leisure, this book allows you to create a workout that you can perform in your hotel room.

Most of us like the idea of getting fit, or becoming fitter, but it's often just too much effort—there are too many decisions to make—Free weights? Swiss Ball? Resistance bands? And then there's the expense of all that equipment—a pair of dumbbells or kettle bells is one thing, but a treadmill? Or a stationary bike? You'll soon be in second-mortgage territory!

The Ultimate Guide to Weight-Free Exercises addresses all those issues and more, enabling you to create a workout routine tailor-made for your specific requirements, and using just a single piece of equipment that you always have with you—your own body! (OK, a chair and a mat or rug will come in handy too...)

Whether you want to increase strength, build mass, burn fat, or define your muscles (or all of the above), *Ultimate Guide to Weight-Free Exercises* is the authoritative resource for sculpting your physique without free weights, machines, or other equipment.

With full-color anatomical illustrations, step-by-step instructions, and expert training advice, this book is designed to be used by the absolute beginner and be of equal use to a seasoned trainer.

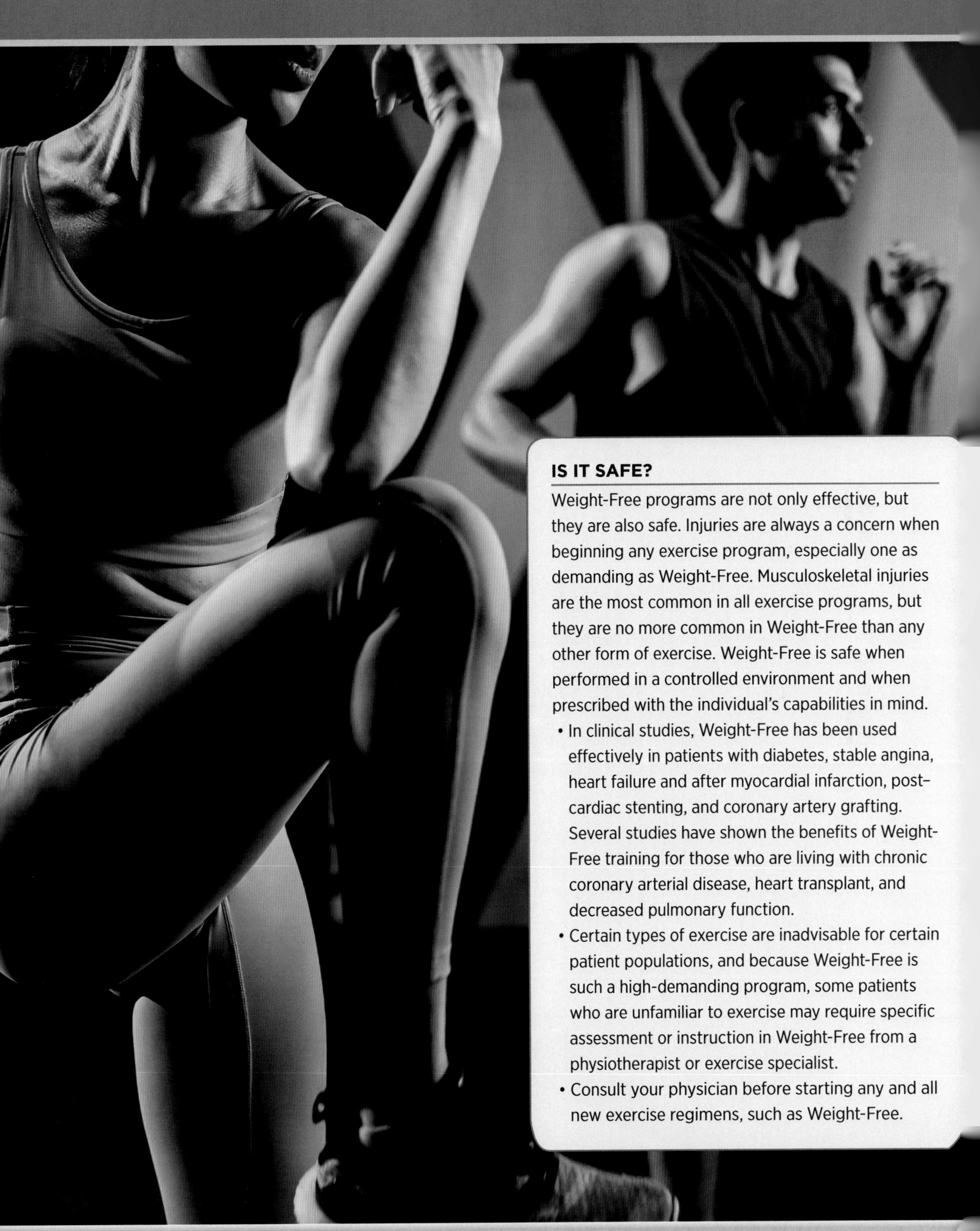

IS IT SAFE?

Weight-Free programs are not only effective, but they are also safe. Injuries are always a concern when beginning any exercise program, especially one as demanding as Weight-Free. Musculoskeletal injuries are the most common in all exercise programs, but they are no more common in Weight-Free than any other form of exercise. Weight-Free is safe when performed in a controlled environment and when prescribed with the individual's capabilities in mind.

- In clinical studies, Weight-Free has been used effectively in patients with diabetes, stable angina, heart failure and after myocardial infarction, post-cardiac stenting, and coronary artery grafting. Several studies have shown the benefits of Weight-Free training for those who are living with chronic coronary arterial disease, heart transplant, and decreased pulmonary function.
- Certain types of exercise are inadvisable for certain patient populations, and because Weight-Free is such a high-demanding program, some patients who are unfamiliar to exercise may require specific assessment or instruction in Weight-Free from a physiotherapist or exercise specialist.
- Consult your physician before starting any and all new exercise regimens, such as Weight-Free.

Total Body Fitness

Structured to target all the muscle zones and primary muscle regions—core, arms, chest, shoulders, back, glutes, thighs, and calves—*Ultimate Guide to Weight-Free Exercises* showcases the most effective exercises that can be performed anytime, anywhere, showing how to combine, modify, and sequence exercises to create the ideal routine, or combination of routines. You will have no excuse not to get into the best shape of your life in the convenience of your own home!

Gyms tend to lean toward increasing strength and bulk—but that's not necessarily the same thing as improving fitness, and unless you're lucky enough to have a personal trainer with you in a gym, there's a likelihood you could do as much damage as good by overstressing joints. *Ultimate Guide to Weight-Free Exercises* shows you how to have perfect form in any given exercise, how to modify it to suit your level of experience or fitness, and how many times you should repeat it for optimal results. Because weight-free exercise, by definition, doesn't use free weights, it involves less joint-stress and instead provides an effective and efficient way to decrease body fat, if that is your intention, increase lean muscle mass, improve endurance, build strength, and it leads to better overall health. In-depth and practical, this book walks you through each exercise with accurate anatomical artwork that displays primary muscles worked along with the utilized ligaments and tendons.

EXERCISE FOR EVERYONE

It doesn't matter how experienced you are, how much time you have, how much money you have, or how much space you have—this book will help you. Experience? As stated above this book can be used by beginners and experts. Time? You can adjust the workout routines to suit your own needs, whether it's a quick five-minute high-intensity routine, or a thorough one-hour workout. Money? You don't need any—with the aid of this book, all you need is you! Space? You could perform most of the exercises in an eight-foot cube. Whether you are just beginning your path to a better body or looking for a routine for training at home or on the road, *Ultimate Guide to Weight-Free Exercises* is the book you need.

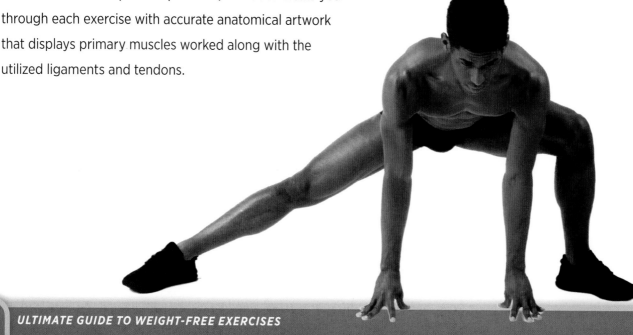

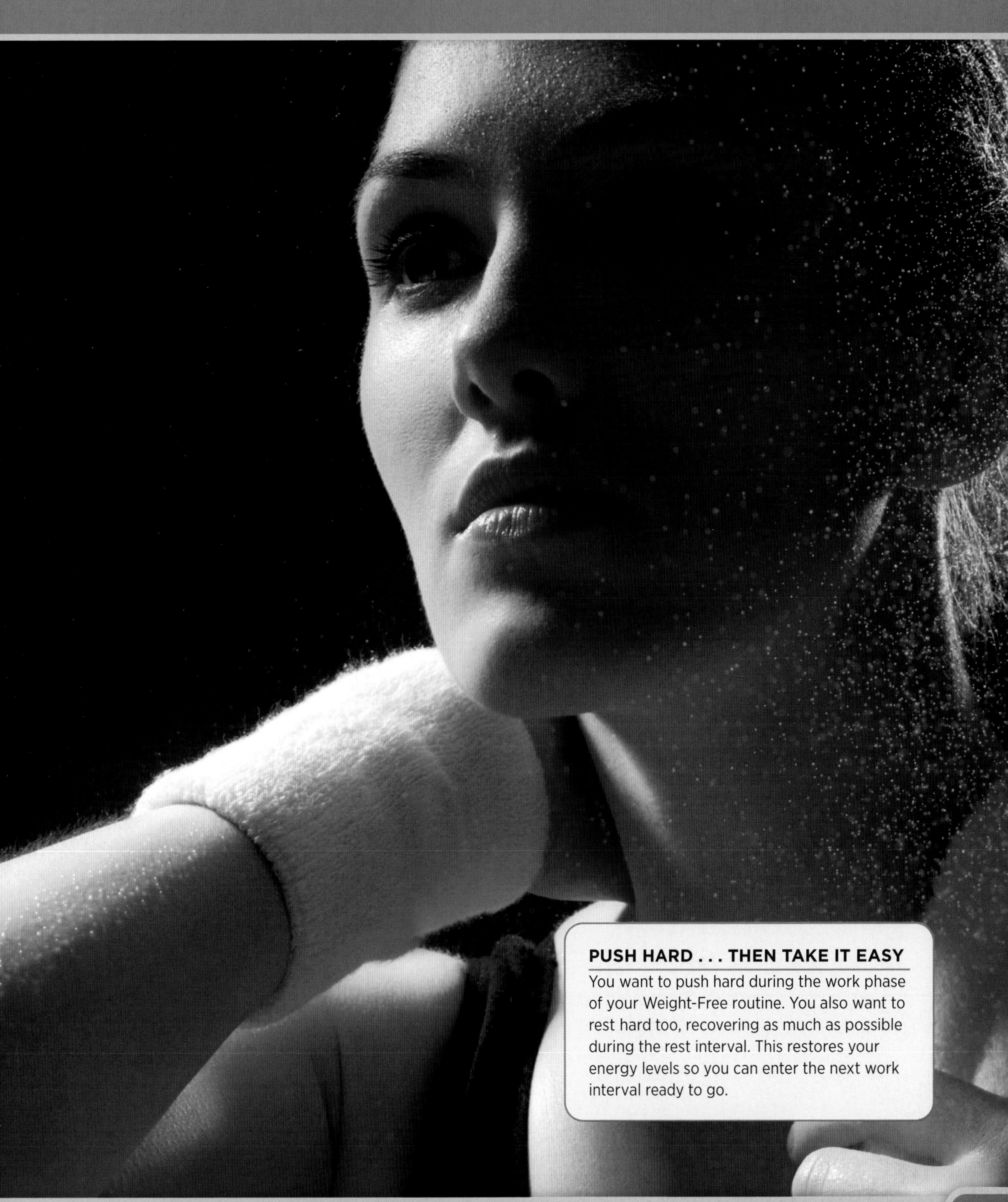

PUSH HARD . . . THEN TAKE IT EASY

You want to push hard during the work phase of your Weight-Free routine. You also want to rest hard too, recovering as much as possible during the rest interval. This restores your energy levels so you can enter the next work interval ready to go.

Weight-Free exercise has been shown to be superior for weight loss in comparison with steady-state aerobic exercise. The weight loss that comes from Weight-Free routines substantially reduces subcutaneous body fat (the fat that sits under the skin) rather than the visceral fat, which surrounds the organs. A Weight-Free program significantly increases the total caloric burn and fat breakdown, compared with spending hours on a treadmill.

HOW TO CREATE A WEIGHT-FREE ROUTINE

For Weight-Free routines, there is no specific number of repetitions or sets to accomplish. Instead, you'll use time as the foundation for building your program. Begin with the total amount of time you will give to a circuit—anything from 5 minutes to an hour. Then, depending on your fitness level, separate that total time into the appropriate work/rest ratio for your fitness level. Consider the complexity of the movements you are performing: for example, compound, complicated exercises may require more time to complete repetitions than relatively simple, quick movements. Resistance can also have an effect, with increased demand also requiring increased work time, as well as rest. You can adjust the resistance or complexity of movements, as well as the work interval, to craft a workout for a desired result.

If your desired outcome is power, for example, a repetition range to strive for is 1 to 3 repetitions to be completed within one work interval. With this example, you would choose an appropriate exercise that is challenging enough so that you can perform it only 1 to 3 times within the work interval. You can lower the intensity if your goal is either hypertrophy or endurance.

On the opposite page are sample charts to help you understand how to create your own Weight-Free routines. Chart A, at right, displays the appropriate repetition range for the desired fitness outcome. Chart B displays an example of a beginner routine for building muscle.

CHART A—FITNESS OBJECTIVES

OBJECTIVE	DEFINITION	REPETITION RANGE	PERCENTAGE OF MAXIMAL EFFORT
Power	Power is the ability to move weight with speed. This is using maximal strength with explosiveness.	1–3	85%–100%
Strength	Muscular strength is the ability of a muscle or muscle group to exert maximal force against resistance.	4–6	75%–85%
Hypertrophy	Muscle hypertrophy describes the process of muscle building, or the actual increase in size of skeletal muscle through a growth in the size of its component cells.	8–12	60%–75%
Endurance	Muscular endurance is the ability of a muscle to exert submaximal force against resistance for an extended period of time.	15+	< 60%

CHART B—HYPERTROPHY ROUTINE

FITNESS LEVEL: BEGINNER (5 exercises)	WORK/REST INTERVAL (1:3)	TOTAL EXERCISE DURATION	SETS (total rotations of circuit completed)	REPS FOR GOAL: HYPERTROPHY
Body-Weight Routine II 1. Squat 2. Triceps Push-Up 3. Arm Hauler 4. Bench Dip 5. Bent-Knee Sit-Up	20 seconds of work: 1 minute of rest	40 minutes	6	8–12 repetitions performed during work interval

How to Use This Book

Ultimate Guide to Weight-Free Exercises features step-by-step instructions to 170 exercises specially selected to fit into a multiplicity of different training regimen.

For each pose, you'll find a short overview of the position, photos with step-by-step instructions, tips on proper form, and anatomical illustrations that highlight the targeted muscles. A quick-read panel features key points.

CHAPTER BREAKDOWNS

Chapter One: Stretches. Here you will find a selection of exercises that you can perform before or after your full Weight-Free routine.

Chapter Two: Balance/Yoga. These yoga-based exercises are good for improving balance, strength and relaxation.

Chapter Three: Cardio. Cardio exercise plays a vital role in how effective our workout routines are.

Chapter Four: Back. Strengthening your back muscles can help prevent injuries and ensure that your entire body works smoothly during daily movement.

Chapter Five: Arms and Shoulders. Muscles essential in pushing, pulling and lifting, and therefore in most everyday activities.

Chapter Six: Chest. Chest exercises help to diminish the pressure, stress and tension on and around the bones and muscles in the chest area.

Chapter Seven: Core. Core exercises train the muscles in your abdomen, lower back, pelvis, and hips to work in harmony, improving balance and stability.

Chapter Eight: Legs. Leg workouts can help you to better engage in cardiovascular exercise and lifting, as stronger legs results in better endurance and core strength.

Chapter Nine: Total Body. These more challenging exercises incorporate a full range of movement, working out the whole body.

Chapter Ten: Workout Routines. Once you've familiarized yourself with the featured exercises, turn to this chapter to learn how to put them together in targeted Weight-Free routines.

KEY

EXERCISE SPREADS

1. **Category**
   Gives the overall body areas targeted: your back, arms, chest, core, legs, or total body.
2. **Exercise Info**
   Gives the name of the exercise and some key details you need to know about it.
3. **How to Do It**
   Step-by-step instructions detailing how to perform the exercise.
4. **Step-by-Step Photos**
   Images of the key steps to the exercise.
5. **Do It Right**
   Tips to help you perfect your form.
6. **Fact File**
   A quick list of key facts: the exercise's main targets, equipment needed to perform it, its principal benefits, and any cautions that may apply.
7. **Anatomical Illustration**
   Highlights the key working muscles. May also include an inset showing muscles not illustrated in the main image.

WORKOUT SPREADS

1. **Routine Info**
   Gives the name of the routine and some key details you need to know about it.
2. **Exercise Info**
   Listed in the order you perform each exercise; shows the name, page number to find it, and how many repetitions to perform.
3. **Photo Icon**
   A quick view of the exercise.
4. **Fact File**
   A quick list of key facts about the routine: its level of difficulty, its objective, the work/rest ratio, and how long it takes.

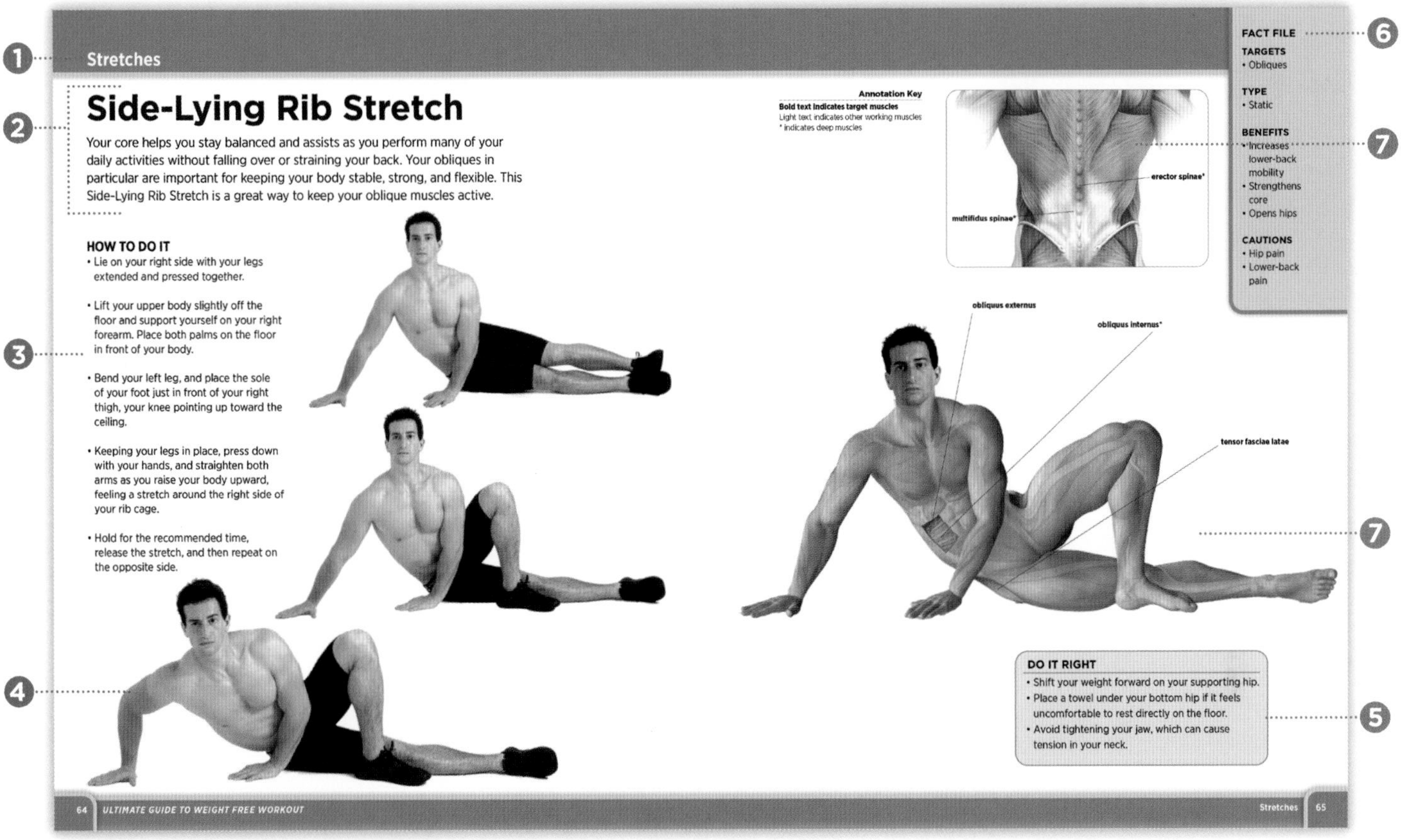

1 Stretches

2 Side-Lying Rib Stretch

Your core helps you stay balanced and assists as you perform many of your daily activities without falling over or straining your back. Your obliques in particular are important for keeping your body stable, strong, and flexible. This Side-Lying Rib Stretch is a great way to keep your oblique muscles active.

HOW TO DO IT

3
- Lie on your right side with your legs extended and pressed together.
- Lift your upper body slightly off the floor and support yourself on your right forearm. Place both palms on the floor in front of your body.
- Bend your left leg, and place the sole of your foot just in front of your right thigh, your knee pointing up toward the ceiling.
- Keeping your legs in place, press down with your hands, and straighten both arms as you raise your body upward, feeling a stretch around the right side of your rib cage.
- Hold for the recommended time, release the stretch, and then repeat on the opposite side.

4

Annotation Key
Bold text indicates target muscles
Light text indicates other working muscles
* indicates deep muscles

7

FACT FILE 6

TARGETS
- Obliques

TYPE
- Static

BENEFITS 7
- Increases lower-back mobility
- Strengthens core
- Opens hips

CAUTIONS
- Hip pain
- Lower-back pain

DO IT RIGHT 5
- Shift your weight forward on your supporting hip.
- Place a towel under your bottom hip if it feels uncomfortable to rest directly on the floor.
- Avoid tightening your jaw, which can cause tension in your neck.

64 ULTIMATE GUIDE TO WEIGHT FREE WORKOUT

Stretches 65

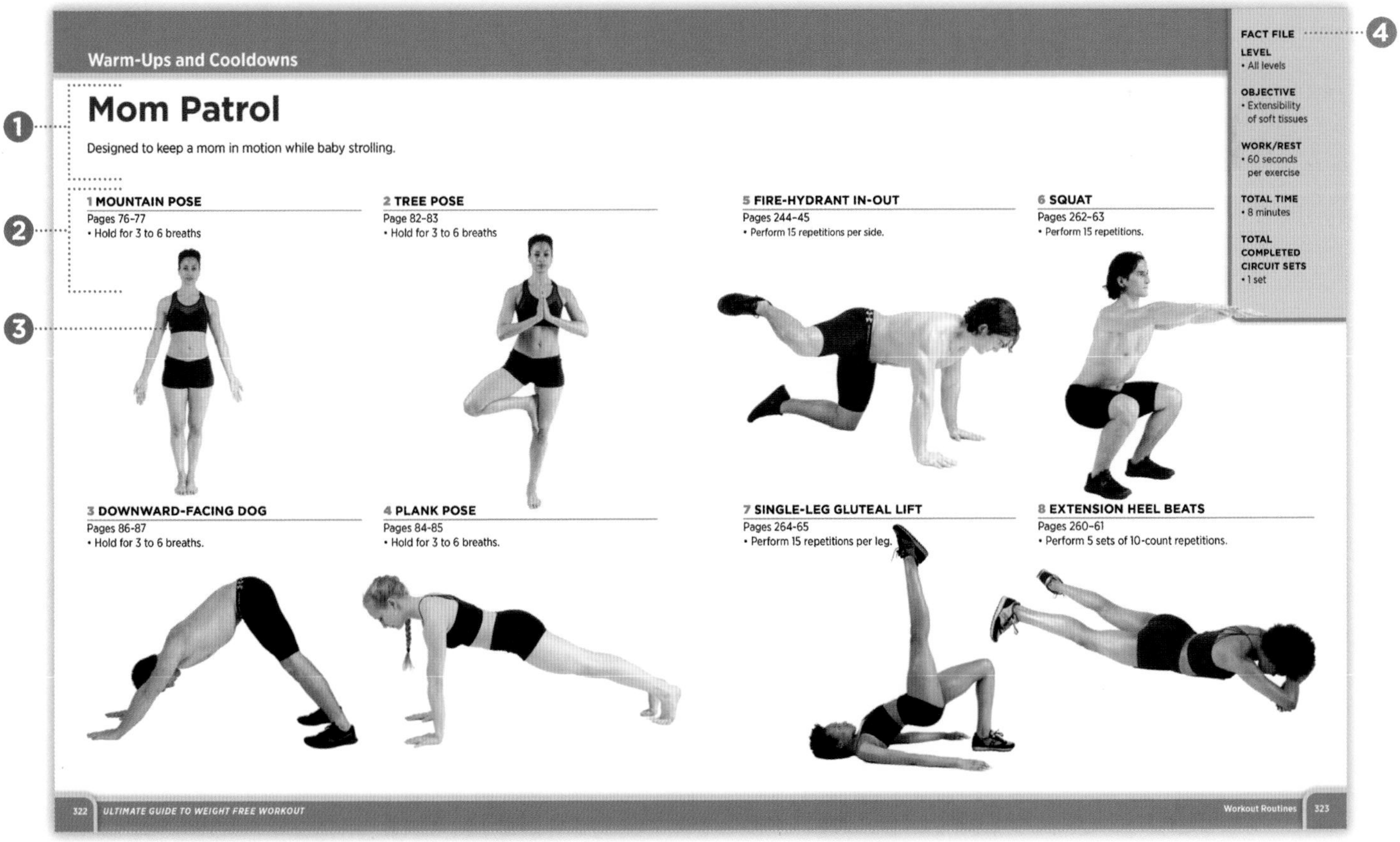

Warm-Ups and Cooldowns

1 Mom Patrol

Designed to keep a mom in motion while baby strolling.

2 **1 MOUNTAIN POSE**
Pages 76–77
- Hold for 3 to 6 breaths

3

2 TREE POSE
Page 82–83
- Hold for 3 to 6 breaths

3 DOWNWARD-FACING DOG
Pages 86-87
- Hold for 3 to 6 breaths.

4 PLANK POSE
Pages 84-85
- Hold for 3 to 6 breaths.

5 FIRE-HYDRANT IN-OUT
Pages 244–45
- Perform 15 repetitions per side.

6 SQUAT
Pages 262–63
- Perform 15 repetitions.

7 SINGLE-LEG GLUTEAL LIFT
Pages 264-65
- Perform 15 repetitions per leg.

8 EXTENSION HEEL BEATS
Pages 260–61
- Perform 5 sets of 10-count repetitions.

FACT FILE 4

LEVEL
- All levels

OBJECTIVE
- Extensibility of soft tissues

WORK/REST
- 60 seconds per exercise

TOTAL TIME
- 8 minutes

TOTAL COMPLETED CIRCUIT SETS
- 1 set

322 ULTIMATE GUIDE TO WEIGHT FREE WORKOUT

Workout Routines 323

Full-Body Anatomy

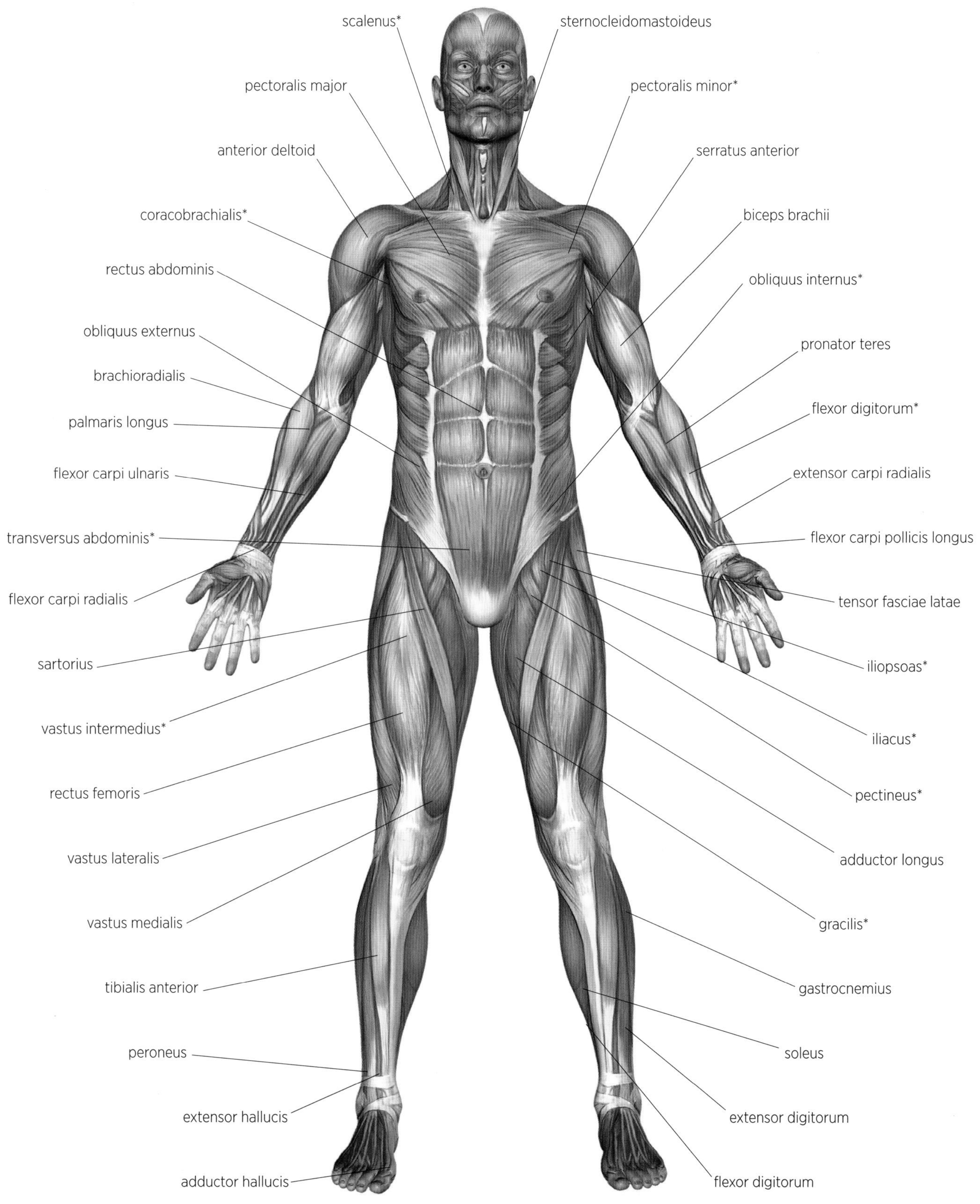
scalenus*
sternocleidomastoideus
pectoralis major
pectoralis minor*
anterior deltoid
serratus anterior
coracobrachialis*
biceps brachii
rectus abdominis
obliquus internus*
obliquus externus
pronator teres
brachioradialis
palmaris longus
flexor digitorum*
flexor carpi ulnaris
extensor carpi radialis
transversus abdominis*
flexor carpi pollicis longus
flexor carpi radialis
tensor fasciae latae
sartorius
iliopsoas*
vastus intermedius*
iliacus*
rectus femoris
pectineus*
vastus lateralis
adductor longus
vastus medialis
gracilis*
tibialis anterior
gastrocnemius
peroneus
soleus
extensor hallucis
extensor digitorum
adductor hallucis
flexor digitorum

Annotation Key
* indicates deep muscles

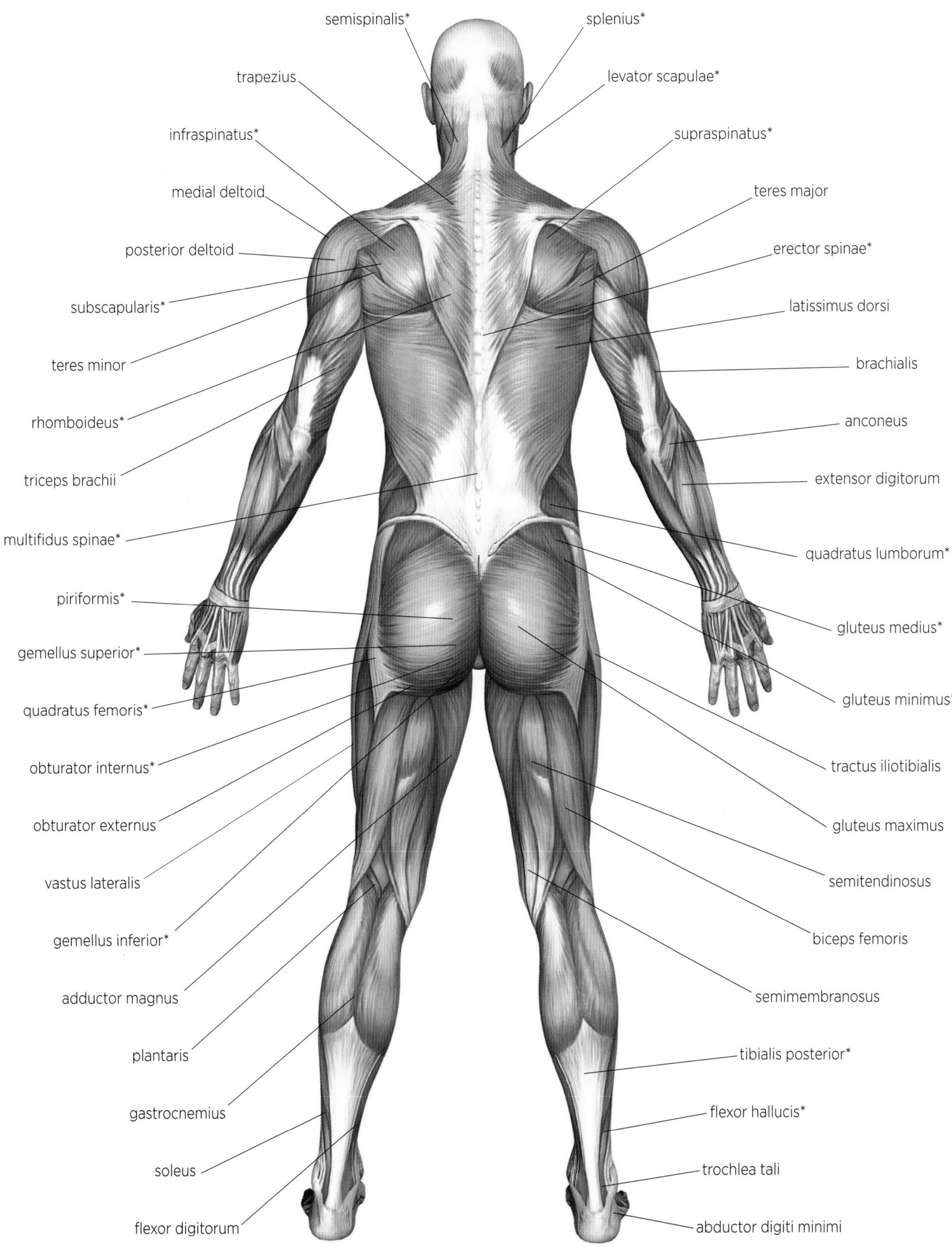
semispinalis*
splenius*
trapezius
levator scapulae*
infraspinatus*
supraspinatus*
medial deltoid
teres major
posterior deltoid
erector spinae*
subscapularis*
latissimus dorsi
teres minor
brachialis
rhomboideus*
anconeus
triceps brachii
extensor digitorum
multifidus spinae*
quadratus lumborum*
piriformis*
gluteus medius*
gemellus superior*
gluteus minimus*
quadratus femoris*
tractus iliotibialis
obturator internus*
gluteus maximus
obturator externus
semitendinosus
vastus lateralis
biceps femoris
gemellus inferior*
semimembranosus
adductor magnus
tibialis posterior*
plantaris
flexor hallucis*
gastrocnemius
trochlea tali
soleus
abductor digiti minimi
flexor digitorum

CHAPTER ONE

STRETCHES

Runners know the importance of stretching their legs before and after their endeavors, but the muscles in your shoulders, arms, and upper back benefit greatly from stretching too; these muscles are key to mobility and posture, and are constantly at work, whether you are in motion or sitting still. They are also frequent victims of localized muscle pain, tightness, and discomfort. Regularly performing stretches that target these areas can help improve mobility throughout the whole body, as well as improve overall range-of-motion and physical health.

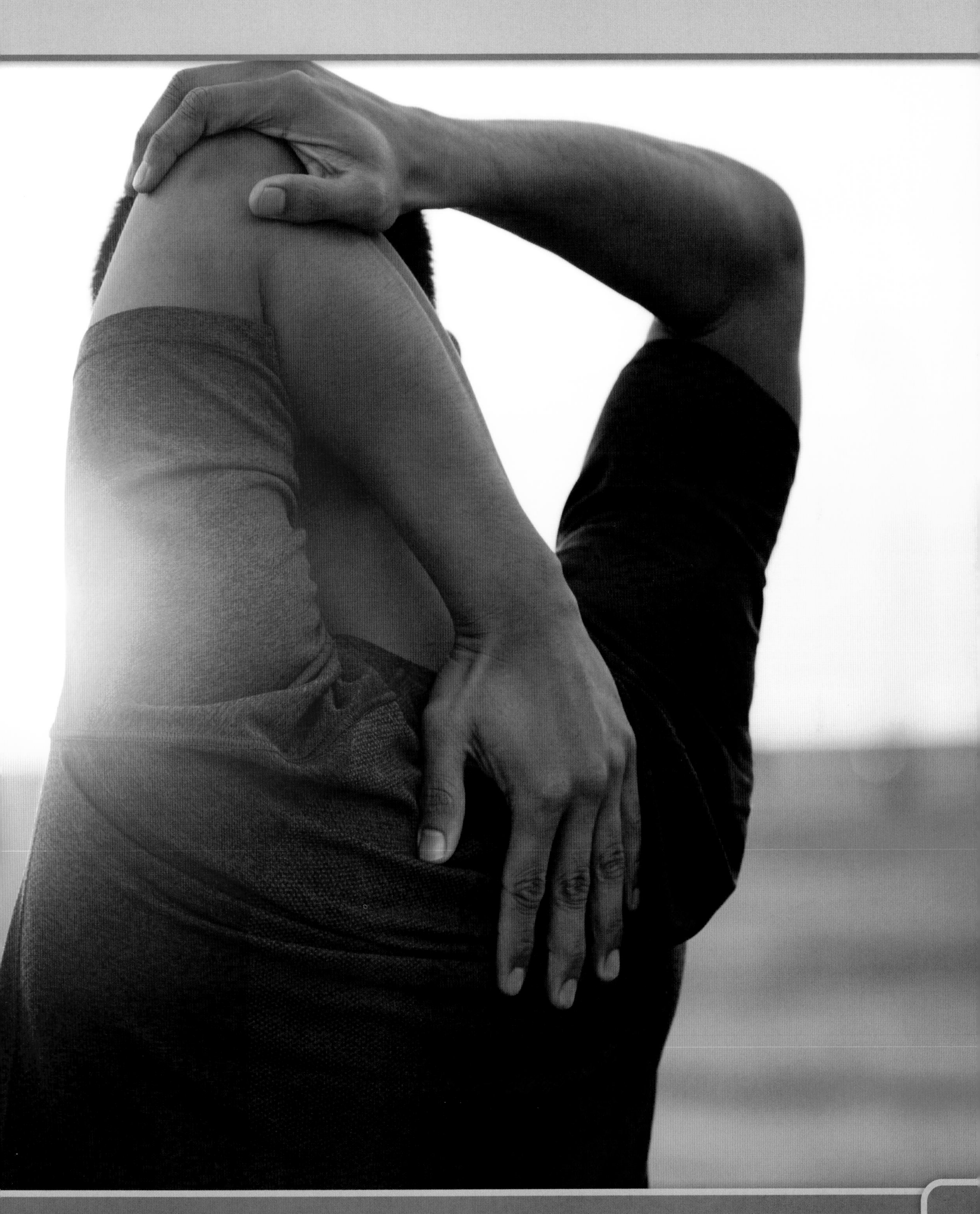

Good Morning Stretch

Perform this invigorating stretch first thing in the morning. It will engage your core and lengthen your spine while relieving any tension in your shoulders and upper back that may result from a bad night's sleep.

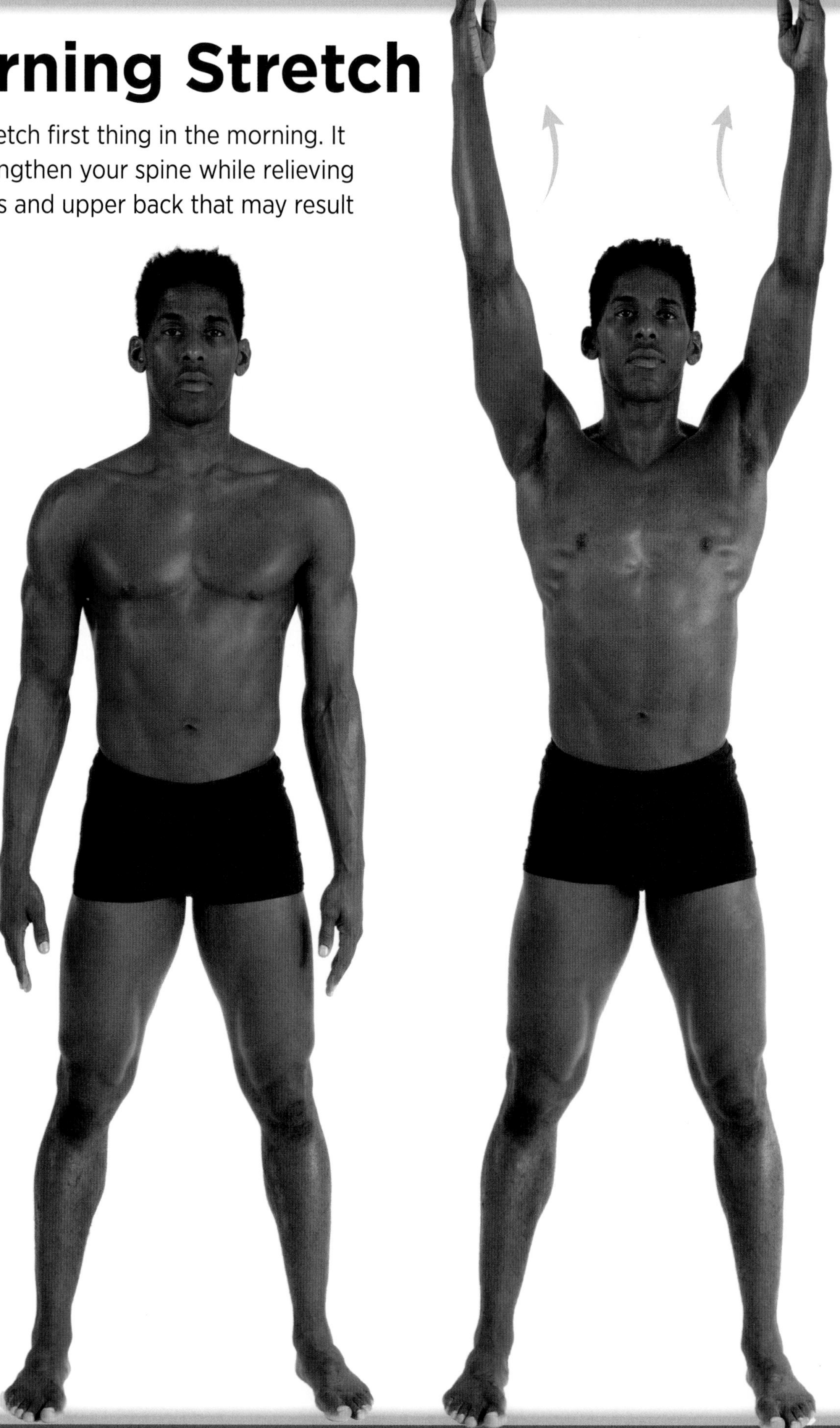

HOW TO DO IT

- Stand with your legs and feet parallel and shoulder-width apart. Bend your knees very slightly, and tuck your pelvis slightly forward.
- Reach your arms up toward the ceiling, keeping them long and in parallel with your body. Focus your energy on the middle of your palms, which should be facing inward, and turn your gaze upward as you stretch.
- Hold for the recommended time, release the stretch, and then repeat for the recommended repetitions.

FACT FILE

TARGETS
- Back
- Neck
- Abdominals
- Obliques
- Palms
- Forearms
- Upper arms

TYPE
- Static

BENEFITS
- Increases upper-back mobility
- Reduces shoulder tightness
- Lengthens spinal column

CAUTIONS
- Neck issues
- Shoulder issues

Annotation Key

Bold text indicates target muscles
Light text indicates other working muscles
* indicates deep muscles

splenius*
levator scapulae*
trapezius
brachialis
brachioradialis
rhomboideus*
latissimus dorsi

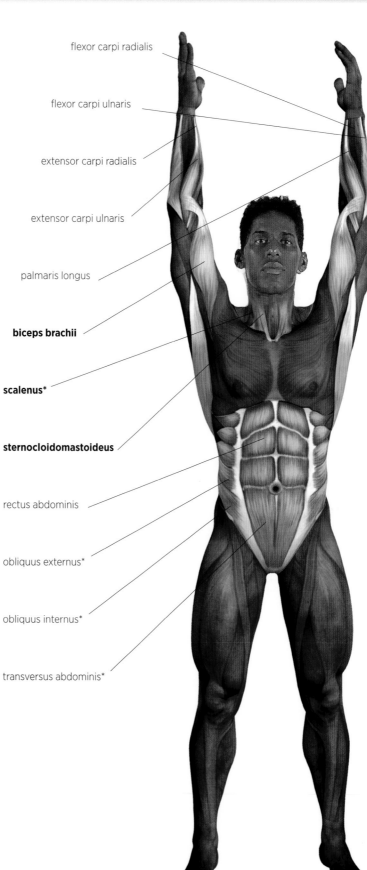

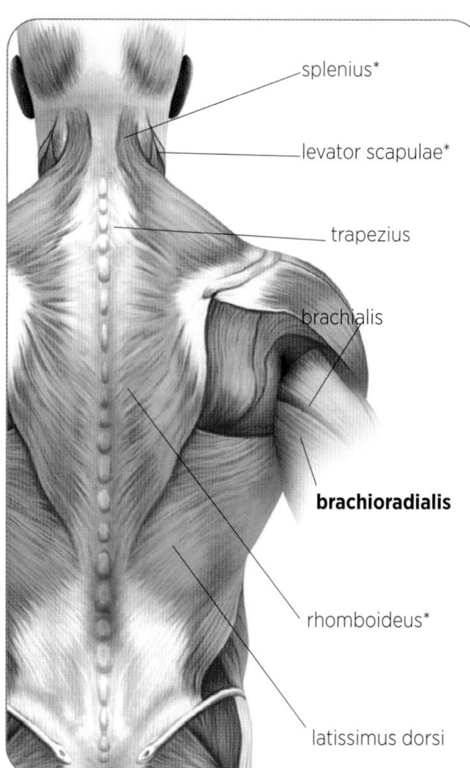

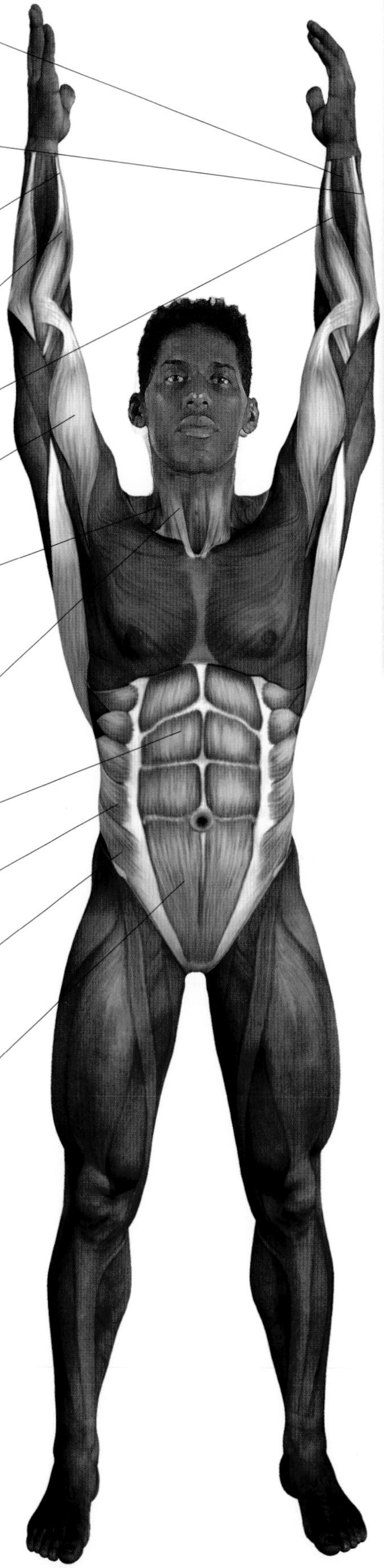

flexor carpi radialis
flexor carpi ulnaris
extensor carpi radialis
extensor carpi ulnaris
palmaris longus
biceps brachii
scalenus*
sternocloidomastoideus
rectus abdominis
obliquus externus*
obliquus internus*
transversus abdominis*

DO IT RIGHT
- Keep your elbows slightly bent.
- Tuck your pelvis.
- Avoid hyperextending either your lower back or elbows.

Cervical Stars

A simple but essential stretch to reduce cervical tightness and increase neck mobility. Cervical Stars effectively targets many different muscles around the neck bone.

HOW TO DO IT

- Sit or stand, keeping your neck, shoulders, and torso straight. Keeping your chin level, gaze straight ahead.
- Imagine that there is a star in front of you with a vertical line, a horizontal line, and two diagonal lines. Trace the star shape with your head and neck by following the vertical line up and down three times.
- Next, follow the horizontal line once.
- Finally, trace the two diagonal lines.
- Return to the starting position, and then repeat for the recommended repetitions.

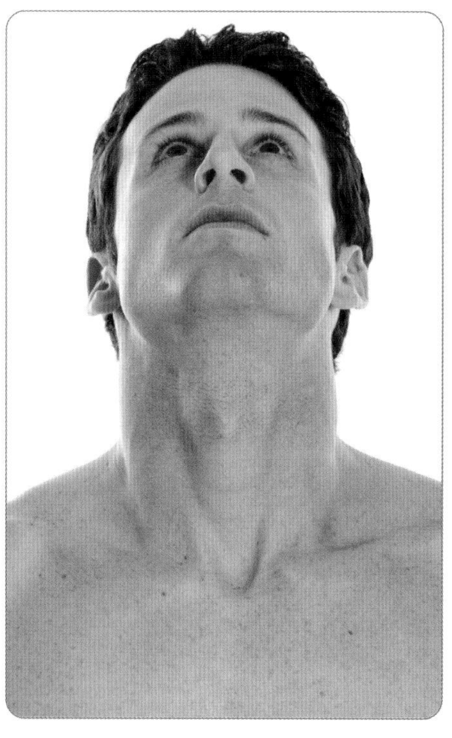

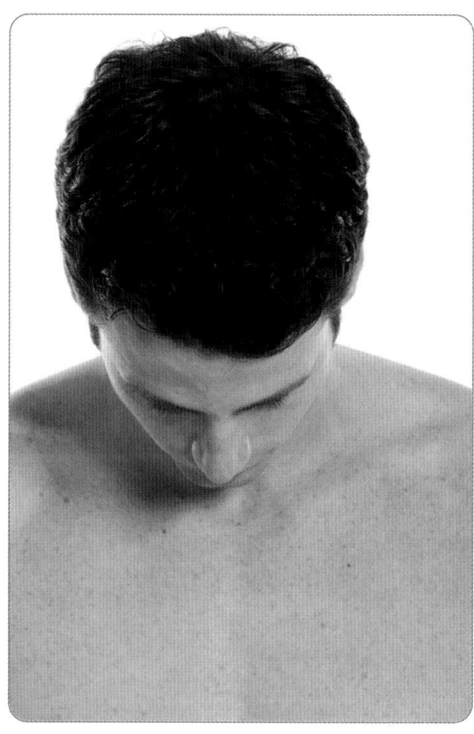

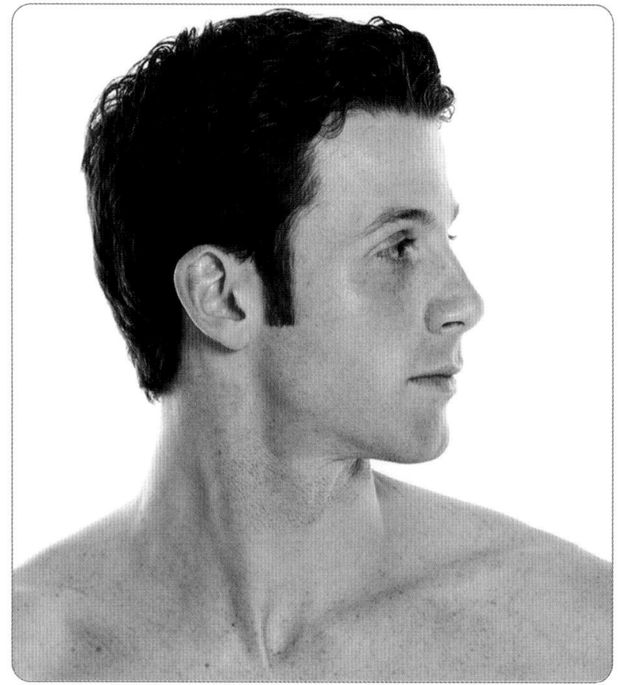

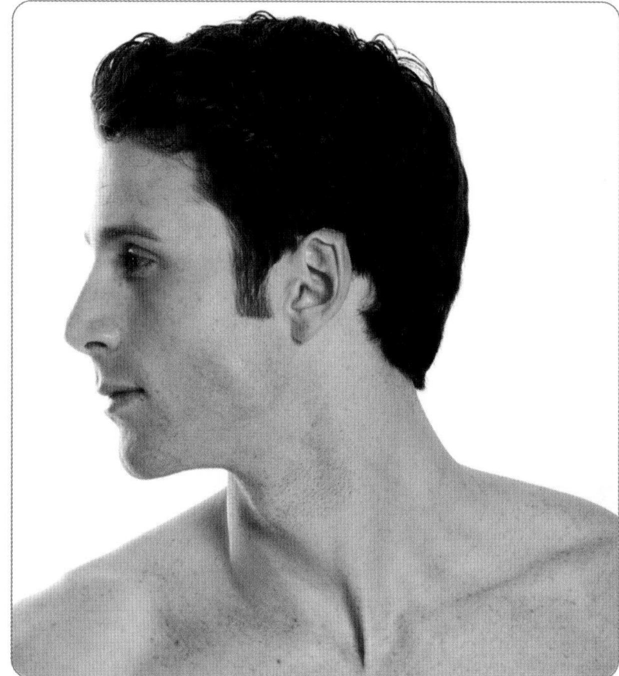

Annotation Key

Bold text indicates target muscles

Light text indicates other working muscles

* indicates deep muscles

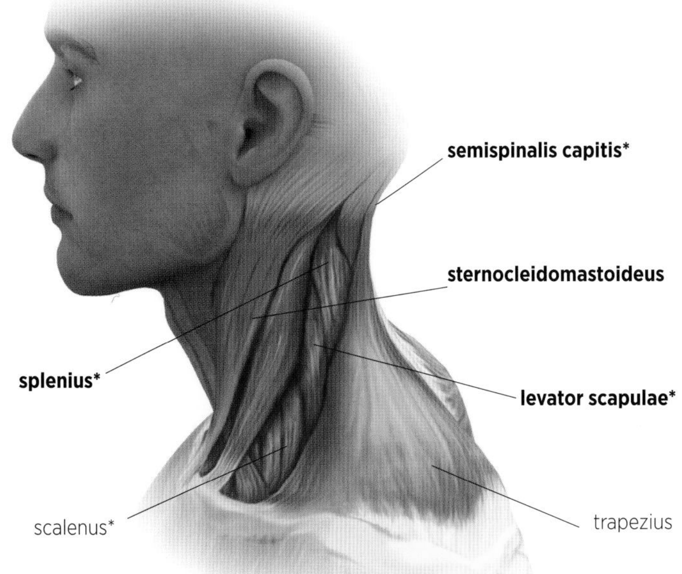

DO IT RIGHT

- Move in a smooth, controlled manner.
- Avoid hunching or tensing your shoulders.

FACT FILE

TARGETS

- Neck rotators
- Neck flexors
- Neck extensors
- Neck lateral flexors

TYPE

- Static

BENEFITS

- Improves range of motion
- Relieves neck pain

CAUTIONS

- Numbness in arms or hands

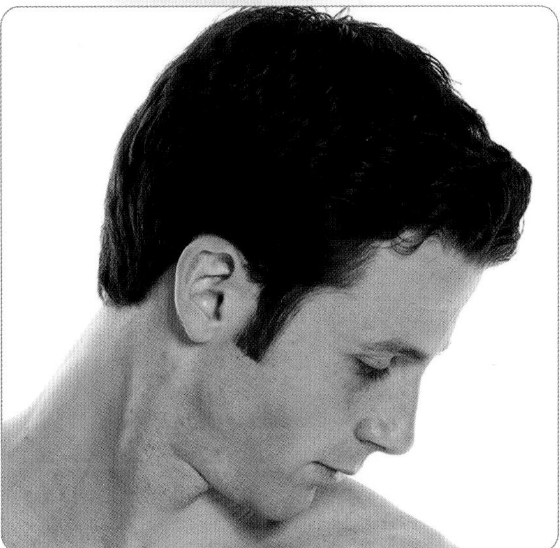

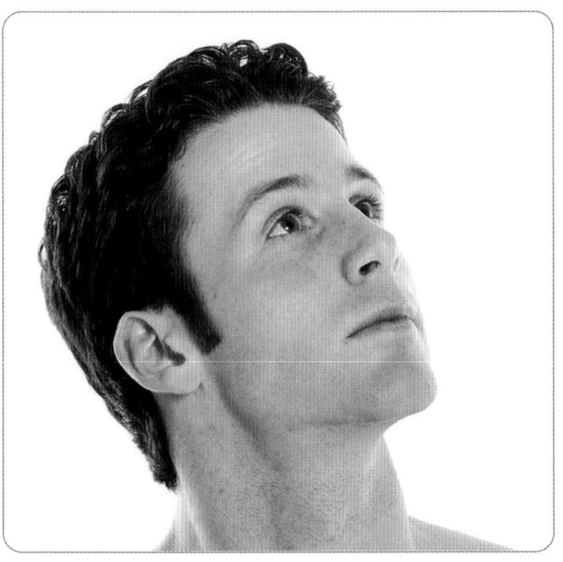

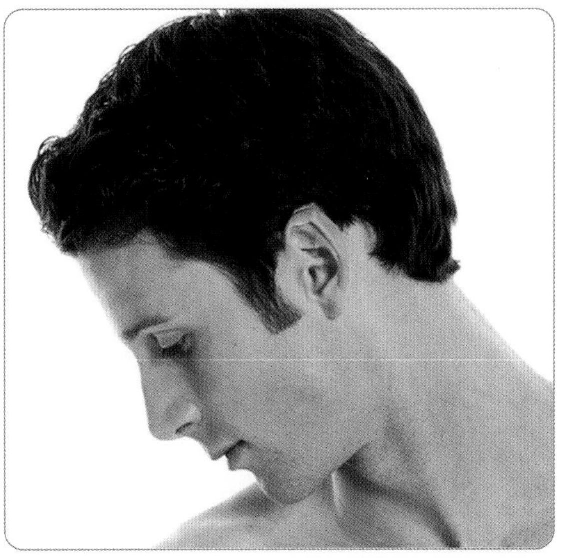

Turtle Neck

A group of muscles known as the neck flexors, which includes the sternocleidomastoid, is responsible for rotating and tilting the head to the side. The Turtle Neck stretch is an effective means of strengthening these important muscles.

HOW TO DO IT

- Sit or stand, keeping your neck, shoulders, and torso straight. Keeping your chin level, look straight ahead.
- Move your chin in as if you were a turtle drawing back into its shell until you feel a stretch in the back of your neck.
- Extend your head forward, this time as if you were a turtle coming out of its shell.
- Hold for five seconds, release the stretch, and then repeat for the recommended repetitions.

DO IT RIGHT

- Move in a smooth, controlled manner.
- Avoid lifting your chin as you move your head back.

FACT FILE

TARGETS
- Neck flexors

TYPE
- Static

BENEFITS
- Improves range of motion
- Corrects forward head protrusion

CAUTIONS
- Numbness in arms or hands

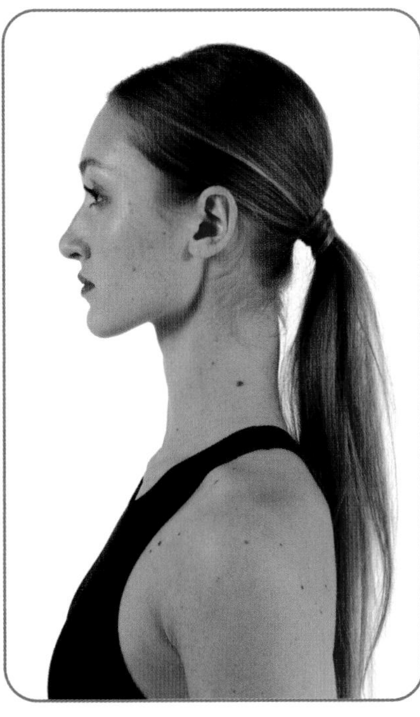

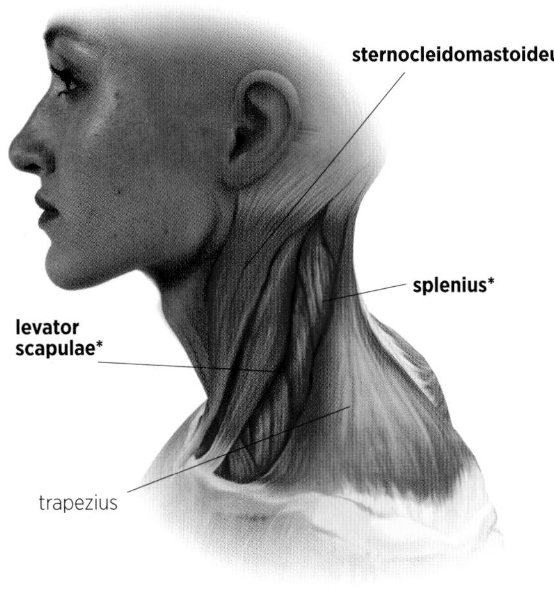

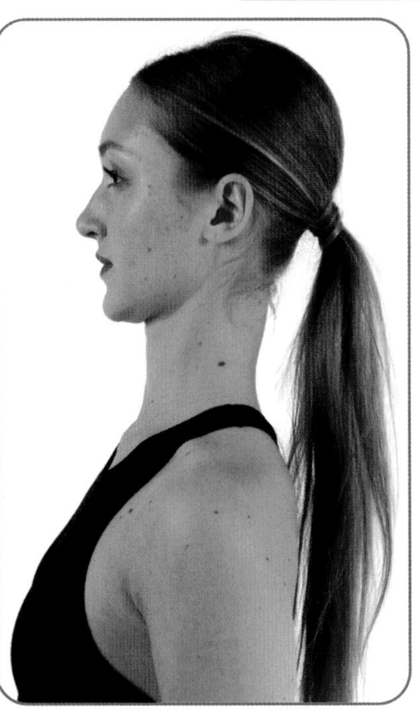

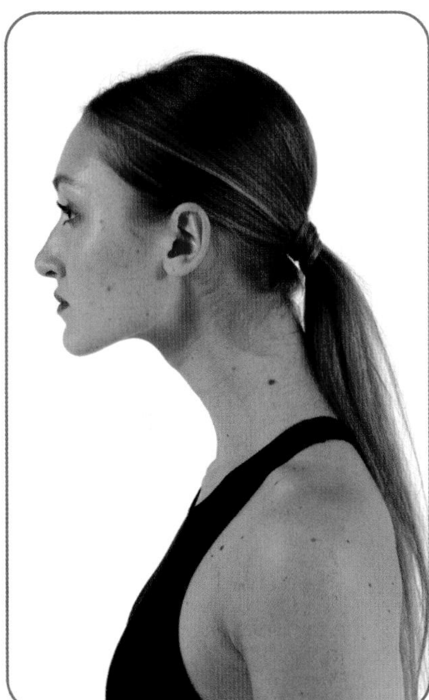

Annotation Key

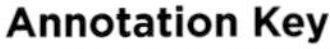

Bold text indicates target muscles
Light text indicates other working muscles
* indicates deep muscles

Shrug

It might seem like we shrug all the time, but purposefully engaging the shrug muscles can be an effective means to strengthen the neck, upper back, and shoulders.

HOW TO DO IT

- Sit on a Swiss ball or chair. Keep your back straight and your head and neck centered over the rest of your spinal column.
- With your arms at your sides, bend your elbows slightly. Hold your hands with the palms up.
- Bring your shoulders down and forward, and then lift them as high as you can.
- Return the starting position, and then repeat for the recommended repetitions.

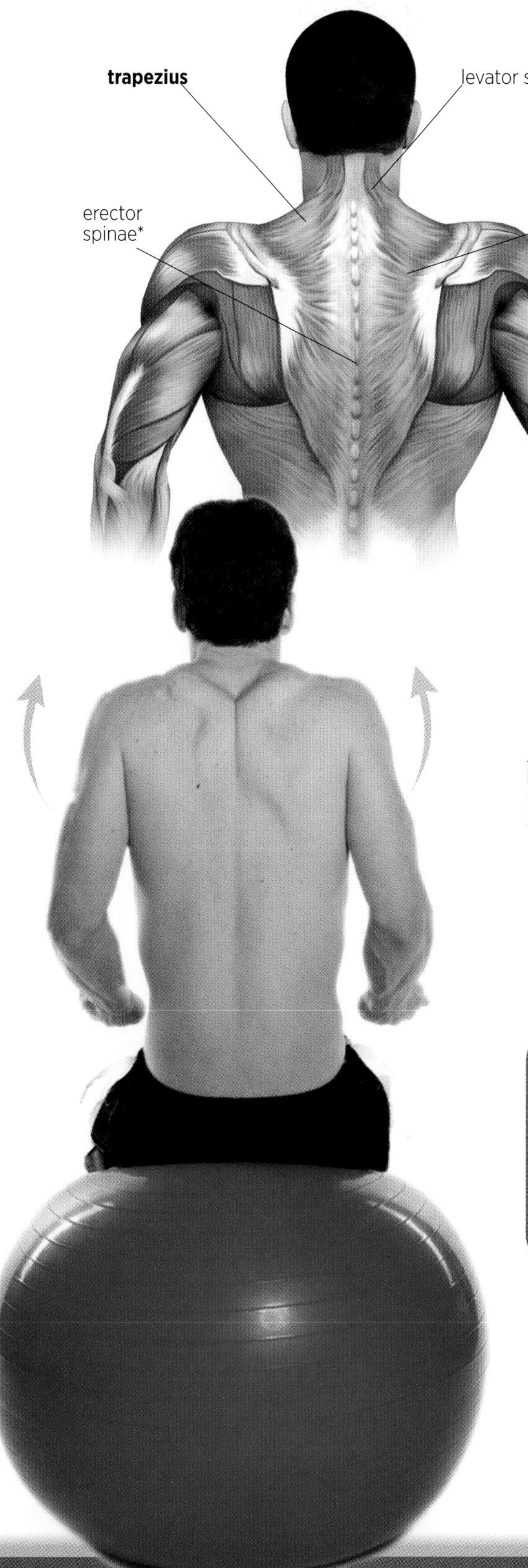

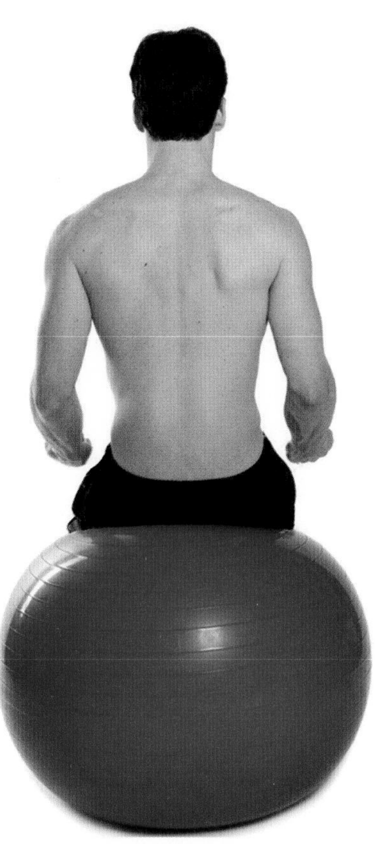

FACT FILE

TARGETS
- Neck
- Shoulders
- Scapulae

TYPE
- Dynamic

BENEFITS
- Improves range of motion
- Relaxes tight neck, shoulders, chest, and upper-back muscles
- Stabilizes your shoulder blades

CAUTIONS
- Numbness in arms or hands
- Severe shoulder or spinal pain

Annotation Key

Bold text indicates target muscles
Light text indicates other working muscles
* indicates deep muscles

DO IT RIGHT
- Move in a smooth, controlled manner.
- Avoid rolling your shoulders.

Flexion Stretch

There are two kinds of neck flexion. The first kind involves flexing the very deep muscles on the front of your neck to tuck your chin down. The second kind of flexion involves bending the whole neck forward from its base on top of the torso. Moves like the Flexion Stretch can help undo the neck stiffness that comes with a head-forward posture.

HOW TO DO IT

- Sit or stand, keeping your neck, shoulders, and torso straight. Place one or both hands behind your head.
- Slowly pull your chin toward your chest until you feel a stretch in the back of your neck.
- Hold for the recommended time, release the stretch, and then repeat for the recommended repetitions.

DO IT RIGHT

- Let your gaze fall downward as you stretch.
- Move slowly and with control.
- Keep your back straight.
- Relax your shoulder muscles.
- Avoid pulling too hard with your hand.

FACT FILE

TARGETS
- Neck

TYPE
- Static

BENEFITS
- Improves range of motion
- Relieves neck pain
- Reduces tension in the shoulders and upper back

CAUTIONS
- Severe neck pain or numbness
- Spinal stenosis
- Numbness in arms or hands

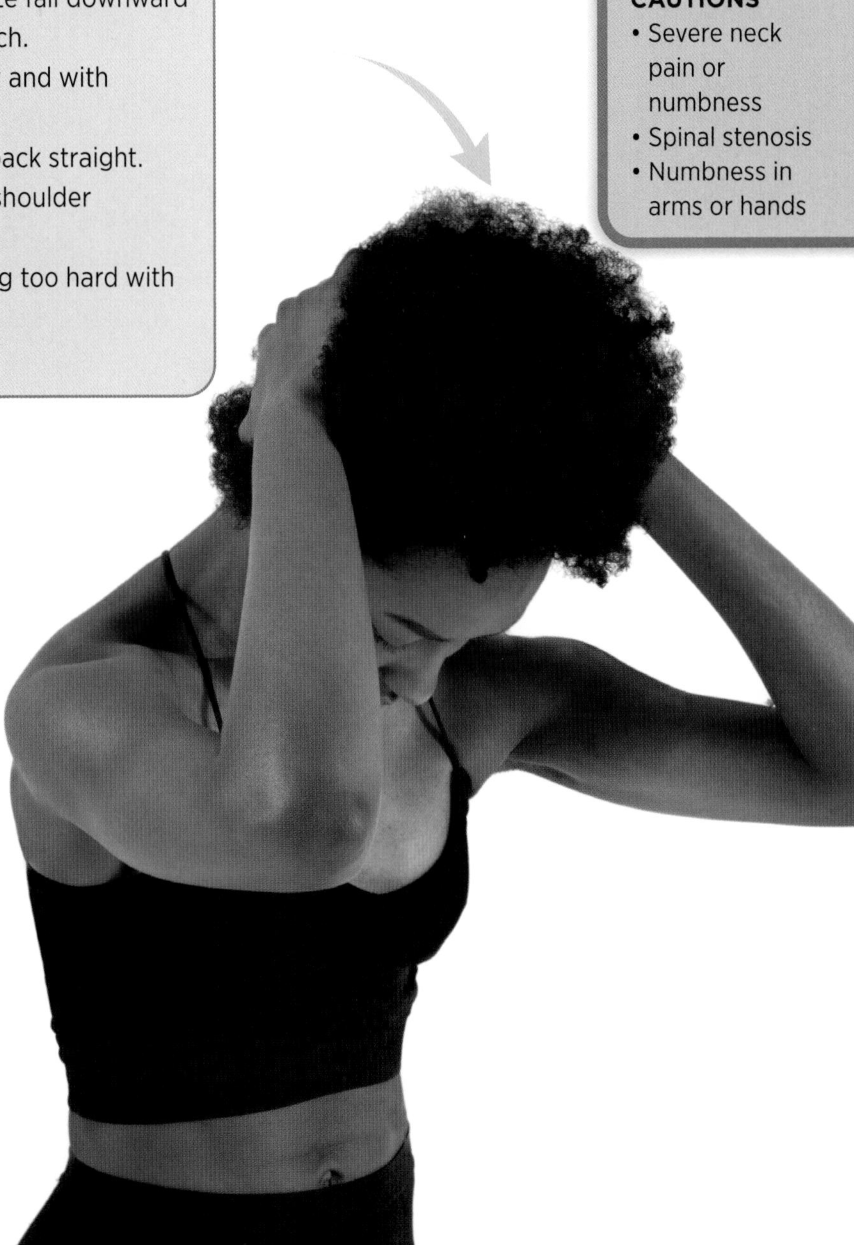

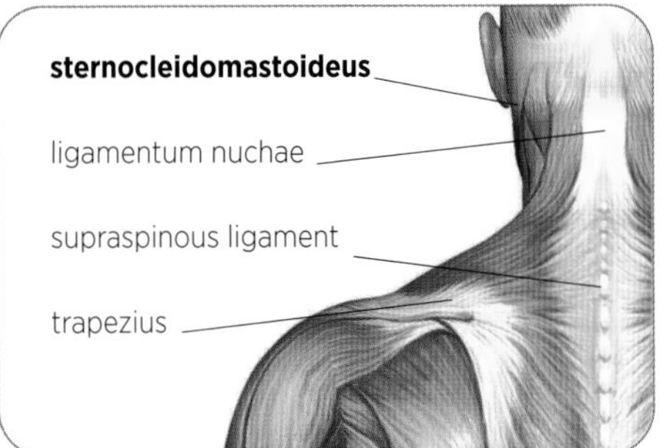

Annotation Key
Bold text indicates target muscles
Light text indicates other working muscles
* indicates deep muscles

Flexion Isometric

This cervical stretch serves as a countermove to the Flexion Stretch (opposite). Isometric exercises serve to strengthen muscles without irritating ligaments, tendons, or joints.

FACT FILE

TARGETS
- Neck flexors

TYPE
- Isometric

BENEFITS
- Strengthens neck flexors

CAUTIONS
- Numbness in arms or hands

DO IT RIGHT

- Apply only a gentle pressure.
- Avoid any movement in the neck.

HOW TO DO IT

- Sit or stand, keeping your neck, shoulders, and torso straight. Slightly flex your neck.
- Place your palm against your forehead, and gently push your forehead into your palm, holding the position static.
- Hold for the recommended time, release the stretch, and then repeat for the recommended repetitions.

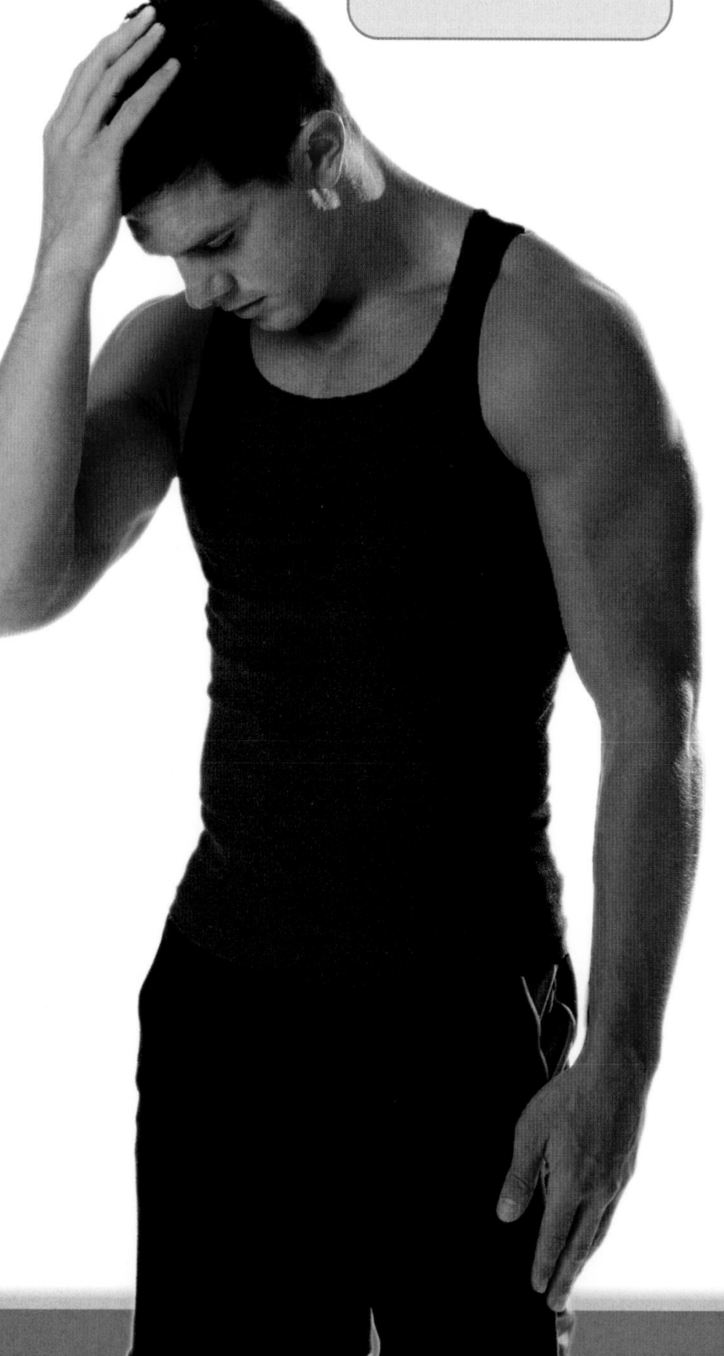

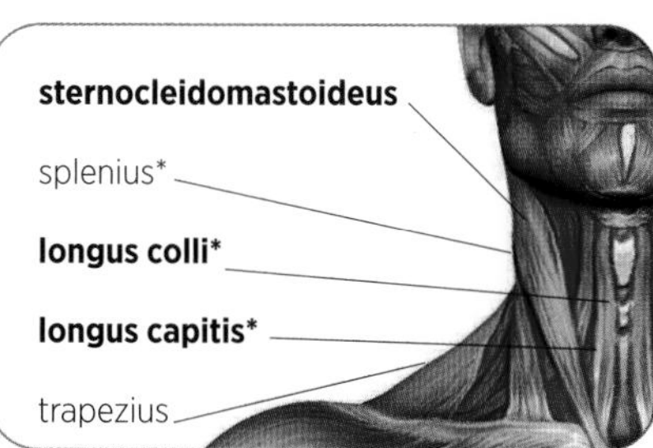

Annotation Key
Bold text indicates target muscles
Light text indicates other working muscles
* indicates deep muscles

Lateral Stretch

In the Lateral Stretch you move your neck from a straight position to a lateral bend in an action called lateral flexion. A group of muscles called the scalenes (or scalenus muscles) help make it happen.

FACT FILE

TARGETS
- Neck lateral flexors

TYPE
- Static

BENEFITS
- Improves range of motion
- Relieves neck pain

CAUTIONS
- Numbness in arms or hands

HOW TO DO IT
- Sit or stand, keeping your neck, shoulders, and torso straight.
- Tilt your head down and to the side. Continue until right ear approaches your right shoulder and you feel a distinct stretch in the left side of your neck.
- Hold for the recommended time, release the stretch, and then repeat on the opposite side. Alternate sides for the recommended repetitions.

rectus capitis lateralis*
rectus capitis*
sternocleidomastoideus
scalenus*
trapezius

DO IT RIGHT
- Relax your shoulder muscles.
- Avoid rotating your head while tilting it.

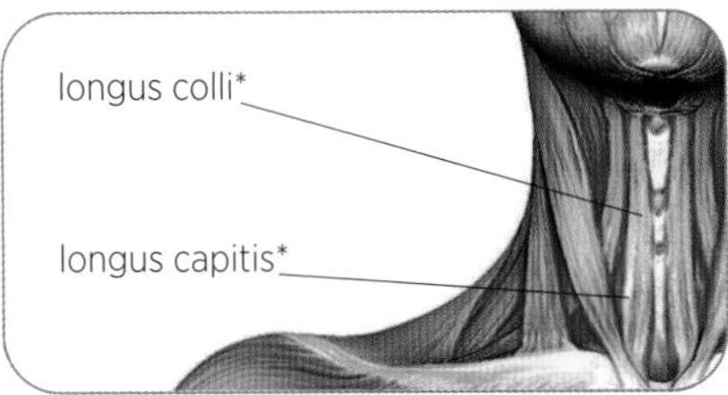

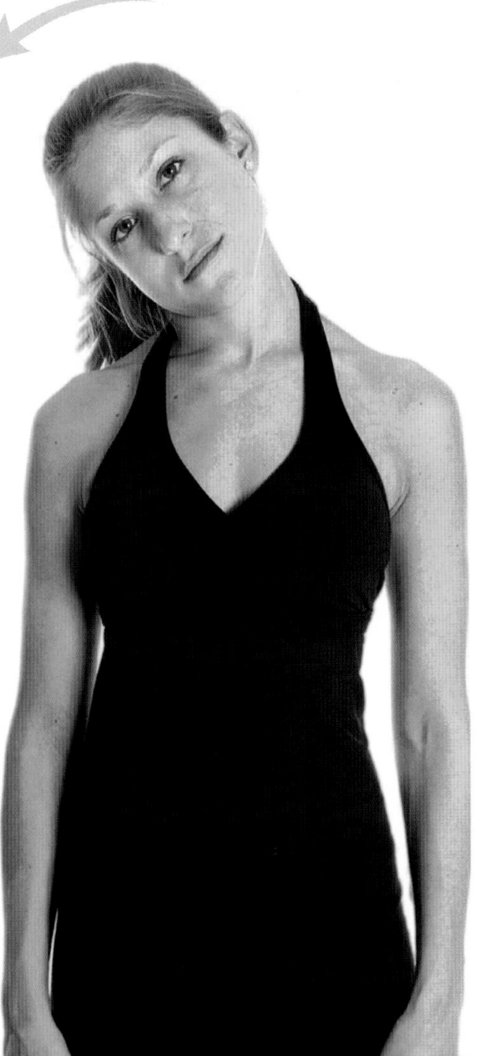

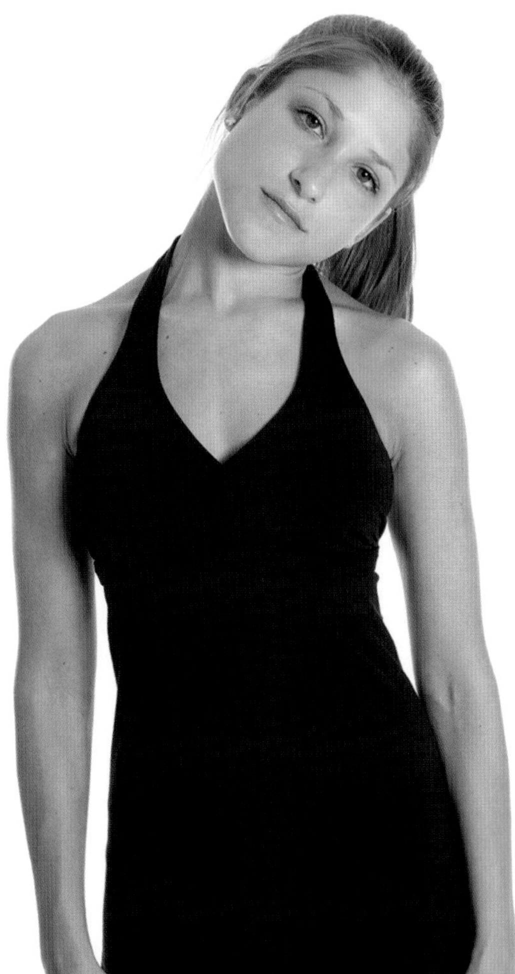

Annotation Key
Bold text indicates target muscles
Light text indicates other working muscles
* indicates deep muscles

Lateral Isometric

This stretch helps you maintain or regain cervical mobility simply by applying pressure while you move your neck through its normal movements. Perform this stretch slowly and gently to ease and release the top of your shoulders and lower-neck muscles.

FACT FILE

TARGETS
- Neck lateral flexors

TYPE
- Isometric

BENEFITS
- Strengthens the lateral flexors

CAUTIONS
- Numbness in arms or hands

HOW TO DO IT

- Sit or stand, keeping your neck, shoulders, and torso straight. Place the palm of your right hand on the top of your head.
- Reach toward the small of your back with your left hand, bending your arm at the elbow.
- Tilt your head toward your raised elbow until you feel the stretch in the side of your neck.
- Press your head into the palm of your hand as you try to tilt your ear to your shoulder.
- Hold for the recommended time, release the stretch, and then repeat on the opposite side. Alternate sides for the recommended repetitions.

Annotation Key
Bold text indicates target muscles
Light text indicates other working muscles
* indicates deep muscles

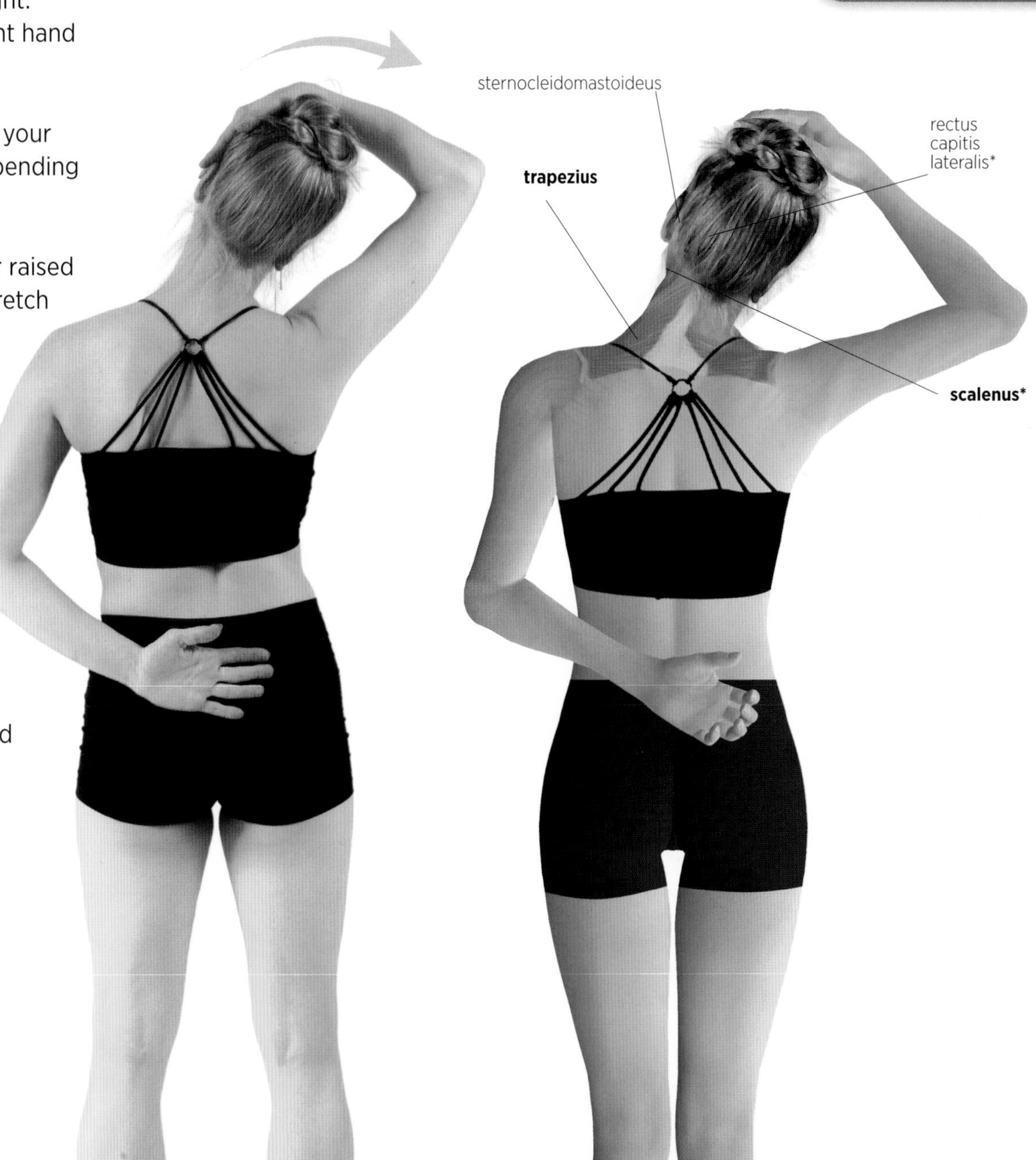

DO IT RIGHT

- Apply only a gentle pressure.
- Avoid any movement in the neck.

Lateral Lunge Stretch

Sideway lunges tone key muscles in your thighs and buttocks, helping to free up movement in your legs and hips as well as stabilizing your knees.

HOW TO DO IT

- Begin bent over, with your feet planted far apart. Allow your arms to dangle toward the floor in front of you.
- Bend your right knee while keeping your left leg straight. Place most of your weight on your bent leg, feeling the stretch in your lengthened leg.
- Hold for the recommended time, release the stretch, and then repeat on the opposite side.

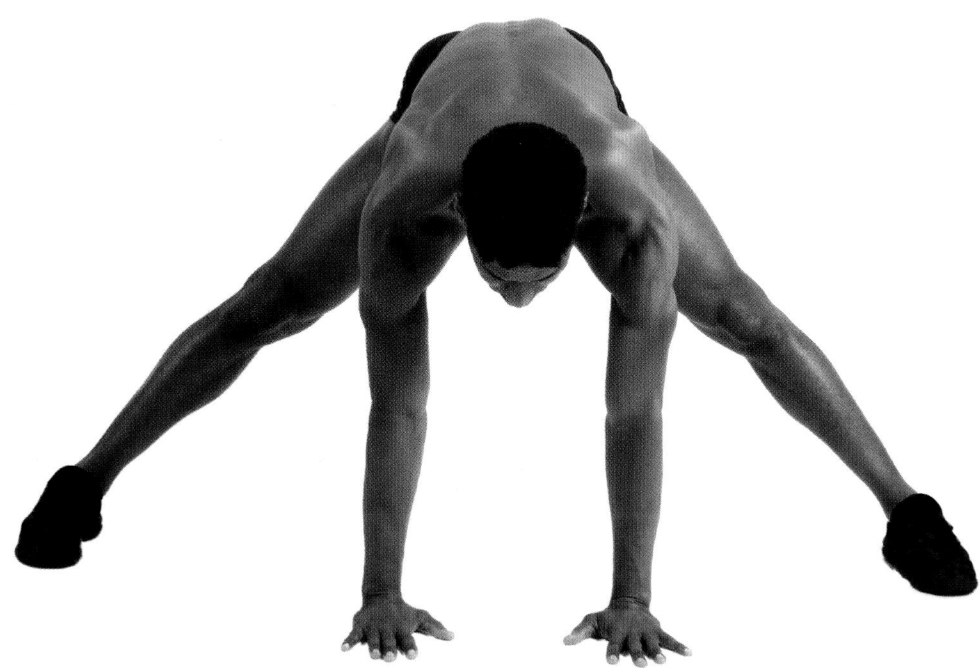

DO IT RIGHT

- Extend your leg fully while in the stretch position.
- Gaze toward the floor throughout the stretch.
- Keep your feet flat on the floor.
- Avoid twisting your torso.
- Avoid curving your back forward.
- Avoid arching your back or neck.

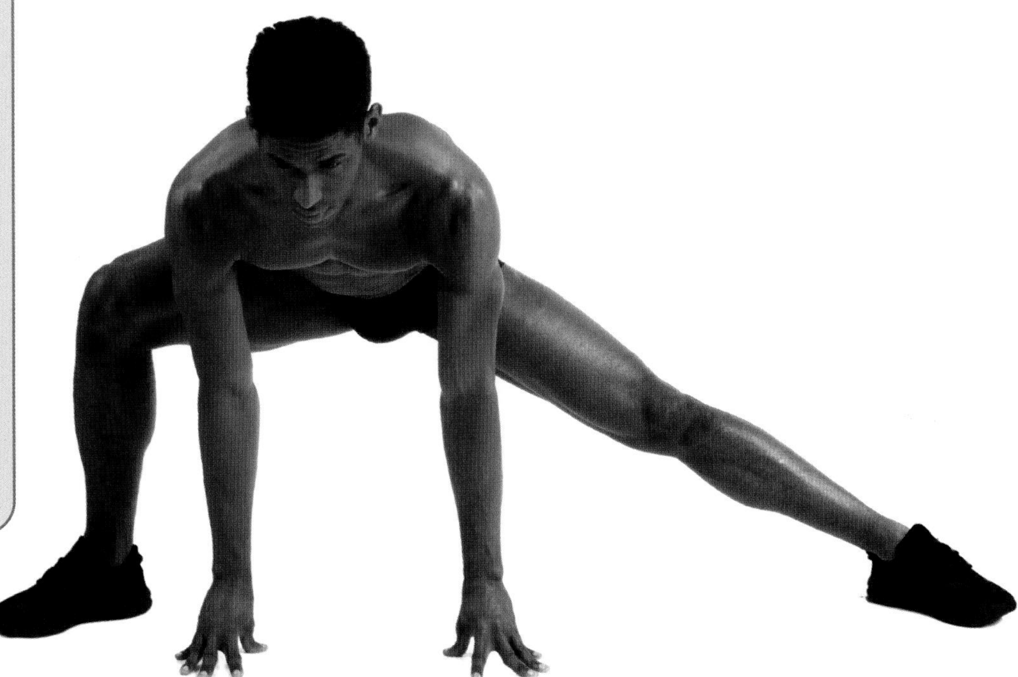

FACT FILE

TARGETS
- Glutes
- Inner thighs
- Quadriceps

TYPE
- Isometric

BENEFITS
- Stretches leg muscles

CAUTIONS
- Knee issues

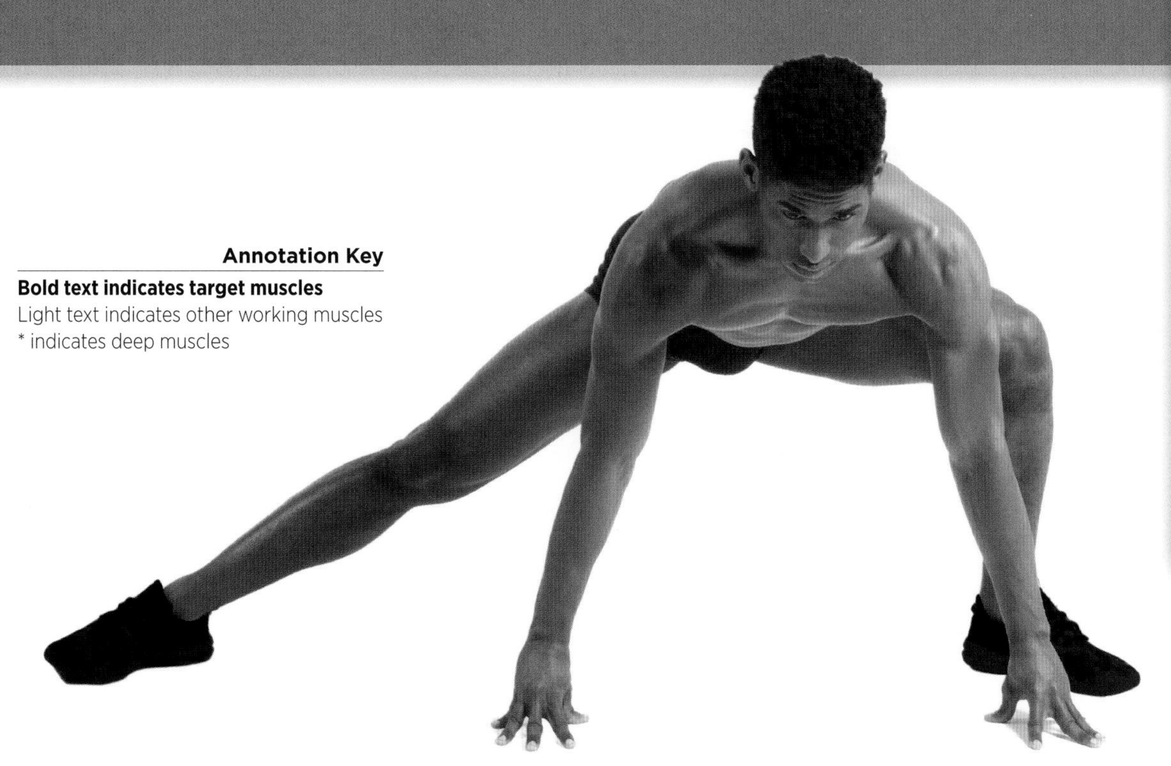

Annotation Key
Bold text indicates target muscles
Light text indicates other working muscles
* indicates deep muscles

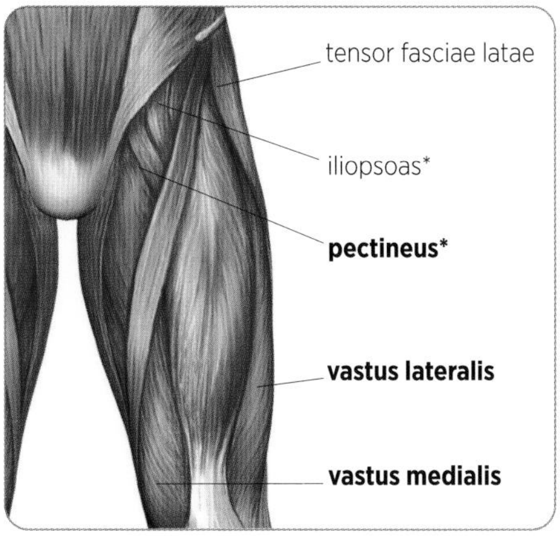

tensor fasciae latae
iliopsoas*
pectineus*
vastus lateralis
vastus medialis

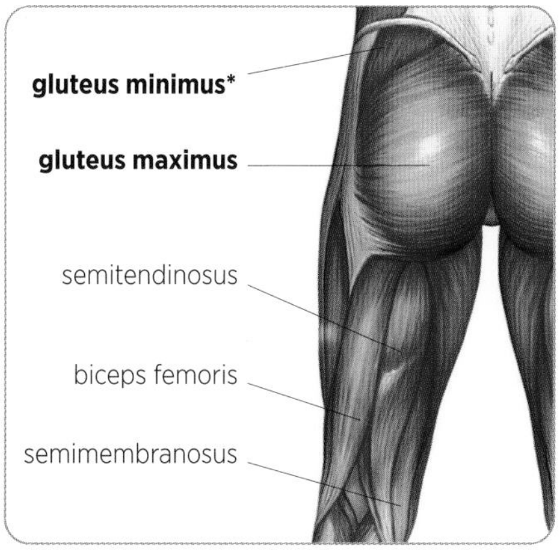

gluteus minimus*
gluteus maximus
semitendinosus
biceps femoris
semimembranosus

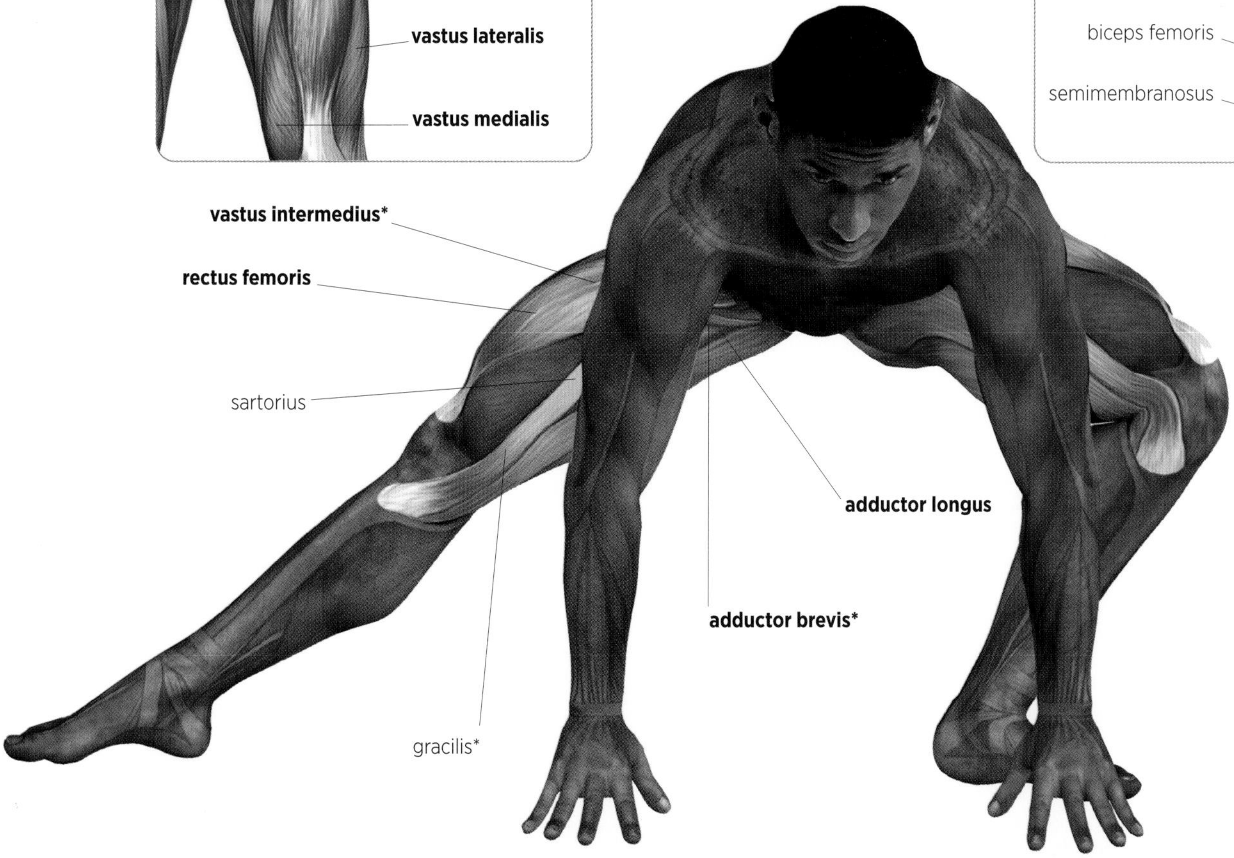

vastus intermedius*
rectus femoris
sartorius
adductor longus
adductor brevis*
gracilis*

Wall-Assisted Chest Stretch

You can practice the Wall-Assisted Chest Stretch almost anywhere. This chest opener is a great exercise for relieving tension in your shoulders and pectoral muscles and for improving your posture.

HOW TO DO IT

- Stand with the left side of your body next to a wall.
- Extend your left arm toward the wall, and place your palm flat against the wall, with your fingers pointing behind you.
- Lunge forward with your left leg. Remain facing forward as you stretch.
- Place your right hand on your ribcage just below your left pectoral muscle to help keep your torso from twisting.
- Hold for the recommended time, return to the starting position, and repeat on the opposite side.

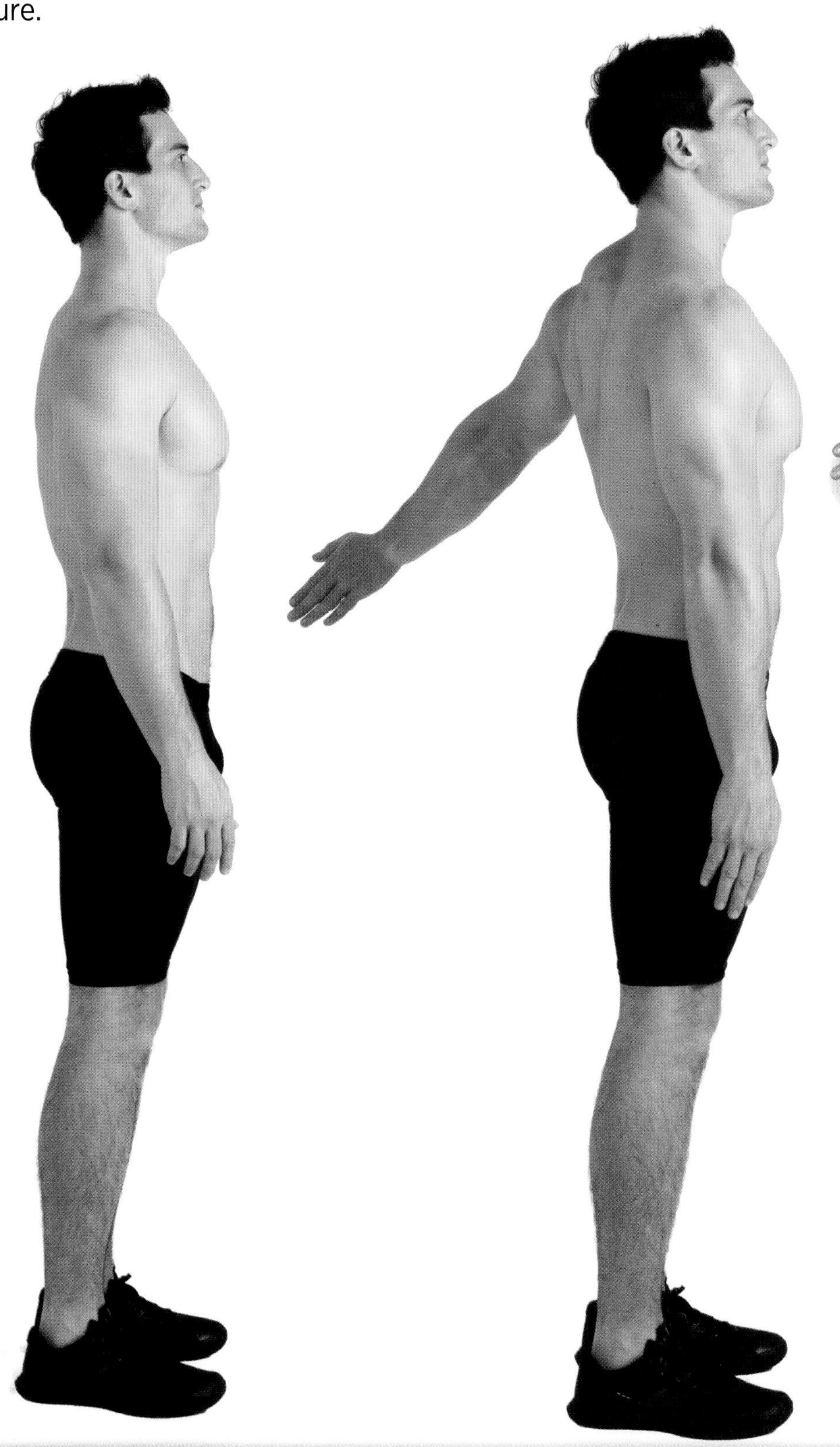

DO IT RIGHT

- Keep your shoulders pressed down and back, away from your ears.
- Position your arm at a slight downward diagonal, with your elbow slightly lower than your shoulder, to protect your rotator cuff from injury.
- Avoid rotating your chest and torso toward the wall when lunging; instead, face forward.

FACT FILE

TARGETS
- Chest
- Shoulders

TYPE
- Static

BENEFITS
- Opens chest
- Increases shoulder mobility

CAUTIONS
- Shoulder issues

Annotation Key

Bold text indicates target muscles

Light text indicates other working muscles

* indicates deep muscles

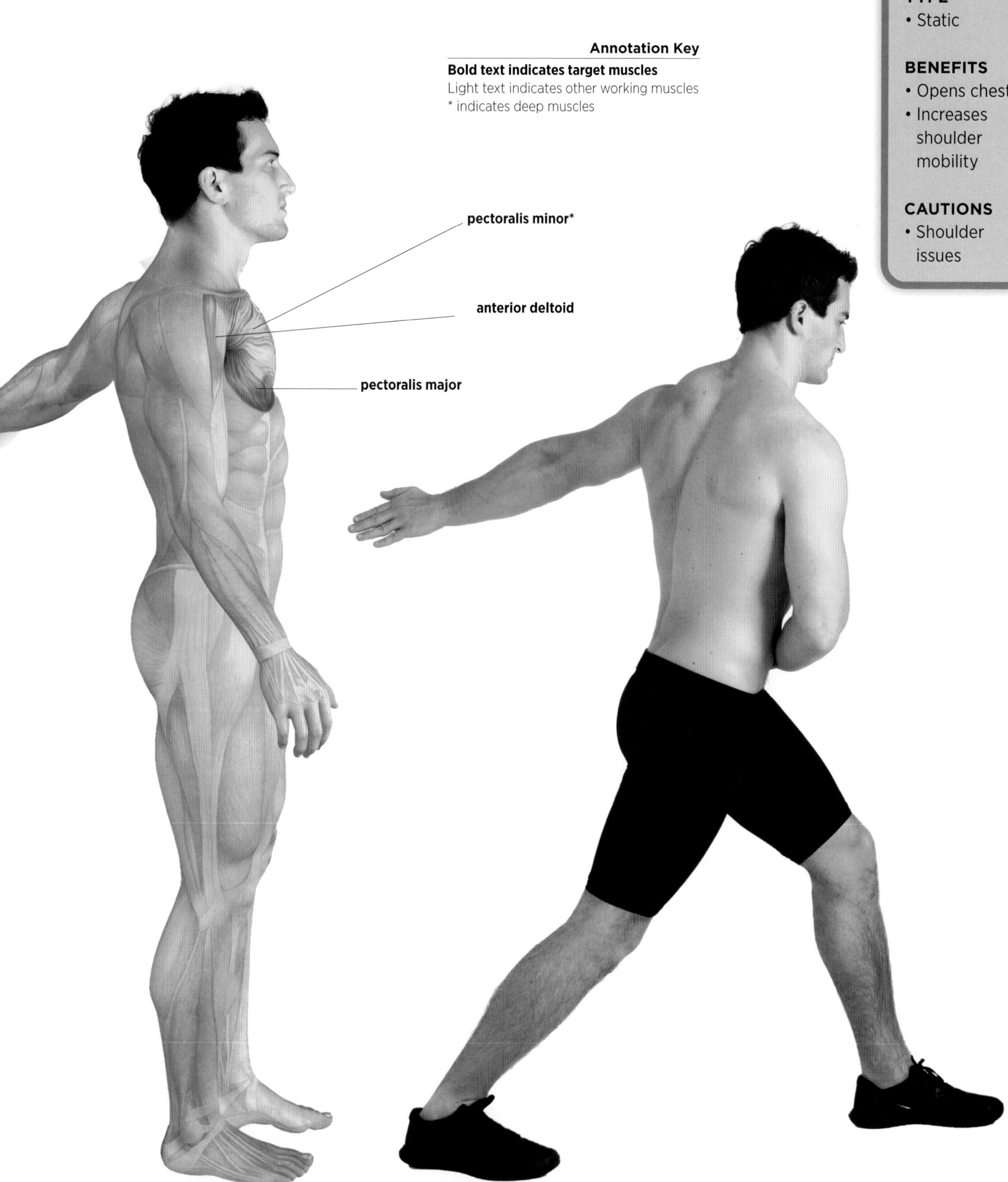

Saw Stretch

This classic Pilates exercise uses oppositional movement to stretch your chest and upper back. The Saw improves flexibility in the spine and strengthens your abdominal obliques. This exercise helps you focus on stabilizing your pelvis during rotation.

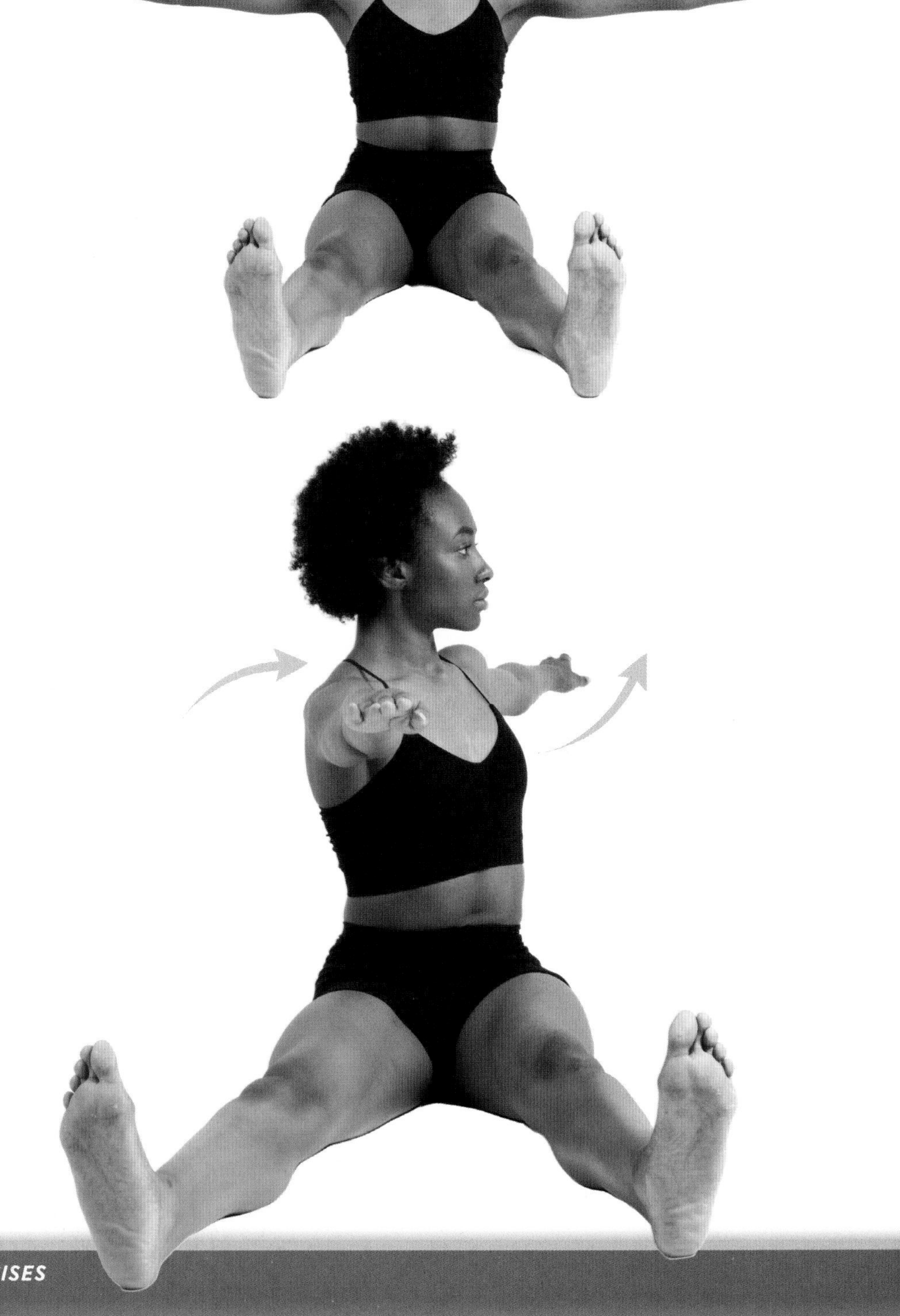

HOW TO DO IT

- Sit upright with your legs forward. Flex your feet, and position them slightly more than hip-width apart.
- Raise your arms out to your sides, with your palms facing down. Twist your torso to your left.
- Reach your right hand over your left foot, as if "sawing" your little toe.
- Return to the starting position, and repeat on the opposite side. Perform the recommended repetitions.

DO IT RIGHT

- Keep your hips planted firmly on the floor.
- Use your legs to anchor your body.
- Lengthen your neck.
- Avoid hunching your shoulders.
- Avoid rolling your hips.

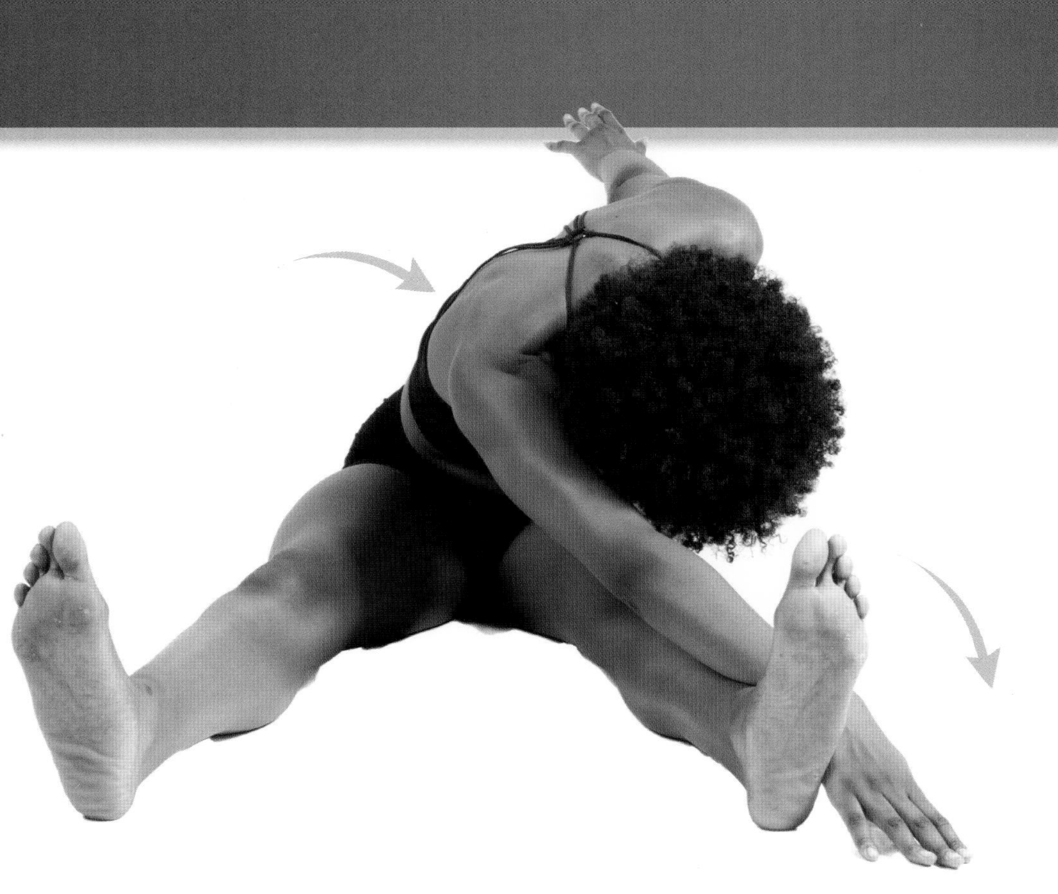

FACT FILE

TARGETS
- Chest
- Upper back
- Obliques

TYPE
- Dynamic

BENEFITS
- Stretches hip flexors, thighs, and abdominals
- Opens shoulders and chest
- Improves posture

CAUTIONS
- Knee issues
- Lower-back issues
- Neck issues

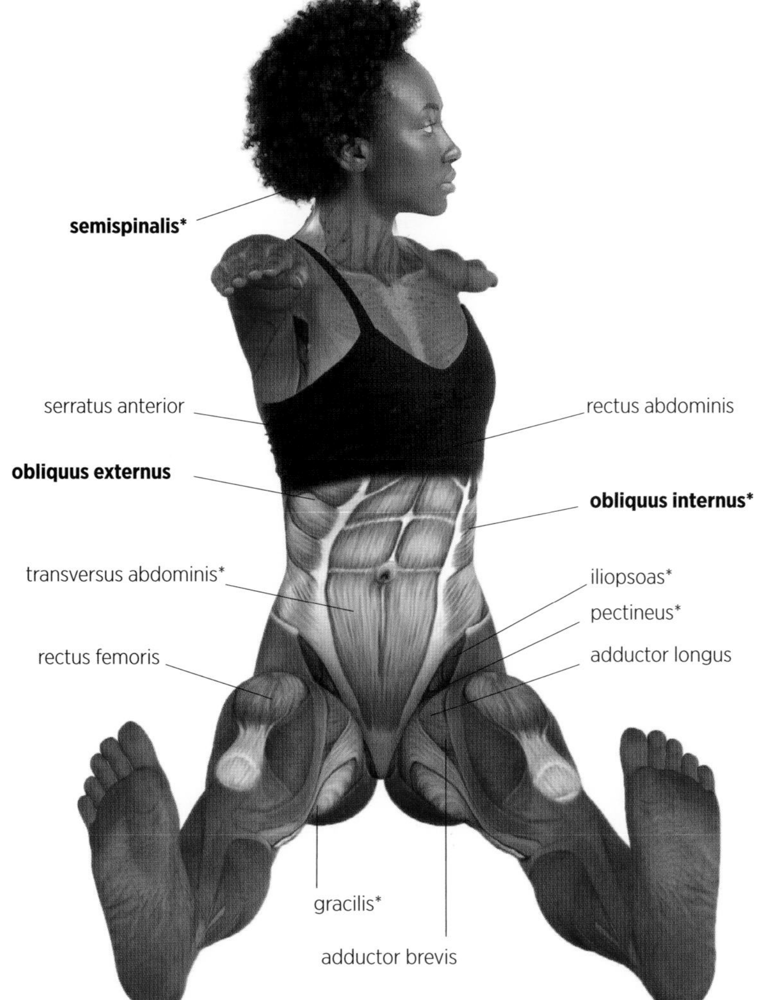

Annotation Key

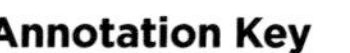

Bold text indicates target muscles
Light text indicates other working muscles
* indicates deep muscles

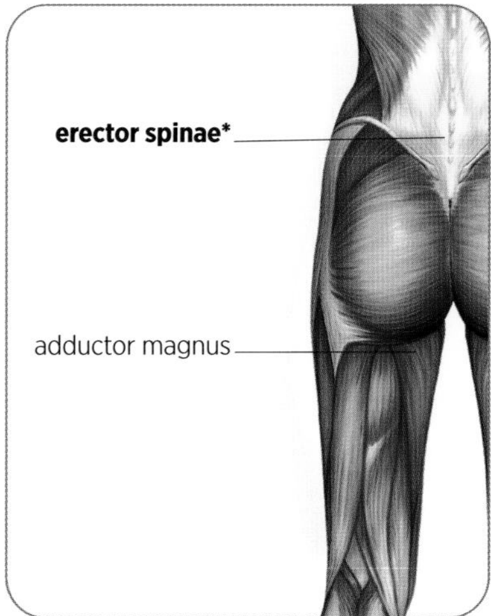

Lying-Down Pretzel Stretch

The Lying-Down Pretzel Stretch increases strength and flexibility in your hips. It can help to improve posture, alleviate lower-back pain, and stabilize your pelvis during everyday activities.

HOW TO DO IT

- Lie on your back, with both legs elongated and parallel. Extend your arms away from your torso, palms facing up. Bend your right leg and place the sole of your foot on the floor.
- Carefully lift your hip bones off the floor, shifting your torso a few inches to your left. Cross your right leg over your left leg, with your knee bent at a right angle.
- Hold for the recommended time, release the stretch, and repeat on the opposite side.

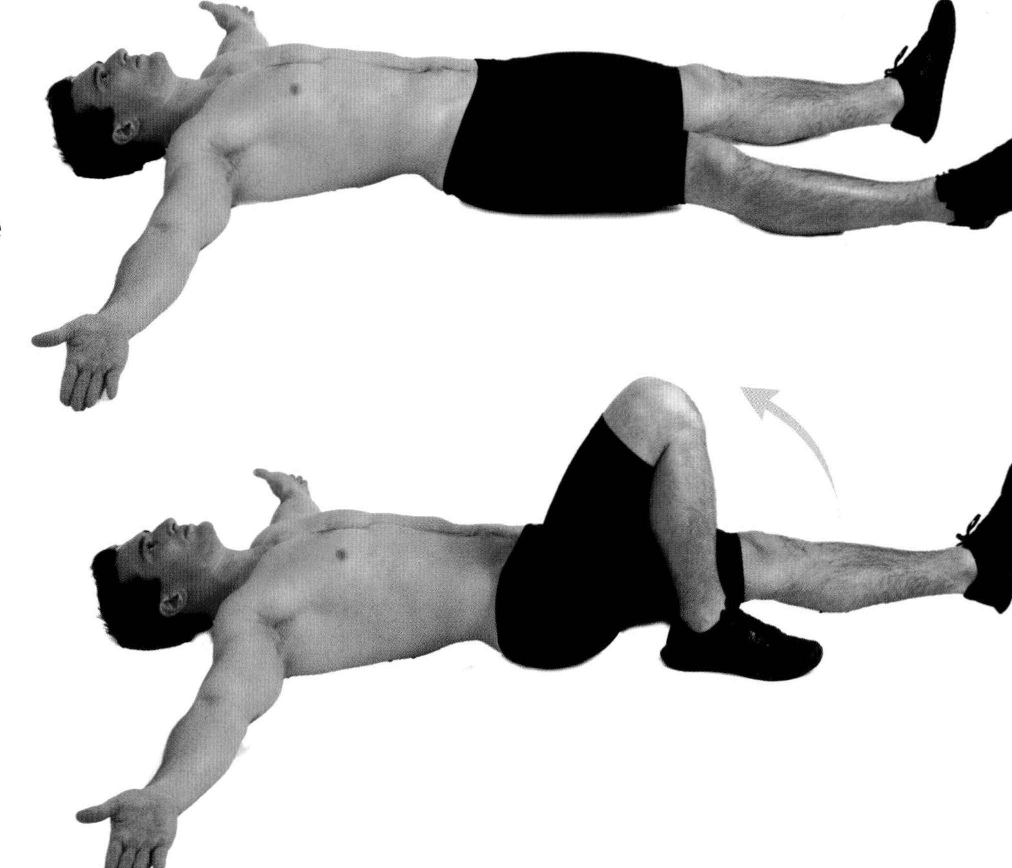

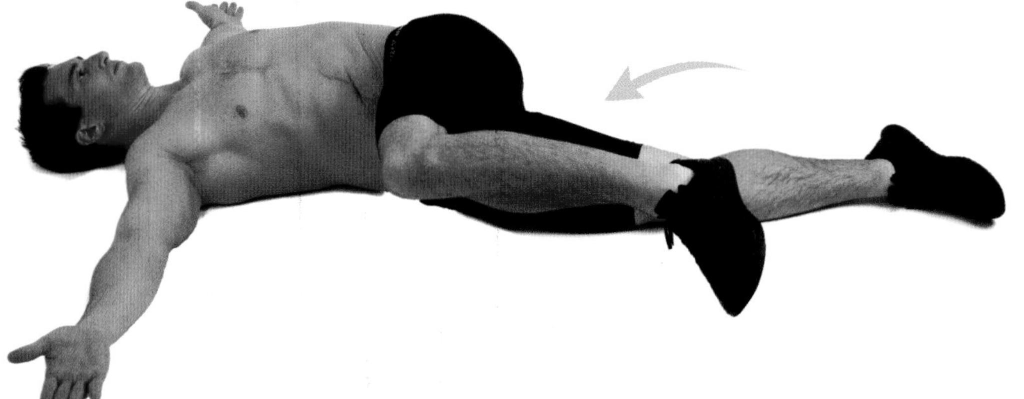

DO IT RIGHT

- Keep your elbows and wrists lower than your shoulders, protecting your rotator cuffs.
- Avoid lifting your shoulders from the floor during this stretch.

FACT FILE

TARGETS
- Chest
- Glutes

TYPE
- Static

BENEFITS
- Opens chest
- Increases hip mobility
- Stretches glutes and spine

CAUTIONS
- Lower-back pain
- Hip issues

Annotation Key
Bold text indicates target muscles
Light text indicates other working muscles
* indicates deep muscles

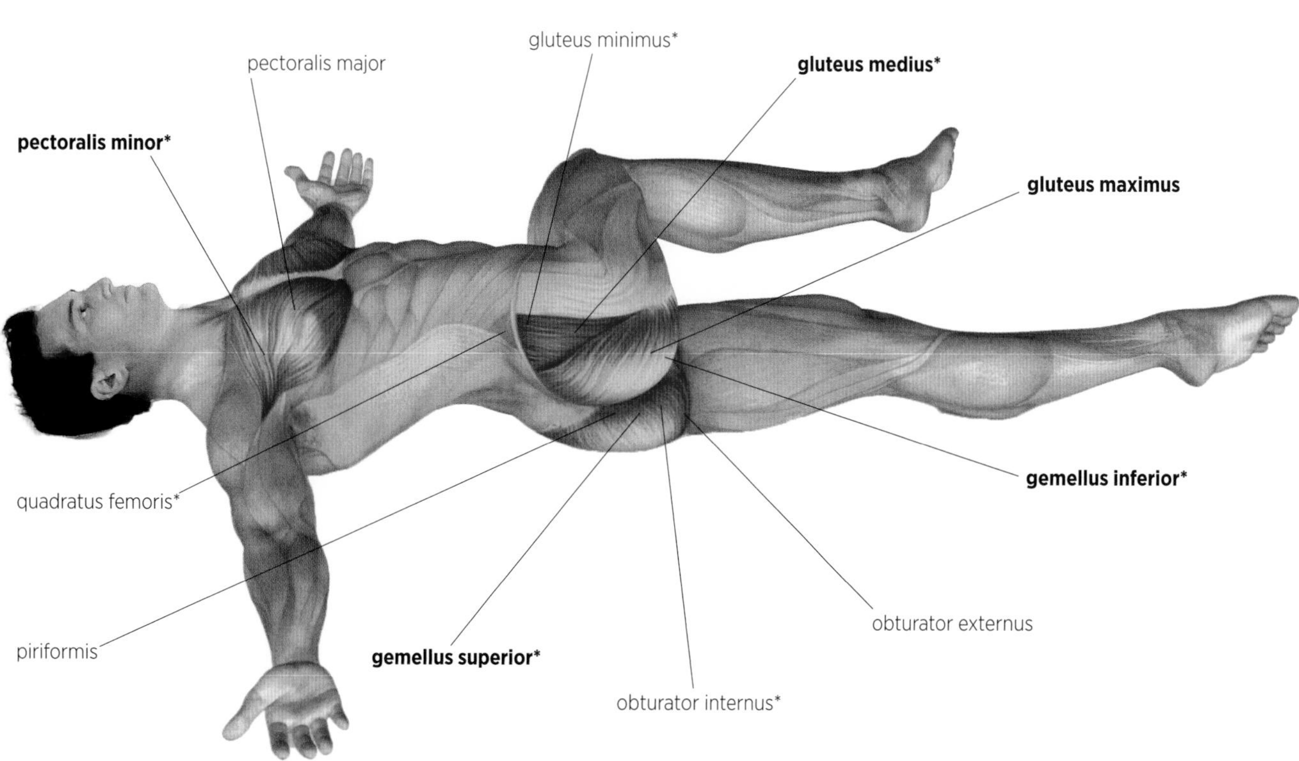

Triceps Stretch

The Triceps Stretch is easy to do anytime, anywhere. It improves shoulder and upper-body flexibility, fends off muscle soreness, and extends your range of motion while building durability.

HOW TO DO IT

- Stand with your legs and feet parallel and shoulder-width apart. Bend your knees very slightly, and shift your pelvis slightly forward.
- Reach your right arm up behind your head. Bend from the elbow, aiming to bring your elbow toward the middle of the back of your head. Your right hand should fall between your shoulder blades.
- Grab your right elbow with your left hand, and gently pull down to intensify the stretch.
- Hold for the recommended time, release the stretch, and then repeat on the opposite side.

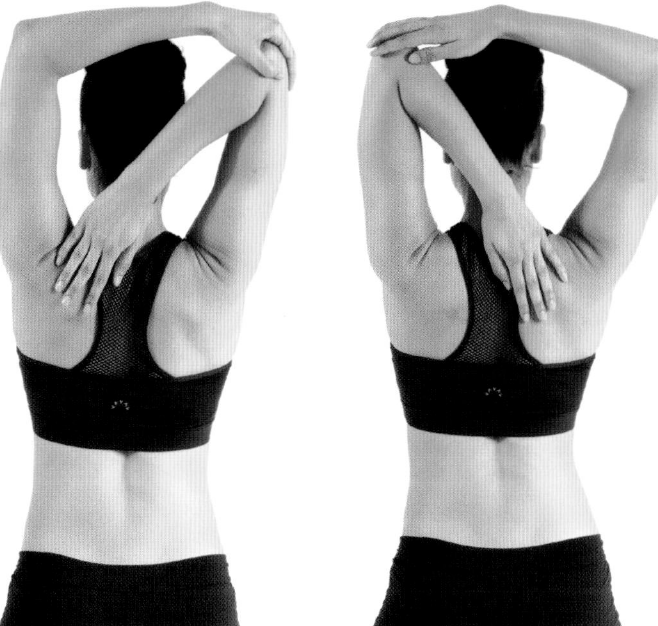

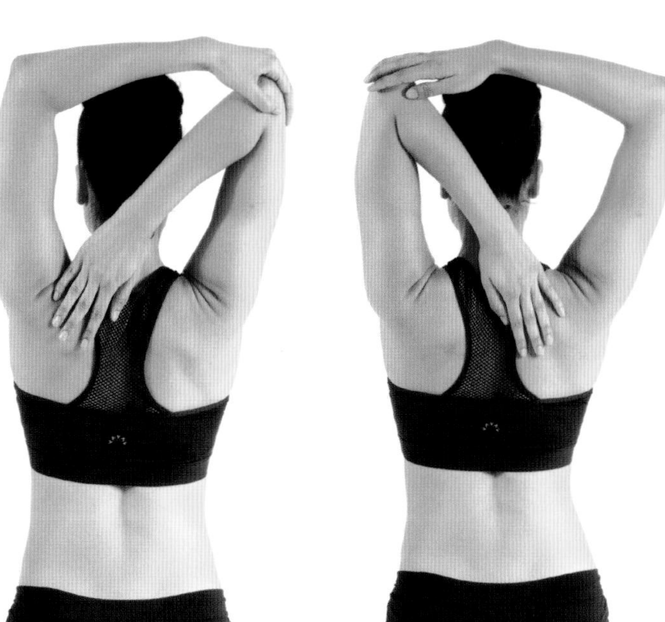

FACT FILE

TARGETS
- Triceps brachii

TYPE
- Isometric

BENEFITS
- Increases upper-arm mobility
- Relaxes tight shoulder joints

CAUTIONS
- Shoulder issues

DO IT RIGHT

- Keep your shoulders pressed down and back, away from your ears.
- Maintain a firm, stable midsection, keeping your pelvis slightly tucked.
- Avoid tilting your head or neck forward.

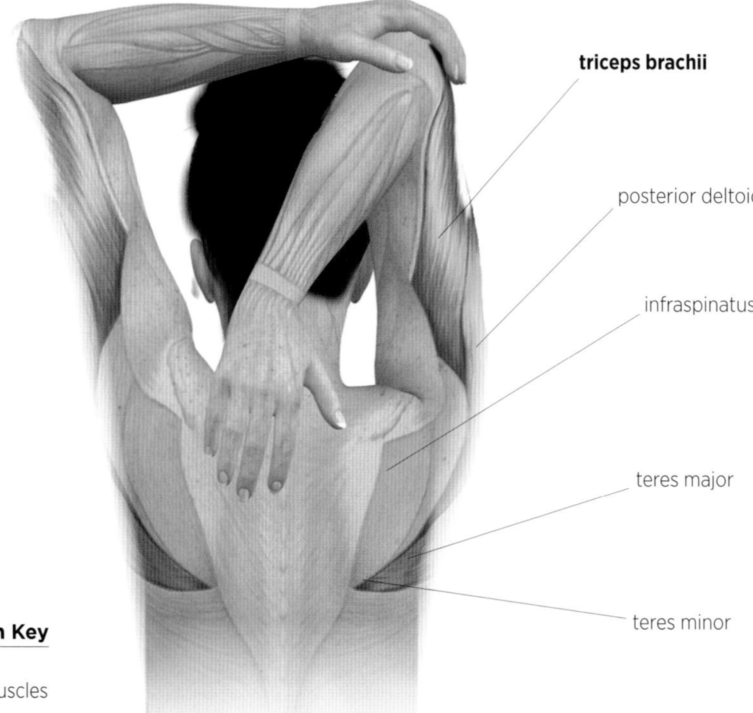

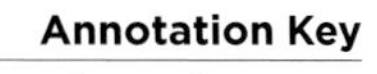

Annotation Key

Bold text indicates target muscles
Light text indicates other working muscles
* indicates deep muscles

Biceps-Pecs Stretch

This stretch opens up the upper-front part of your body. Working the chest and upper arms together, it counteracts tightening caused by bad habits such as slouching.

FACT FILE

TARGETS
- Biceps brachii
- Shoulders
- Chest

TYPE
- Isometric

BENEFITS
- Stretches and strengthens arms
- Opens chest

CAUTIONS
- Shoulder issues
- Wrist issues

HOW TO DO IT

- Stand with your legs and feet parallel and shoulder-width apart. Shift your pelvis slightly forward.
- Clasp your hands together behind your back with your fingers interwoven. If you want an extra stretch, twist your hands and wrists so that your palms are pulled in toward your buttocks and your thumbs point downward.
- Hold for the recommended time, release the stretch, and then repeat for the recommended repetitions.

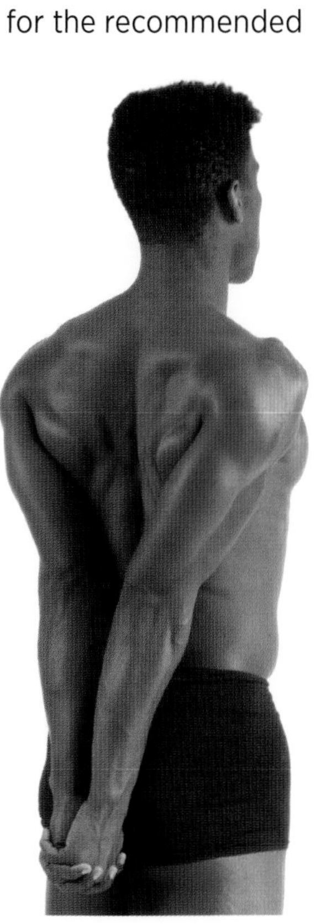

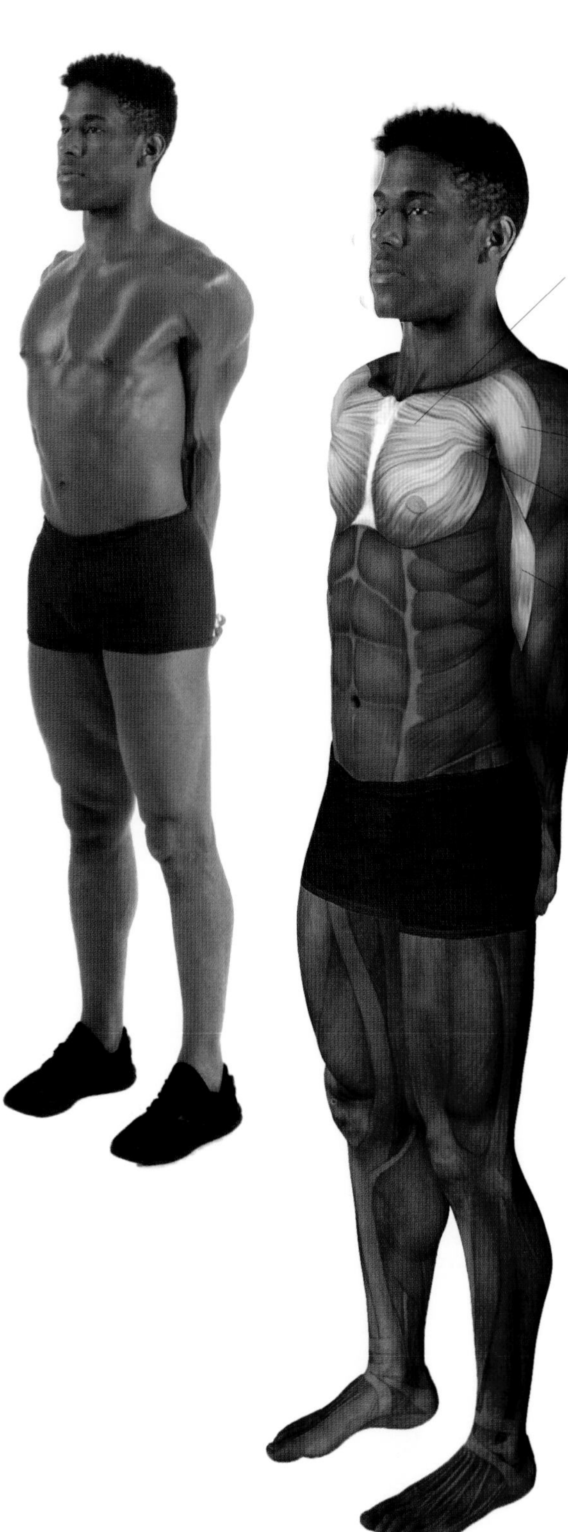

DO IT RIGHT

- Keep your shoulders pressed down and back, away from your ears.
- Avoid collapsing your chest forward.

Annotation Key

Bold text indicates target muscles
Light text indicates other working muscles
* indicates deep muscles

Hip and Iliotibial Band Stretch

The Hip and Iliotibial Band Stretch improves flexibility in your hips and keeps your iliotibial band supple. It also provides a full spinal and abdominal twist and boosts your overall mobility. If you're a runner or biker, this stretch can also help prevent sports-related injuries.

HOW TO DO IT

- Sit on the floor as straight as possible with your back flat and your legs extended in front of you. Your feet should be slightly flexed.
- Bend your right knee and cross it over to the outside of your left thigh. Keep your right foot flat on the floor.
- Wrap your left arm around your bent knee for stability as you rotate your torso.
- Hold this pose for the recommended amount of time. Slowly release, and then repeat on the opposite side.

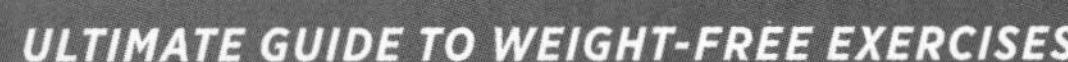

FACT FILE

TARGETS
- Hips
- Iliotibial band
- Spine

TYPE
- Static

BENEFITS
- Stretches hip extensors and flexors
- Stretches obliques

CAUTIONS
- Severe lower-back pain

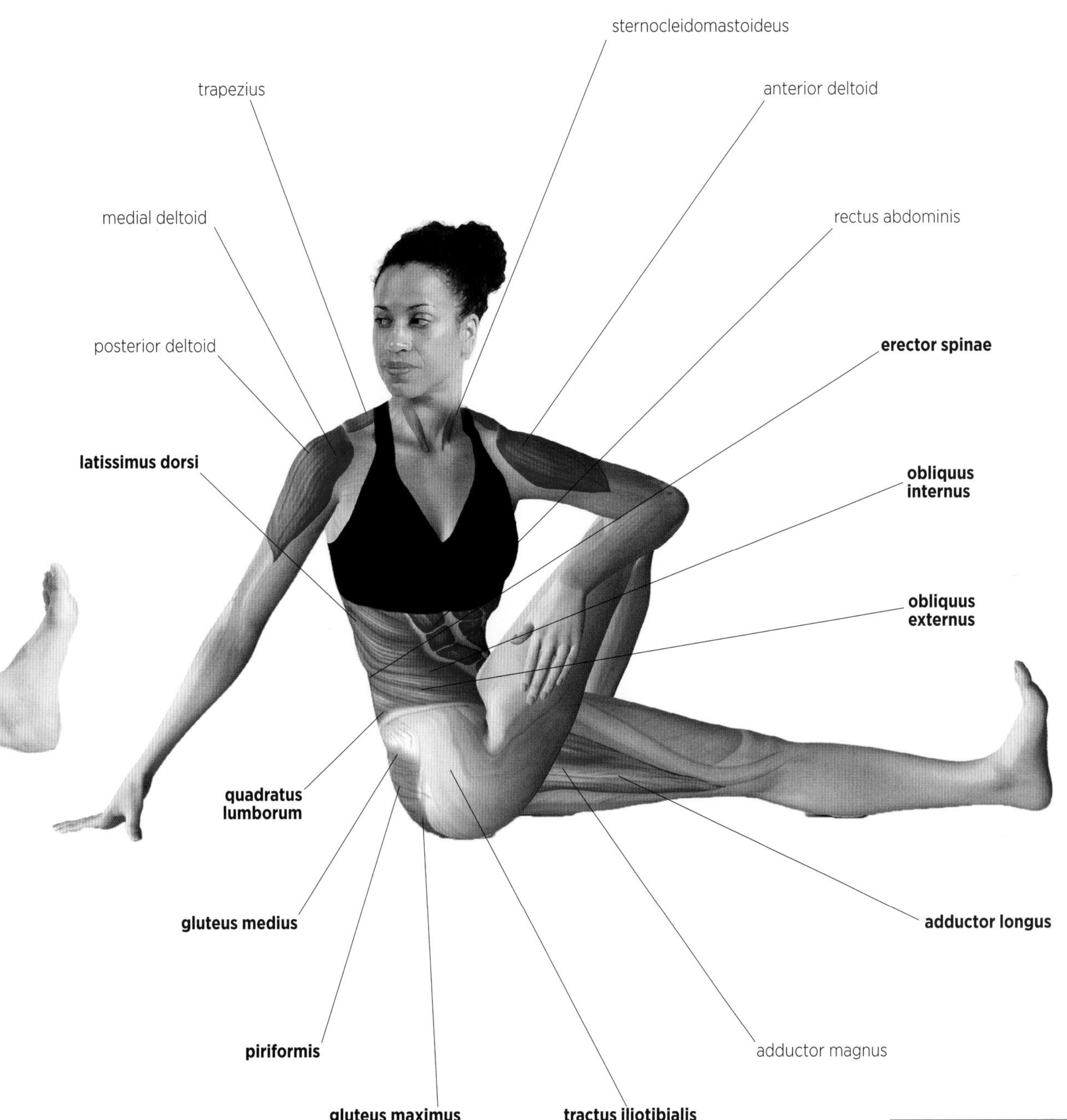

Annotation Key

Bold text indicates target muscles

Light text indicates other working muscles

* indicates deep muscles

DO IT RIGHT
- Apply even pressure to your leg with your active hand.
- Keep your torso upright as you pull your knee and torso together.
- Avoid lifting the foot of your bent leg off the floor.

Standing Quadriceps Stretch

The Standing Quadriceps Stretch relieves stiffness by giving the front and sides of your thighs a strong stretch while also releasing hip flexor muscles and improving balance and posture.

FACT FILE

TARGETS
- Quadriceps

TYPE
- Static

BENEFITS
- Helps to keep thigh muscles flexible

CAUTIONS
- Knee issues

HOW TO DO IT

- Stand with your legs and feet parallel and shoulder-width apart. Tuck your pelvis slightly forward, lift your chest, and press your shoulders downward and back.
- Bend your right knee behind you so that your ankle is raised toward your buttocks.
- Reach down with your right hand to grab your foot just below your ankle, and gently pull as you stretch.
- Hold for the recommended time, release the stretch, and then repeat on the opposite side

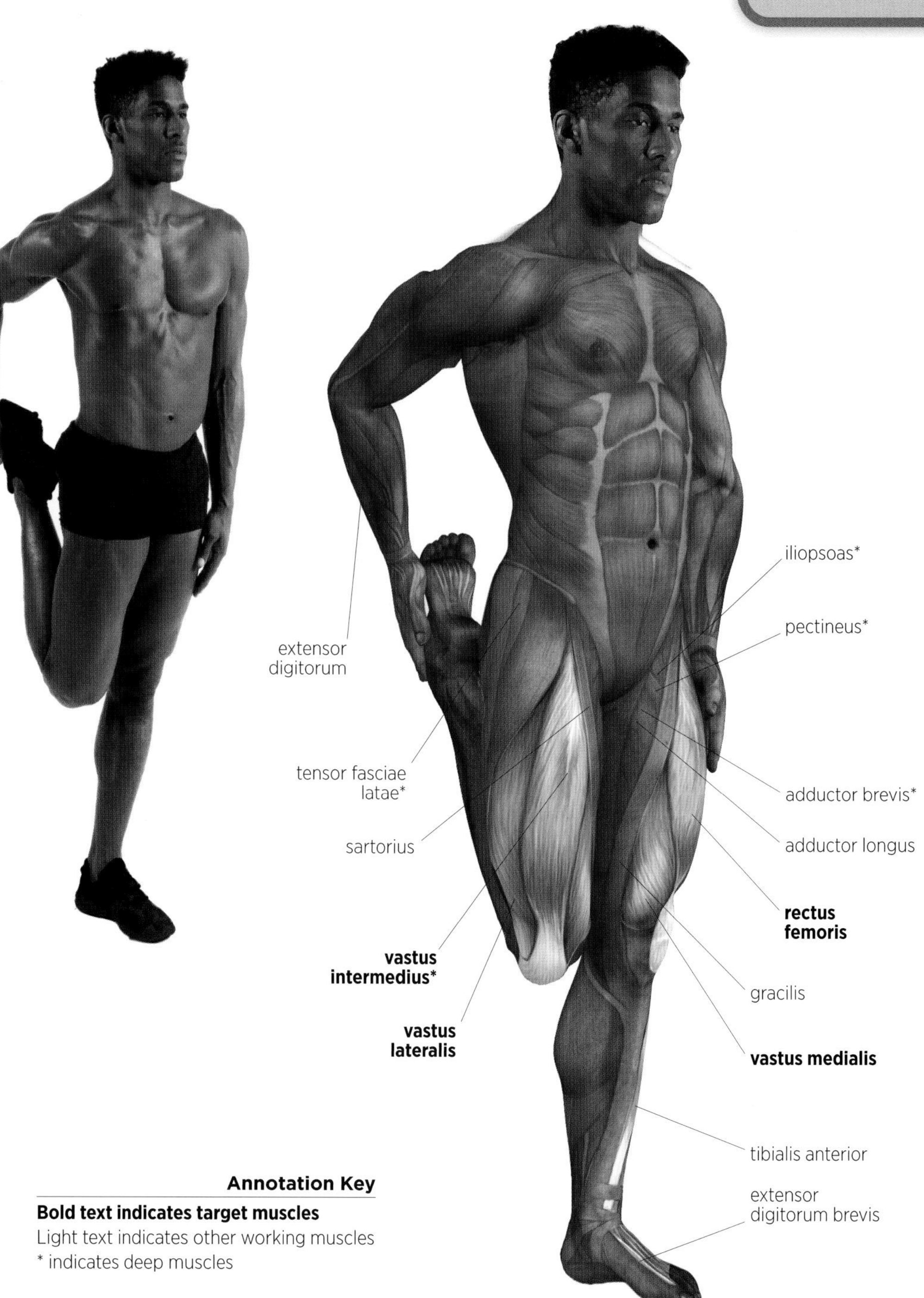

DO IT RIGHT

- Keep your torso upright.
- Pull your foot toward your buttocks gently, stretching only as far as you feel comfortable.
- Gaze forward.
- Avoid leaning forward.
- Avoid arching your back.
- Avoid hunching your shoulders.

Annotation Key

Bold text indicates target muscles

Light text indicates other working muscles

* indicates deep muscles

Standing Hamstrings Stretch

A simple, effective way to counteract the common problem of tight muscles at the back of the thigh, this stretch should benefit both your calves and your lower back.

HOW TO DO IT

- Stand with your right leg bent and your left leg extended in front of you with the heel on the floor.
- Lean over your left leg, resting both hands above your knee. Place the majority of your body weight on your front heel while feeling the stretch in the back of your thigh.
- Hold for the recommended time, release the stretch, and then repeat on the opposite side.

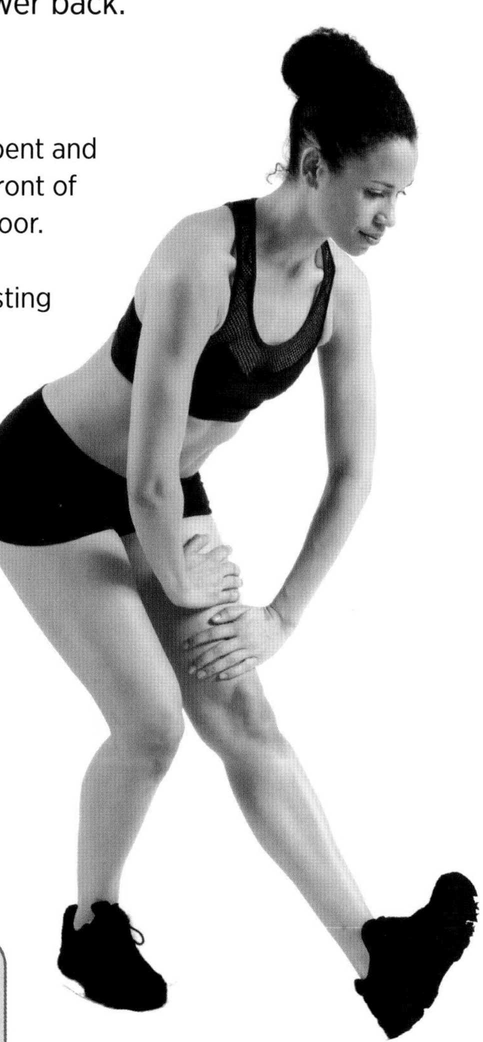

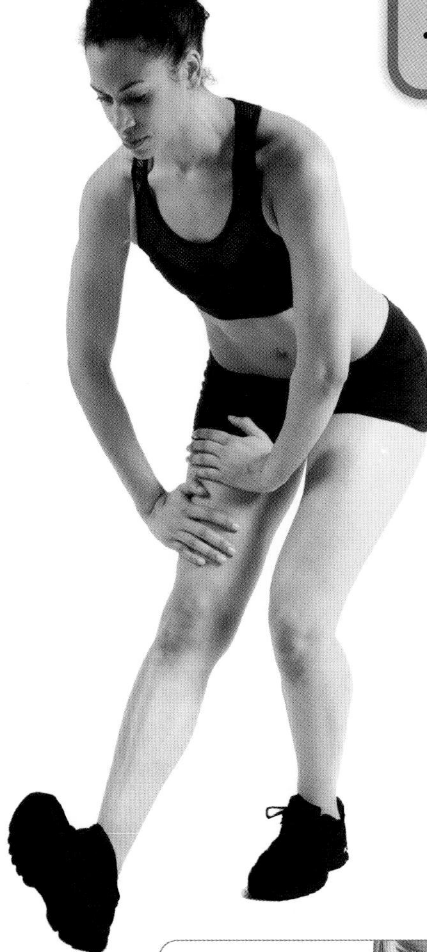

FACT FILE

TARGETS
- Hamstrings

TYPE
- Static

BENEFITS
- Helps to keep hamstring muscles flexible

CAUTIONS
- Lower-back issues
- Knee issues

DO IT RIGHT

- Keep your front leg straight.
- Flex the foot of your front leg as you stretch.
- Avoid arching your back or rounding it forward.
- Avoid hunching your shoulders.

Annotation Key
Bold text indicates target muscles
Light text indicates other working muscles
* indicates deep muscles

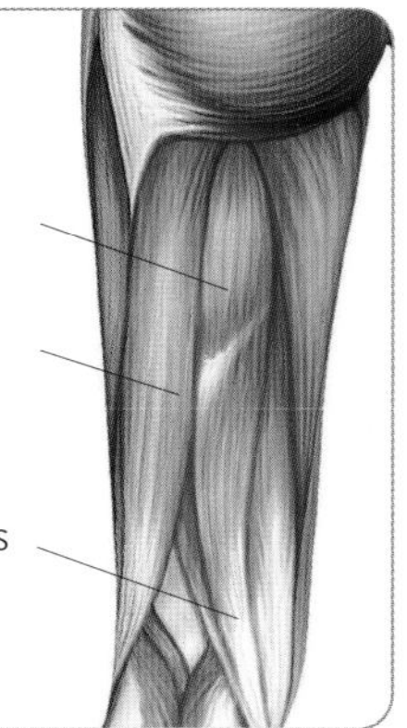

Garland Yoga Stretch

The Garland Yoga Stretch is a popular pose in many yoga routines that provides a more intense stretch than a traditional squat. This challenging position is a deep hip opener that also lengthens your spine and strengthens your core. It improves your balance as well.

HOW TO DO IT

- Stand with your feet turned out and wider than hip-width apart.
- Bend your knees as deeply as you can, squatting down until your hips are lower than your knees.
- Join your hands in prayer position in front of your heart. Hold for the recommended breaths.

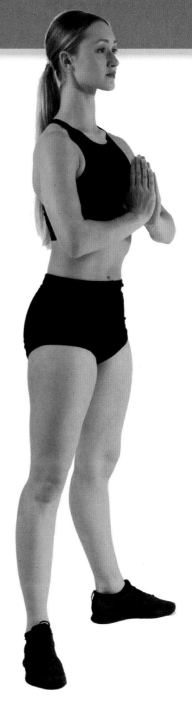

DO IT RIGHT

- Apply gentle pressure between your elbows and your knees, encouraging your knees to open farther and deepening the inner-thigh stretch.
- Lengthen your spine, keeping your back straight.
- Broaden across your collarbones.
- Avoid rounding your shoulders forward.

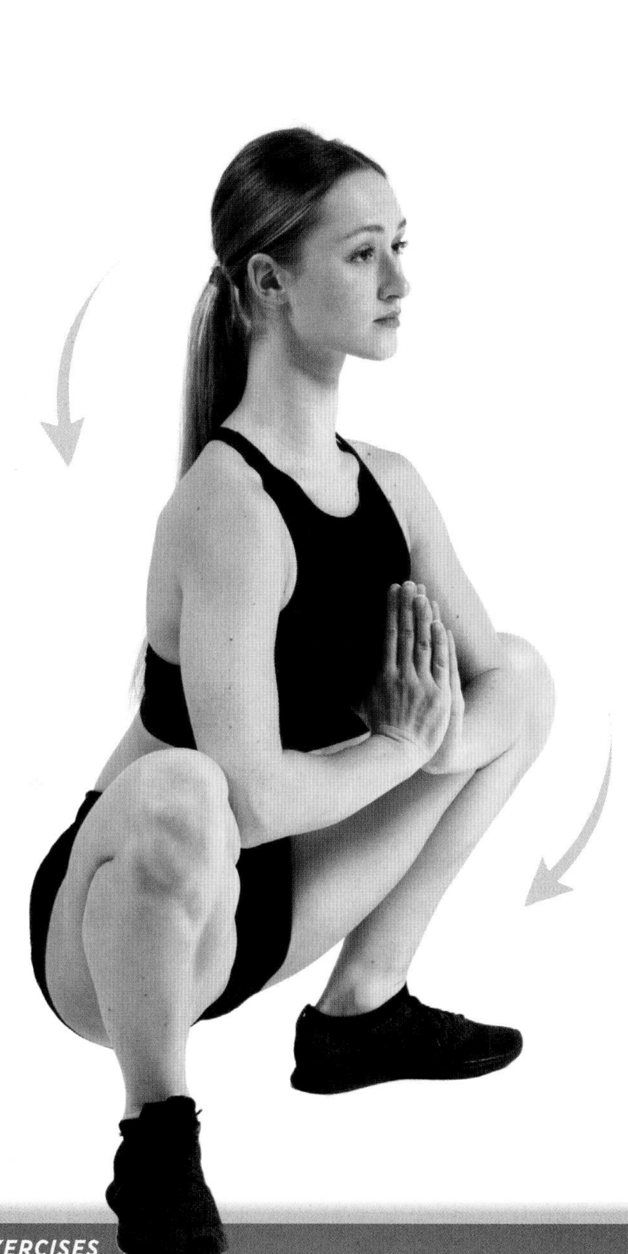

FACT FILE

TARGETS
- Inner thighs

TYPE
- Static

BENEFITS
- Stretches hips, groin, and ankles
- Lengthens spine
- Engages quadriceps and adductors

CAUTIONS
- Knee issues
- Lower-back issues

Annotation Key
Bold text indicates target muscles
Light text indicates other working muscles
* indicates deep muscles

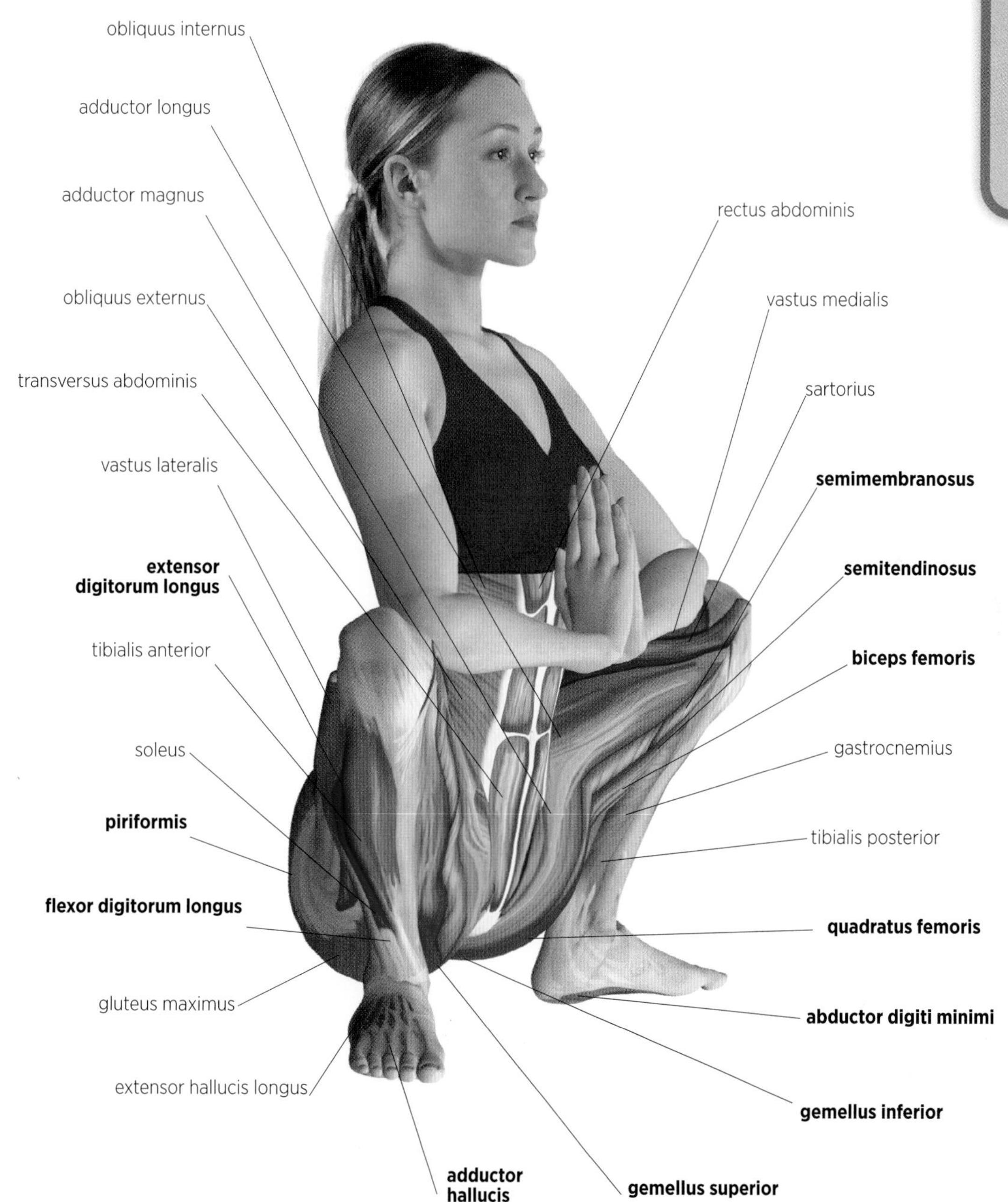

Iliotibial Band Stretch

The tractus iliotibialis, commonly called the iliotibial band or ITB, is a band of tissue linking your hips and shins and interconnecting with major muscles. This stretch counters common problems in the knees, hips, or thighs.

HOW TO DO IT

- Stand upright, with your arms along your sides. Cross your right foot in front of your left.
- Bending at your waist, gradually reach toward the floor with your hands.
- Hold for the recommended time, release the stretch, and then slowly roll up to the starting position. Repeat on the opposite side.

DO IT RIGHT

- Keep your knees straight, yet soft, throughout the exercise.
- Let your head drop.
- Avoid bending or locking your knees.
- Avoid twisting your neck, shoulders, or torso to either side.

MODIFICATION

EASIER: If you find it difficult to reach the floor with your hands while maintaining your form, hold the stretch when your hands are only partway to the floor, or hold onto your straight leg. Try to reach slightly lower each time you stretch.

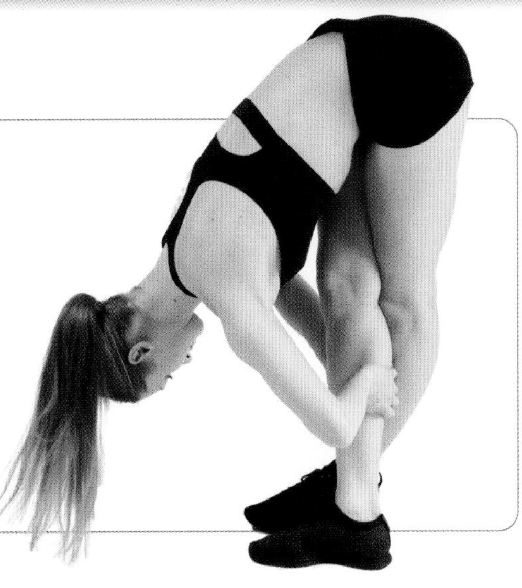

FACT FILE

TARGETS
- Iliotibial band
- Glutes
- Hamstrings

TYPE
- Static

BENEFITS
- Stretches IT band
- Counteracts effects of wearing high heels
- Boosts performance in running, skiing, and cycling

CAUTIONS
- Neck issues
- Lower-back pain

Annotation Key

Bold text indicates target muscles

Light text indicates other working muscles

* indicates deep muscles

Half-Kneeling Rotation

This warm-up stretch brings important benefits to your general spinal mobility, improves both your posture and balance, and boosts your core rotation.

HOW TO DO IT

- Kneel on your left leg with your right leg bent at 90 degrees in front of you, foot on the floor. Place your hands beside your head so that your elbows flare outward.
- Keeping your back straight, rotate your left shoulder so that your upper body turns to the right.
- Hold for the recommended time, release the stretch, and then repeat on the opposite side.

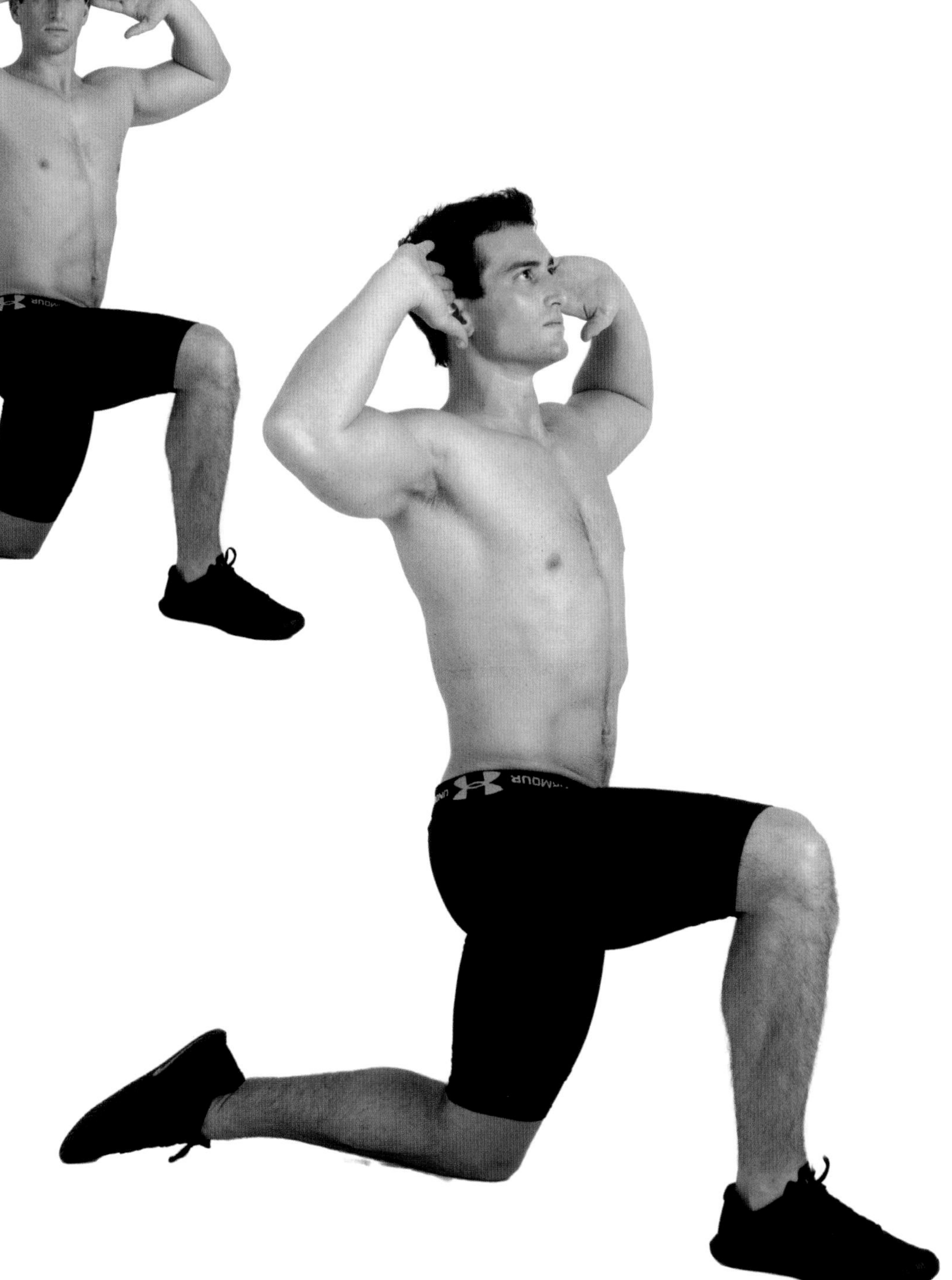

DO IT RIGHT

- Keep your back straight.
- Avoid rotating too far.
- Avoid letting your stomach bulge outward as your upper body rotates from one side to the other.

FACT FILE

TARGETS
- Obliques
- Spine

TYPE
- Static

BENEFITS
- Increases spinal rotation
- Improves posture

CAUTIONS
- Knee issues

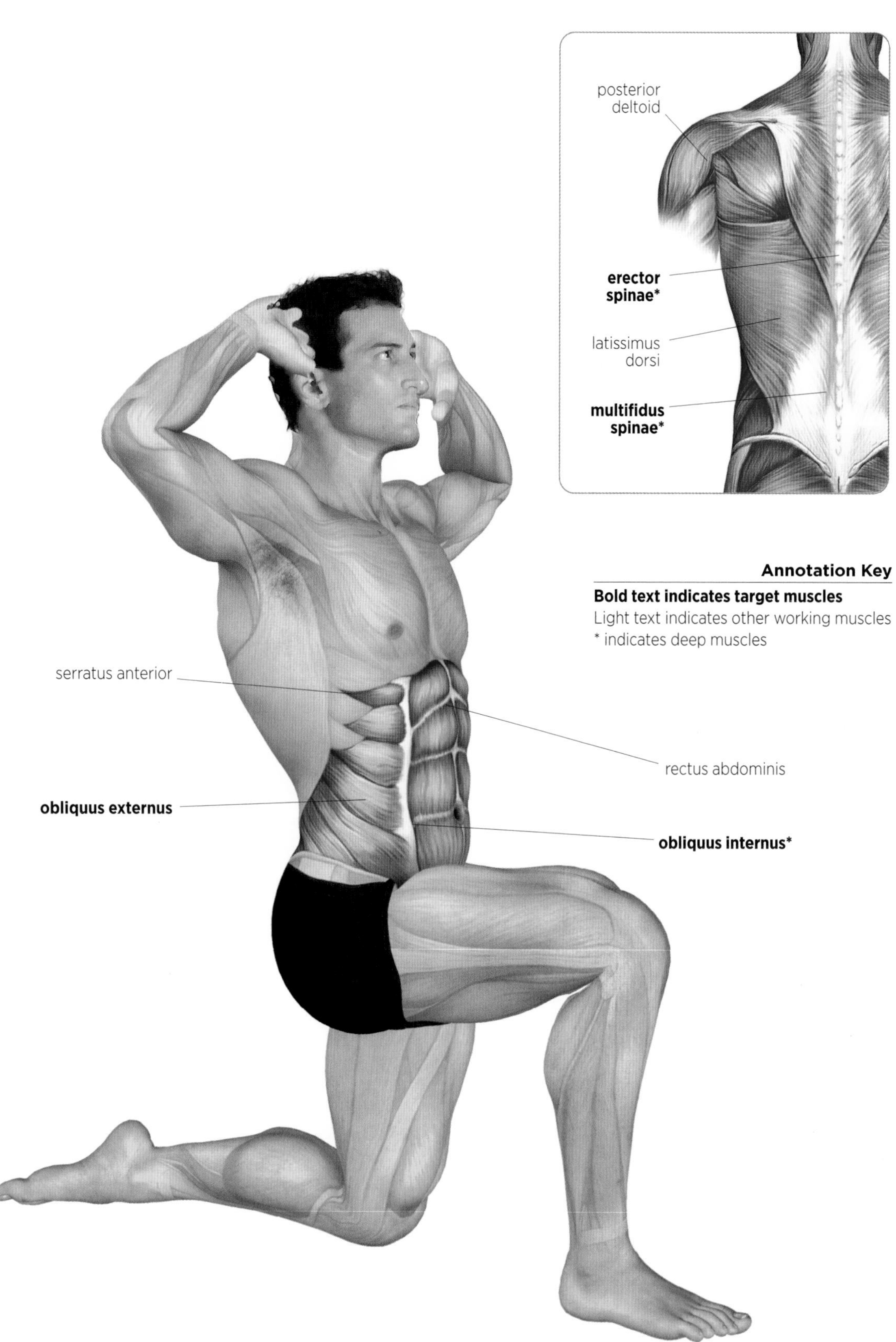

Annotation Key

Bold text indicates target muscles
Light text indicates other working muscles
* indicates deep muscles

Side Bending

This straightforward standing exercise stretches out the top half of your body and helps to counteract the poor, hunched posture that comes with sedentary lifestyles.

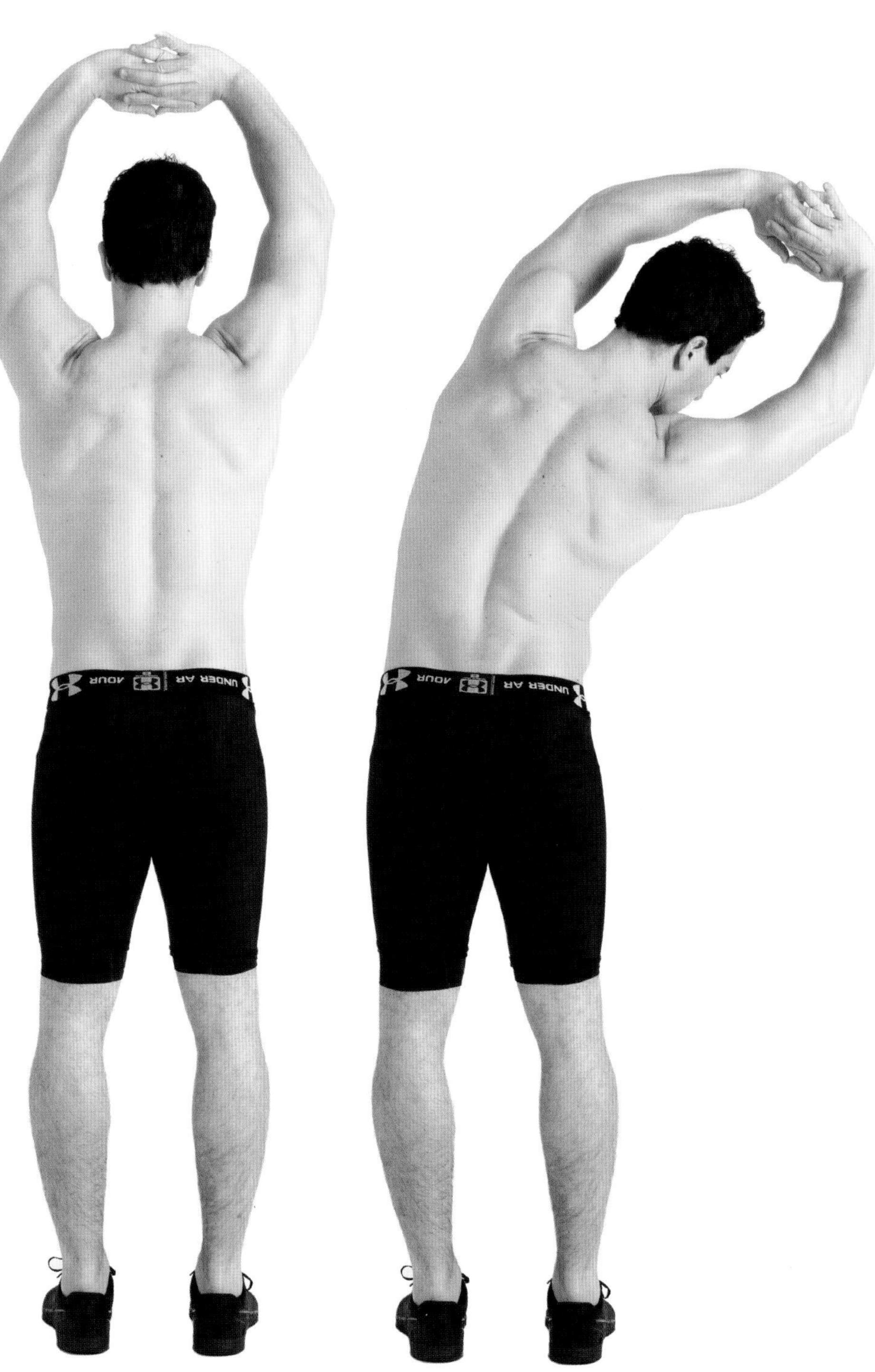

HOW TO DO IT

- Stand, keeping your neck, shoulders, and torso straight.
- Raise both arms above your head, and clasp your hands together, with your fingers interlocked and palms facing upward.
- Leaning from the hips, slowly drop your torso to the right.
- Keeping a smooth flow, lean your torso to the left.
- Continue alternating sides for the recommended repetitions.

DO IT RIGHT

- Elongate your arms and shoulders as much as possible.
- Avoid dropping to the side too quickly.

FACT FILE

TARGETS
- Upper back
- Obliques

TYPE
- Static

BENEFITS
- Increases upper-body mobility
- Improves posture

CAUTIONS
- Lower-back pain

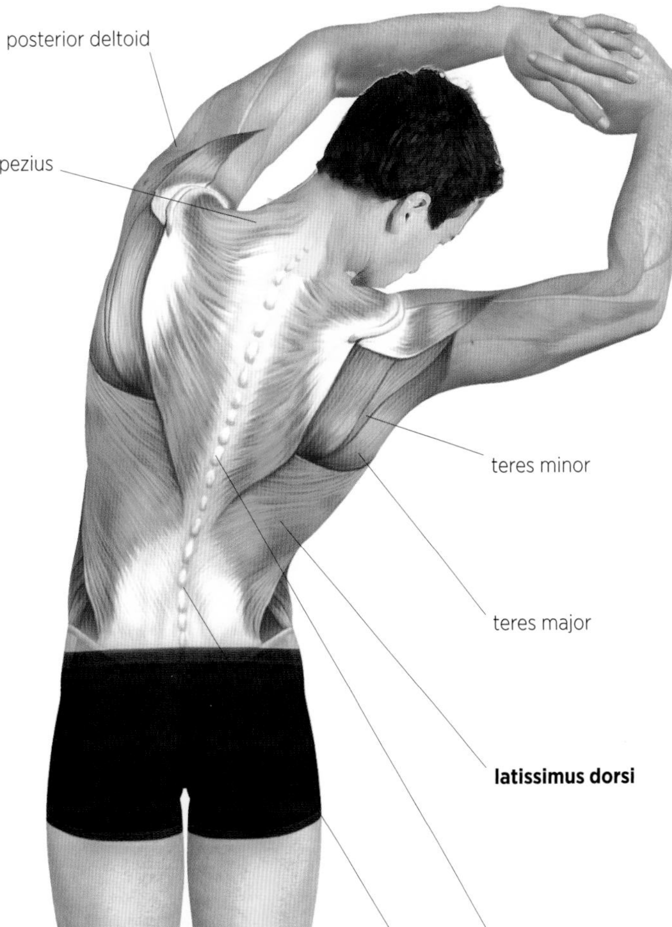

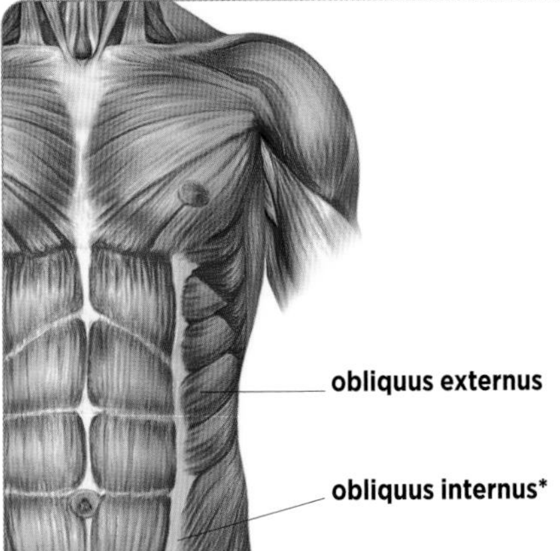

Annotation Key

Bold text indicates target muscles
Light text indicates other working muscles
* indicates deep muscles

Cobra Stretch

As well as promoting spinal flexibility, this yoga-inspired stretch builds strength in your back and shoulders and also in your abdominals, buttocks, and chest.

HOW TO DO IT

- Lie facedown. Bend your elbows, placing your hands flat on the floor beside your chest. Extend your legs, and press down into the floor with your thighs and the tops of your feet.
- Inhaling, lift your chest off the floor, pressing your palms downward.
- Continue lifting your chest as you straighten your arms.
- Hold for the recommended time, and then, on an exhalation, lower yourself to the floor.

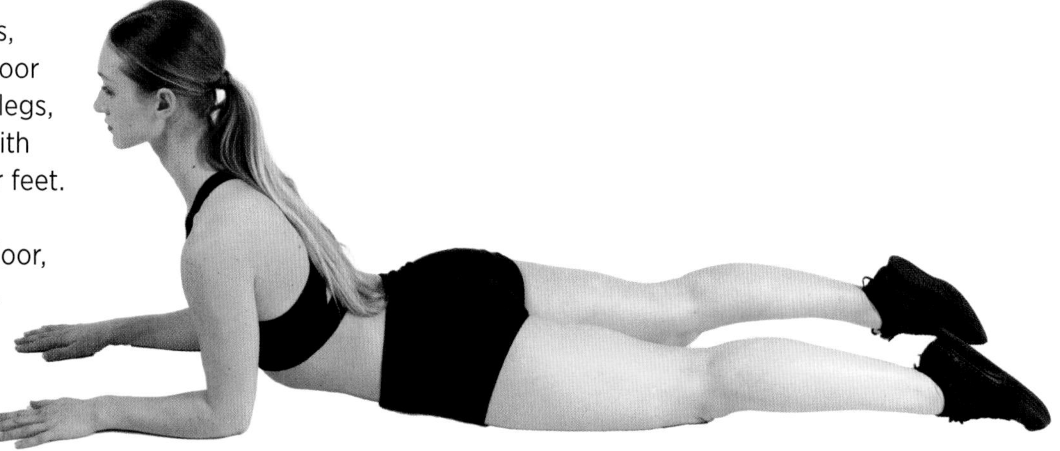

DO IT RIGHT

- Gaze forward.
- Keep your elbows pulled in toward your body.
- Lift from your chest and back, rather than depending too much on your arms to create the arch in your back.
- Keep your shoulders and elbows pressed back.
- Press your pubic bone into the floor as you lift.
- Avoid tensing your buttocks.
- Avoid splaying your elbows out to the sides.
- Avoid lifting your hips off the floor.
- Avoid twisting your neck.

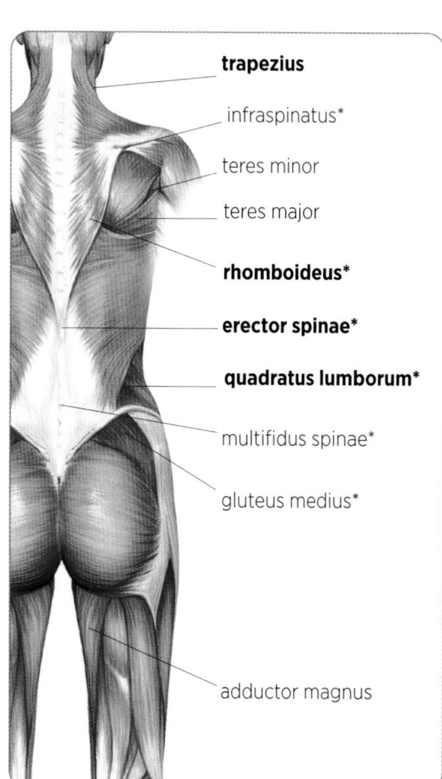

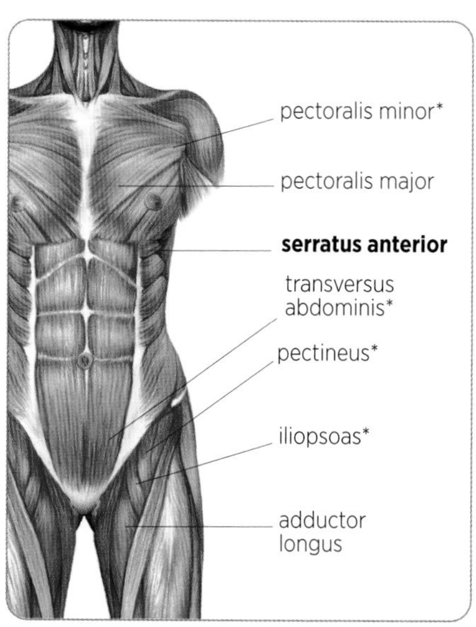

Annotation Key
Bold text indicates target muscles
Light text indicates other working muscles
* indicates deep muscles

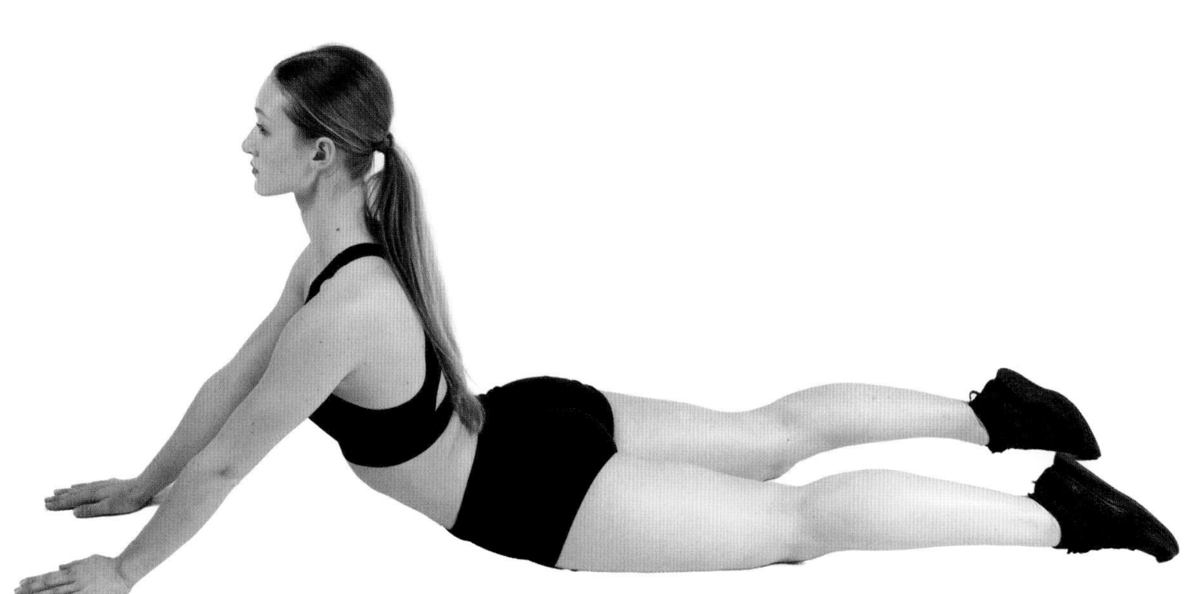

FACT FILE

TARGETS
- Abdominals
- Back
- Chest
- Glutes
- Shoulders
- Triceps

TYPE
- Static

BENEFITS
- Strengthens spine and glutes
- Stretches chest, abdominals, and shoulders
- Boosts performance in all sports

CAUTIONS
- Lower-back issues/pain

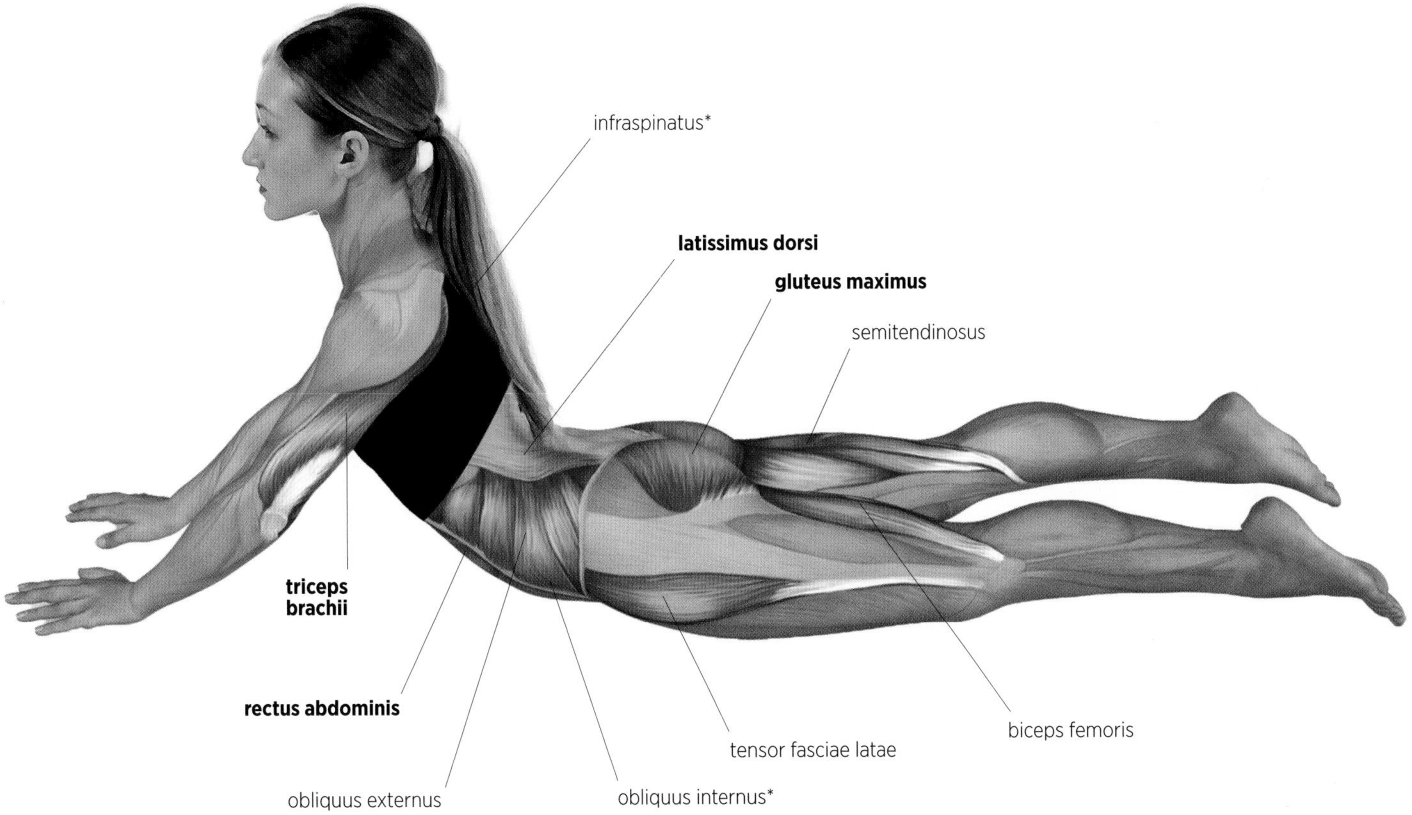

infraspinatus*

latissimus dorsi

gluteus maximus

semitendinosus

triceps brachii

rectus abdominis

tensor fasciae latae

biceps femoris

obliquus externus

obliquus internus*

Standing Back Roll

The Standing Back Roll is a great stretch to include in your flexibility workouts, providing an easy, flowing movement from a standing forward bend to an upright posture. On its own, it is a dynamic upper-back stretch that effectively reduces tightness and tension in the rhomboid muscles.

HOW TO DO IT

- Stand with your legs and feet parallel and shoulder-width apart. Bend your knees very slightly.
- Slowly round your spine downward, from your neck through your lower back, and lower your arms down the sides of your legs. Continue bending at the waist, letting the weight of your body draw your head toward the floor as you stretch.
- Slowly roll up halfway to the point at which you feel your gluteal muscles above your hips and thighs.
- Cross your forearms to place your hands on the opposite thighs, and round your shoulders forward. Feel the heaviness of your head as you stretch your upper back between the shoulder blades.
- Slowly rise to the starting position, and then repeat for the recommended repetitions.

DO IT RIGHT

- Keep your knees slightly bent.
- Tuck your pelvis forward slightly, allowing your upper body to contract.
- Avoid allowing your knees to turn inward.

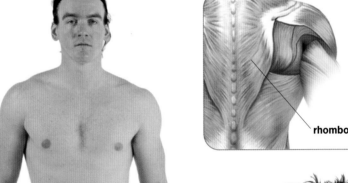

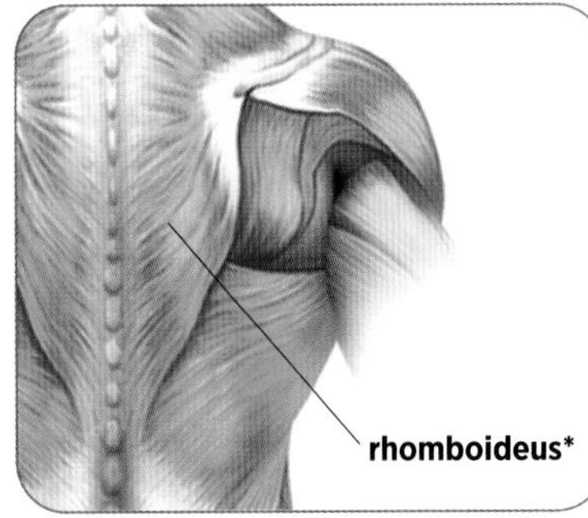

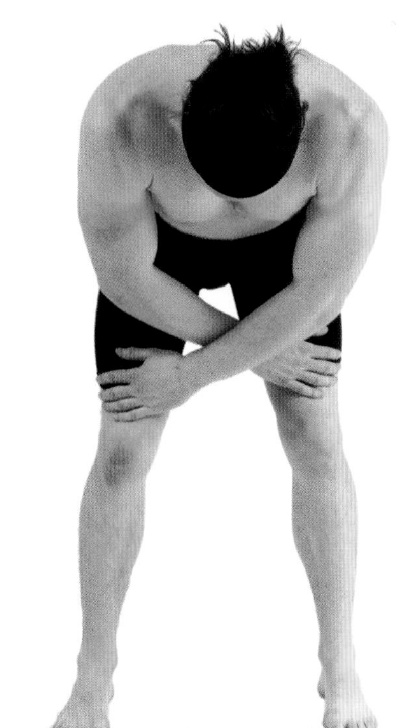

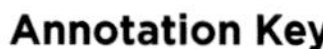

Annotation Key

Bold text indicates target muscles
Light text indicates other working muscles
* indicates deep muscles

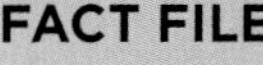

FACT FILE

TARGETS
- Upper back
- Middle back

TYPE
- Dynamic

BENEFITS
- Increases upper-back mobility
- Reduces shoulder tightness
- Lengthens spinal column

CAUTIONS
- Spinal injury
- Shoulder issues
- Hip issues

Scoop Rhomboids

Located in the middle of the back, the rhomboid muscles retract your shoulder blades. These deep muscles are phasic, meaning they weaken with disuse. This upper-back and shoulder stretch will reduce tension in the shoulder blades, while keeping the rhomboids healthy and engaged.

FACT FILE

TARGETS
- Upper back

TYPE
- Static

BENEFITS
- Increases upper-back mobility
- Reduces shoulder tightness
- Lengthens spinal column

CAUTIONS
- Shoulder issues
- Back issues

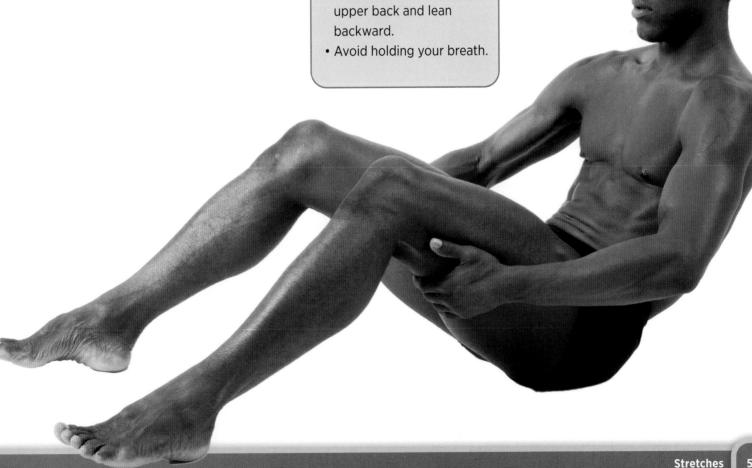

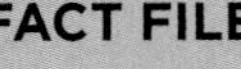

HOW TO DO IT

- Sit up tall with your legs extended in front of you. Bend your knees slightly, keeping your heels on the floor, and then grasp your legs behind your knees.
- Keeping your head straight, lean back whilst still grasping your legs.
- Hold for the recommended time, and then slowly roll back up to the starting position. Repeat for the recommended repetitions.

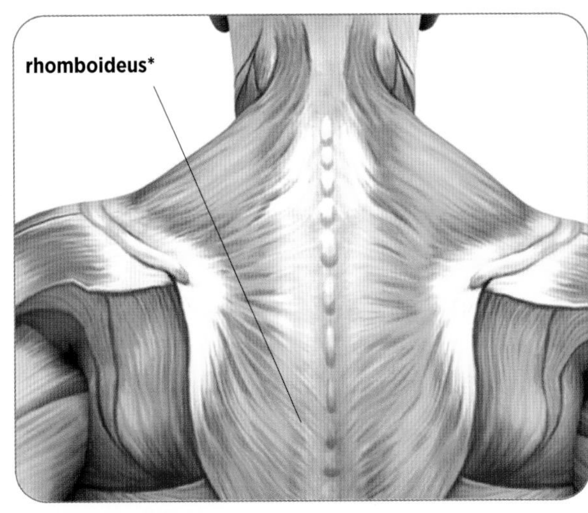

DO IT RIGHT

- Exhale as you round your upper back and lean backward.
- Avoid holding your breath.

Spine Stretch Forward

The Spine Stretch Forward is a great beginner exercise that improves flexibility along your spine and in your hamstrings. As you perform this simple stretch, focus on articulating your spine as you slowly curl your body forward.

DO IT RIGHT

- Create a C-curve along your spine, from head to tailbone.
- Feel your ribcage expand outward as you inhale.
- Avoid shifting your pelvis or rolling your knees inward.

HOW TO DO IT

- Sit up tall with your legs extended in front of you slightly more than one hip-width apart.
- Flex your feet, place your palms on the floor by your hips, and inhale.
- Exhale as you curl forward, beginning with your head, neck, and upper back.
- Reach your arms forward, with palms facing up, and try to touch your feet.
- Hold for the recommended time, slowly roll back to an upright position to release the stretch, and then repeat for the recommended repetitions.

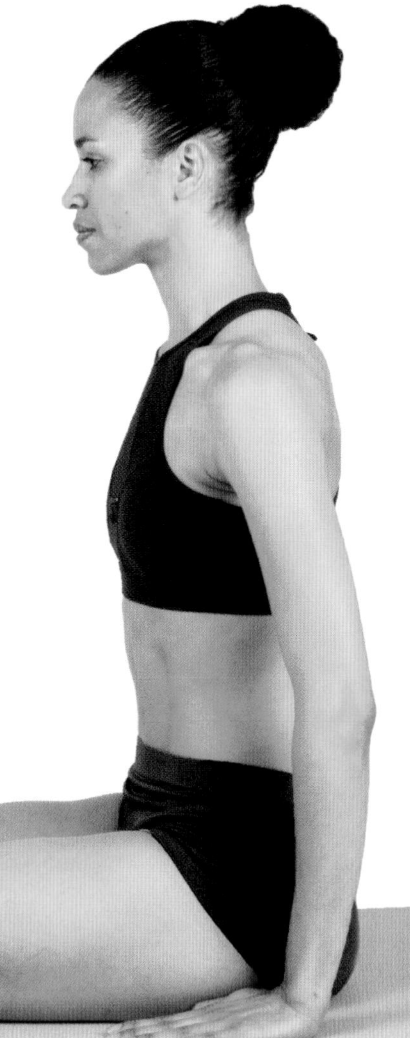

FACT FILE

TARGETS
- Spine
- Obliques
- Thighs

TYPE
- Static

BENEFITS
- Improves back flexibility
- Strengthens and lengthens torso
- Lengthens calf and hamstring muscles

CAUTIONS
- Back issues
- Hip issues

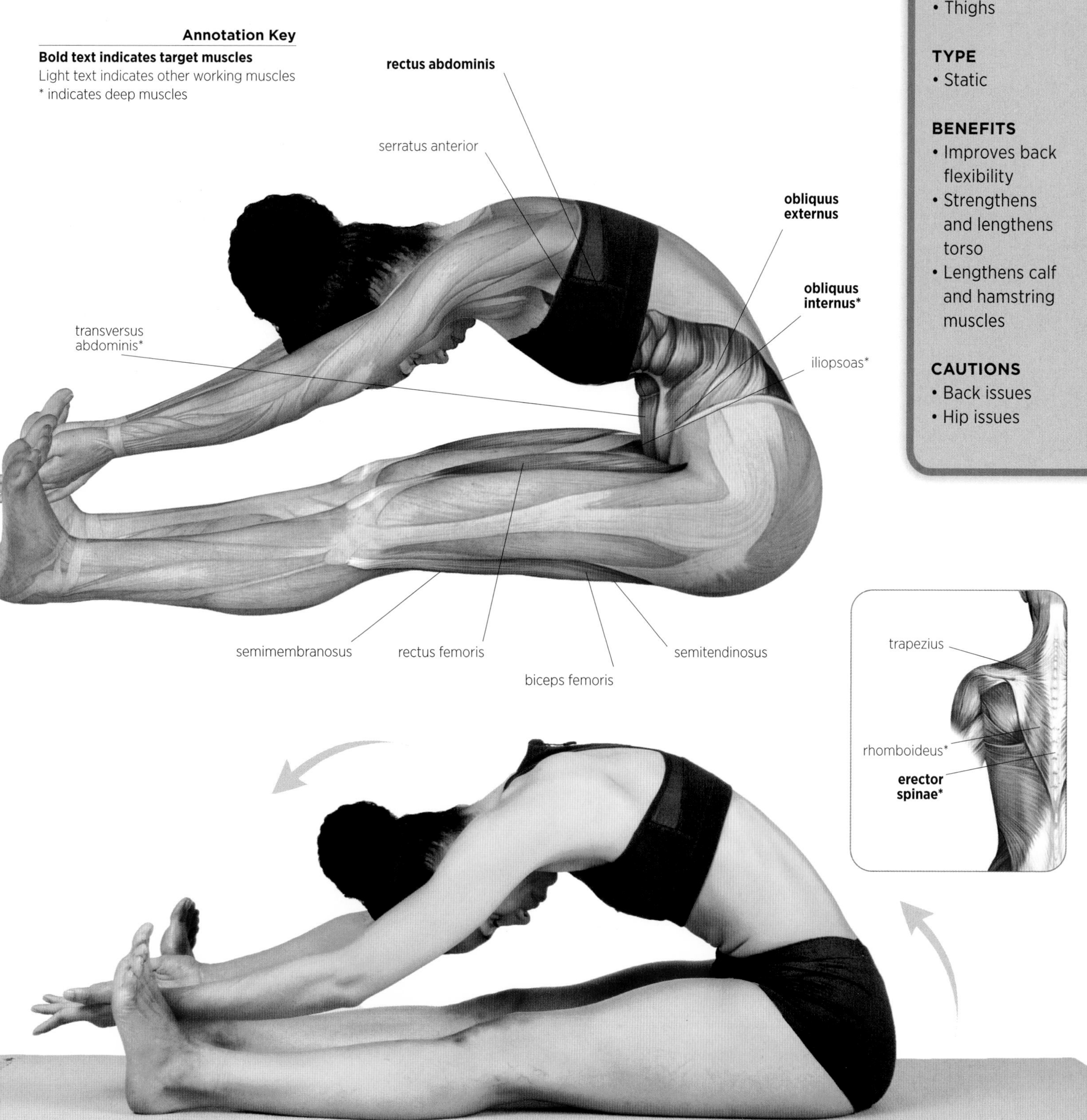

Front Deltoid Towel Stretch

This stretch improves mobility in people who regularly perform repetitive shoulder and arm motions. Gripping the end of a short towel with either hand is a great way to target these specific shoulder muscles.

HOW TO DO IT

- Sit up tall with your legs extended in front of you. Bend your knees slightly, keeping your heels on the floor.
- Grip either end of a small towel behind your back, with your palms facing behind you.
- Gently slide your buttocks forward along the floor until you feel a comfortable stretch in your front deltoids.
- Hold for the recommended time, and then slide back up to the starting position. Repeat for the recommended repetitions.

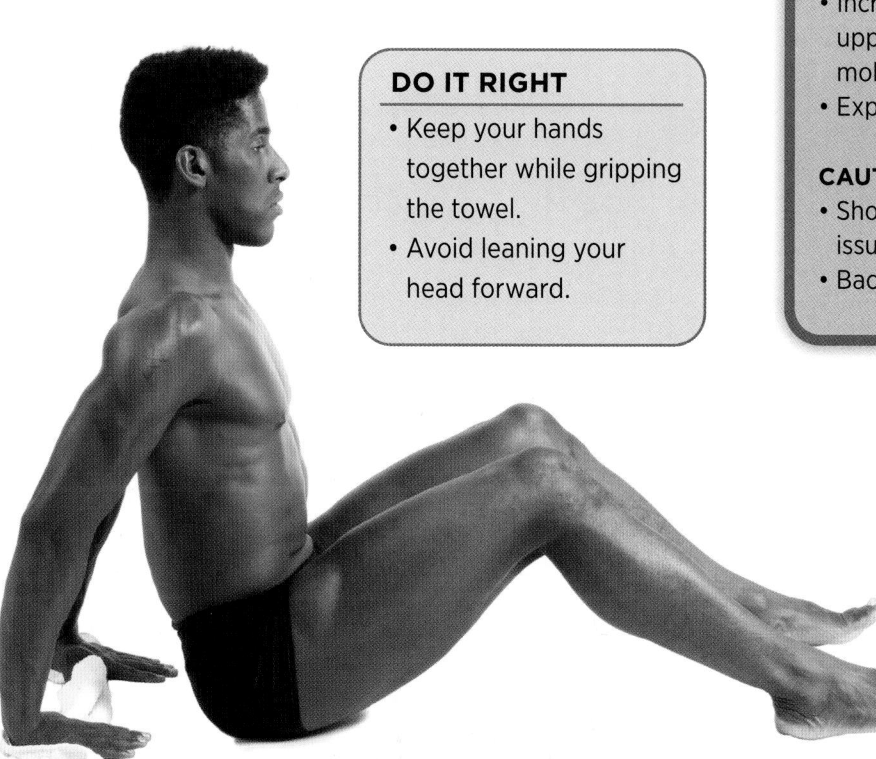

DO IT RIGHT

- Keep your hands together while gripping the towel.
- Avoid leaning your head forward.

FACT FILE

TARGETS
- Anterior deltoids

TYPE
- Static

BENEFITS
- Reduces shoulder tightness
- Increases upper-back mobility
- Expands chest

CAUTIONS
- Shoulder issues
- Back issues

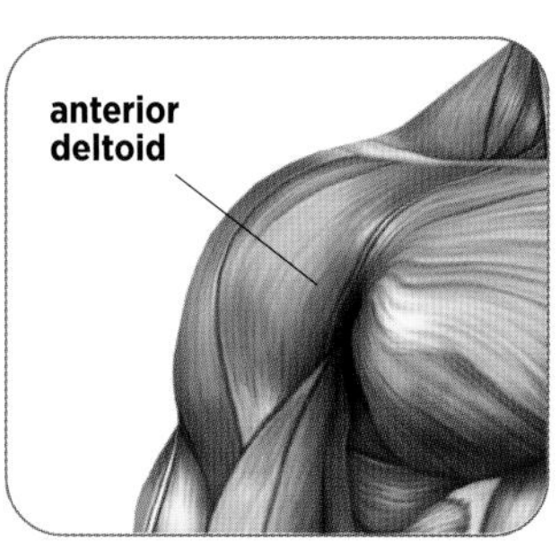

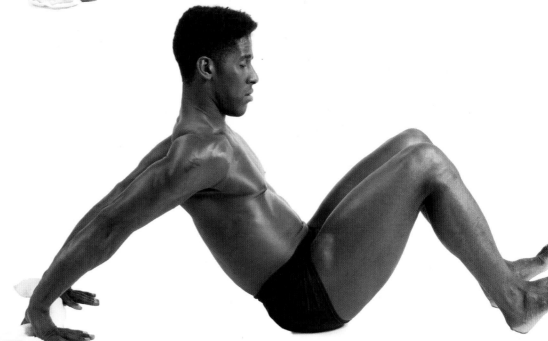

Annotation Key
Bold text indicates target muscles
Light text indicates other working muscles
* indicates deep muscles

Spine Stretch Reaching

Spine Stretch Reaching eases your muscles into a full forward bend. This exercise provides a great opportunity for you to practice lengthening your shoulder blades and upper spinal column.

HOW TO DO IT

- Sit up tall with your legs extended in front of you slightly more than one hip-width apart.
- Flex your feet, place your palms on the floor by your hips, and then inhale.
- Raise your arms overhead, palms facing inward, forming a straight line with your back.
- Inhale to prepare, and then exhale as you curl forward. Reach your arms forward keeping them at shoulder height.
- Hold for the recommended time, slowly roll back to an upright position to release the stretch, and then repeat for the recommended repetitions.

DO IT RIGHT

- Keep your arms straight and at shoulder-height as you fold forward.
- Keep your feet flexed.
- Avoid hunching your shoulders.
- Breath steadily throughout the stretch.

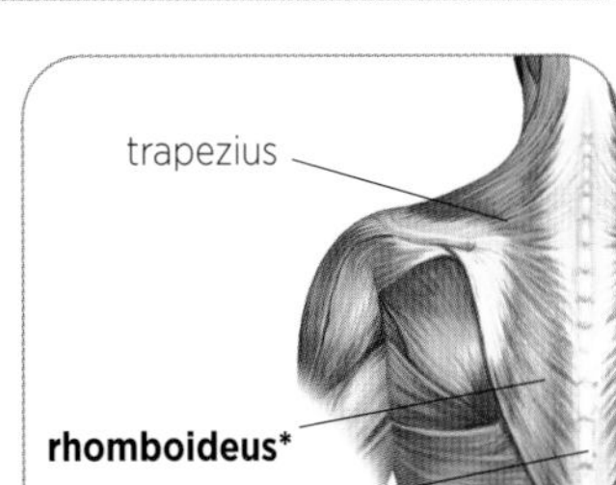

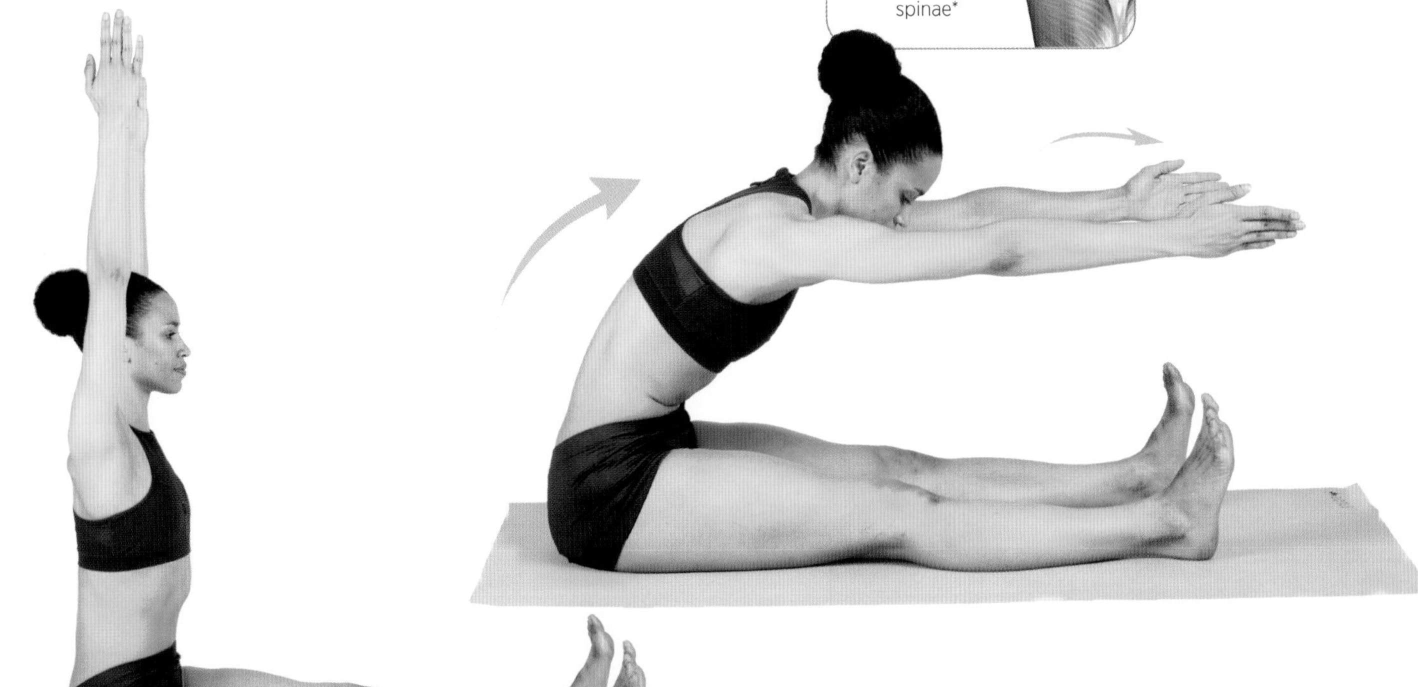

Annotation Key

Bold text indicates target muscles

Light text indicates other working muscles

* indicates deep muscles

FACT FILE

TARGETS
- Shoulders
- Neck
- Upper back
- Middle back

TYPE
- Static

BENEFITS
- Improves spinal mobility
- Relieves shoulder tightness
- Strengthens and lengthens torso
- Engages calf and hamstring muscles

CAUTIONS
- Back issues
- Hip issues

Knee-to-Chest Hug

The Knee-to-Chest Hug is an easy-to-do stretch that is great for releasing tightness in the lower back and increasing range of motion along the spine. Perform it to reduce stiffness associated with spinal arthritis or spinal stenosis.

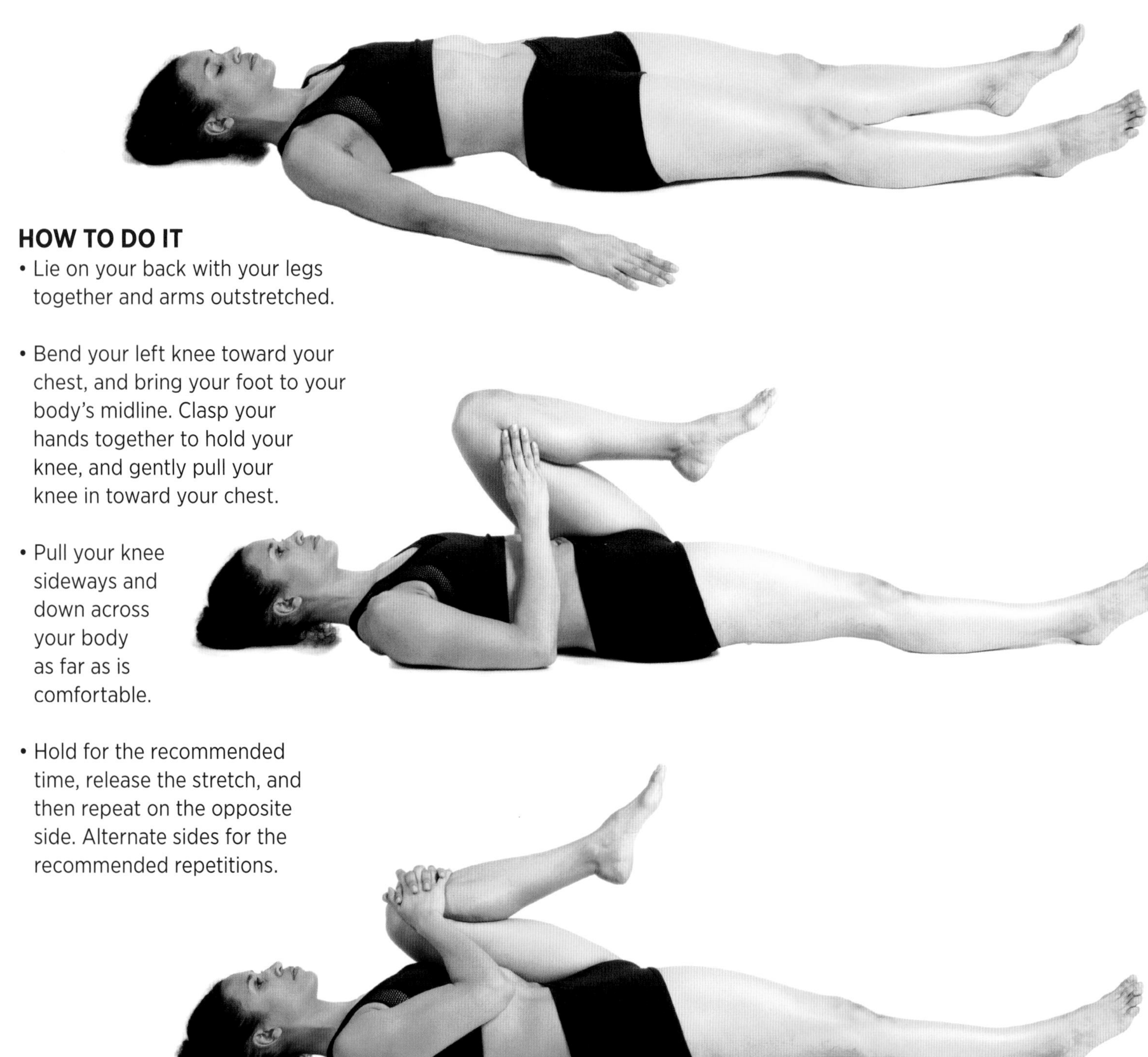

HOW TO DO IT

- Lie on your back with your legs together and arms outstretched.
- Bend your left knee toward your chest, and bring your foot to your body's midline. Clasp your hands together to hold your knee, and gently pull your knee in toward your chest.
- Pull your knee sideways and down across your body as far as is comfortable.
- Hold for the recommended time, release the stretch, and then repeat on the opposite side. Alternate sides for the recommended repetitions.

FACT FILE

TARGETS
- Lower back
- Groin muscles
- Glutes
- Hamstrings

TYPE
- Static

BENEFITS
- Reduces upper-back and shoulder stress
- Stretches lower back, hip extensors, and hip rotators

CAUTIONS
- Knee issues
- Shoulder issues

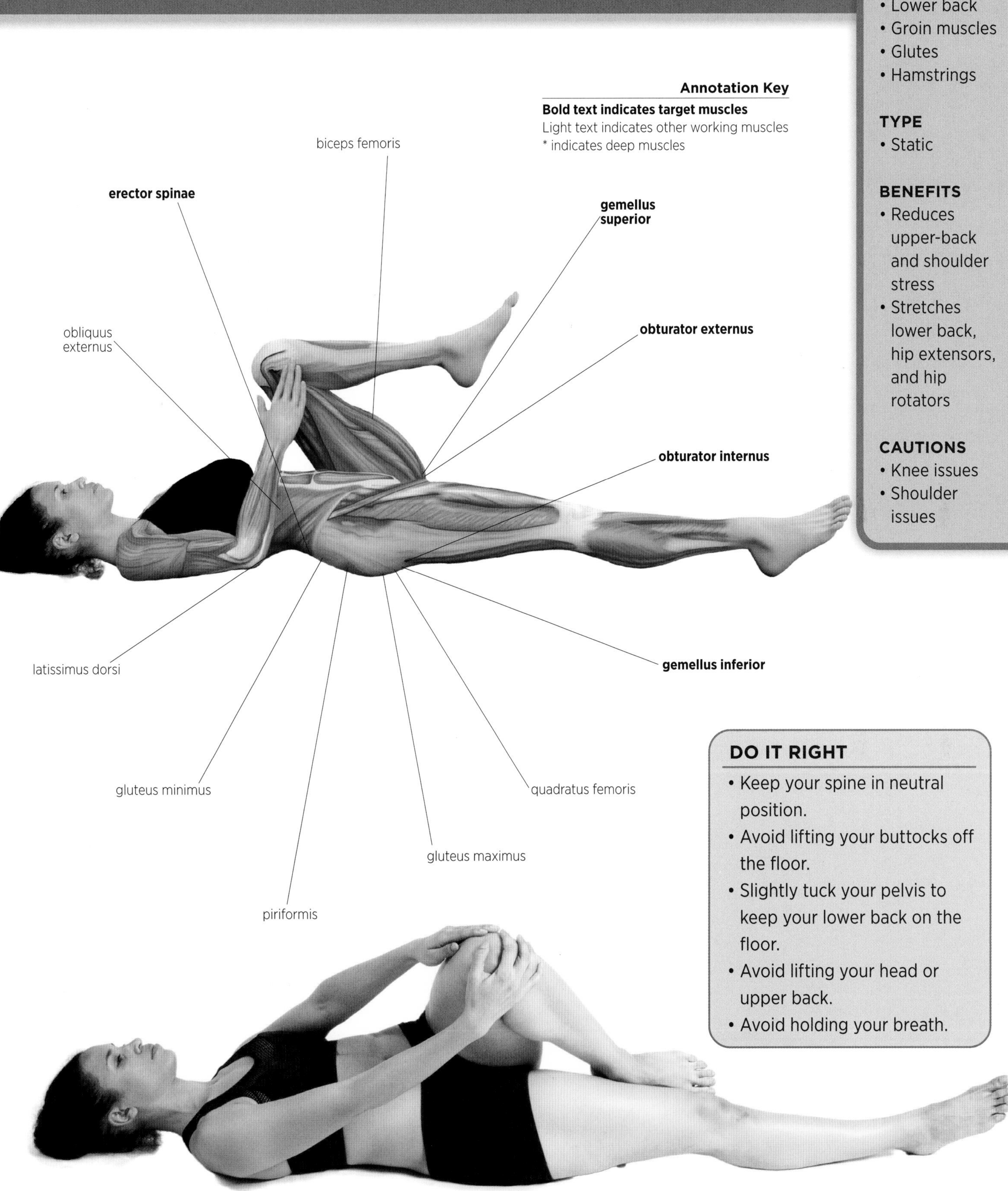

DO IT RIGHT
- Keep your spine in neutral position.
- Avoid lifting your buttocks off the floor.
- Slightly tuck your pelvis to keep your lower back on the floor.
- Avoid lifting your head or upper back.
- Avoid holding your breath.

Half Straddle Stretch

The Half Straddle Stretch benefits your lower torso and your legs, opening your hips and lengthening your obliques, thighs, quads, and calves.

HOW TO DO IT

- Sit upright with your knees bent.
- Keeping your right knee bent, lower it to the floor, and draw your right foot in toward your groin.
- Extend your left leg straight out to your left side.

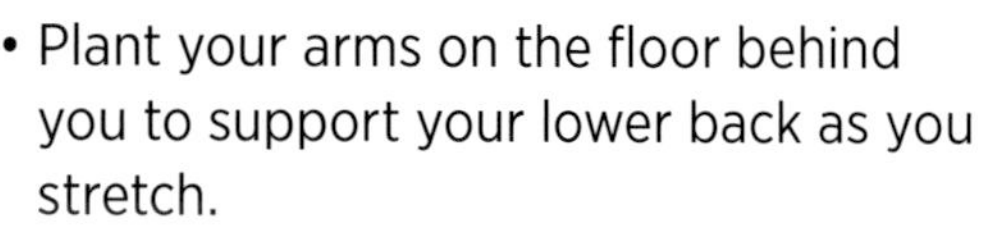

- Plant your arms on the floor behind you to support your lower back as you stretch.
- Hold for the recommended time, release the stretch, and then repeat on the opposite side.

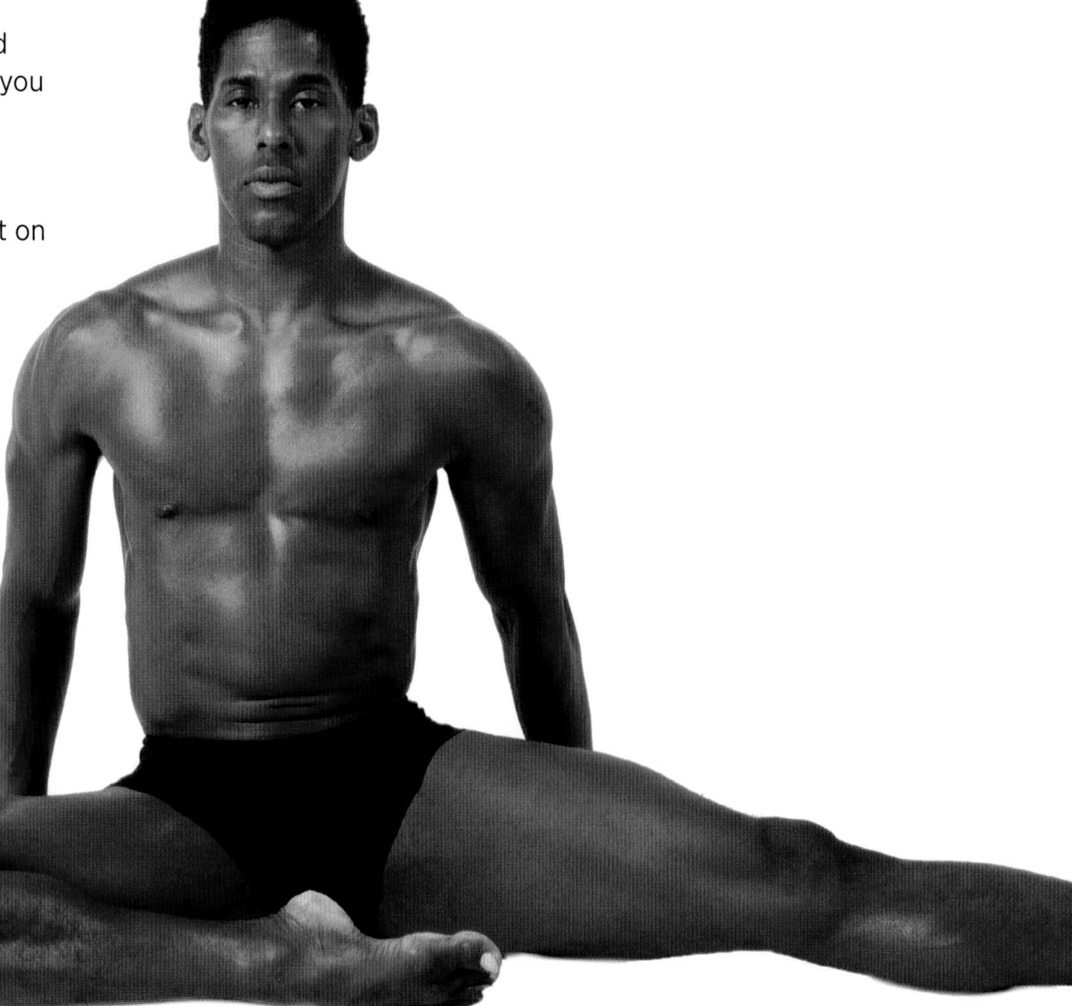

FACT FILE

TARGETS
- Hamstrings
- Quadriceps
- Inner thighs
- Calves
- Obliques

TYPE
- Static

BENEFITS
- Stretches obliques, quads, and hamstrings
- Improves lower-body flexibility

CAUTIONS
- Groin injury
- Lower-back issues

Annotation Key

Bold text indicates target muscles
Light text indicates other working muscles
* indicates deep muscles

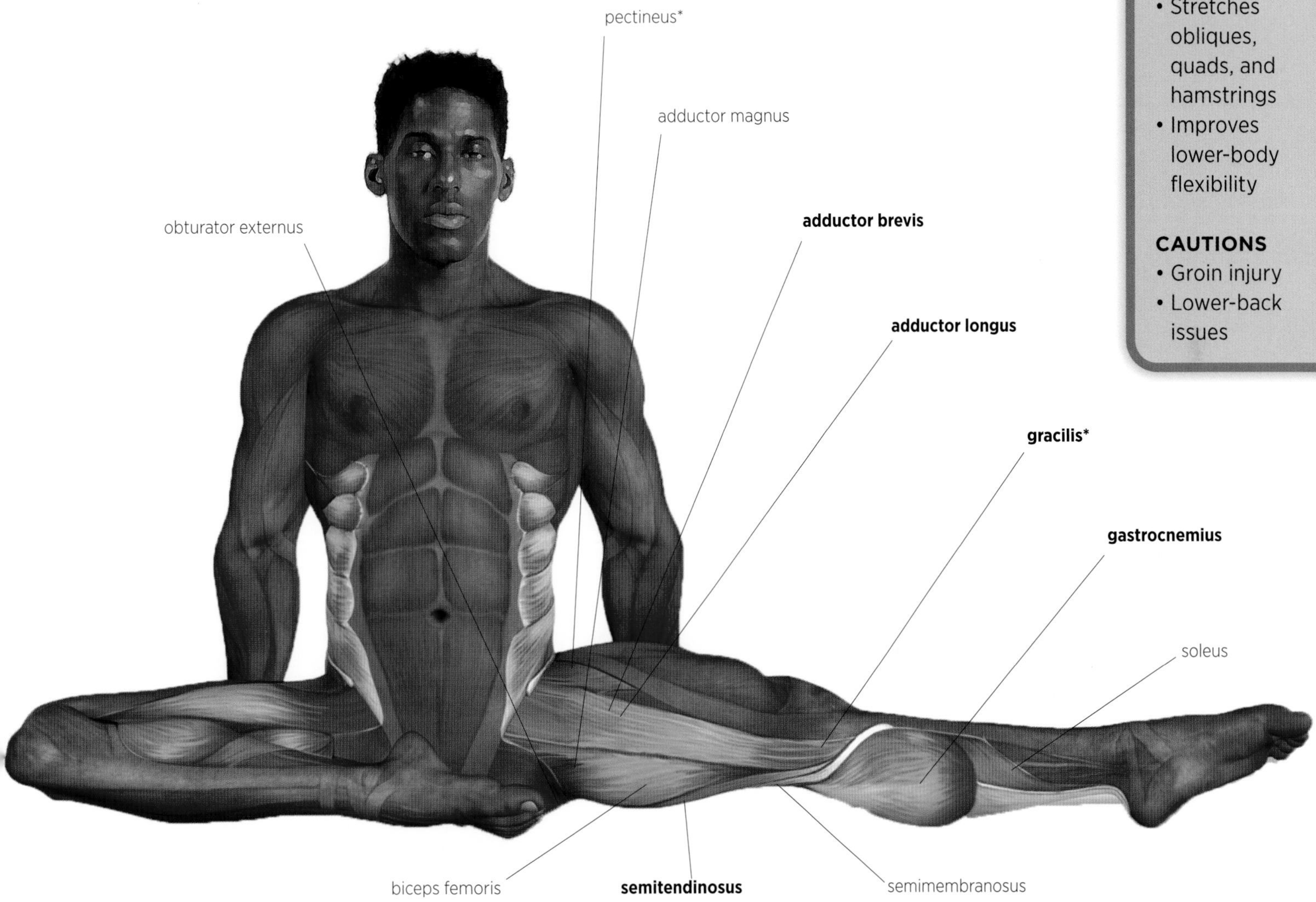

pectineus*

adductor magnus

obturator externus

adductor brevis

adductor longus

gracilis*

gastrocnemius

soleus

biceps femoris

semitendinosus

semimembranosus

DO IT RIGHT
- Lean your back against a sofa, if necessary, to stabilize yourself and to correctly align your hip bones on the floor.
- Avoid raising your grounded thigh from the floor.

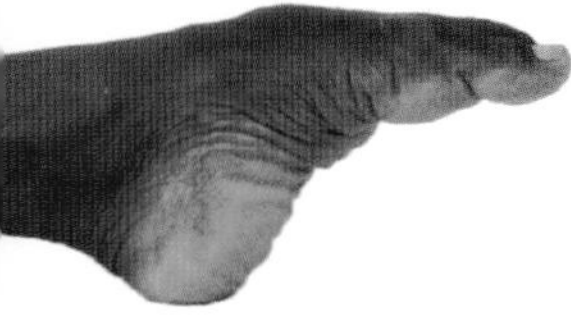

Side-Lying Rib Stretch

Your core helps you stay balanced and assists as you perform many of your daily activities without falling over or straining your back. Your obliques in particular are important for keeping your body stable, strong, and flexible. This Side-Lying Rib Stretch is a great way to keep your oblique muscles active.

HOW TO DO IT

- Lie on your right side with your legs extended and pressed together.
- Lift your upper body slightly off the floor and support yourself on your right forearm. Place both palms on the floor in front of your body.
- Bend your left leg, and place the sole of your foot just in front of your right thigh, your knee pointing up toward the ceiling.
- Keeping your legs in place, press down with your hands, and straighten both arms as you raise your body upward, feeling a stretch around the right side of your rib cage.
- Hold for the recommended time, release the stretch, and then repeat on the opposite side.

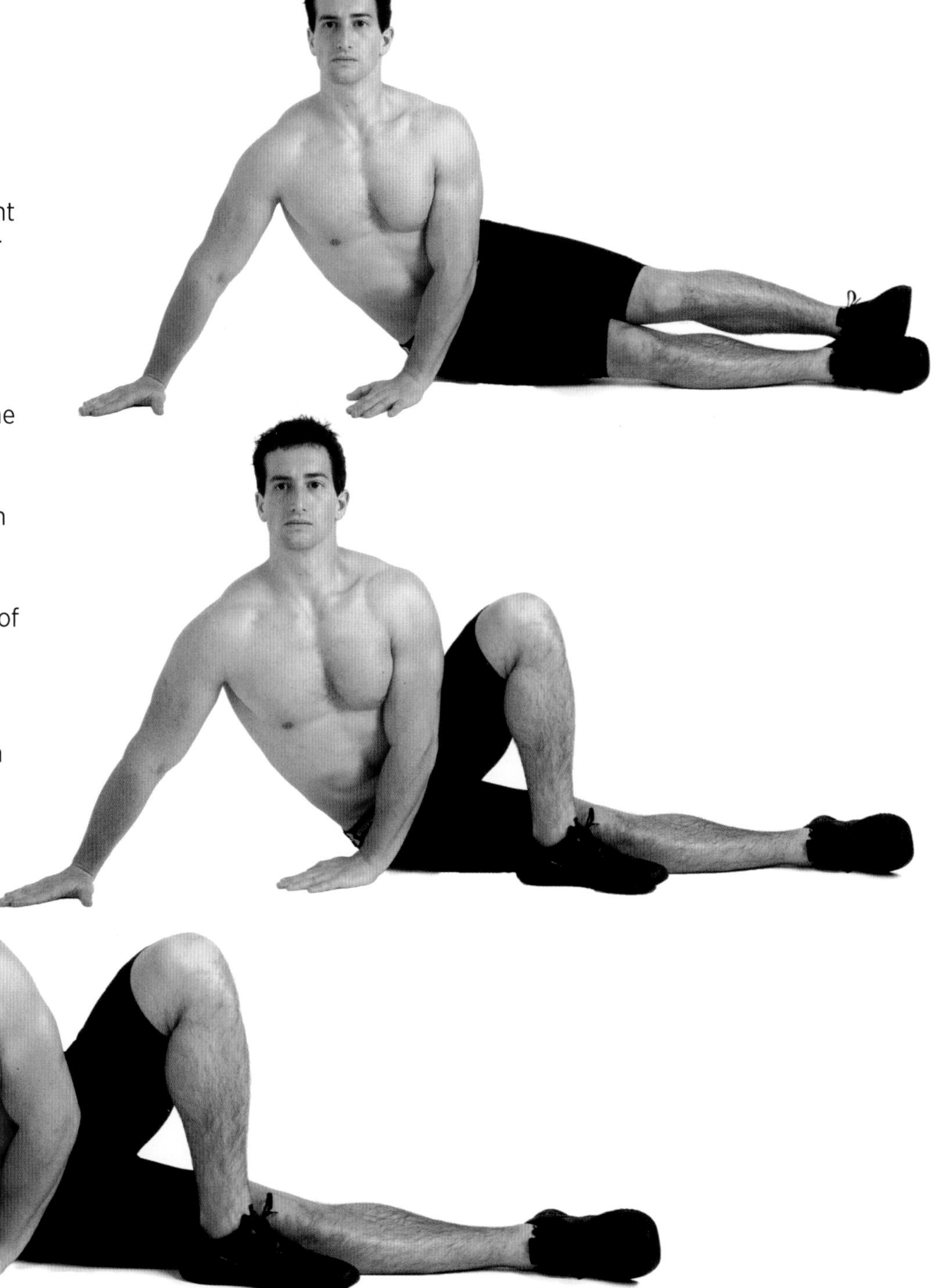

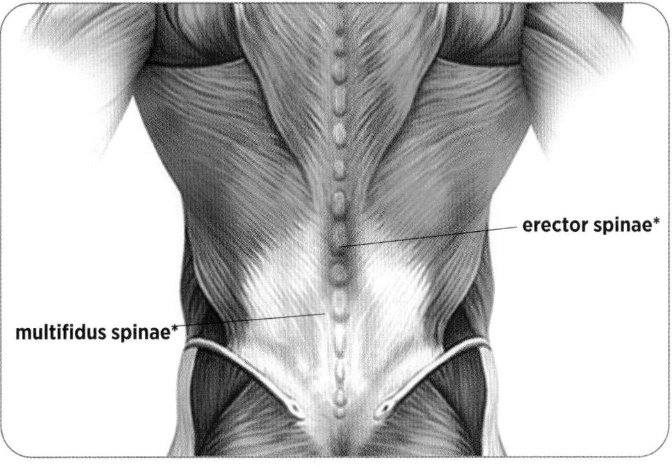

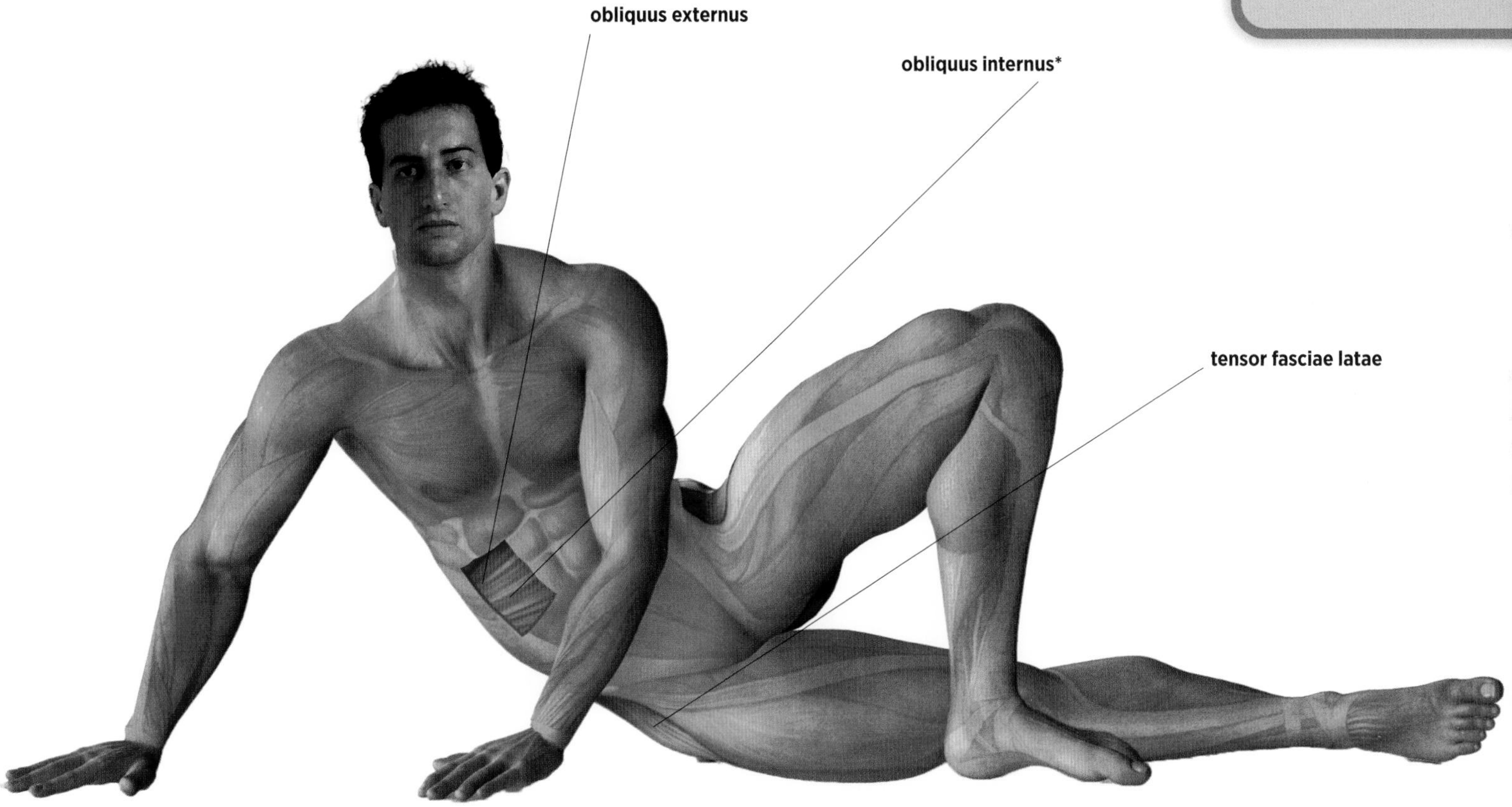

FACT FILE

TARGETS
- Obliques

TYPE
- Static

BENEFITS
- Increases lower-back mobility
- Strengthens core
- Opens hips

CAUTIONS
- Hip pain
- Lower-back pain

Annotation Key

Bold text indicates target muscles
Light text indicates other working muscles
* indicates deep muscles

erector spinae*
multifidus spinae*

obliquus externus
obliquus internus*
tensor fasciae latae

DO IT RIGHT
- Shift your weight forward on your supporting hip.
- Place a towel under your bottom hip if it feels uncomfortable to rest directly on the floor.
- Avoid tightening your jaw, which can cause tension in your neck.

Seated Russian Twist

This seated exercise works your abdominal muscles as you rotate from your midriff. This twisting motion is an effective way to relieve pain and tightness in your lower-back. The Seated Russian Twist also engages your obliques, which are crucial for rotational strength in your torso.

HOW TO DO IT

- Sit with your knees bent and your feet flat on the floor.
- Lift up through your torso.
- Extend your arms in front of you with your hands above your knees.
- Rotate your upper body to the right, keeping your arms parallel to the floor.
- Return to the center and rotate to the left.
- Repeat twisting from side to side for the recommended repetitions.

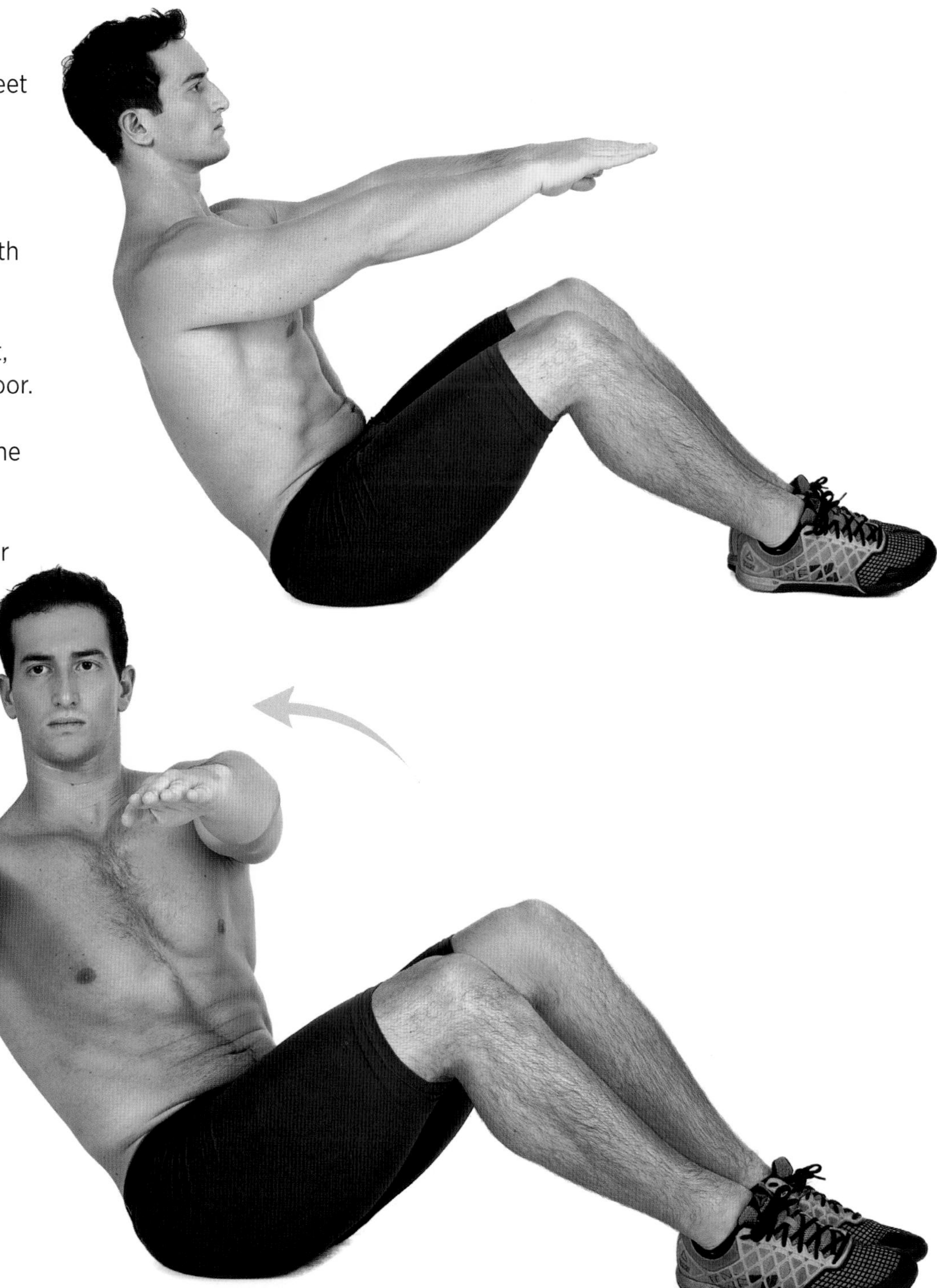

FACT FILE

TARGETS
- Abdominals
- Obliques

TYPE
- Dynamic

BENEFITS
- Increases abdominal endurance

CAUTIONS
- Shoulder pain
- Lower-back issues

Annotation Key
Bold text indicates target muscles
Light text indicates other working muscles
* indicates deep muscles

rectus abdominis
transversus abdominis*
tibialis anterior
latissimus dorsi
obliquus internus*
obliquus externus
vastus intermedius*
iliacus*
iliopsoas*
rectus femoris
vastus lateralis
tensor fasciae latae

DO IT RIGHT

- Keep your back straight.
- Use your abs to perform the movement.
- Avoid shifting your feet or knees to the sides as you twist.

Rollover Stretch

Borrowed from Pilates, the Rollover requires a strong core and a controlled, fluid progression. With time and practice, you can perfect this spinal stretch and core strengthener by engaging your abs, articulating your spine, and breathing deeply.

HOW TO DO IT

- Lie on your back with knees bent and arms at your sides.
- Inhale and elongate your spine.
- On exhale, raise your legs straight up and squeeze them together.
- Peel your spine off the mat and press into your palms for stability as you pull your legs overhead, parallel to the floor.
- Roll back down slowly.

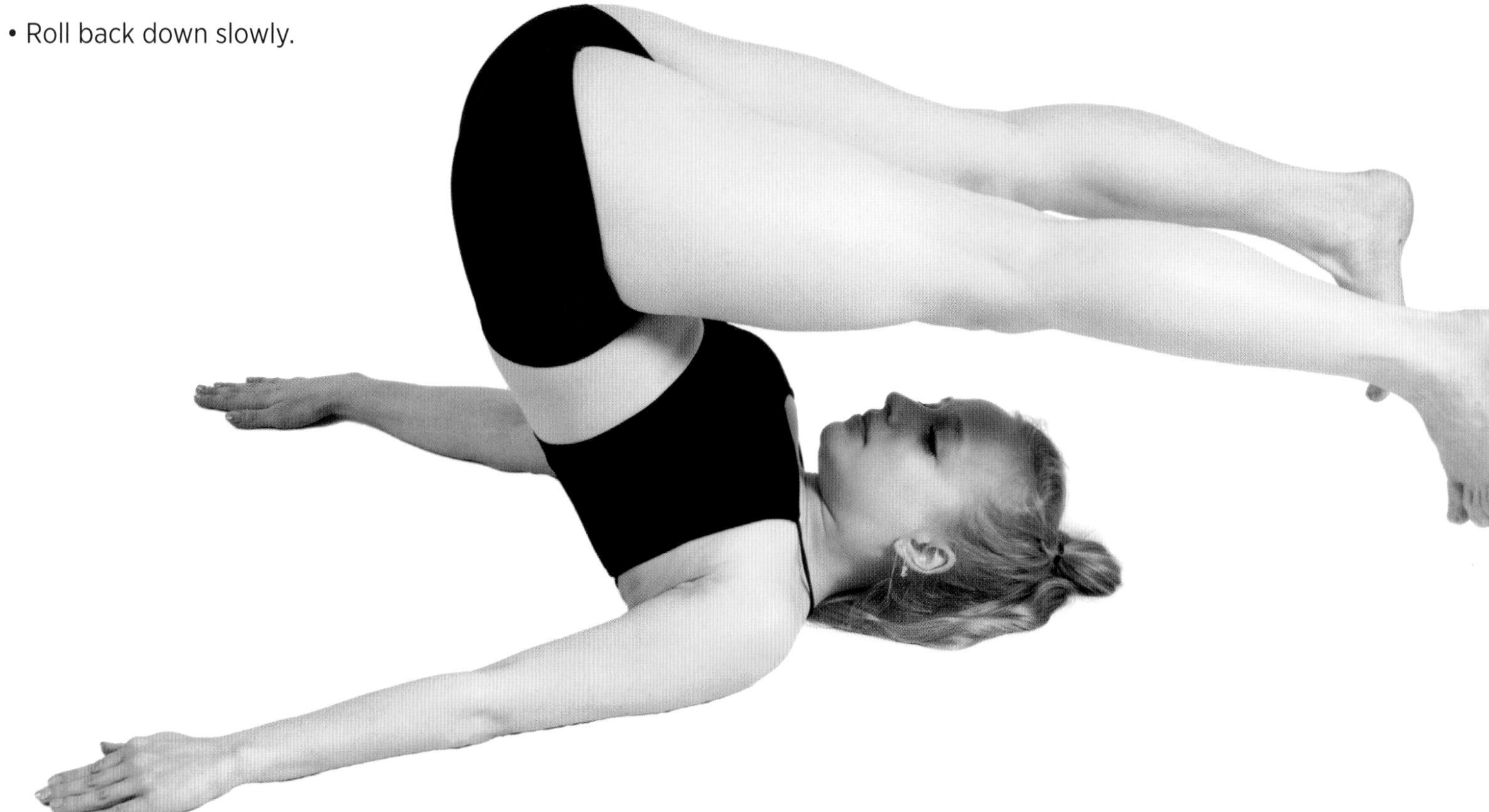

Annotation Key

Bold text indicates target muscles
Light text indicates other working muscles
* indicates deep muscles

rectus abdominis
obliquus internus*
transversus abdominis*
tensor fasciae latae
iliopsoas
pectineus
sartorius
adductor longus
rectus femoris

DO IT RIGHT

- If you're having difficulty rolling over, bend your knees slightly or place a rolled-up towel under your hips.
- Avoid using momentum to push through the movement.

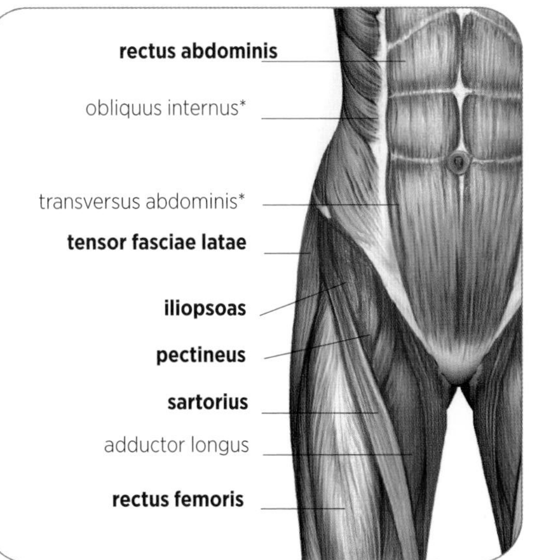

FACT FILE

TARGETS
- Back
- Hamstrings
- Calves
- Abdominals

TYPE
- Dynamic

BENEFITS
- Hip strengthener
- Lower-back relief
- Core strength

CAUTIONS
- Neck pain
- Hip pain
- Lower-back problems

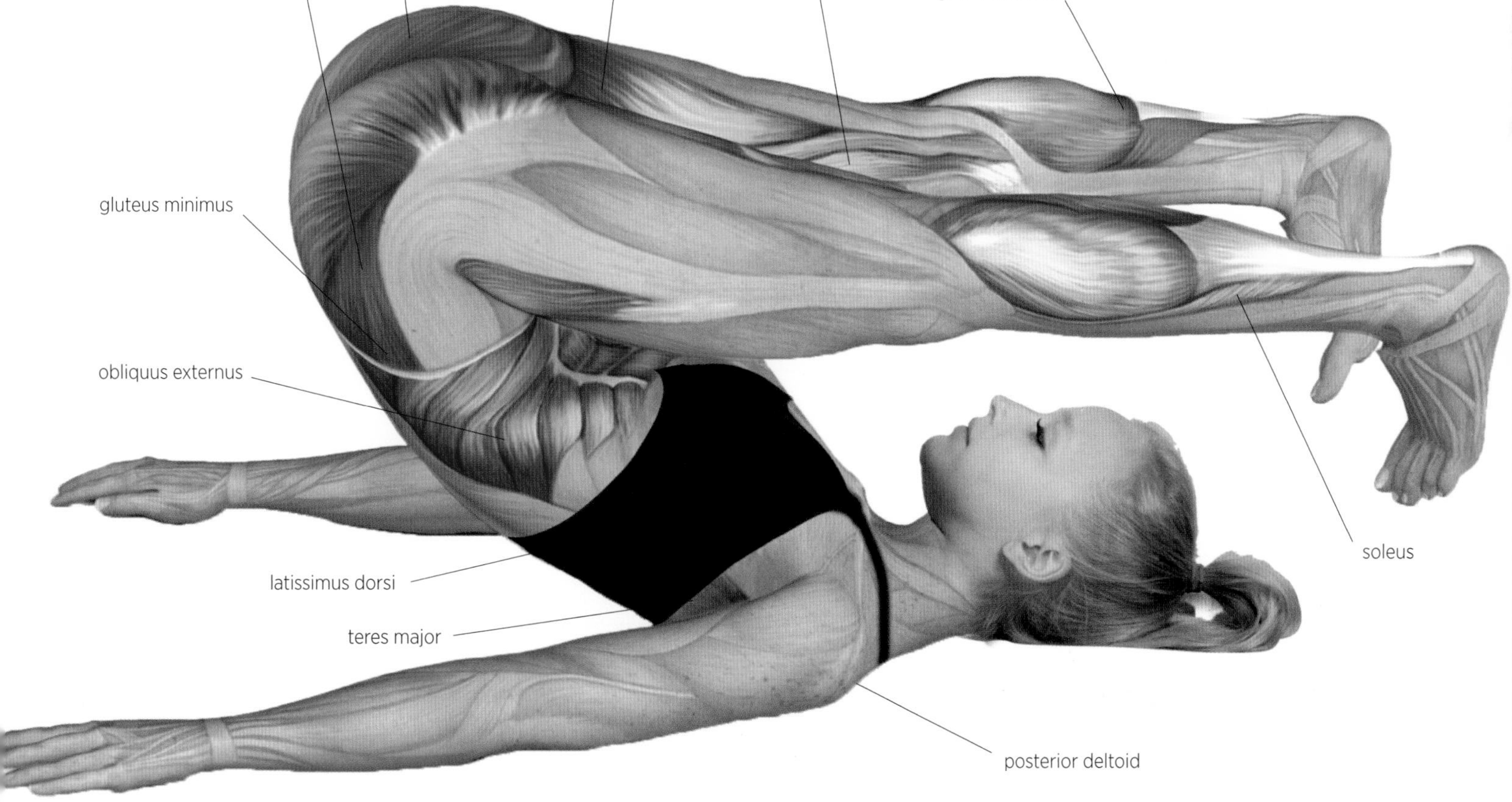

gluteus maximus
adductor magnus
gracilis*
gluteus medius*
gastrocnemius
gluteus minimus
obliquus externus
soleus
latissimus dorsi
teres major
posterior deltoid

Standing Forward Bend

The Standing Forward Bend lengthens your hamstrings and calves and stretches your entire back. This basic inversion exercise, a common first step in many yoga sequences, also benefits your circulation as you lower your head below your heart.

HOW TO DO IT

- Stand straight with your feet together and arms at your sides. Inhale, and raise your arms toward the ceiling. Exhale, as you hinge at your hips to fold forward, bringing your arms down. Try to reach your fingertips to the floor in line with your toes.
- Straighten your legs and arms as you draw in your abdominals. Press your heels into the floor as you lift your tailbone up toward the ceiling, keeping your hips in line with your heels.
- Inhale, and lengthen your spine, as you fold further from your hips and rest your palms on the floor.
- Lengthen your torso as you bring your belly closer to your thighs.
- Hold for the recommended time, inhaling to lengthen your spine and exhaling to fold deeper.

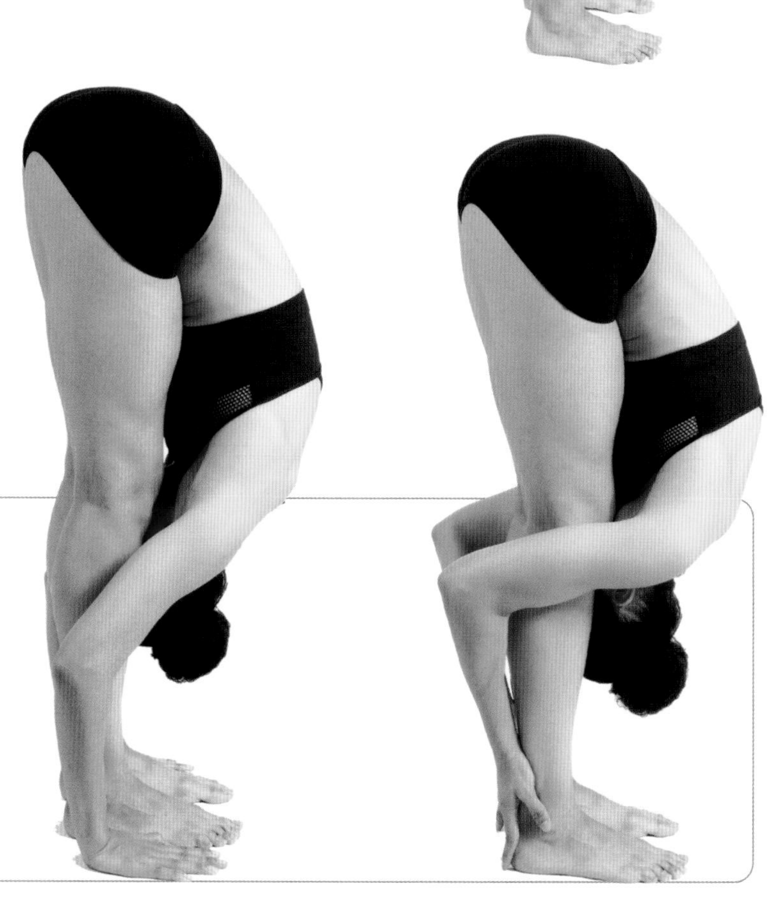

MODIFICATION

HARDER: Bend forward so your head is between your knees and your palms down flat to the floor—or reach behind your ankles for stability.

FACT FILE

TARGETS
- Spine
- Core
- Lower body

TYPE
- Static

BENEFITS
- Stretches hamstrings, hips, and spine
- Strengthens thighs and knees
- Improves circulation
- Reduces stress
- Improves posture
- Aids digestion

CAUTIONS
- Lower-back issues
- Neck pain
- Osteoporosis

Annotation Key

Bold text indicates target muscles
Light text indicates other working muscles
* indicates deep muscles

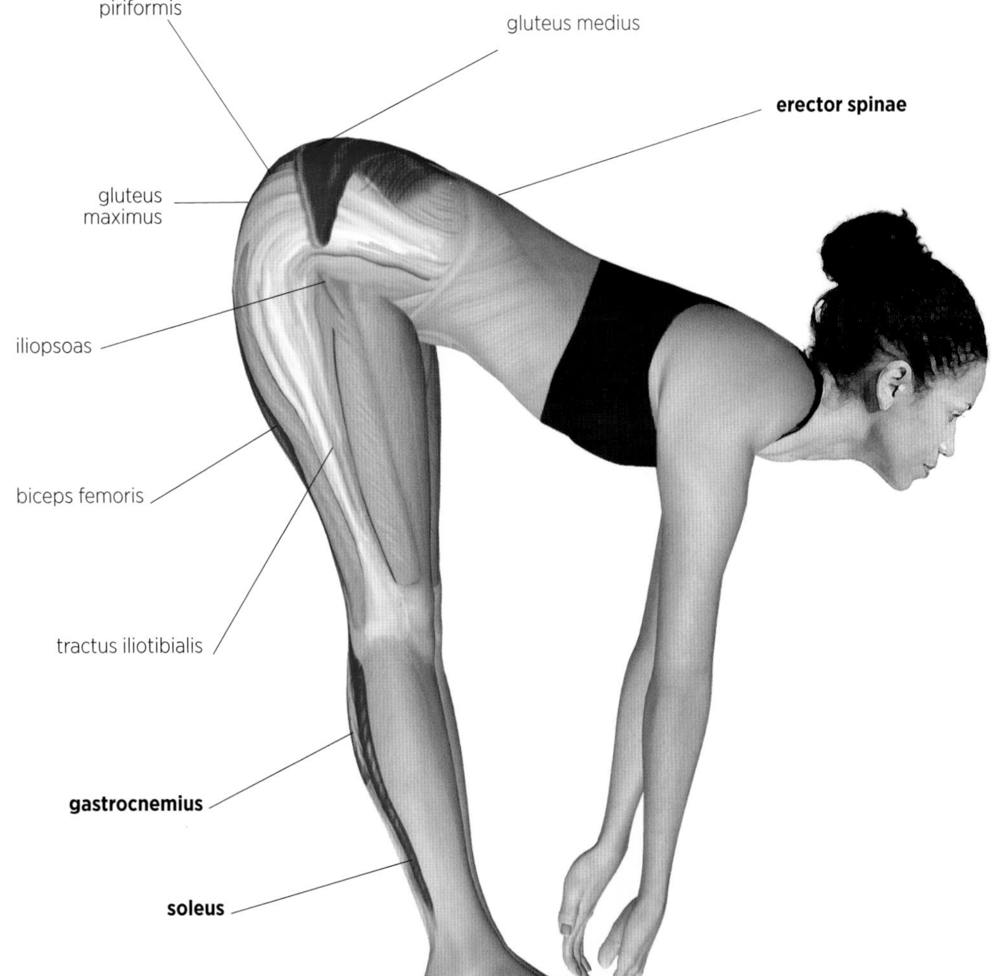

DO IT RIGHT
- Bend from your hips, not your waist.
- Keep a slight bend in your knees if your lower back or hamstrings are tight.
- If you cannot reach your fingertips to the floor, place your hands on your shins or cross your arms.
- Avoid shifting your weight backward and positioning your hips behind your heels.
- Avoid compressing your neck.
- Avoid rolling your spine into or out of the pose.

Backward Ball Stretch

An effective exercise that enhances your coordination, the Backward Ball Stretch combines an abdominal and back stretch with a core-strengthening exercise. You must fully engage your core, using steady, balanced movement to stretch your back over the Swiss ball.

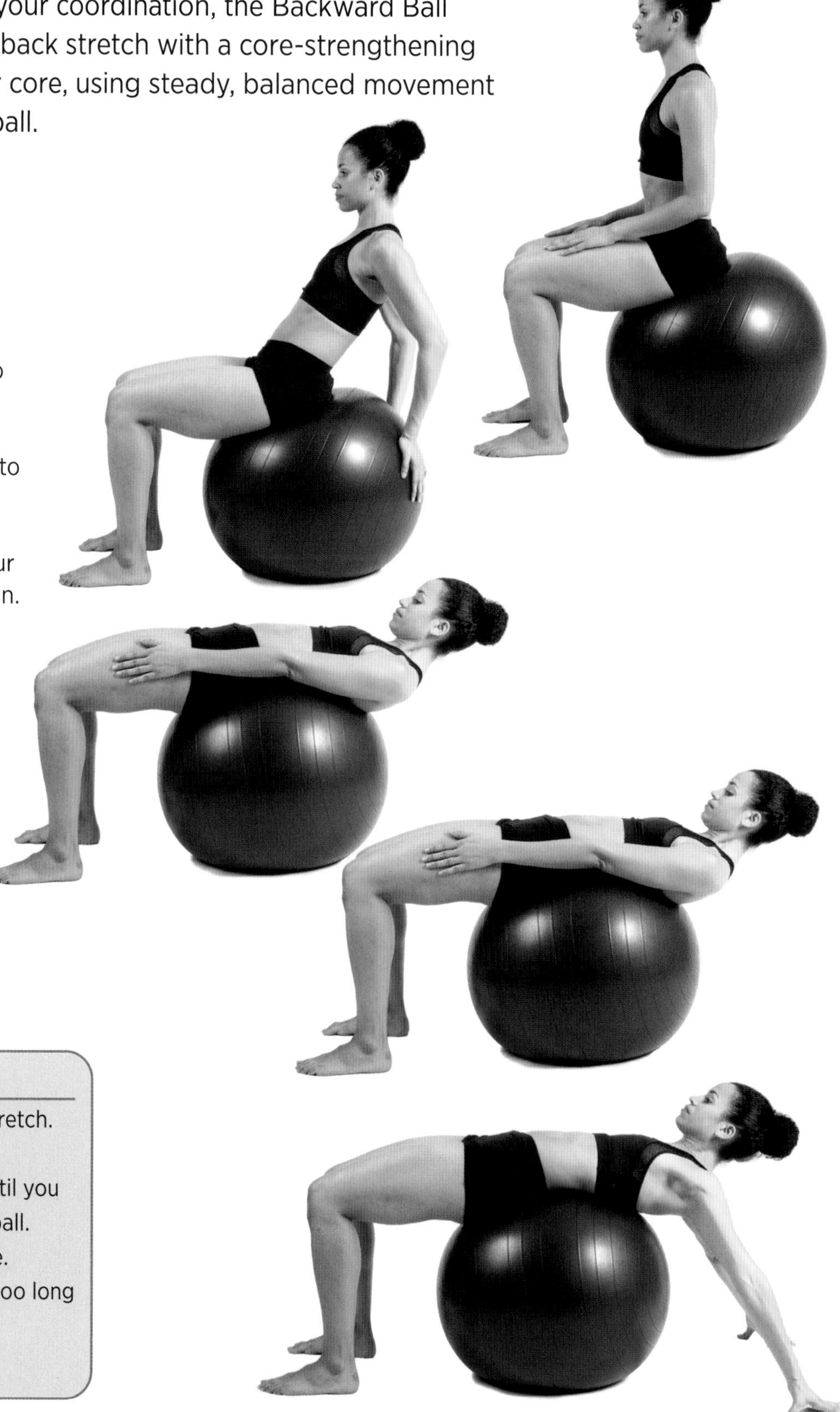

HOW TO DO IT

- Sit on a Swiss ball in a well-balanced, neutral position, with your hips directly over the center of the ball.
- While maintaining good balance, begin to extend your arms behind you.
- Walk your feet forward, allowing the ball to roll up your spine.
- As your hands touch the floor, extend your legs as far forward as you comfortably can. Hold this position for about 10 seconds.
- To deepen the stretch, extend your arms, and walk your legs and hands closer to the ball. Hold this position for about 10 seconds.
- To release the stretch, bend your knees, drop your hips to the floor, lift your head off the ball, and then walk back to the starting position. Repeat for the recommended repetitions.

DO IT RIGHT

- Maintain good balance throughout the stretch.
- Move slowly and with control.
- Keep your head supported on the ball until you feel your torso is fully supported by the ball.
- Avoid allowing the ball to shift to the side.
- Avoid holding the extended position for too long or until you feel dizzy.

FACT FILE

TARGETS
- Thoracic spine
- Shoulders
- Middle back
- Chest

TYPE
- Static-dynamic

BENEFITS
- Stretches thoracic spine
- Increases spinal extension
- Stretches abdominals and large back muscles

CAUTIONS
- Lower-back issues
- Balancing difficulty
- Wrist issues

Annotation Key

Bold text indicates target muscles
Light text indicates other working muscles
* indicates deep muscles

CHAPTER TWO

BALANCE/ YOGA

Yoga poses—standing poses in particular—can help you improve your body's balance, muscular engagement and alignment. Many standing poses may seem simple, but they become more challenging, and therefore more beneficial, as you engage more muscles across your body. With regular practice, you can develop a heightened bodily awareness, which in turn can improve posture. The balance exercises in this chapter are also beneficial for strength—some are quite challenging, so build up to them slowly.

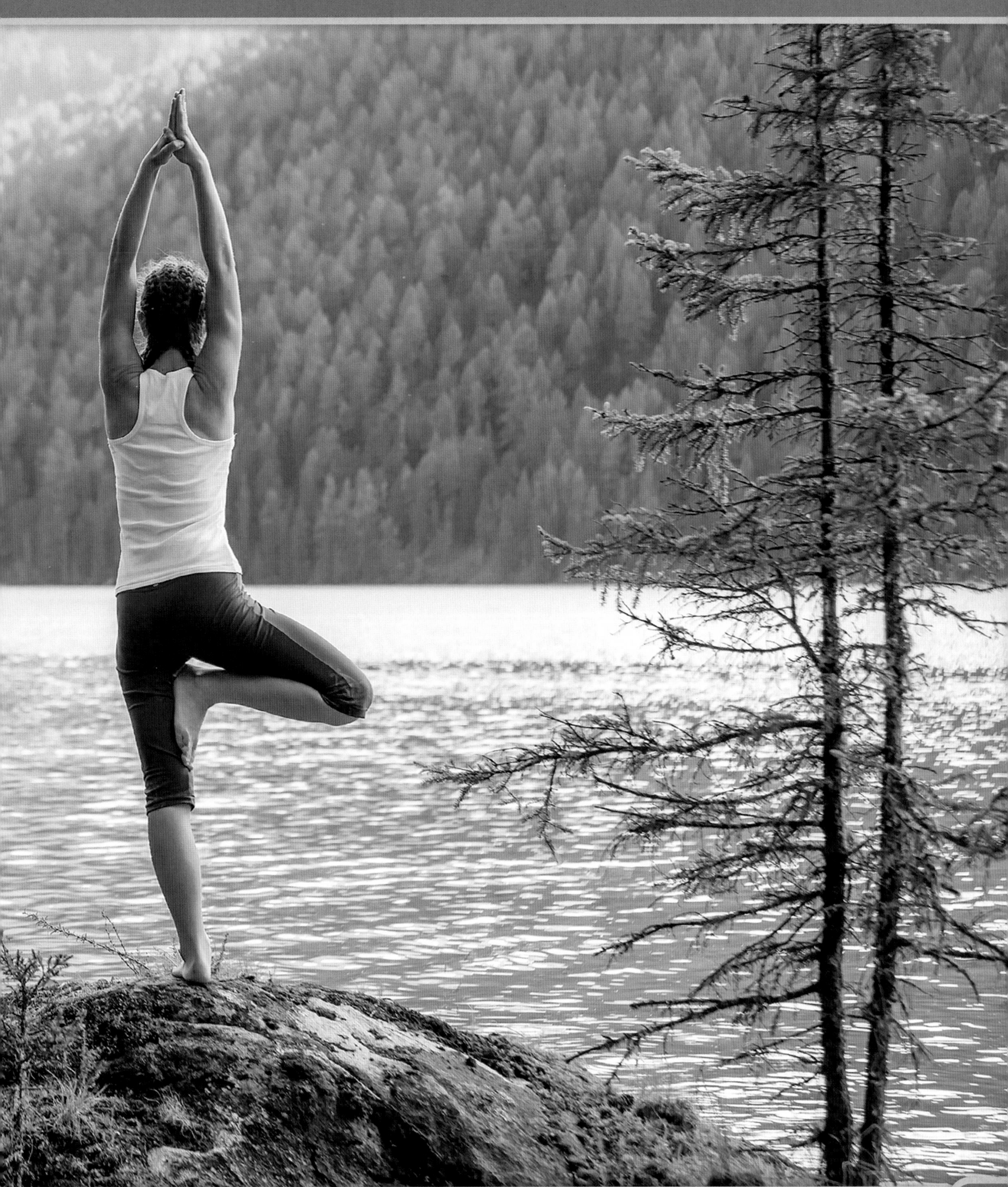

Mountain Pose

Mountain Pose forms the base for all standing poses. This posture may seem simple, but it can actually be quite challenging to achieve the correct alignment. Once you have mastered your form, you will be ready to experiment with more complicated standing poses.

HOW TO DO IT

- Stand with your feet together, with both heels and toes touching.
- Keeping your back straight and both arms pressed slightly against your sides, face your palms outward.
- Lift all your toes and let them fan out, and then gently drop them down to create a wide, solid base.
- Rock from side to side until you gradually bring your weight evenly onto all four corners of both feet.
- While balancing your weight evenly on both feet, slightly contract the muscles in your knees and thighs, rotating both thighs inward to create a widening of the sit bones.
- Tighten your abdominals, drawing them in slightly, maintaining a firm posture.
- Widen your collarbones, making sure your shoulders are parallel to your pelvis.
- Lengthen your neck, so that the crown of your head rises toward the ceiling, and your shoulder blades slide down your back.
- Hold for the recommended breaths.

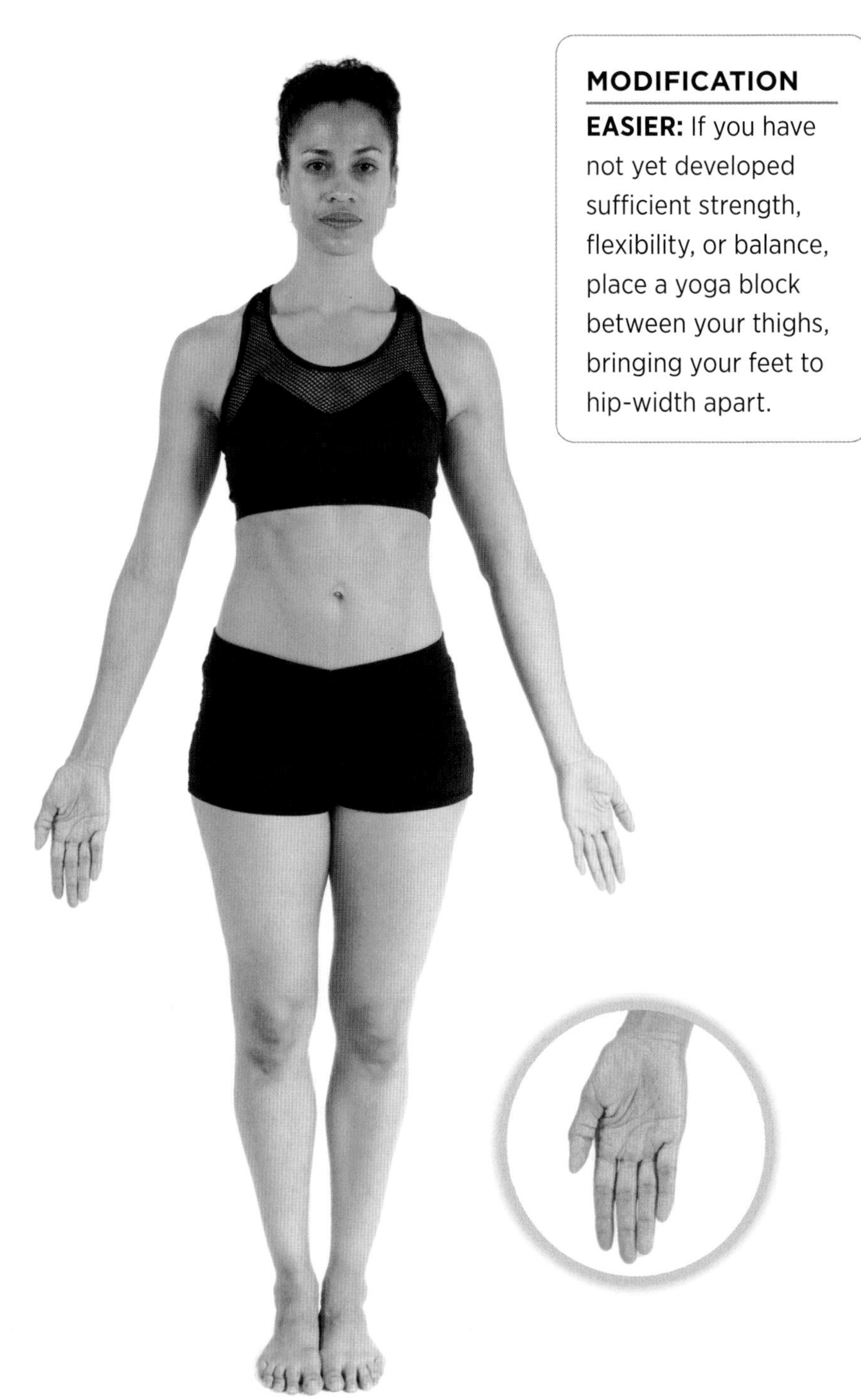

MODIFICATION

EASIER: If you have not yet developed sufficient strength, flexibility, or balance, place a yoga block between your thighs, bringing your feet to hip-width apart.

Annotation Key

Bold text indicates target muscles

Light text indicates other working muscles

* indicates deep muscles

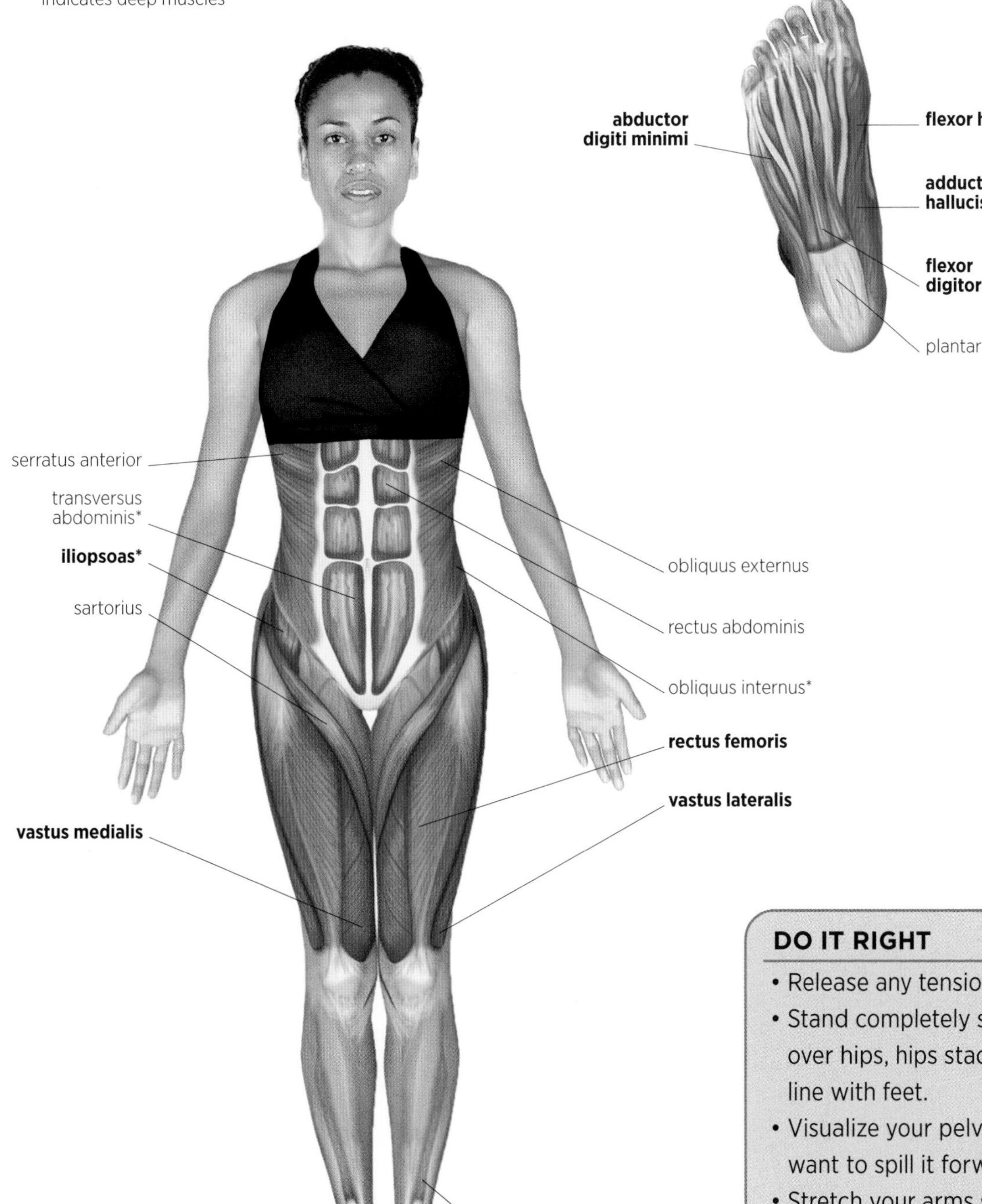

FACT FILE

SANSKRIT
- Tadasana

SANSKRIT
- Samasthiti

TARGET
- Entire body

TYPE
- Static

BENEFITS
- Improves posture
- Strengthens thighs, knees, and ankles
- Tones abdomen and buttocks
- Relieves sciatica
- Helps to treat flat feet

CAUTIONS
- Headache
- Insomnia
- Low blood pressure

DO IT RIGHT

- Release any tension in your facial area.
- Stand completely straight with shoulders stacked over hips, hips stacked over knees, and knees in line with feet.
- Visualize your pelvis as a bowl of soup—you don't want to spill it forward or backward.
- Stretch your arms straight, with energy reaching out of your fingertips.
- Keep your chin parallel to the floor and the crown of your head pressing upward.
- Avoid arching your lower back.
- Avoid pushing your ribs forward.
- Avoid overtucking your pelvis.
- Avoid holding your breath.

Chair Pose

Also known as Awkward Pose, Chair Pose is an element of many yoga flows. It takes quite a bit of strength, but you can easily control its intensity, bending your knees just a few inches or all the way down so that your hips are in line with your knees.

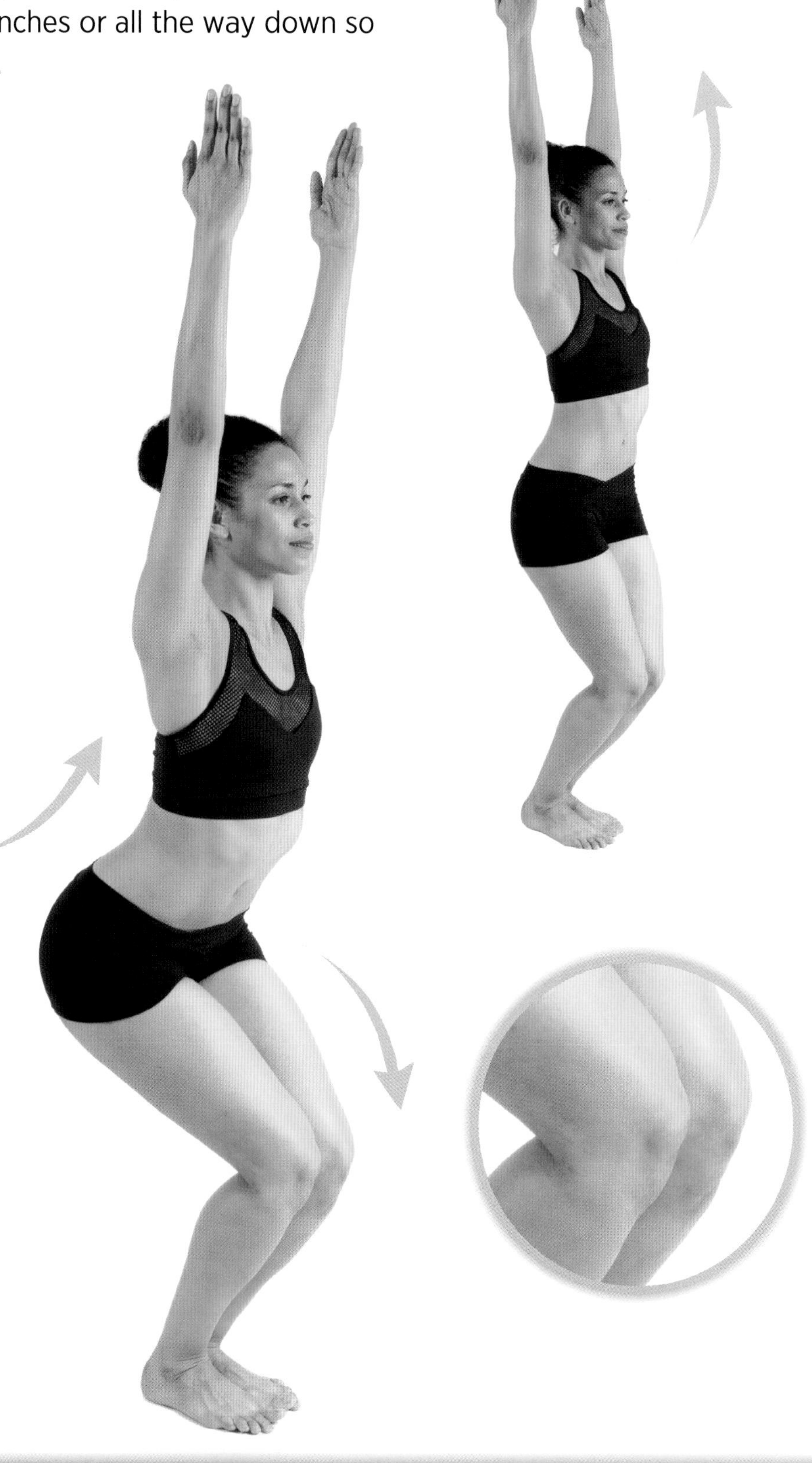

HOW TO DO IT

- Stand in Mountain Pose (pages 74–75), with your feet together and arms by your sides.
- Inhale as you raise your arms, reaching above your head so that your arms are parallel to each other. Rotate your outer upper arms inward and reach up through your fingertips.
- Exhale and bend your knees. Both ankles, inner thighs, and knees should be touching. Bring your weight onto your heels, shift your hips back, and draw your knees right above your ankles. Hold for the recommended breaths.

DO IT RIGHT

- Find a neutral position by drawing your tailbone down as you roll your inner thighs toward the floor.
- Keep your feet together.
- Keep your heels on the floor.
- Avoid overtucking your pelvis.
- Avoid overarching your lower back.
- Avoid knocking your knees inward.

Annotation Key

Bold text indicates target muscles

Light text indicates other working muscles

* indicates deep muscles

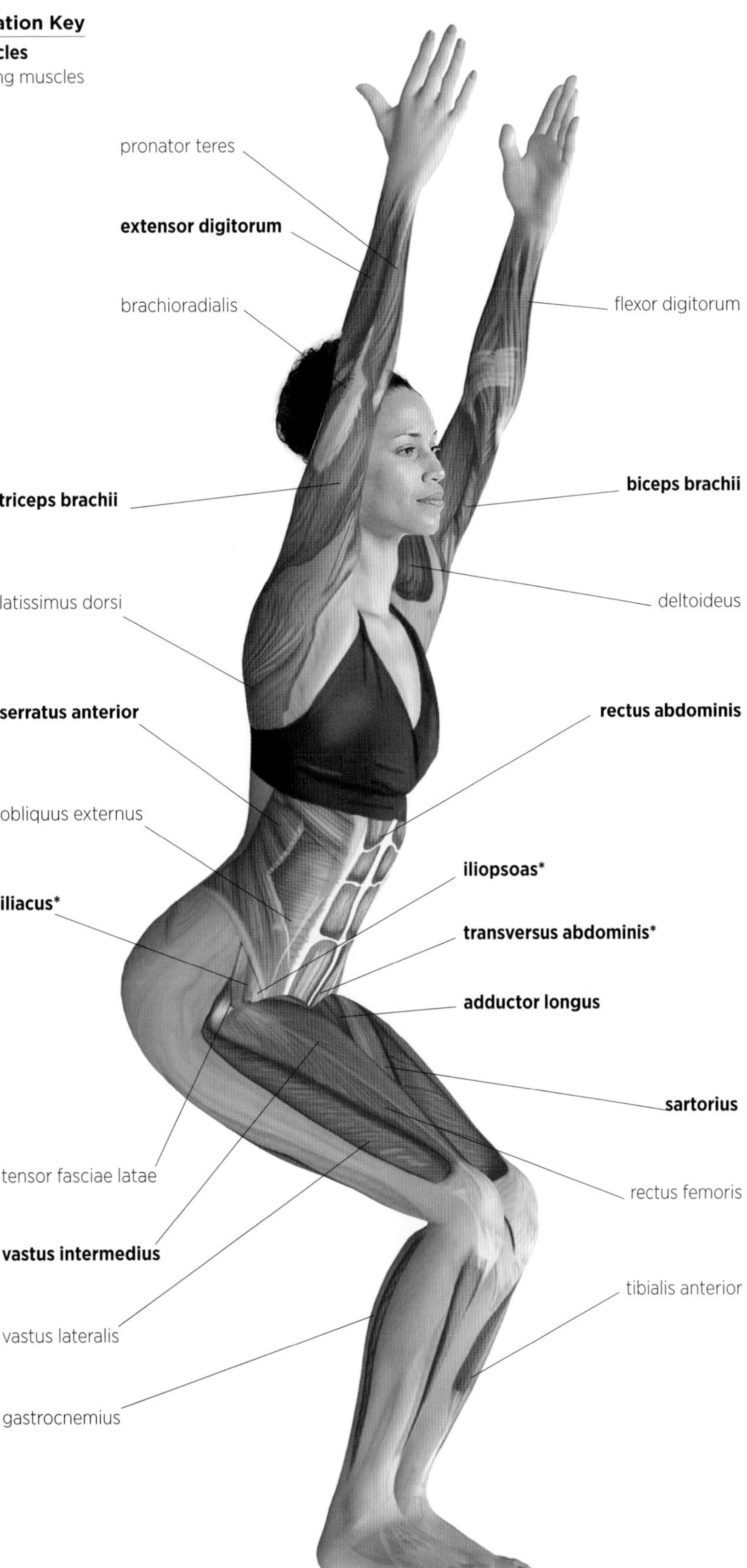

FACT FILE

SANSKRIT
- Utkatasana

TARGETS
- Legs
- Back
- Arms

TYPE
- Static

BENEFITS
- Strengthens thighs, ankles, spine, and arms
- Stretches shoulders and chest

CAUTIONS
- Knee issues

Twisting Chair Pose

Perform Twisting Chair Pose to improve digestion and elimination. Imagine wringing out your stomach as if it were a sponge, twisting a little deeper with each breath.

HOW TO DO IT

- Begin in Chair Pose (pages 76-77), with your arms parallel to each other above your head and your knees bent deeply.
- Inhale as you lengthen your spine and join your hands in a prayer position in front of your heart.
- Keep your hips square as you exhale and twist to the right, bringing your left elbow to the outside of your right thigh. Press your left elbow into your right knee and your knee into your elbow.
- Inhale to lengthen the spine, letting your abdomen move outward, and then exhale to twist as your navel draws strongly back toward your spine.
- Hold for the recommended breaths, and then inhale as you return to the center and reach your arms upward. Repeat on the other side.

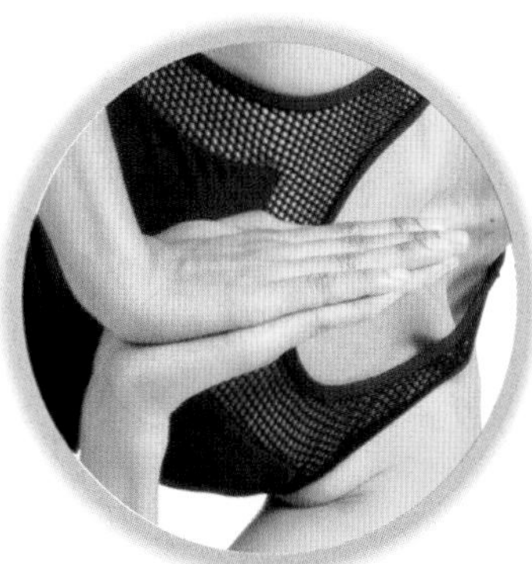

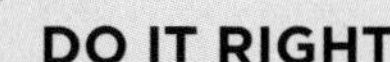

DO IT RIGHT

- Keep your hands in prayer position at the center of your chest, even though they will want to move toward one of your shoulders.
- Try to find a small bend in your upper back as you broaden across your collarbones.
- Twist from your torso, and keep your hips square; this will keep your knees in line with each other.
- Avoid rounding your shoulders as you twist.
- Avoid letting your left knee jut forward as you twist to the right, or vice versa.

FACT FILE

SANSKRIT
- Parivrtta Utkatasana

TARGETS
- Lower body
- Back
- Obliques

TYPE
- Static

BENEFITS
- Strengthens thighs, ankles, spine, buttocks, and arms
- Stretches spine and obliques
- Tones abdomen
- Stimulates digestion

CAUTIONS
- Knee issues
- Back issues
- Pregnancy

Annotation Key

Bold text indicates target muscles
Light text indicates other working muscles
* indicates deep muscles

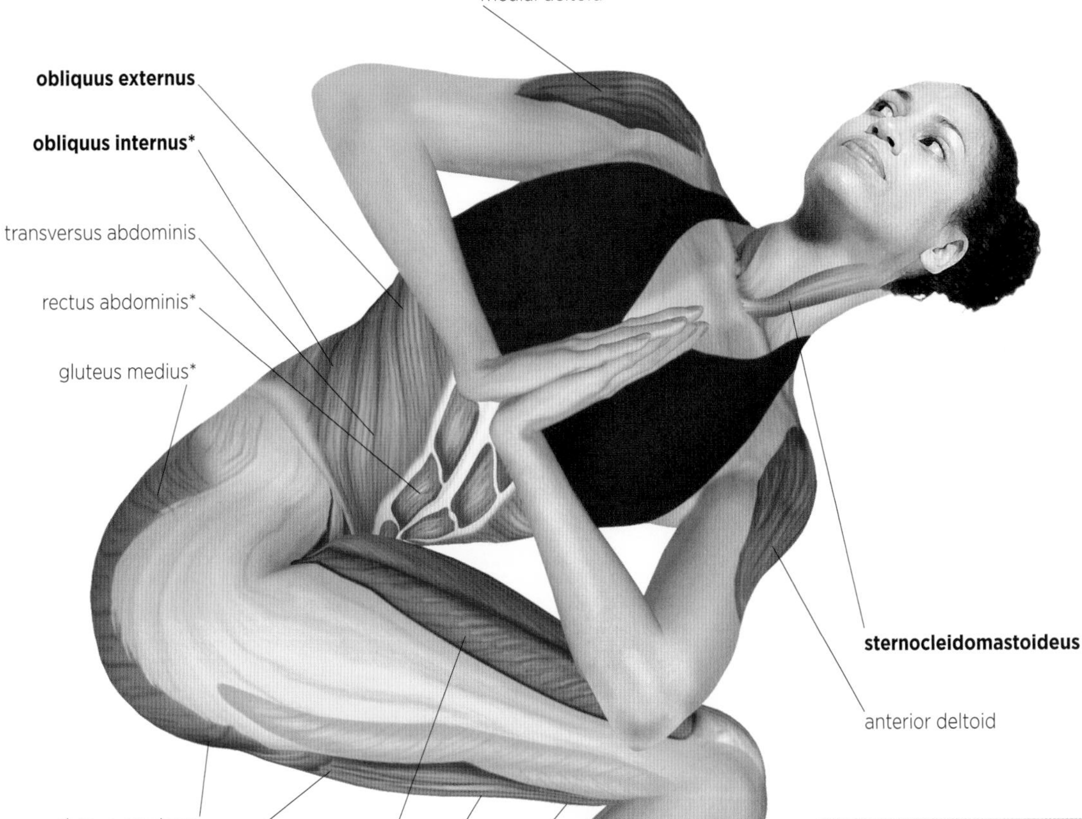

trapezius
medial deltoid
infraspinatus
teres minor
subscapularis
teres major
latissimus dorsi
quadratus lumborum
erector spinae*

Tree Pose

Tree Pose tests your balance. To perform it correctly, think of yourself as a tree, rooting your standing foot to the floor and reaching your head up toward the ceiling, so that you feel energy moving down and up at the same time.

HOW TO DO IT

- Stand in Mountain Pose (pages 74–75), with your feet together and arms by your sides.
- Bend your right knee, and bring your foot up to your left inner thigh, with toes pointing to the floor.
- Externally rotate your right thigh, allowing your right knee to point out to the right while keeping your hips level.
- Continue to open your right hip, rotating your inner thigh clockwise as you draw your tailbone down toward your left heel to neutralize your pelvis. Press your right foot into your left inner thigh as you draw your left outer hip in for stability.
- Find your balance, exhale, and draw your hands together into prayer position at the heart.
- Hold for the recommended breaths, and then inhale as you return to Mountain Pose. Repeat on the other side.

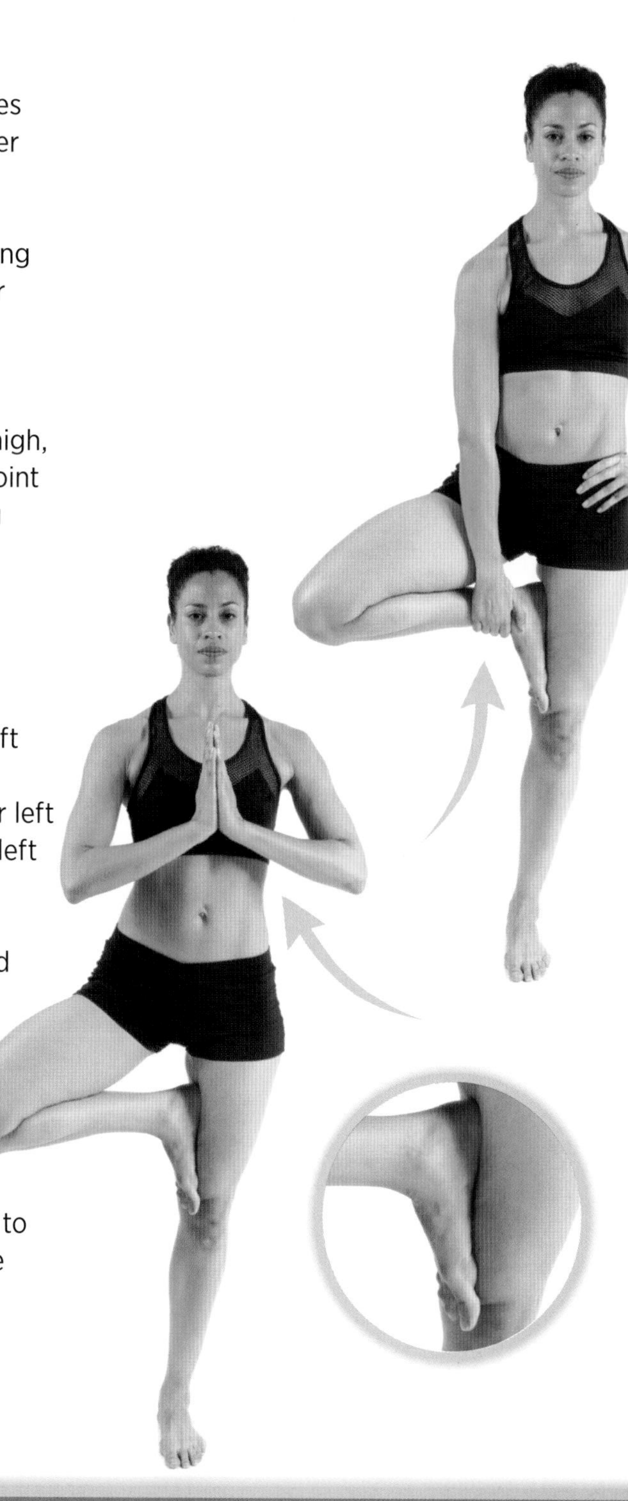

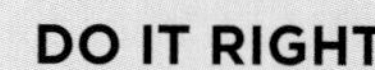

DO IT RIGHT

- Keep your standing leg in place with the foot facing straight ahead.
- If you need help placing your foot at your thigh, grasp your ankle with your hand; alternatively, you can rest your foot on the side of your shin instead.
- Ground down through all four corners of the raised foot to help you maintain balance.
- To assist in balancing, place your heel at your ankle with the ball of the foot on the floor, or lean against a wall.
- Avoid resting your foot on the sensitive kneecap area.

FACT FILE

SANSKRIT
- Vrksasana

TARGETS
- Legs
- Groin
- Feet

TYPE
- Static

BENEFITS
- Improves balance
- Strengthens legs, ankles, and feet
- Stretches groin and inner thighs

CAUTIONS
- Groin issues
- Lower-back issues

Annotation Key

Bold text indicates target muscles

Light text indicates other working muscles

* indicates deep muscles

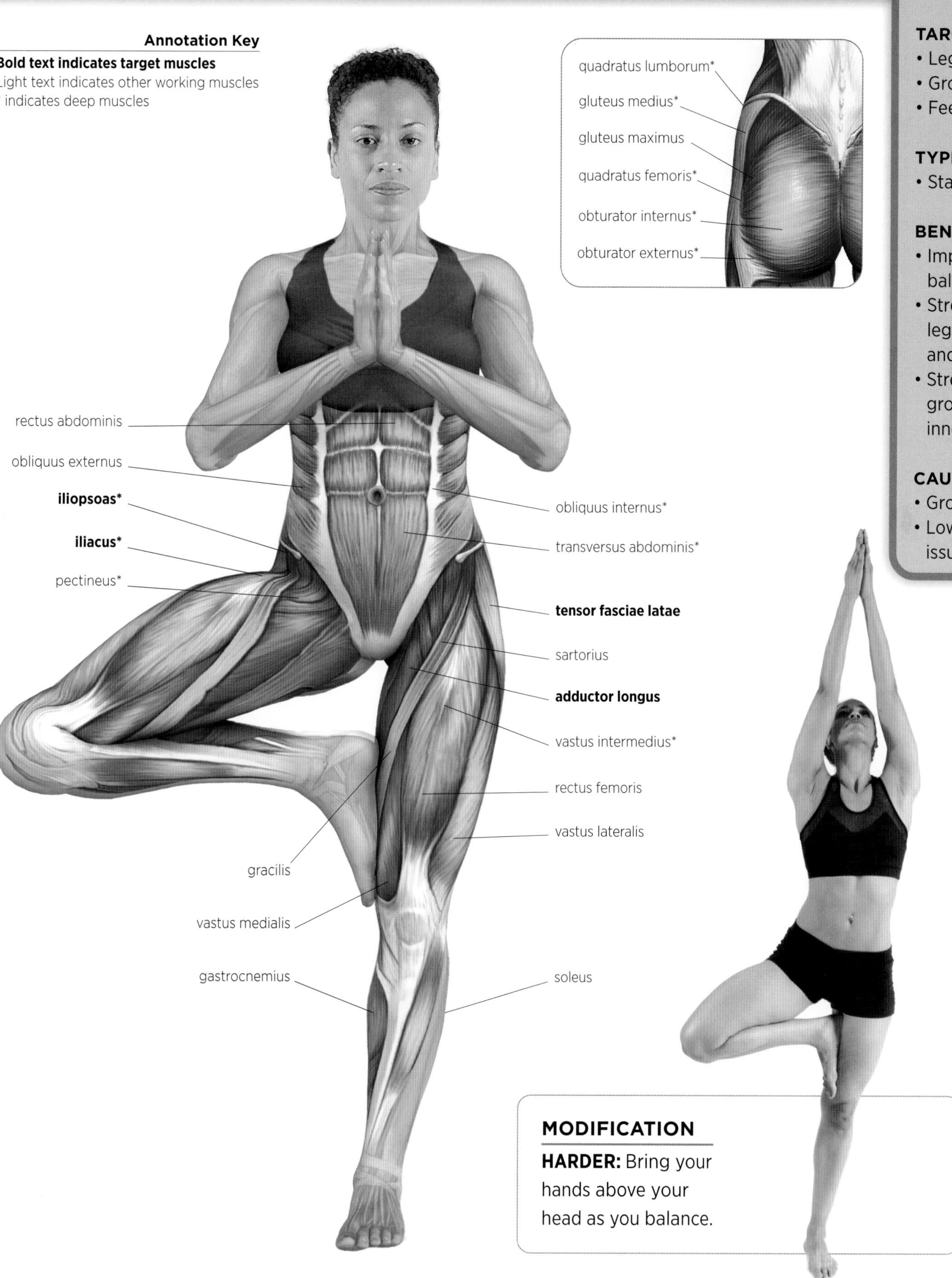

MODIFICATION

HARDER: Bring your hands above your head as you balance.

Plank Pose

A classic across disciplines, Plank Pose strengthens and tones the arms, abdominals, and wrists. It plays a part in many yoga sequences and is also a good precursor to more challenging arm balances.

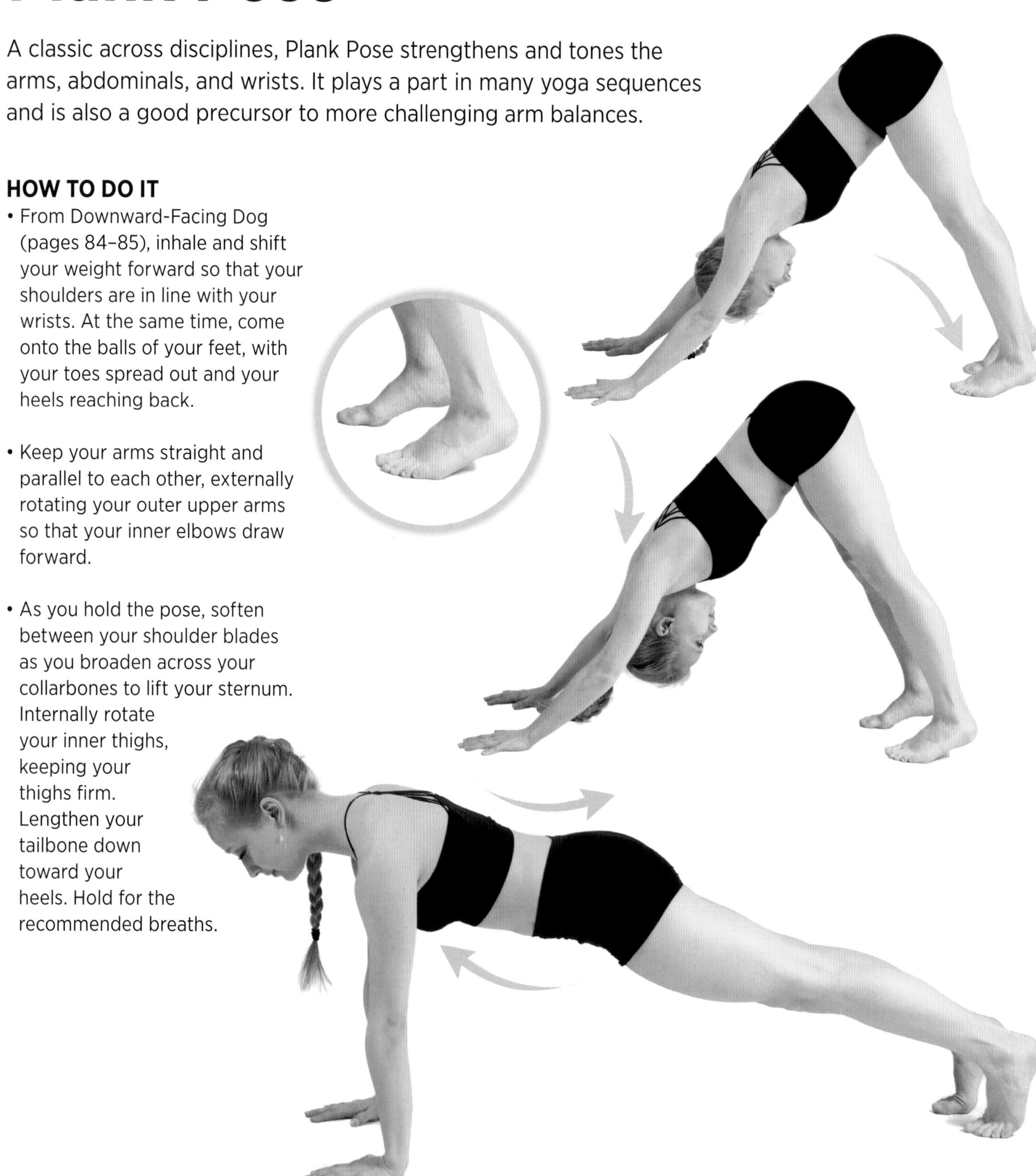

HOW TO DO IT

- From Downward-Facing Dog (pages 84–85), inhale and shift your weight forward so that your shoulders are in line with your wrists. At the same time, come onto the balls of your feet, with your toes spread out and your heels reaching back.
- Keep your arms straight and parallel to each other, externally rotating your outer upper arms so that your inner elbows draw forward.
- As you hold the pose, soften between your shoulder blades as you broaden across your collarbones to lift your sternum. Internally rotate your inner thighs, keeping your thighs firm. Lengthen your tailbone down toward your heels. Hold for the recommended breaths.

DO IT RIGHT

- Make sure your wrist creases are parallel to the front of your mat.
- Spread your fingers wide, and ground down through every knuckle.
- Use your breath to get you through holding the pose.
- Avoid lifting your fingers off the floor.
- Avoid rounding your upper back.

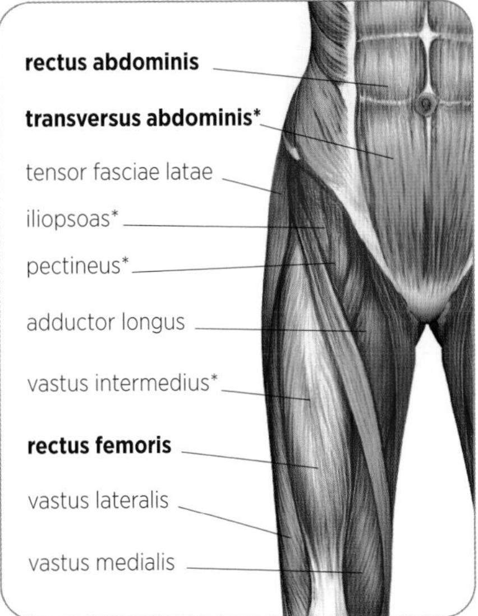

Annotation Key

Bold text indicates target muscles

Light text indicates other working muscles

* indicates deep muscles

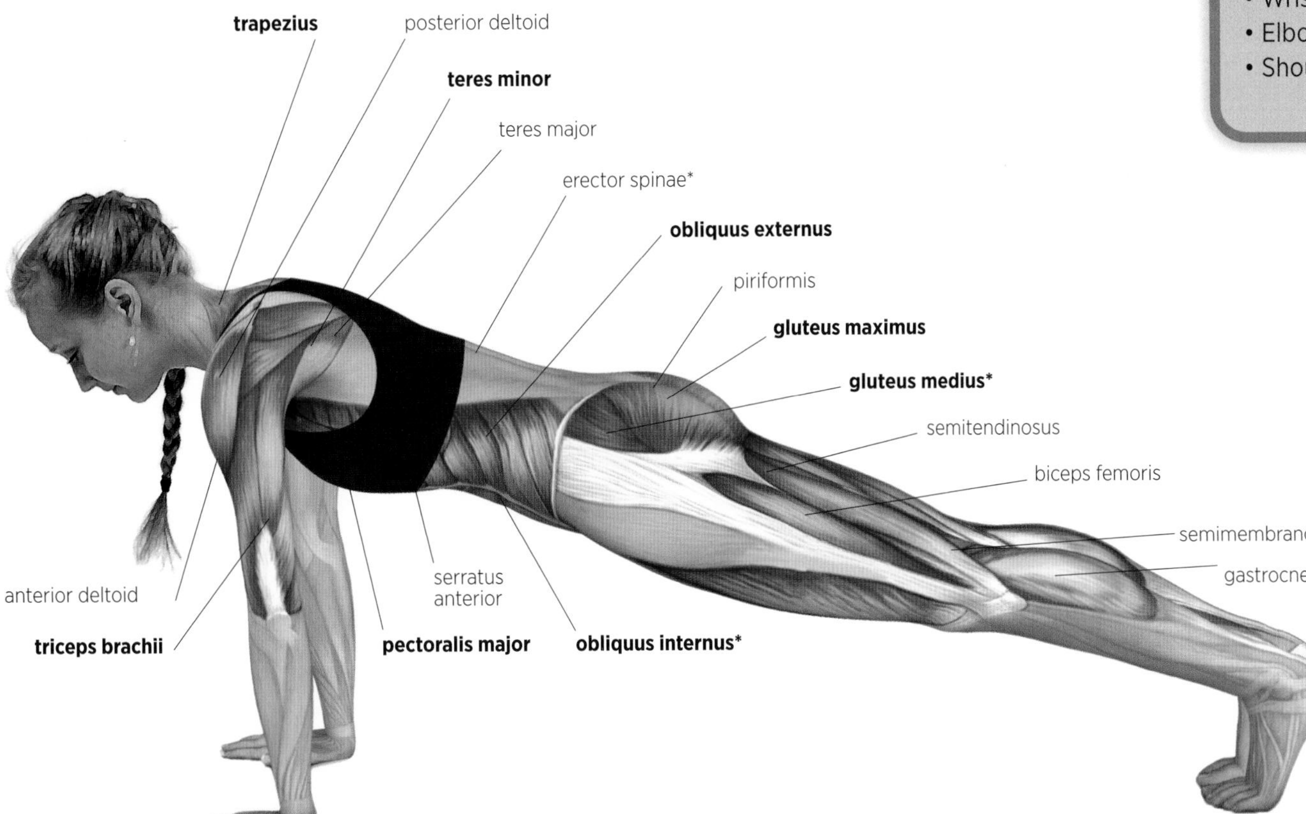

FACT FILE

SANSKRIT

- Phalakasana
- Also Adho Mukha Dandasana, Santolasana, or Kumbhakasana

TYPE

- Dynamic

TARGETS

- Spine
- Chest
- Neck

BENEFITS

- Strengthens arm and core muscles
- Develops core stability
- Prepares the body for other arm balances

CAUTIONS

- Wrist injuries
- Elbow injuries
- Shoulder issues

Downward-Facing Dog

This well-known asana is among the most frequently performed yoga poses—one you'll come into time and again. "Down Dog," as it is often called, stretches and strengthens the entire body.

HOW TO DO IT

- Begin on all fours, with your hands planted directly below your shoulders and your knees aligned beneath your hips.
- Tuck your toes under, and "walk" your hands forward about a palm's distance in front of your shoulders. With your hands and toes firmly planted, lift your hips up as you straighten your legs and draw your heels toward the floor.
- Press your chest toward your thighs, and bring your head between your arms. Lengthen up through your tailbone and keep your thighs slightly internally rotated, finding a neutral pelvis. Gaze between your feet or toward your navel. Hold for the recommended breaths.

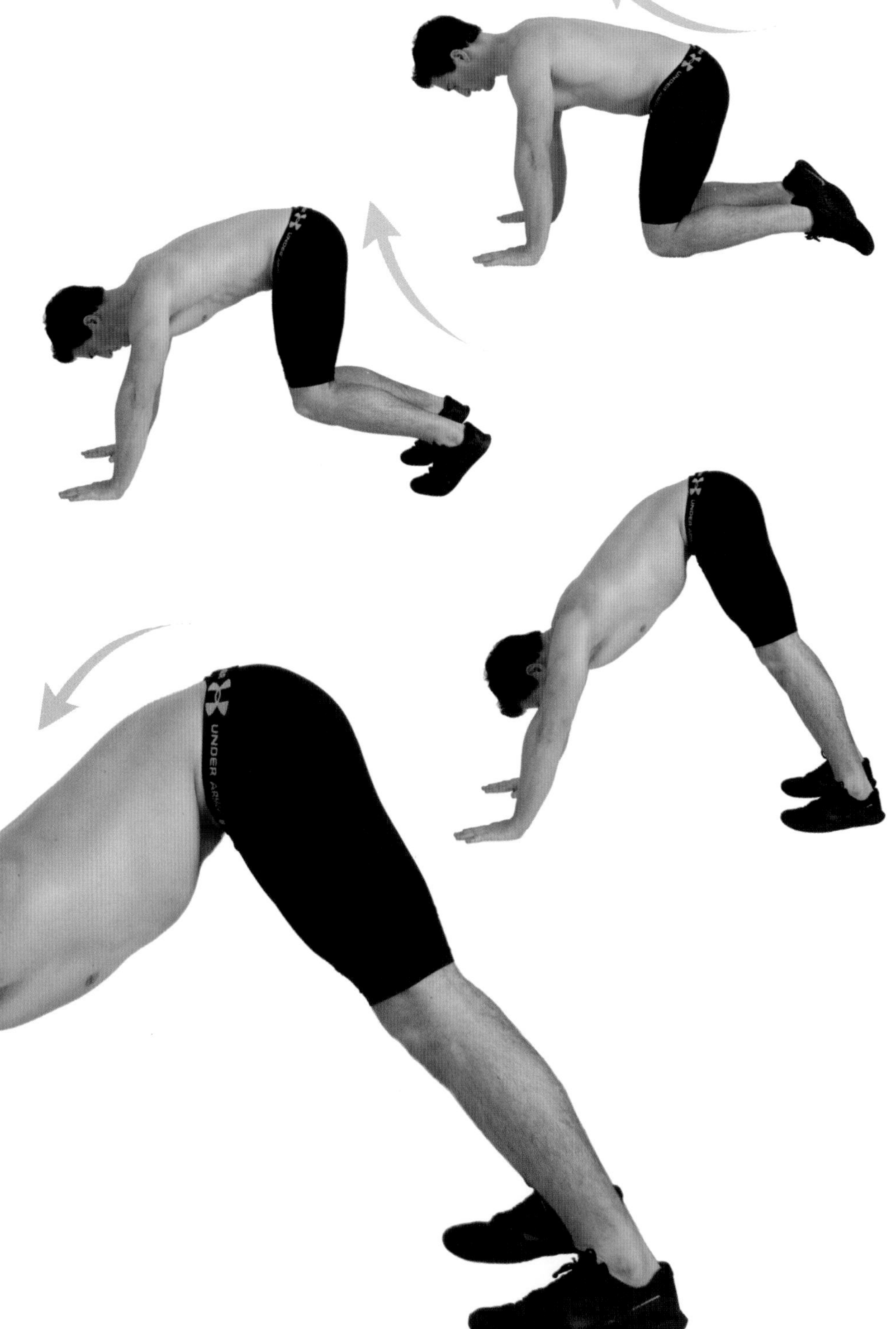

DO IT RIGHT

- Engage your entire hand fully into the floor at all times to avoid excess strain on your wrist joint.
- Keep your head in line with your spine.
- Keep your back flat and your chest elevated.
- Avoid holding your breath: relax your jaw slightly and breathe normally.

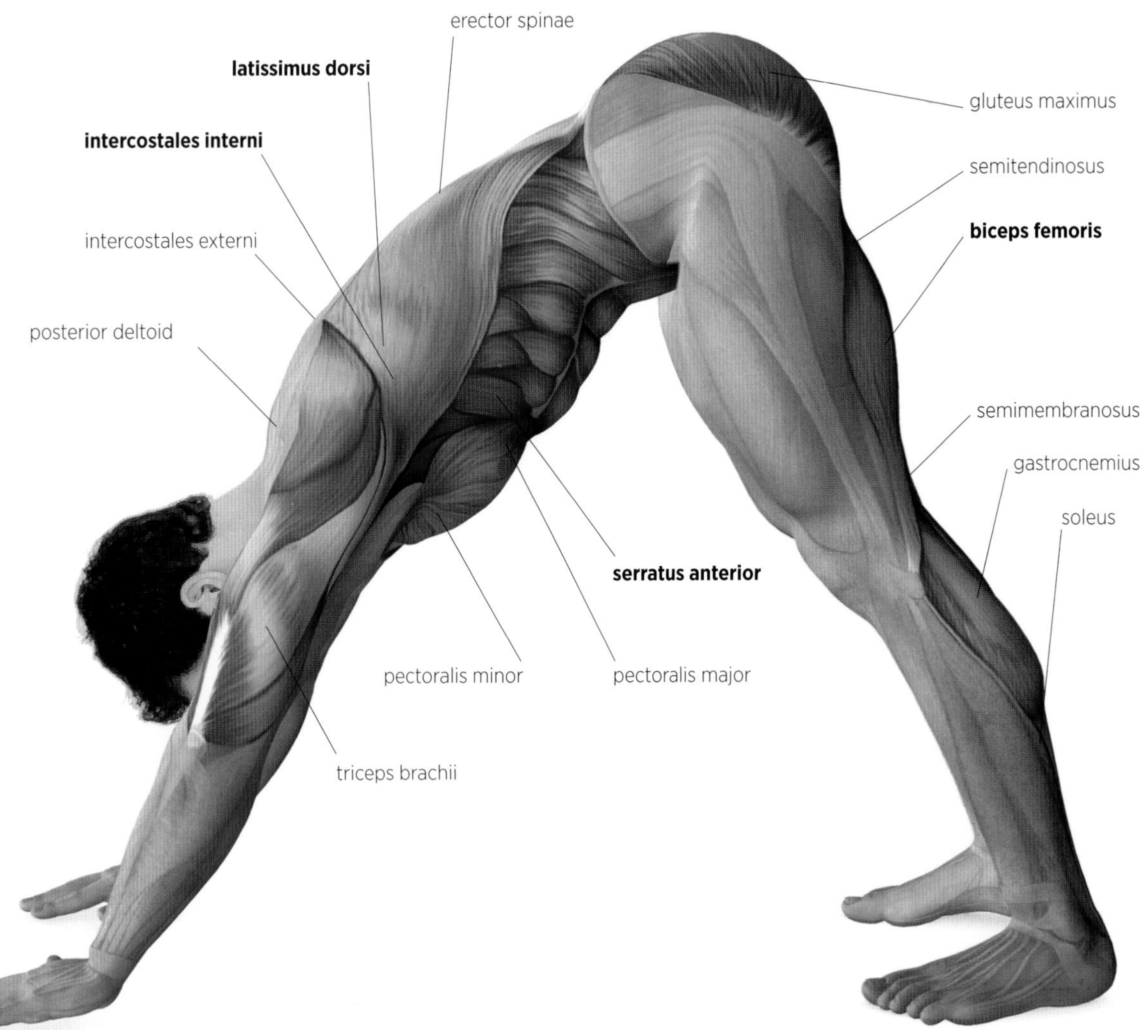

Annotation Key

Bold text indicates target muscles

Light text indicates other working muscles

* indicates deep muscles

FACT FILE

SANSKRIT
- Adho Mukha Svanasana

TARGETS
- Shoulders and arms
- Hamstrings
- Calves

TYPE
- Dynamic

BENEFITS
- Strengthens arms and legs
- Stretches spine, hamstrings, calves, and arches of feet
- Aids digestion
- Helps relieve menstrual cramps
- Helps relieve headaches

CAUTIONS
- Low blood pressure
- Shoulder issues
- Hamstring issues
- Carpal tunnel syndrome

One-Legged Plank

The intermediate One-Legged Plank can be challenging to line up and maintain. Muscle length, strength, and movement flow are all worked thoroughly during this pose.

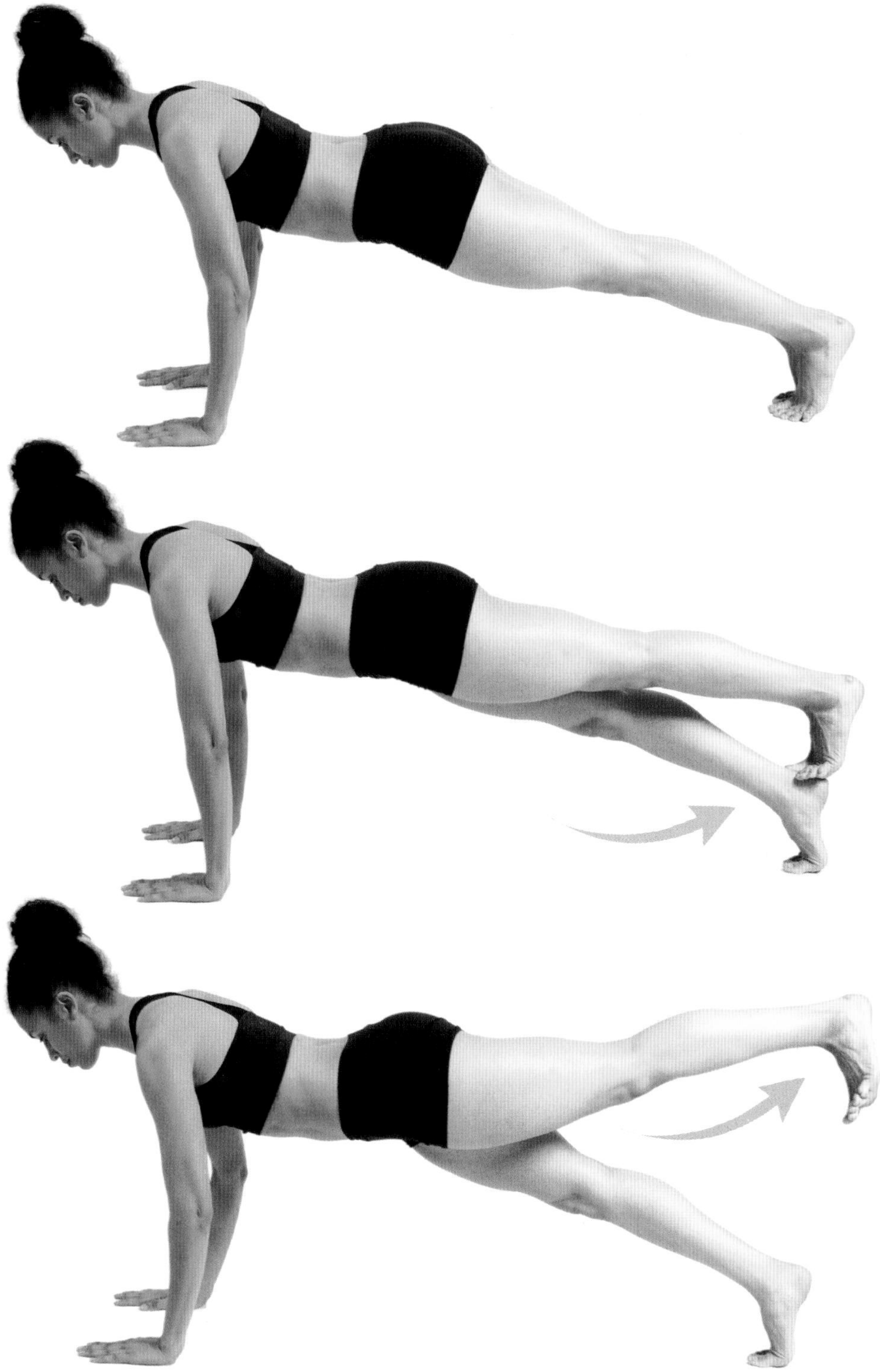

HOW TO DO IT

- Start in Plank Pose (pages 82–83), with the front of your body facing the mat in one long line. Position your arms directly under your shoulders with your fingers pointing forward. Extend your legs parallel and hip-width apart, with your weight on the balls of your feet.

- Inhale to prepare, and press your shoulder blades down your back for stabilization.

- Exhale as you push your left foot gently onto your right heel then lift your left leg to hip height, keeping your left foot flexed. Hold for the recommended breaths.

- Inhale, lower your leg, and repeat on the opposite side. Perform the recommended repetitions.

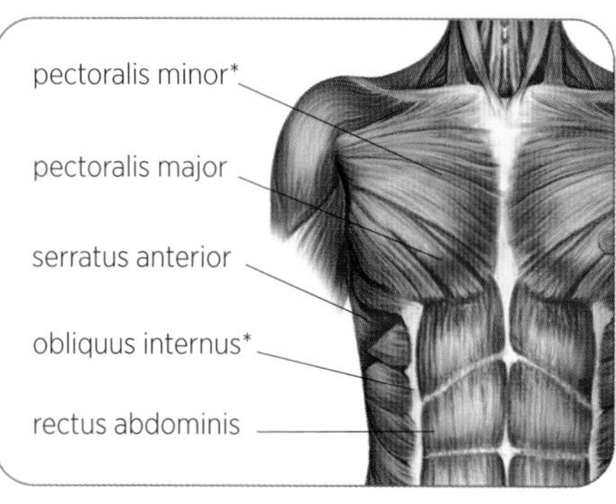

FACT FILE

SANSKRIT
- Eka Pada Phalakasana

TARGETS
- Shoulders
- Abdominals
- Obliques
- Glutes

BENEFITS
- Stretches Achilles tendon
- Strengthens upper limbs and shoulder girdle
- Stabilizes major muscles

CAUTIONS
- Elbow issues
- Toe joint stiffness
- Wrist weakness

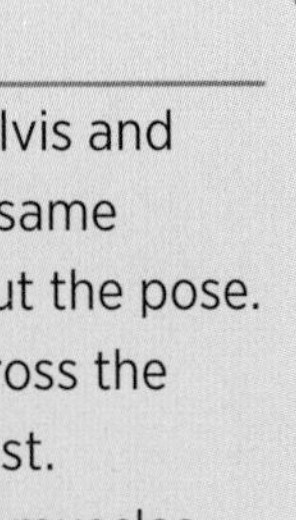

DO IT RIGHT

- Maintain your pelvis and abdomen at the same height throughout the pose.
- Remain open across the front of your chest.
- Keep your major muscles engaged.
- Avoid raising your shoulders toward your ears.
- Do not arch your neck or allow your head to hang.
- Avoid twisting your hips as you move your leg.

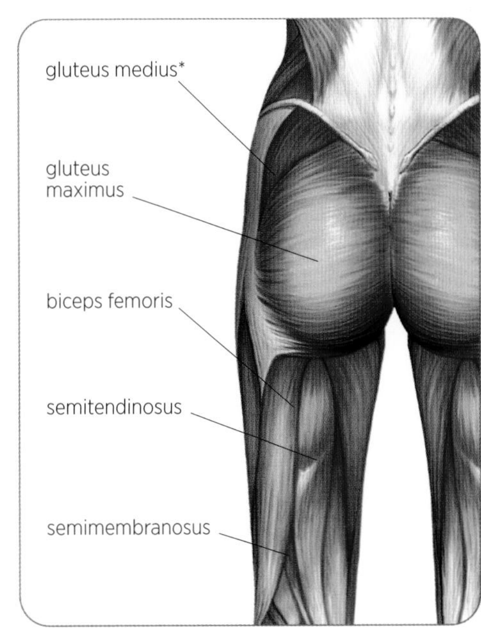

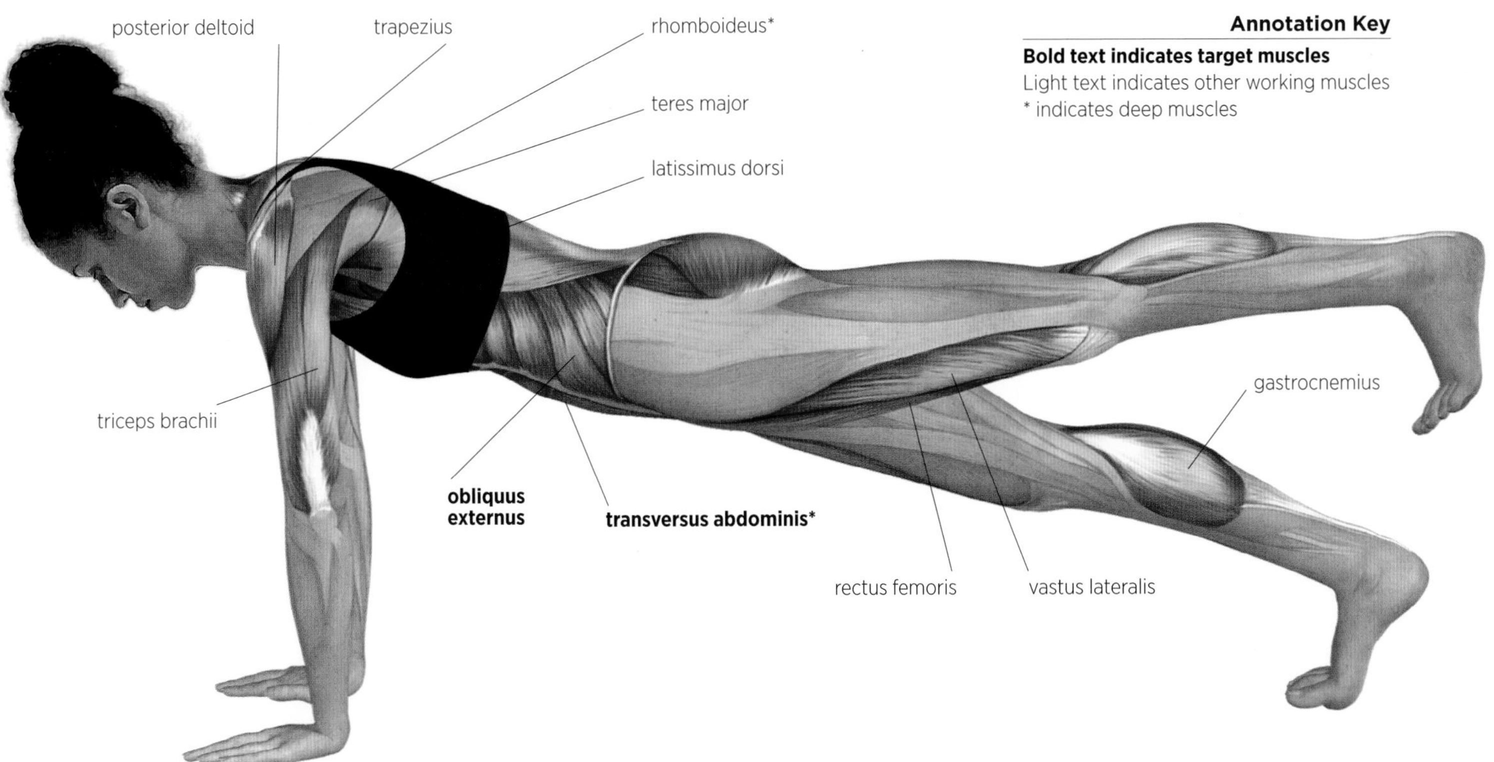

Annotation Key

Bold text indicates target muscles
Light text indicates other working muscles
* indicates deep muscles

Bird Dog Pose

Bird Dog Pose, which resembles a dog pointing at a game bird, stabilizes your upper and lower back as well as your shoulders. The Bird Dog may look simple, but it really challenges your sense of balance and coordination. As an isometric exercise, you contract and hold specific muscles in a static position. This offers the added benefit of stabilizing the associated joints.

HOW TO DO IT

- Squat down and place your hands on the mat, making sure that they are aligned under your shoulders, with your fingers facing the front of the mat.

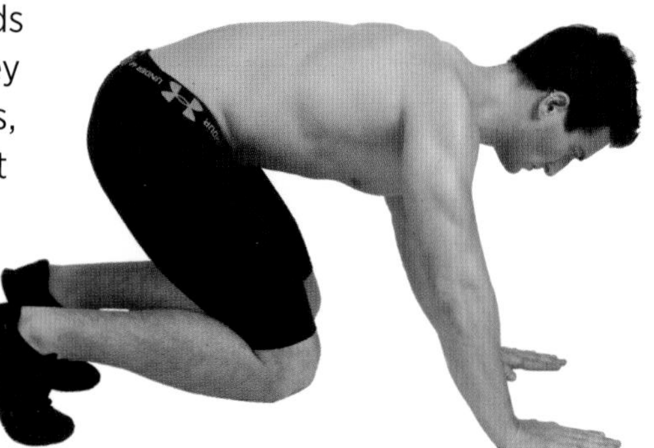

- Extend your legs parallel and hip-width apart, with your weight on the balls of your feet, so that your body forms one long line from your shoulders to your heels.

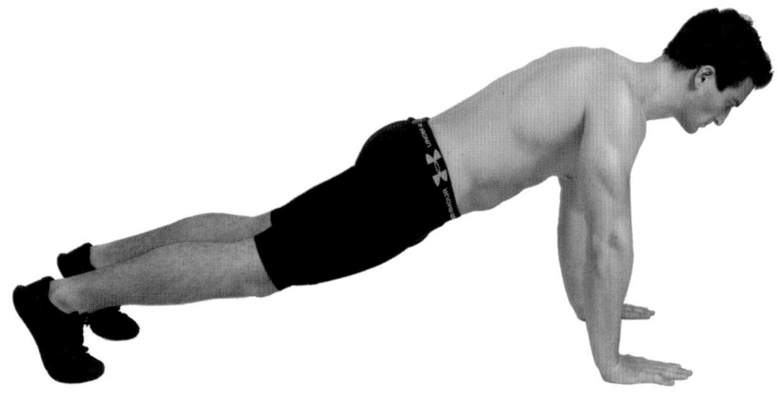

- Extend your left arm forward and parallel to the floor, while lifting your right leg and extending it behind you.
- Hold for the recommended breaths, and then repeat on the opposite side.

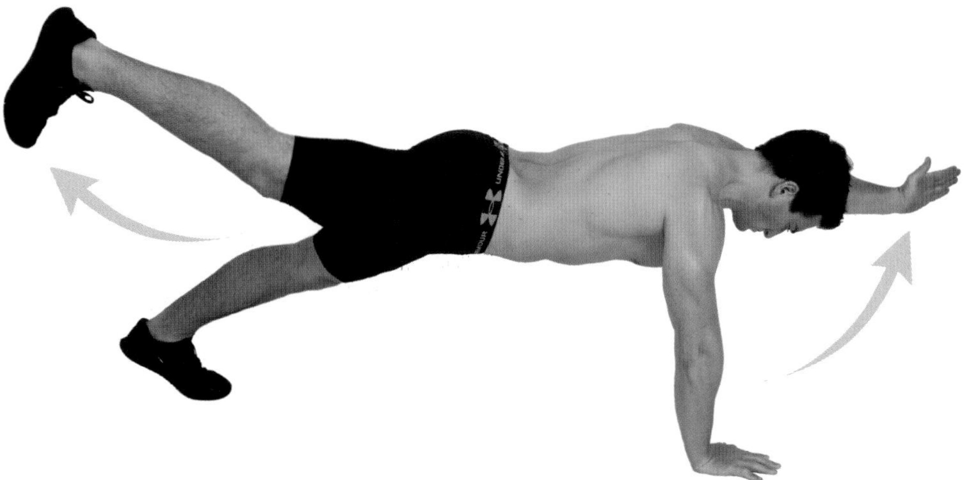

DO IT RIGHT

- Be sure to raise both the extended arm and leg high enough so that they are parallel to the floor.
- Engage your abdominals by drawing your navel toward your spine.
- You may wobble a bit at first—it will take you a few tries to get your balance.
- Avoid allowing your lower back to sag.

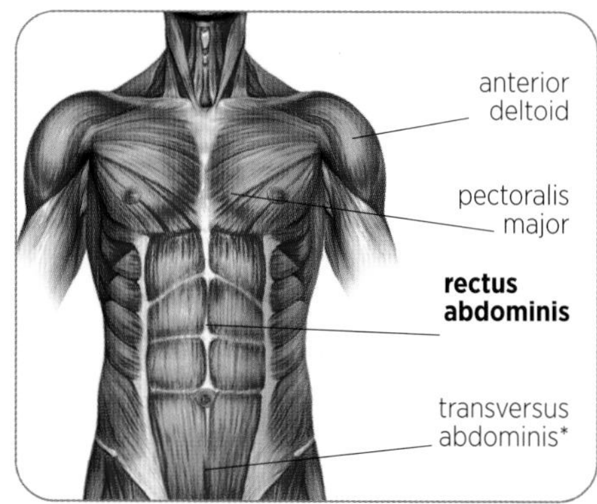

FACT FILE

SANSKRIT
- Parsva Balasana

TARGETS
- Upper arms
- Core
- Glutes
- Hamstrings

TYPE
- Dynamic

BENEFITS
- Stabilizes upper and lower back
- Stabilizes shoulders
- Strengthens abdomen and obliques
- Improves balance and coordination

CAUTIONS
- Shoulder issues
- Wrist injuries
- Lower-back injuries

MODIFICATION

EASIER: Start on all fours, making sure that your hands are under your shoulders and your knees are under your hips. Extend one arm parallel to the floor, while lifting your opposite leg and extending it behind you. Hold for the recommended time, and then repeat on the opposite side.

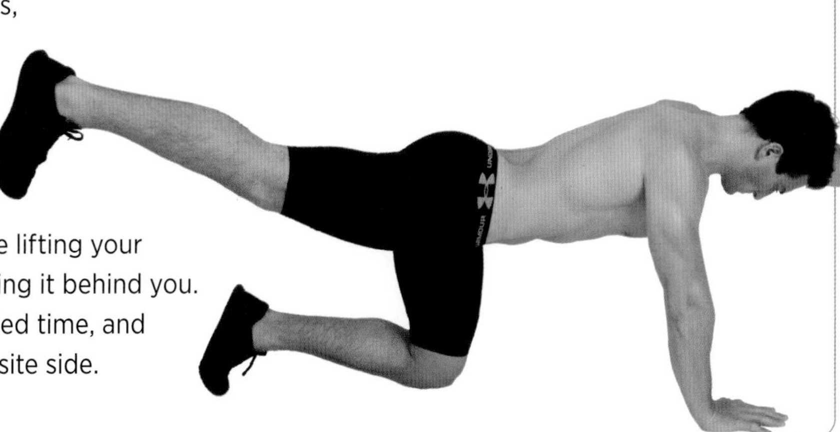

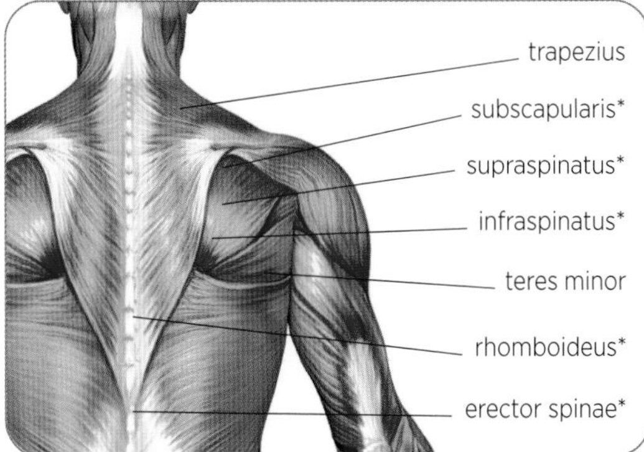

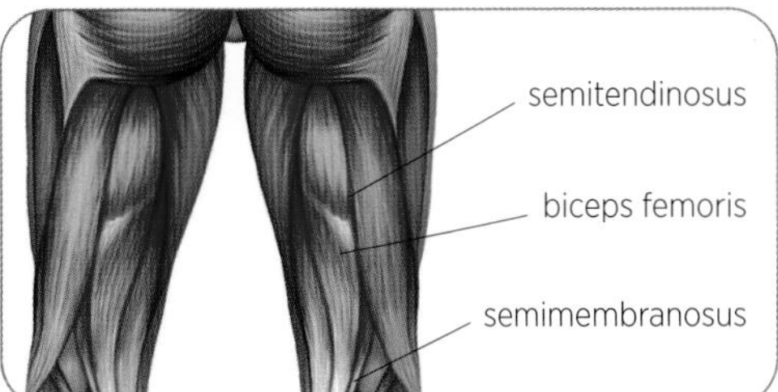

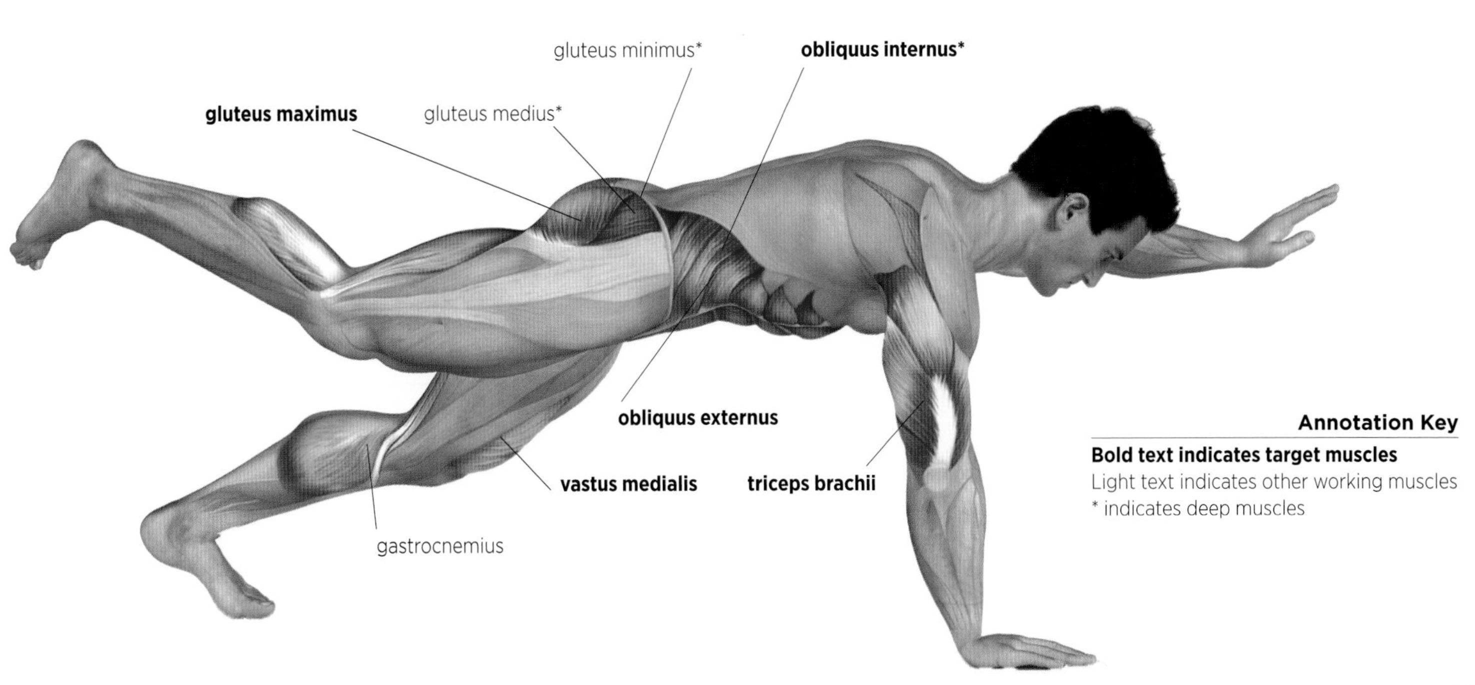

Annotation Key
Bold text indicates target muscles
Light text indicates other working muscles
* indicates deep muscles

Upward Plank Pose

This pose has much to offer: it builds up the muscles of your arms, legs, and spine and stretches your chest, abdominals, ankles, and feet. Upward Plank Pose also helps hone your sense of balance.

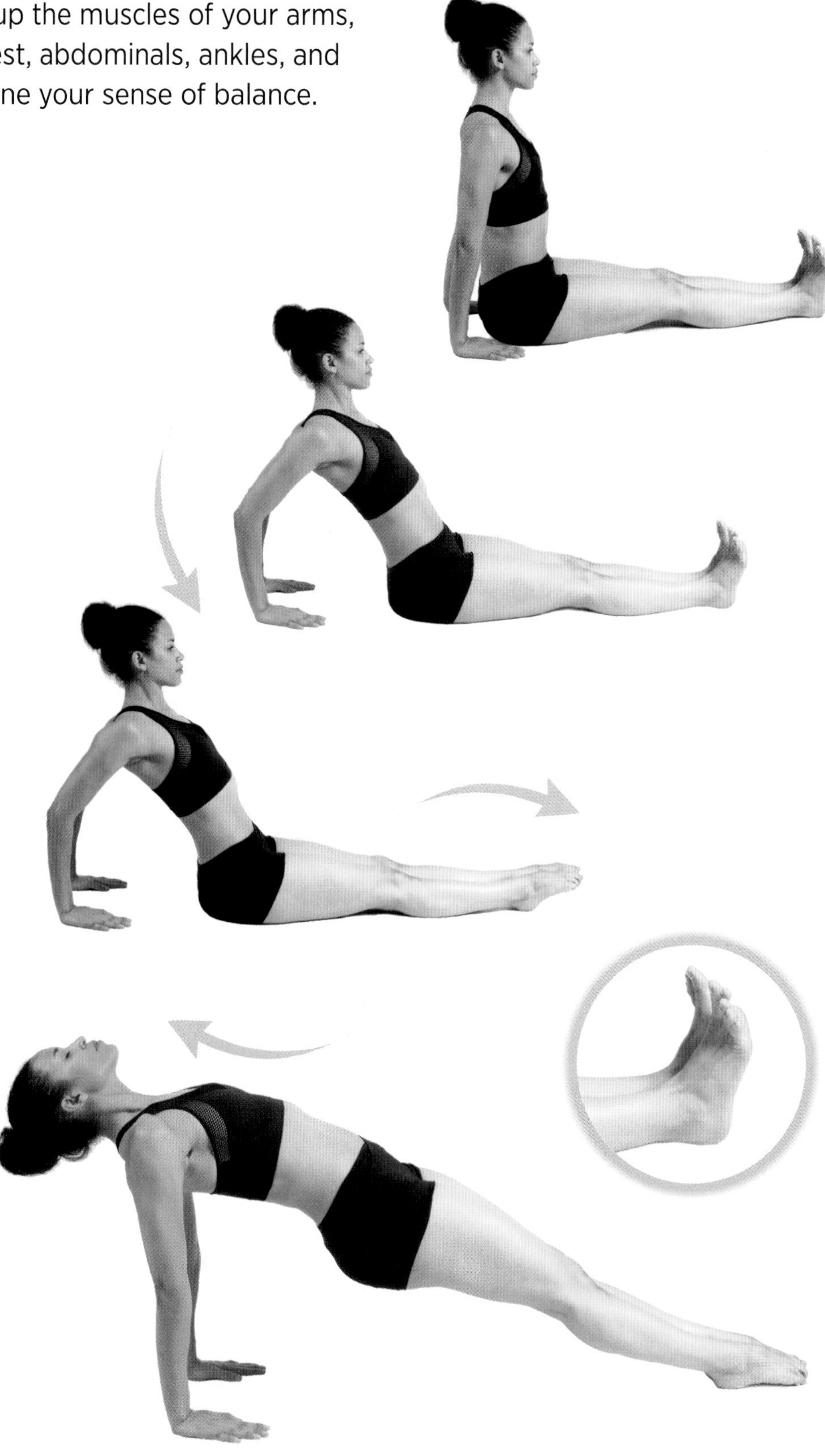

HOW TO DO IT

- Sit with your legs extended in front of you and your hands on the floor at your sides.
- Bring your hands several inches behind your hips, and rotate your palms so that your fingertips point forward, keeping your hands shoulder-width apart.
- Bend your knees and place your fleet flat on the floor, turning your big toes slightly inward and placing your heels at least a foot away from your buttocks.
- Exhale and press down with your hands and feet, lifting your hips until your back and thighs are parallel to the floor. Keep your shoulders directly above your wrists.
- Without lowering your hips, straighten your legs one at a time.
- Lift your chest, and bring your shoulder blades together while pushing your hips higher, creating a slight arch in your back. Do not squeeze your buttocks to create the lift.
- Slowly elongate your neck, and let it drop back gently. Hold for the recommended breaths, and then return to your original position.

FACT FILE

SANSKRIT
- Purvottanasana

TARGETS
- Spine
- Arms and wrists
- Hamstrings

TYPE
- Dynamic

BENEFITS
- Strengthens the spine, arms, and hamstrings
- Extends the hips and chest

CAUTIONS
- Wrist injuries
- Elbow injuries
- Shoulder issues
- Neck issues

DO IT RIGHT

- Be careful not to overextend your back; instead, use your hamstrings and shoulders to open your hips and chest.
- If you have weak hamstrings, widen your legs while holding your hips elevated.
- Deepen the extension of your upper back by breathing steadily.

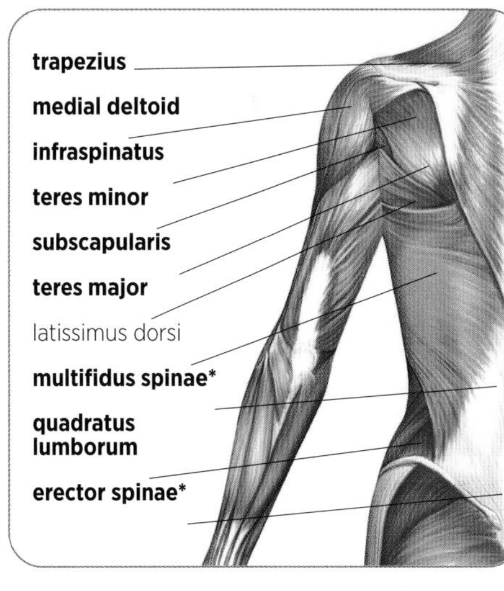

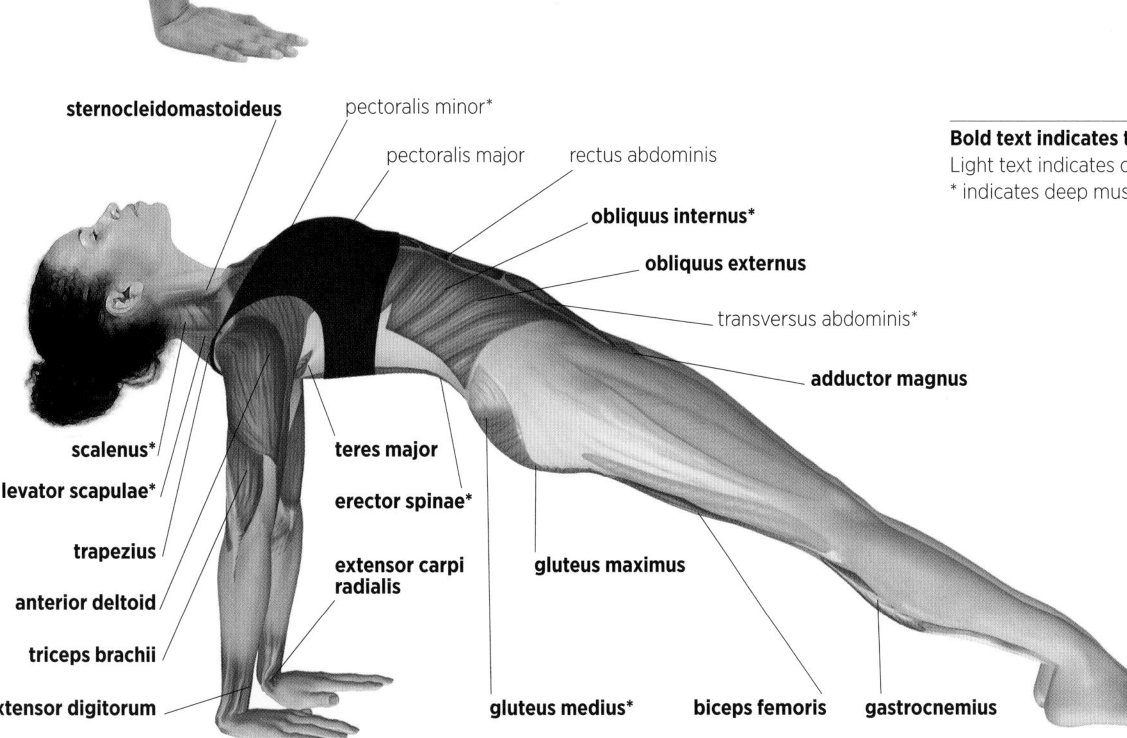

Annotation Key

Bold text indicates target muscles

Light text indicates other working muscles

* indicates deep muscles

Upward Plank with Lifted Leg

Like other plank poses, this variation works many parts of the body—your shoulders, abdominals, sides, hips, glutes, thighs, and lower legs. It also helps improve your balance.

HOW TO DO IT

- Sit with your legs parallel and extended in front of you. Place your hands on the floor behind you, with your fingers pointed toward your feet.

- Press up through your arms and lift up your chest, squeezing your buttocks and lifting your hips while pressing your heels into the floor. Continue lifting your pelvis until your body forms a long straight line from your shoulders to your feet.

- Without allowing your pelvis to drop, raise your right leg to about shoulder height.

- Hold for the recommended breaths, slowly lower your foot to the mat, and repeat on the opposite side. Perform the recommended repetitions.

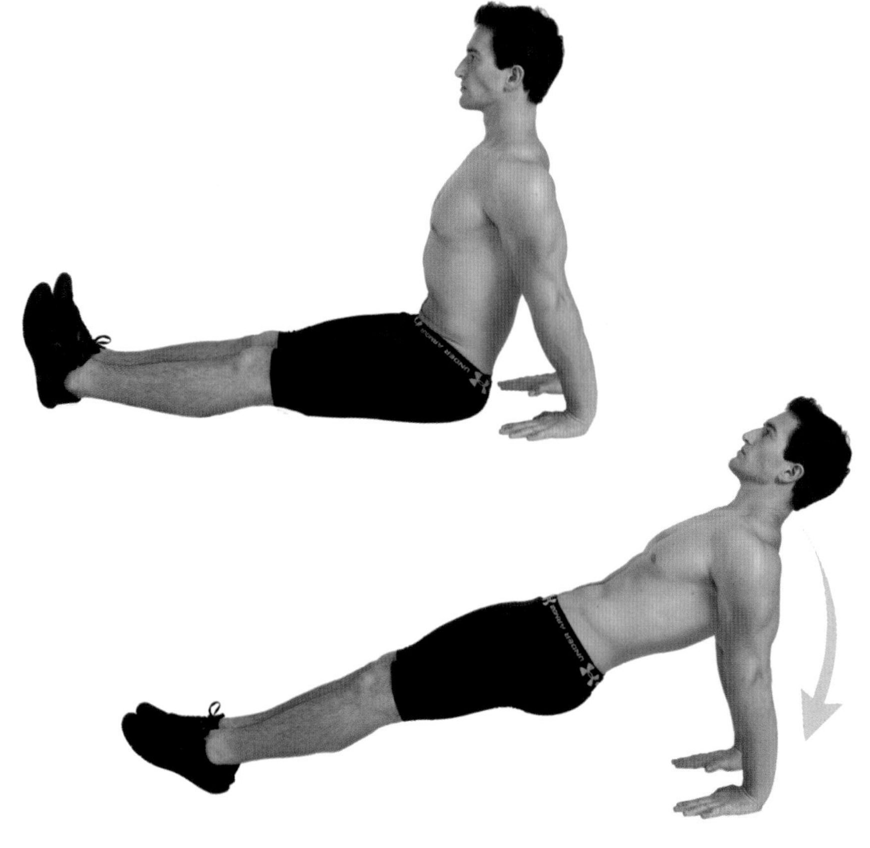

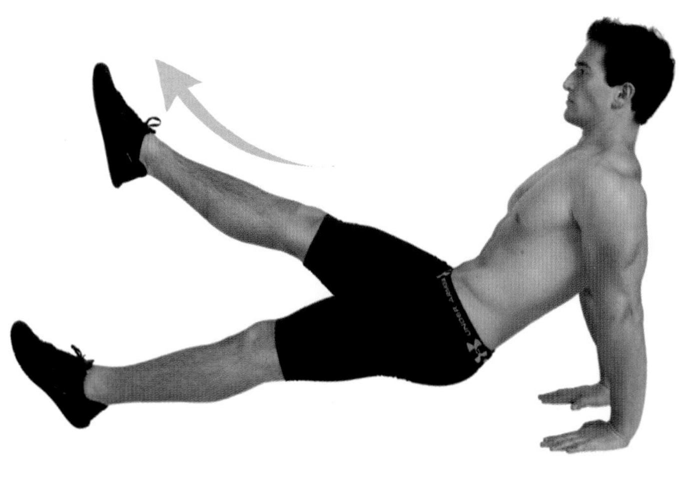

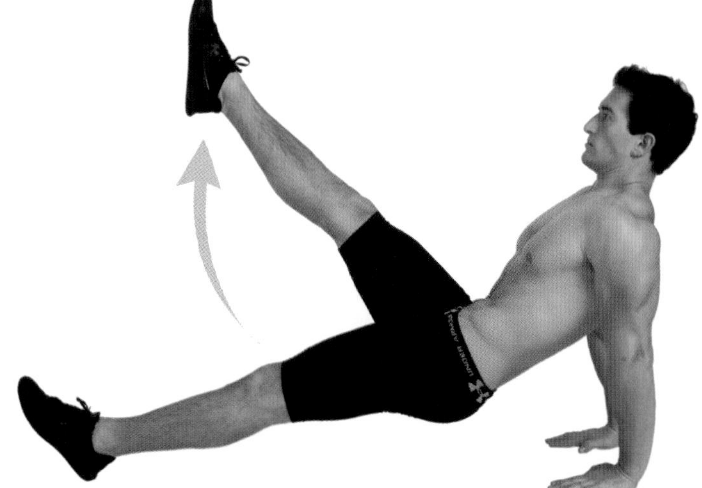

FACT FILE

SANSKRIT
- None

TARGETS
- Hip extensor muscles
- Core stabilizers
- Arms
- Legs

TYPE
- Dynamic

BENEFITS
- Strengthens shins and calves
- Stretches quadriceps and hamstrings
- Targets abdomen and obliques

CAUTIONS
- Wrist pain
- Knee pain
- Shoulder injuries
- Shooting pains down leg

DO IT RIGHT
- Your pelvis should remain elevated throughout the exercise.
- Avoid allowing your shoulders to sink into their sockets. If your legs do not feel strong enough to support your body, slightly bend your knees.

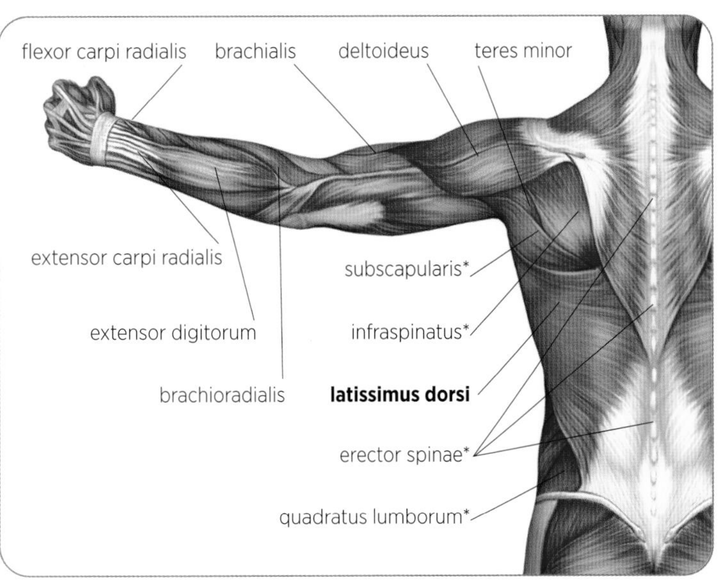

Annotation Key
Bold text indicates target muscles
Light text indicates other working muscles
* indicates deep muscles

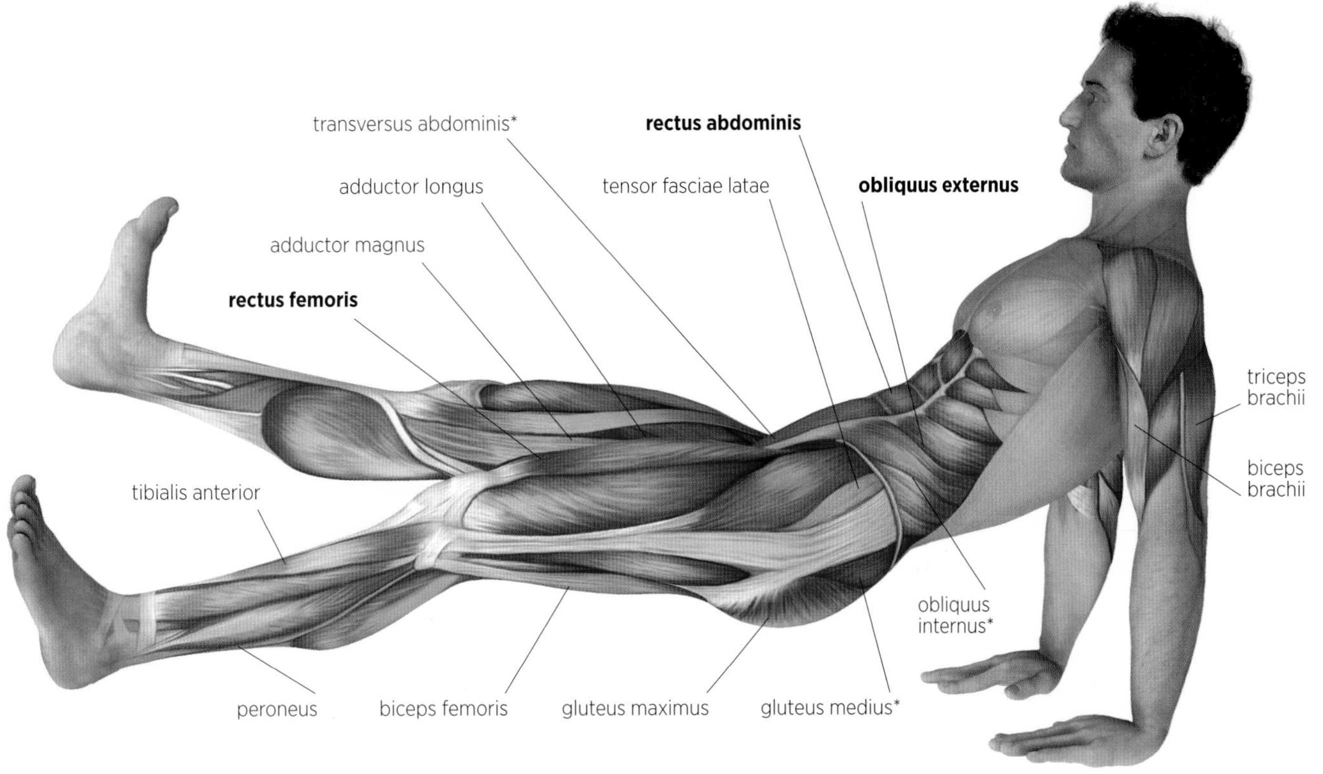

Dolphin Pose

Dolphin Pose is known to strengthen both your upper and lower body—your shoulders, arms, abdominals, and spine, as well as your thighs and calves. This energizing posture also helps you improve your balance.

HOW TO DO IT

- Kneel on the floor with your hips lifted off your heels.
- Bend forward and place your hands on the mat in front of you; lower your elbows to the floor, keeping them tucked in at your sides and aligned with your shoulders.
- Straighten your legs as you lift your sit bones toward the ceiling. Tuck your tailbone toward your pubis, and squeeze your legs together.
- Push through your forearms, and extend the stretch through your shoulders. Keep your head and chest lifted off the mat.
- Hold for the recommended breaths.

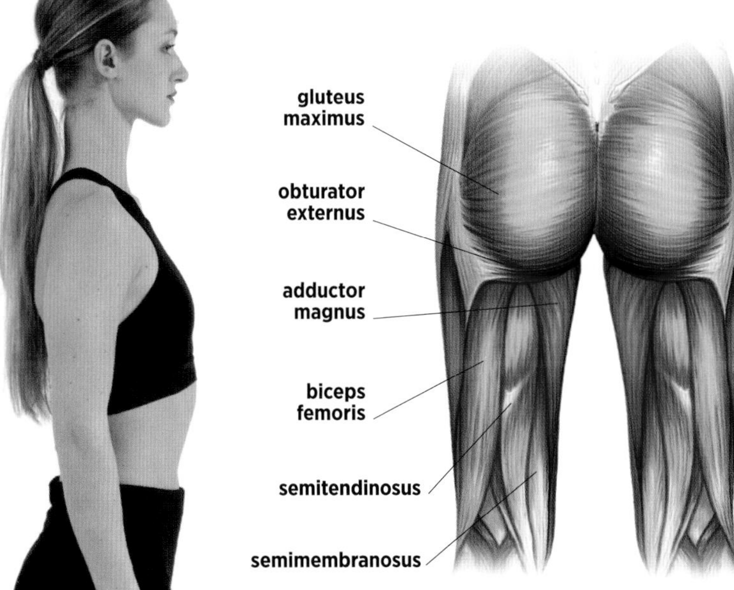

FACT FILE

SANSKRIT
- Ardha Pincha Mayurasana

TARGETS
- Abdominals
- Glutes
- Back
- Hamstrings

TYPE
- Dynamic

BENEFITS
- Strengthens and tones abdomen
- Engages arms, legs, and spine
- Improves balance
- Invigorates and energizes by increasing blood flow to the brain

CAUTIONS
- Back injuries
- Neck injuries
- Headache
- High blood pressure

Annotation Key

Bold text indicates target muscles
Light text indicates other working muscles
* indicates deep muscles

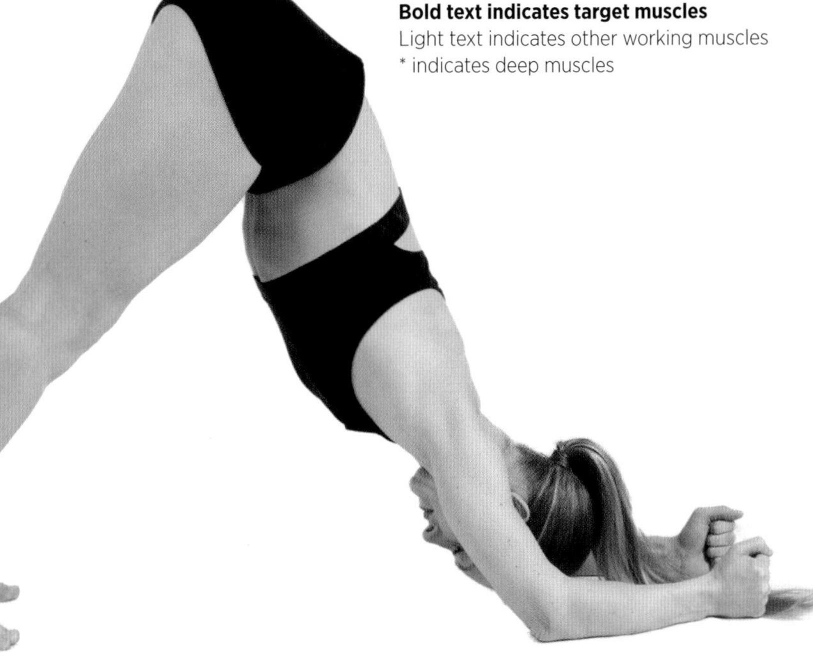

DO IT RIGHT

- While holding Dolphin Pose, keep your back straight. If you cannot straighten your legs without sagging or rounding your spine, keep your knees slightly bent.
- Avoid raising your heels off the mat.

Dolphin Plank Pose

Like all plank poses, this modification strengthens your abdominals and benefits your shoulders, upper arms, and obliques. The isometric hold also helps to build lean muscle.

HOW TO DO IT

- Begin on all fours, with your toes curled forward and facing the front of your mat.
- Plant your forearms on the floor, shoulder-width apart and parallel to each other. Raise your knees off the mat and extend your legs until they are in line with your arms. Do not let your hips or buttocks sink too low or rise too high. Your body should form a straight line from your shoulders to your heels.
- Hold this position for the recommended breaths.

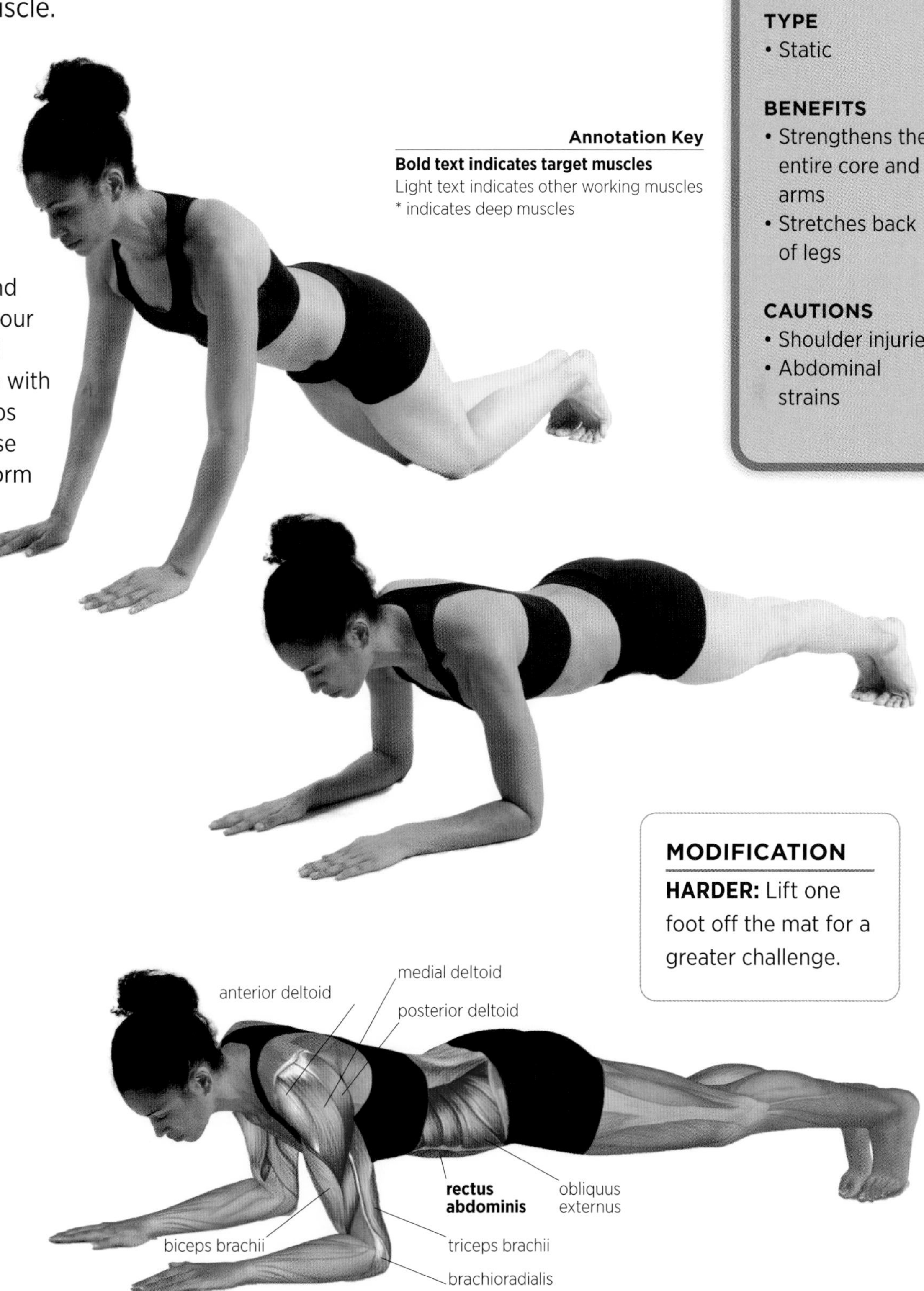

FACT FILE

SANSKRIT
- Makara Adho Mukha Svanasana

TARGETS
- Abdominals
- Shoulders
- Obliques

TYPE
- Static

BENEFITS
- Strengthens the entire core and arms
- Stretches back of legs

CAUTIONS
- Shoulder injuries
- Abdominal strains

DO IT RIGHT

- Keep your abdominal muscles tight and your body in a straight line.
- Keep your shoulder blades and collarbone wide. This prepares you for other balance poses, such as Crow Pose.
- Avoid bridging too high, since this can take stress off your working muscles.

MODIFICATION

HARDER: Lift one foot off the mat for a greater challenge.

Dolphin Plank with Arm Reach

This more challenging variation of Plank Pose (pages 82–83) is effective in strengthening your forearms, upper arms, shoulders, and back. It also improves your stamina and posture by building up the muscles that support your spine. Swimmers, gymnasts, and dancers can all benefit from this pose.

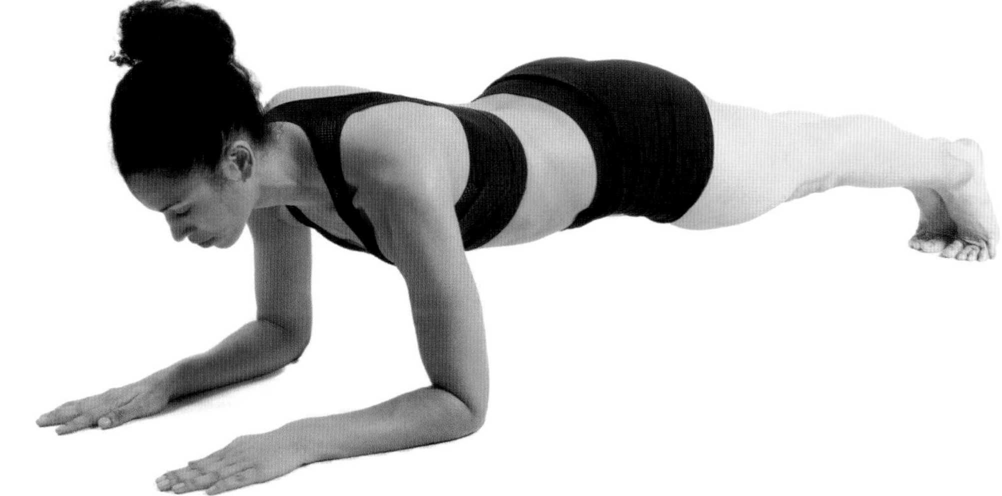

HOW TO DO IT

- Begin on all fours with your toes curled forward and facing the front of your mat.
- Plant your forearms on the floor parallel to each other. Raise your knees off the mat and lengthen your legs until they are in line with your arms. Your body should form a straight line from your shoulders to your heels.
- Maintaining proper plank form, slowly raise your right arm off the mat and extend it away from your shoulder, fingers outstretched.
- Hold for the recommended breaths, release the pose, and then repeat on the opposite side.

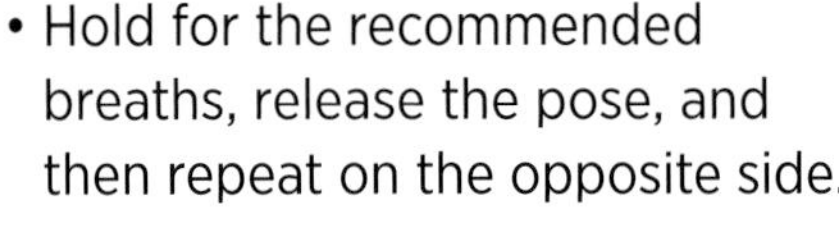

DO IT RIGHT

- Keep your abdominal muscles tight and your body in a straight line.
- Your neck should be in a neutral position, not extended or crunched.
- Avoid letting your hips or buttocks sink too low or rise too high.

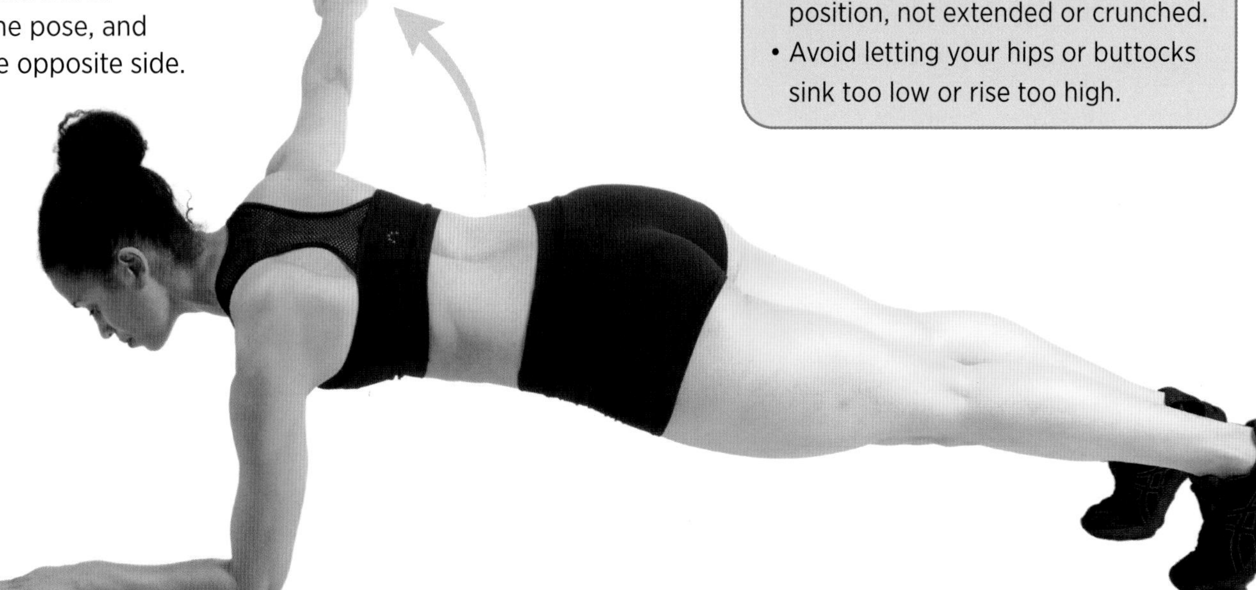

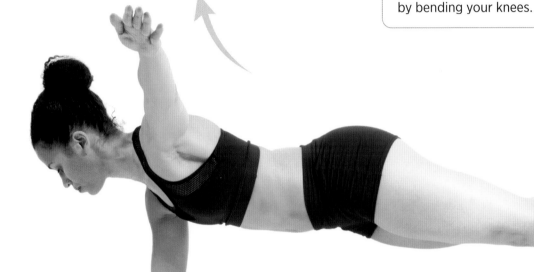

Annotation Key

Bold text indicates target muscles
Light text indicates other working muscles
* indicates deep muscles

MODIFICATION

EASIER: Instead of extending your arm out to your sides, raise only your forearm a few inches off the mat. You can also make the pose less taxing by bending your knees.

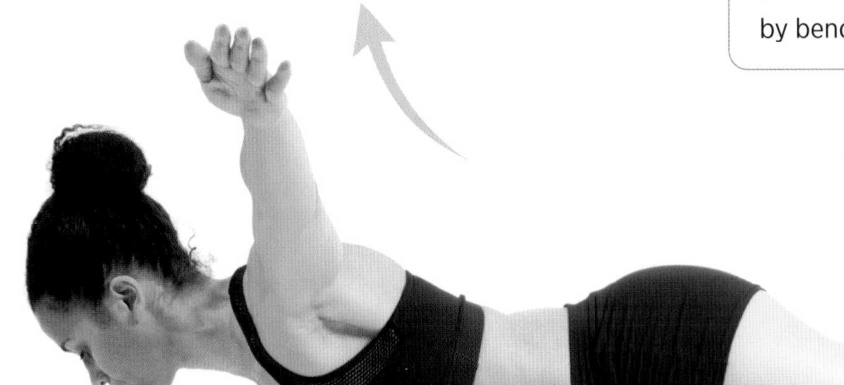

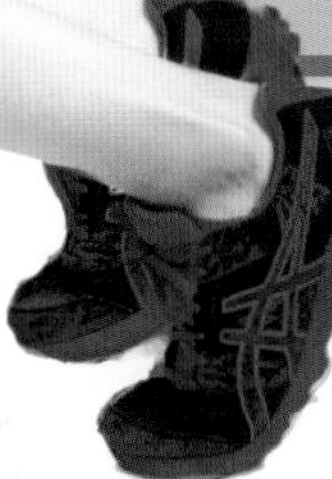

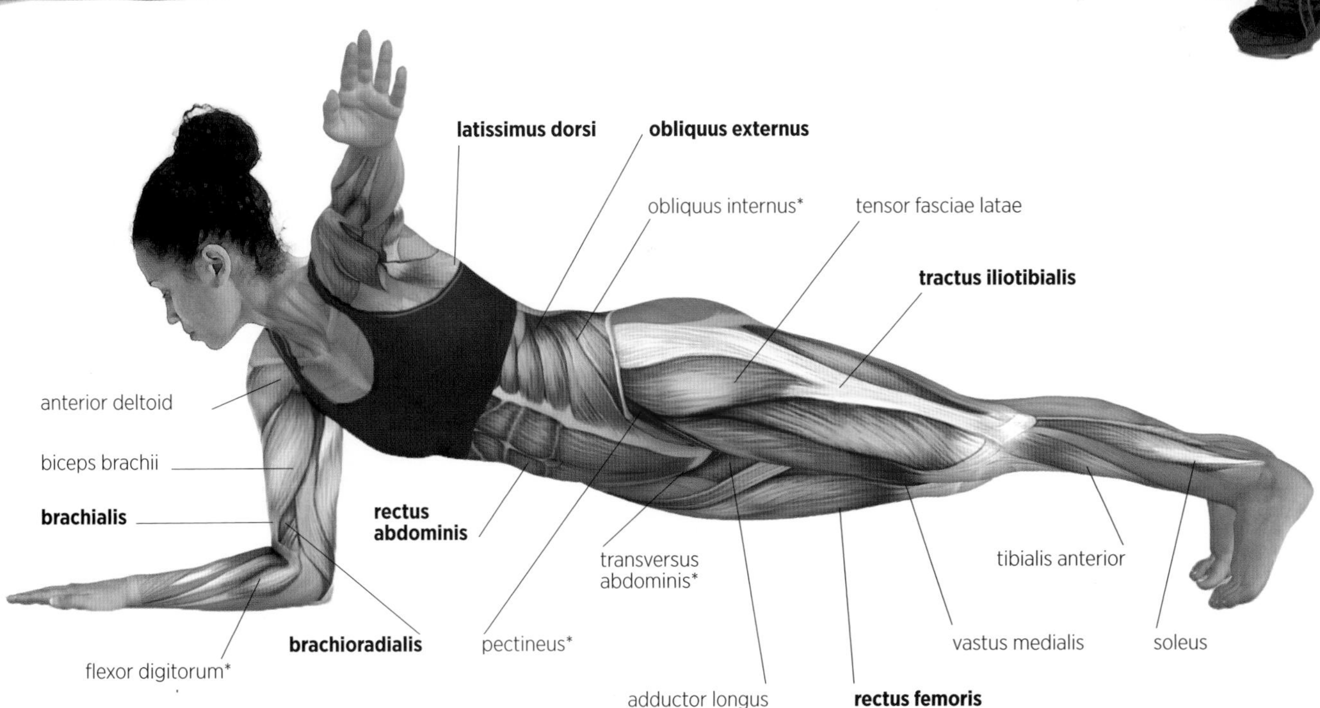

FACT FILE

SANSKRIT
- None

TARGETS
- Abdominals
- Thighs
- Shoulders

TYPE
- Dynamic

BENEFITS
- Strengthens the entire core
- Stretches the hamstrings
- Opens the chest and shoulders
- Improves posture

CAUTIONS
- Groin injuries
- Shoulder issues
- Ankle injuries

Reverse Tabletop Pose

Reverse Tabletop Pose, also called Half Upward Plank Pose, provides a great counterpose after performing forward bends, but it also has many benefits of its own. It stretches the front of your body and your shoulders, and strengthens your arms, wrists, and legs. This energizing chest opener also improves your posture.

HOW TO DO IT

- Begin with your arms straight and the palms flat on the floor on either side of your hips to support your spine, sitting with your legs straight in front of you. Place your palms flat on the mat at your hips, with your fingers pointing toward your feet.

- Bend your knees and place your feet flat on the mat. Leave some space between your hips and feet, so that when you come up into position, your knees are perpendicular to the floor.

- Pressing firmly into your hands and feet, inhale and squeeze your buttocks and thighs as you lift your hips up to knee height.

- Straighten your arms, and check that your thighs and torso are parallel to the floor.

- Your wrists should be directly beneath your shoulders. Draw your shoulder blades together, and open your chest. Keep your neck neutral, or gently begin to drop your head if this feels comfortable. Try to relax your buttocks, and hold the pose only with the strength of your legs.

- Hold for the recommended breaths, then release your hips back to the mat, and straighten your legs.

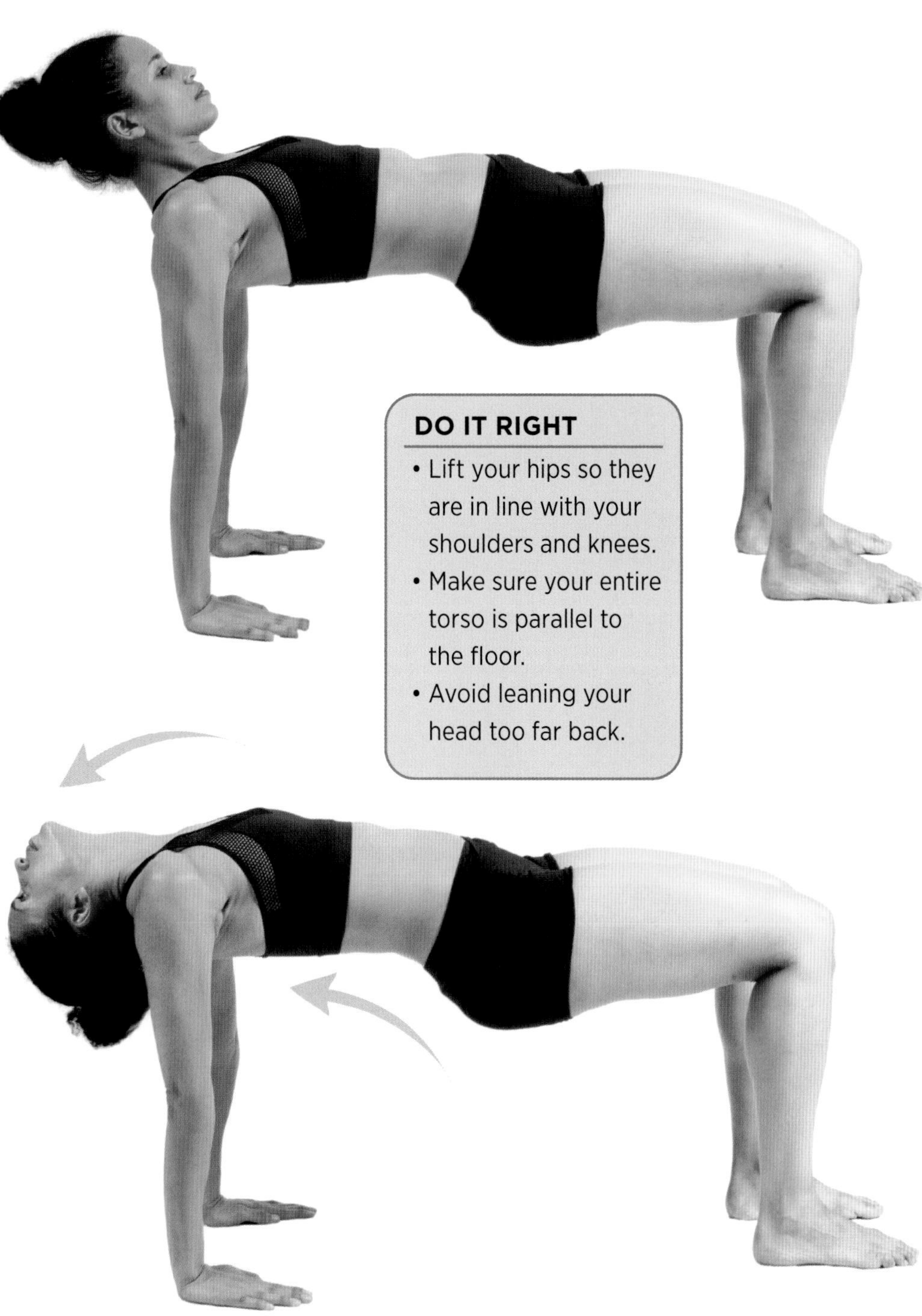

DO IT RIGHT

- Lift your hips so they are in line with your shoulders and knees.
- Make sure your entire torso is parallel to the floor.
- Avoid leaning your head too far back.

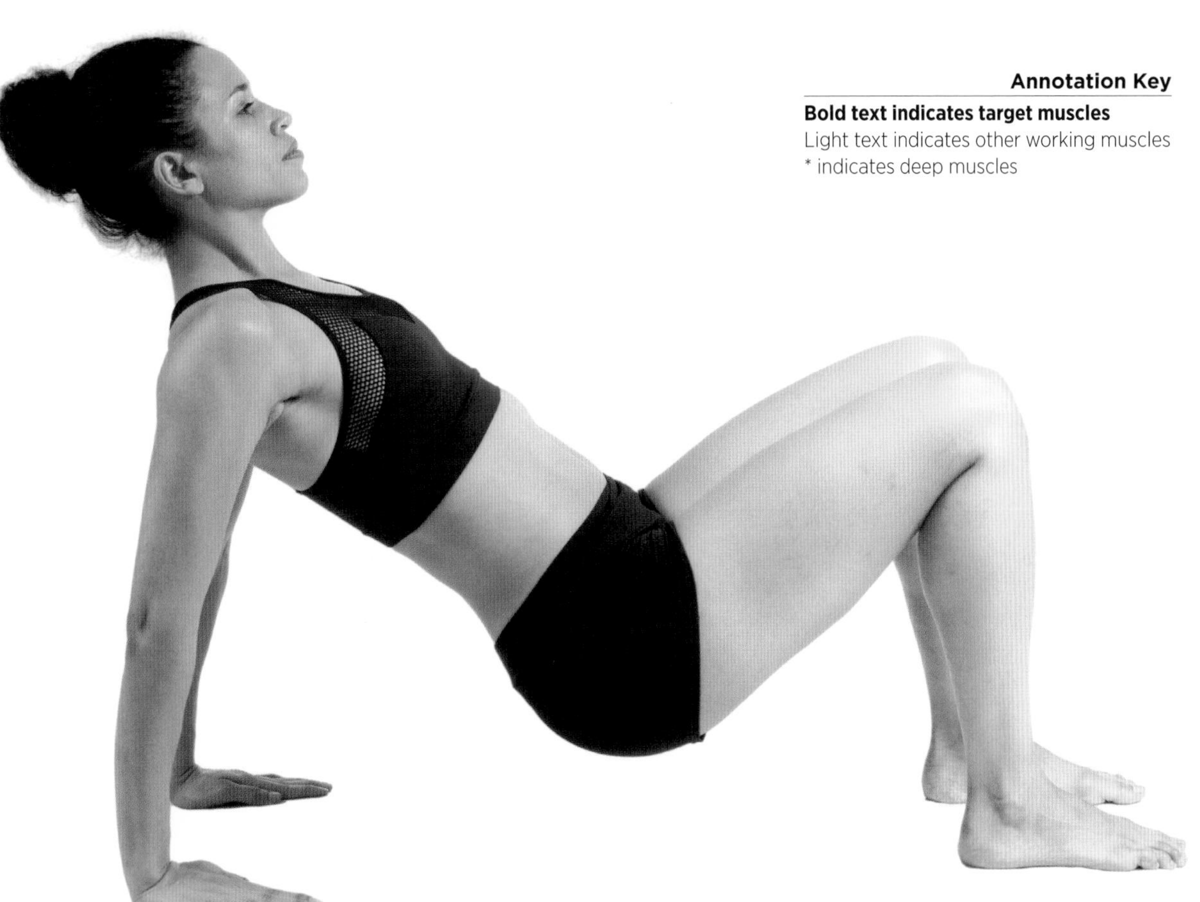

Annotation Key

Bold text indicates target muscles

Light text indicates other working muscles

* indicates deep muscles

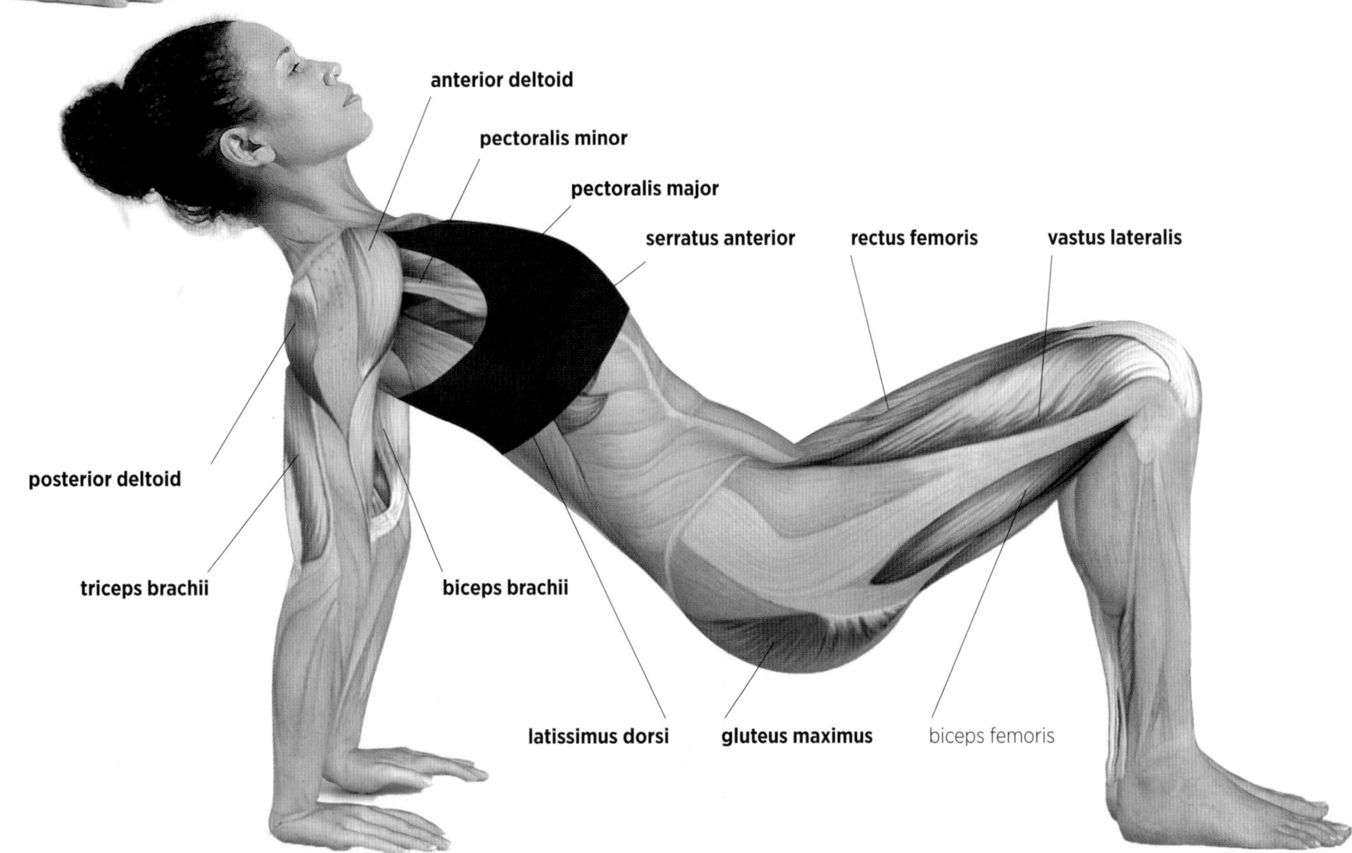

FACT FILE

SANSKRIT
- Ardha Purvottanasana

TARGETS
- Thighs
- Glutes
- Chest
- Shoulders

TYPE
- Static

BENEFITS
- Opens chest
- Stretches quads and hamstrings
- Strengthens glutes and upper back

CAUTIONS
- Lower-back issues
- Wrist injuries

Celibate's Pose

This demanding pose requires arm and shoulder strength as well as a powerful core. In Sanskrit, the name of this empowering pose means "having control over your senses and your lower limbs."

HOW TO DO IT

- Sit with your arms straight and the palms flat on the floor on either side of your hips to support your spine, with your legs together and outstretched.
- Place your palms on the floor beside your hips, with your elbows straight and your fingers facing the front of the mat.
- Adjust your hand position slightly forward, until you find your center of gravity.
- Inhale and push down with your arms, simultaneously using your abdominals to lift your hips, legs, and feet from the mat. Your legs should be horizontal and straight, and your spine slightly curved.
- Hold for the recommended breaths, then slowly lower your hips and legs to the mat.

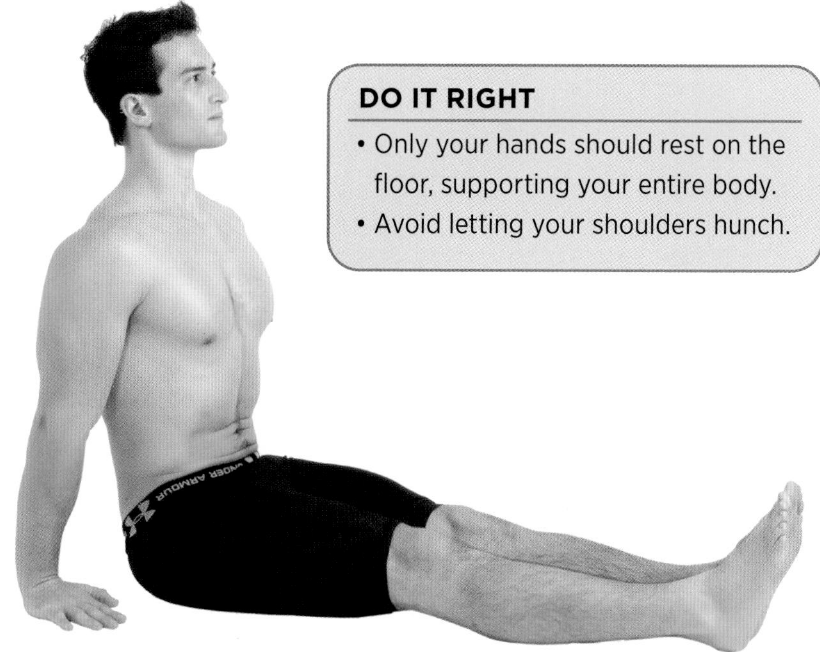

DO IT RIGHT

- Only your hands should rest on the floor, supporting your entire body.
- Avoid letting your shoulders hunch.

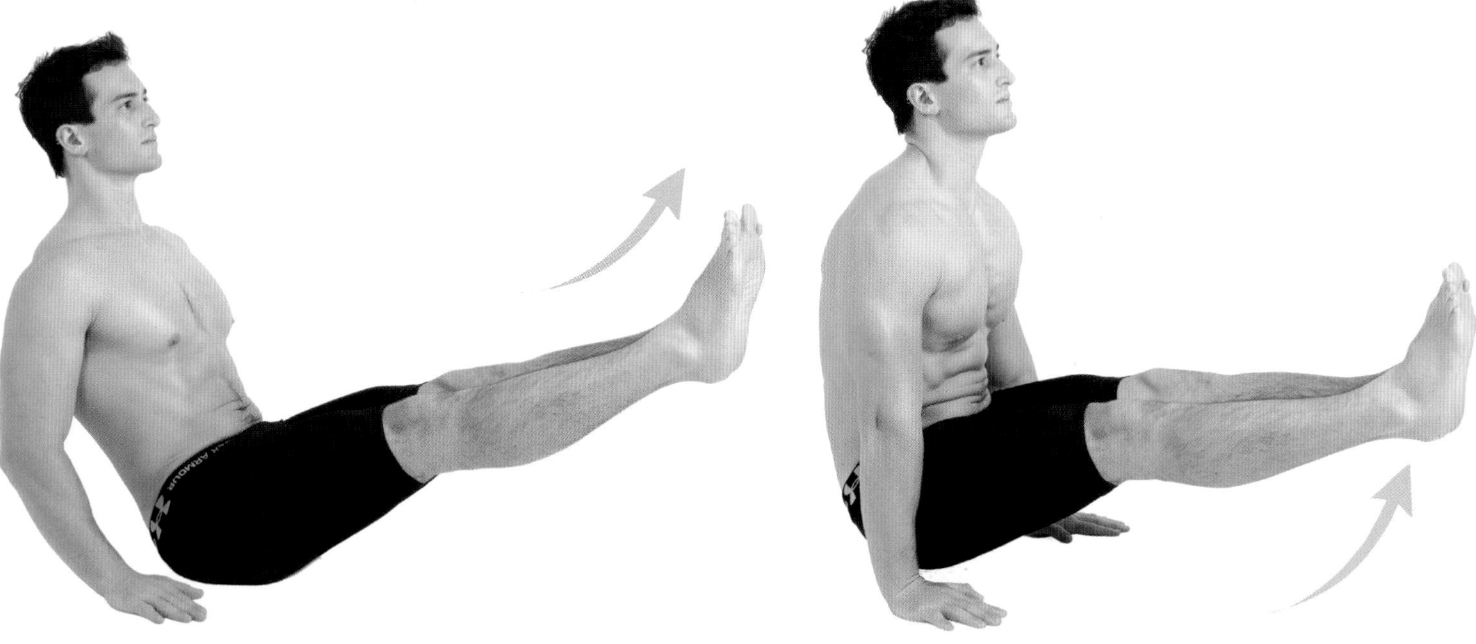

FACT FILE

SANSKRIT
- Brahmacharyasana

TARGETS
- Abdominals
- Shoulders
- Thighs

TYPE
- Dynamic

BENEFITS
- Increases core, pelvic, and shoulder stability
- Strengthens quads
- Improves balance

CAUTIONS
- Wrist pain
- Shoulder pain

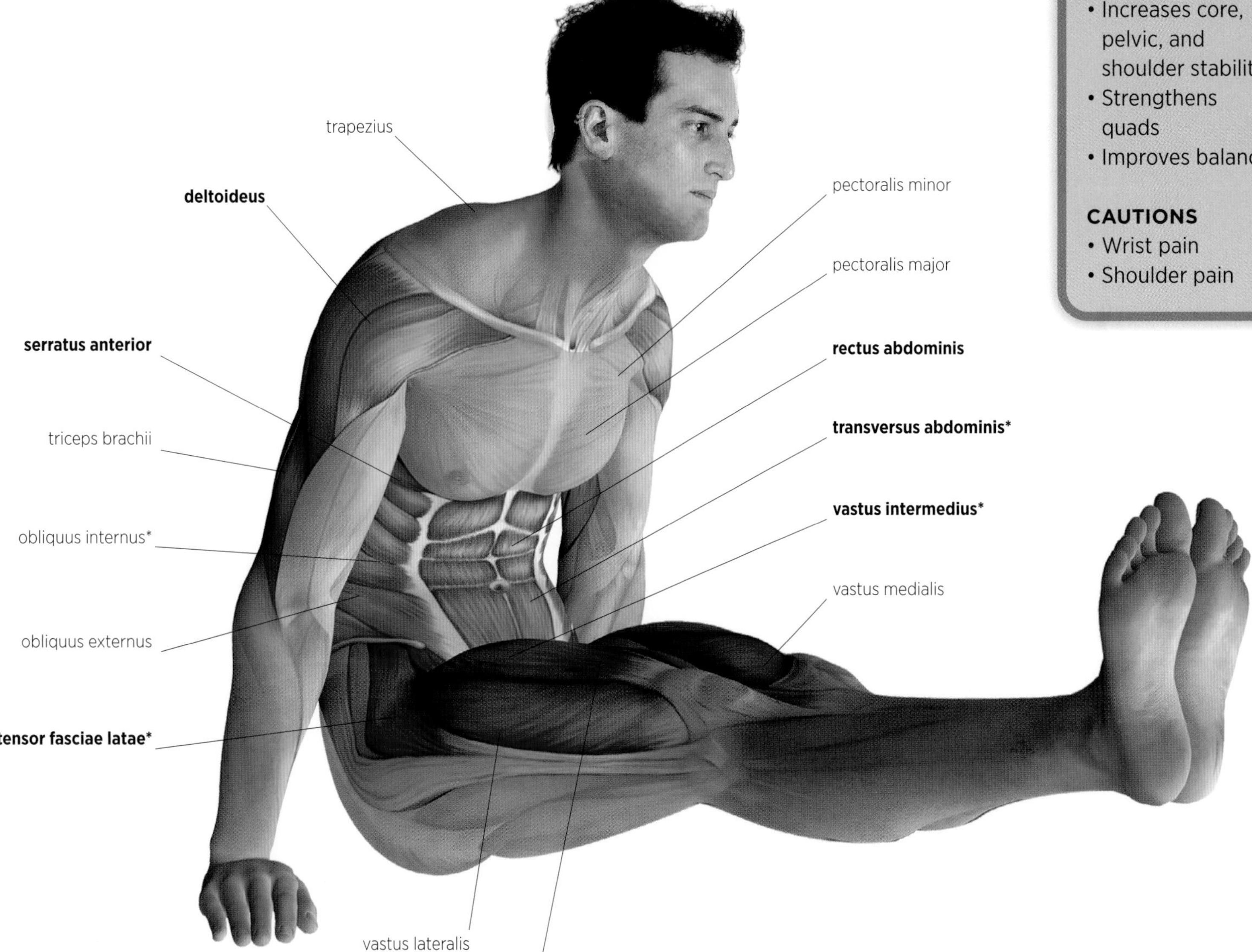

Annotation Key

Bold text indicates target muscles

Light text indicates other working muscles

* indicates deep muscles

Crow Pose

A graceful asana, Crow Pose strengthens and tones your upper body and serves as an introductory stretch to even more advanced arm balances. Crow Pose is often confused with Crane Pose (Pages 296–97). The key difference between the two is in your arms: bend your elbows to perform Crow, and keep them straight to perform Crane.

HOW TO DO IT

- Begin by squatting with your feet and knees more than hip-width apart.
- Lean your torso forward, and place your hands in front of you on the mat, facing slightly inward, fingers spread.
- Bend your elbows, and rest your knees against your upper arms.
- Lifting up on the balls of your feet and leaning forward with your torso, bring your thighs toward your chest and your shins to your upper arms. Round your back as you feel your weight transfer to your wrists. Hold for the recommended breaths.

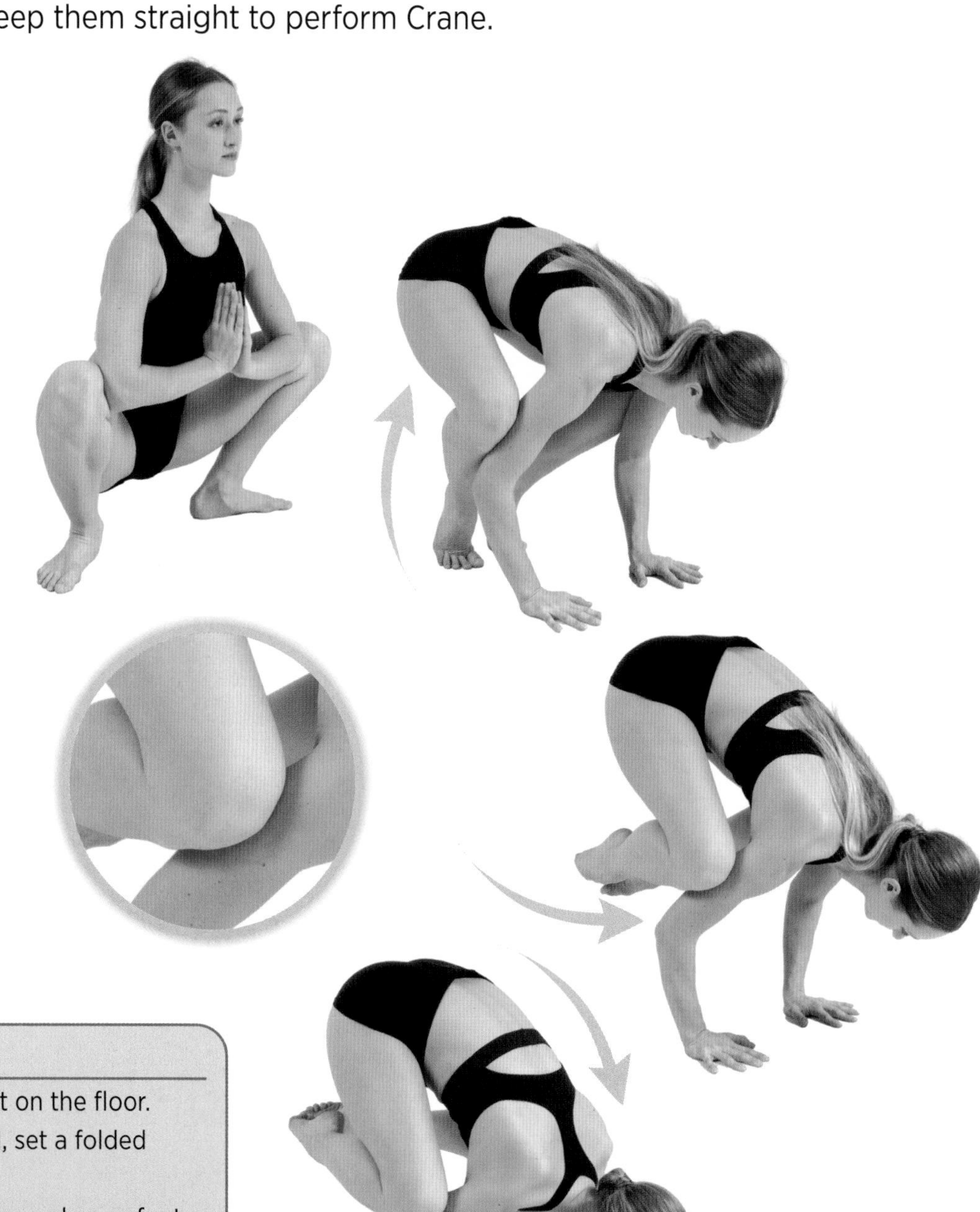

DO IT RIGHT

- To maintain balance, gaze at a spot on the floor.
- If you are afraid of tipping forward, set a folded blanket or cushion in front of you.
- Avoid "jumping" into the pose—raise only one foot at a time.
- Do not lower your head; keep it in a neutral position.

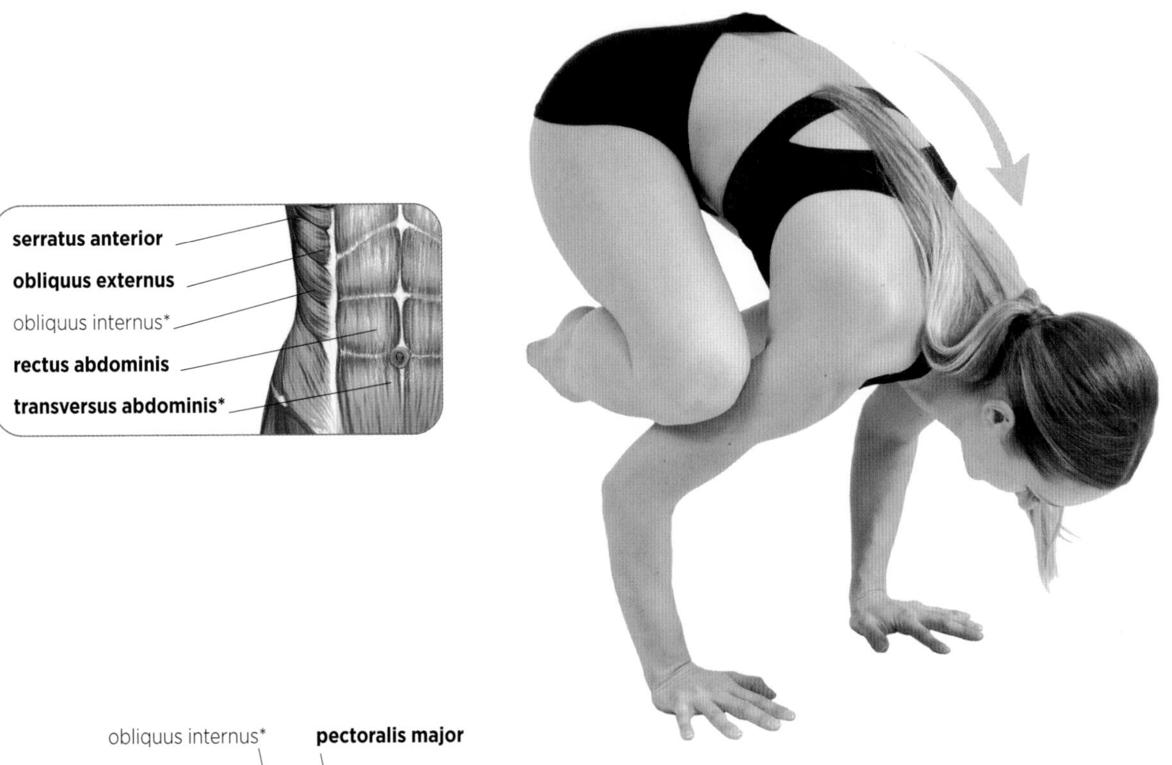

FACT FILE

SANSKRIT
- Kakasana

TARGETS
- Arms
- Shoulders
- Abdominals

TYPE
- Dynamic

BENEFITS
- Strengthens and tones arms and abdomen
- Strengthens wrists
- Improves balance

CAUTIONS
- Wrist injuries

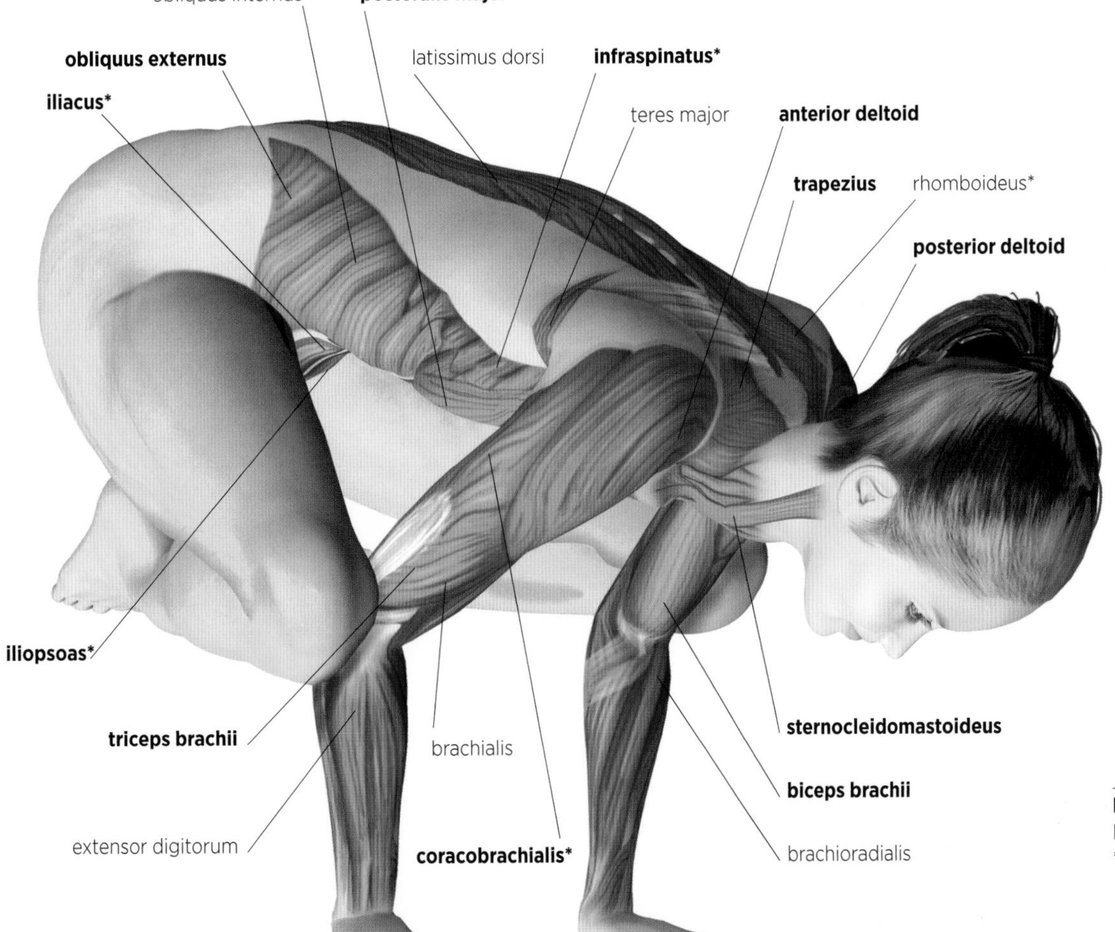

Annotation Key

Bold text indicates target muscles
Light text indicates other working muscles
* indicates deep muscles

Supported Headstand

This advanced inversion pose, often called the "king of asanas," allows you to find clarity of mind while targeting your back, shoulders, and sides. If you are new to this pose, start by performing it against a wall. Once you feel more secure, you can balance on your own.

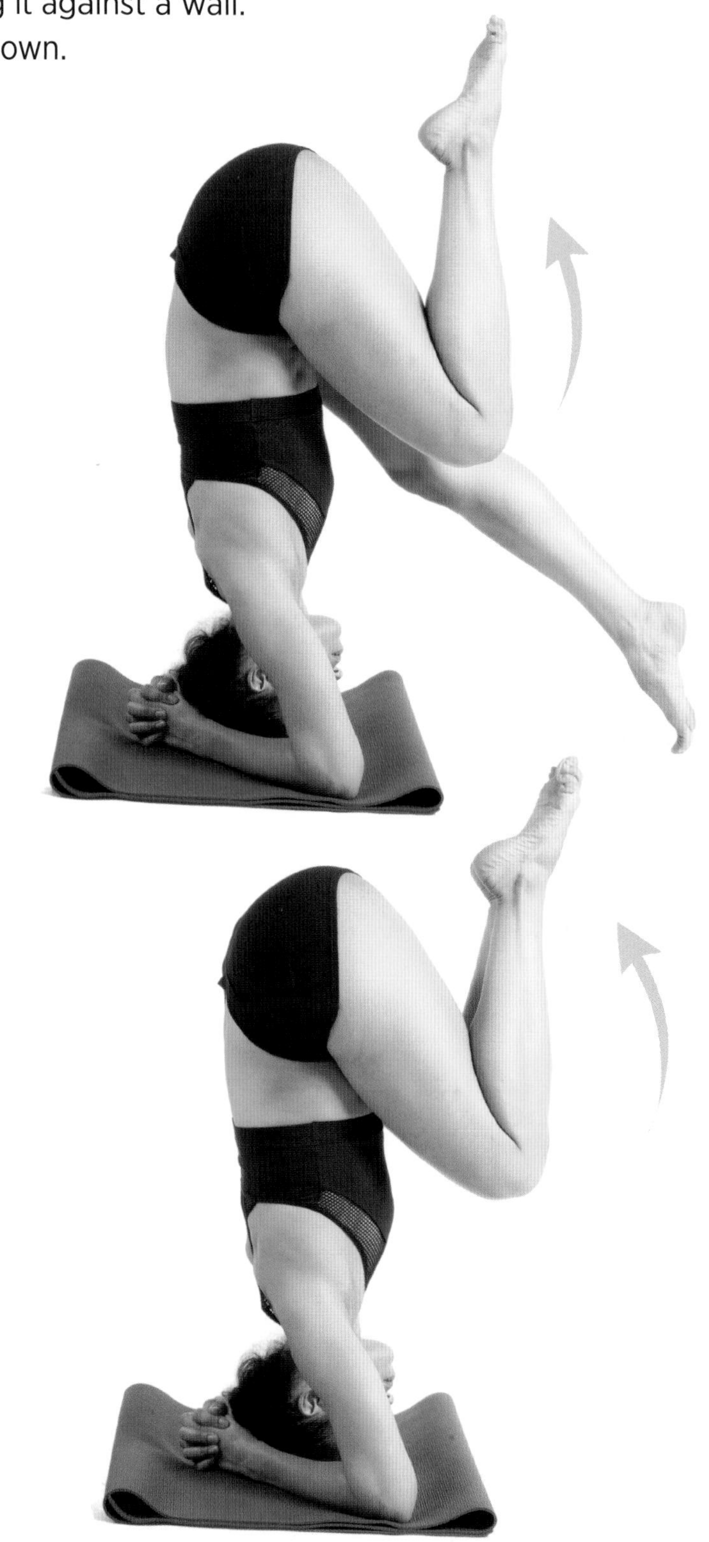

HOW TO DO IT

- Place your mat against a wall, if desired. Begin on all fours. Place your forearms on the floor, shoulder-width apart, externally rotating your outer upper arms and interlacing your fingers. Tuck your toes under and lift your hips upward. This position is called Dolphin Pose (page 94), which is great prep for Headstand.

- Maintaining your alignment, slightly release the grip of your fingers so that your palms are more open while your fingers stay interlaced. Place the top of your head on the floor and the back of your head on your hands. Find a solid foundation, with your forearms and outer wrists pressing down.

- Allowing your heels to lift off the floor, walk your feet toward your head until your hips are directly above your shoulders. At the same time, press your chest toward your thighs. This will help you lift up into the full pose and protect your neck from compression.

- Bend one knee and then the other into your chest. Begin to straighten both legs up toward the ceiling. Alternately, you can rest your feet against a wall before straightening your legs. Hold this pose for as long as you can maintain your form.

- Find a slight internal rotation in your thighs as you lengthen your tailbone up toward your heels. Reach the balls of your feet toward the ceiling to help activate the backs of your legs and your gluteal muscles.

- Hold for the recommended breaths, which should increase as you become more proficient. Release the pose by bending your knees into your chest and slowly lowering your legs to the mat.

FACT FILE

SANSKRIT
- Salamba Sirsasana

TARGETS
- Legs
- Shoulders
- Sides

TYPE
- Dynamic

BENEFITS
- Strengthens legs, arms, and spine
- Calms mind and body
- Relieves stress
- Increases circulation
- Improves digestion

CAUTIONS
- Back issues
- High blood pressure
- Neck issues
- Glaucoma

Annotation Key

Bold text indicates target muscles

Light text indicates other working muscles

* indicates deep muscles

DO IT RIGHT
- Press your forearms firmly and evenly into the mat.
- Avoid placing your forehead on the floor, because this can cause compression in your neck.

gluteus medius*

transversus abdominis*

latissimus dorsi

rectus abdominis

infraspinatus

trapezius

medial deltoid

triceps brachii

Wheel Pose

The invigorating and energizing Wheel Pose is a deep, challenging backbend that strengthens the entire body, and stretches the chest and rib cage. It is excellent for the heart, liver, and kidneys, and can be beneficial to those who suffer from asthma and osteoporosis.

HOW TO DO IT

- Begin by lying on your back, with your knees bent and your feet hip-width apart. Inhale and stretch your arms straight up to the ceiling, with your palms facing away from you. Then, bend your arms and place your hands on the floor next to your ears, shoulder-width apart, with your fingers facing the same direction as your toes.

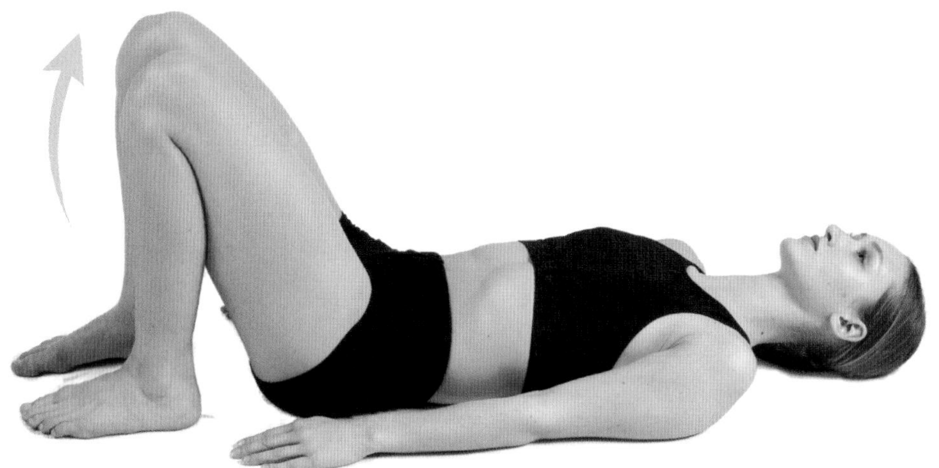

- Press your hands and feet into the floor as you lift your hips up, as if you were coming into Bridge Pose (pages 256–57).

- Lift yourself onto the crown of your head. Pause and press your palms into the floor, spreading your fingers wide and grounding down through every knuckle and through the base of your thumb and index finger.

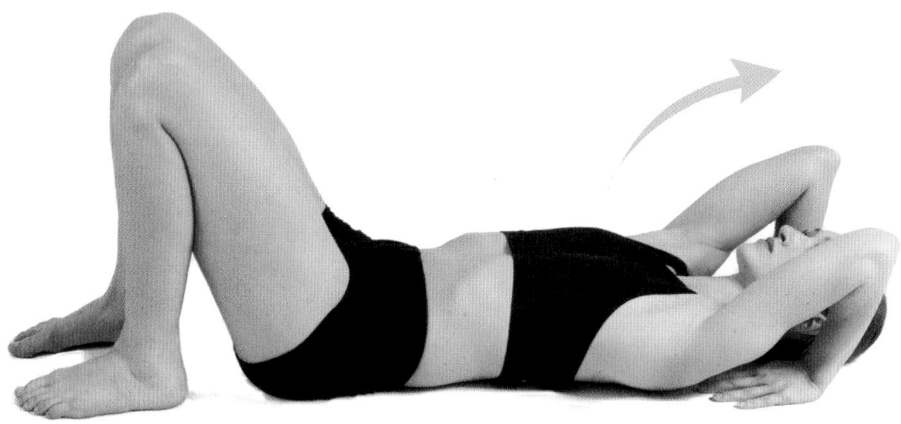

- Straighten your arms, and move your outer upper arms inward to find external rotation. Press down through all four corners of your feet, shifting your weight onto your heels. Roll your inner thighs toward the floor as you firm your outer hips inward. Let your head fall between your shoulders in a comfortable position. Hold for the recommended breaths.

- To come out of the pose, bend your arms and shift your body weight toward your shoulders as you slowly descend, landing on the back of your head and your shoulder blades.

DO IT RIGHT

- Keep your feet parallel, even as you transition into and out of the pose.
- After lifting yourself onto the crown of your head, squeeze your elbows toward each other to keep them positioned over your wrists.
- While holding the pose, draw your tailbone down toward your knees and lift your frontal hip bones up toward your ribs.
- Avoid letting your thighs externally rotate, which can cause compression in your lower back.

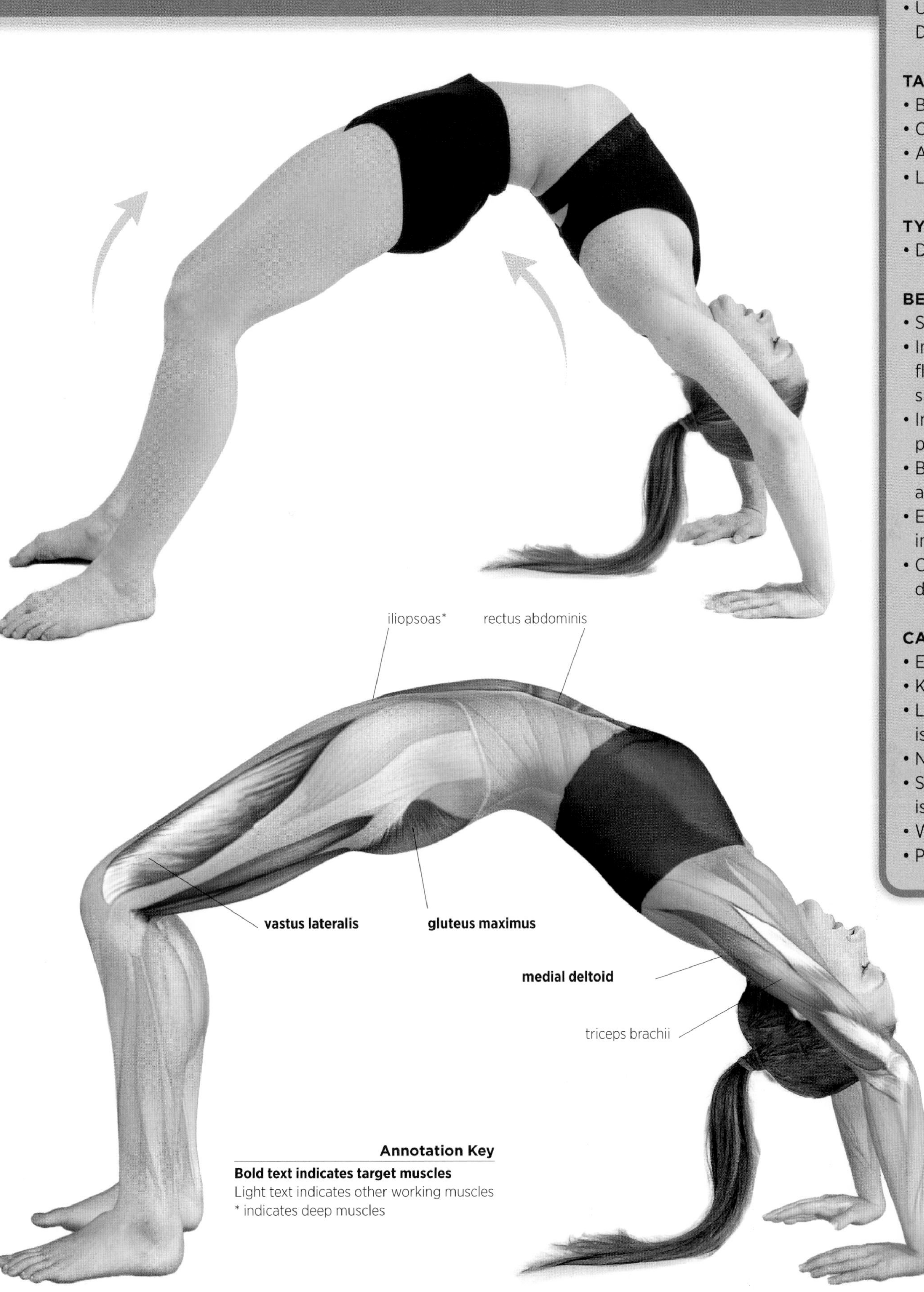

Annotation Key

Bold text indicates target muscles
Light text indicates other working muscles
* indicates deep muscles

FACT FILE

SANSKRIT
- Urdhva Dhanurasana

TARGETS
- Back
- Chest
- Arms
- Legs

TYPE
- Dynamic

BENEFITS
- Stretches chest
- Increases flexibility in spine
- Improves posture
- Builds stamina and strength
- Energizes and invigorates
- Counteracts depression

CAUTIONS
- Elbow issues
- Knee issues
- Lower-back issues
- Neck issues
- Sacroiliac joint issues
- Wrist issues
- Pregnancy

Half Moon Pose

Open your hips and hone your balance and coordination with Half Moon Pose. This posture will also strengthen your entire core.

HOW TO DO IT

- Stand with your left palm or fingertips resting on your shin or on the floor. Gaze down toward your left foot, and bring your right hand onto your hip.
- Bend your left knee slightly, keeping it extended over your middle toe. At the same time, shift more weight onto your left leg, and step your right foot in about 12 inches.
- Straighten your left leg, opening the thigh while lifting your right leg to hip height. Keep your right leg in a neutral position, and flex your ankle.
- Once you have found your balance, extend your right arm straight up toward the ceiling, opening up across the front of your chest.
- Hold for the recommended breaths, and then repeat on the other side.

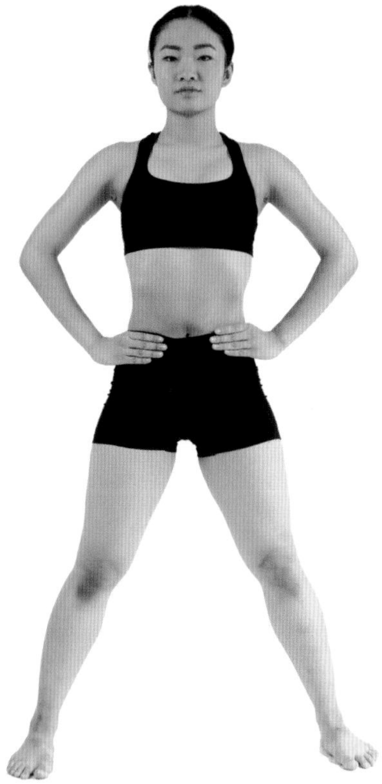

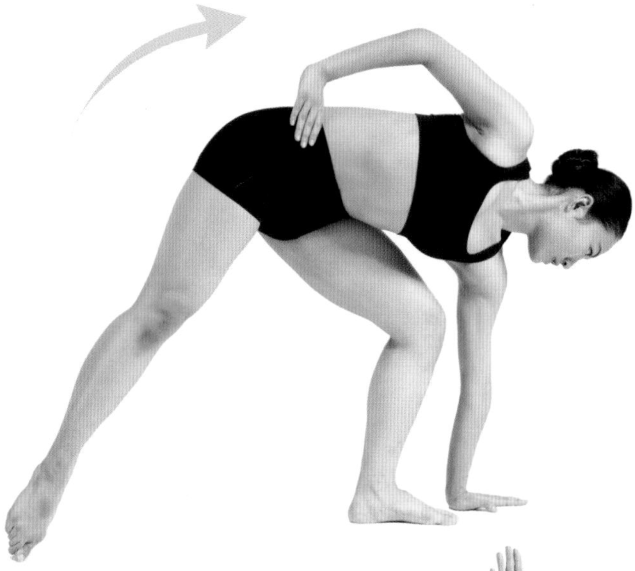

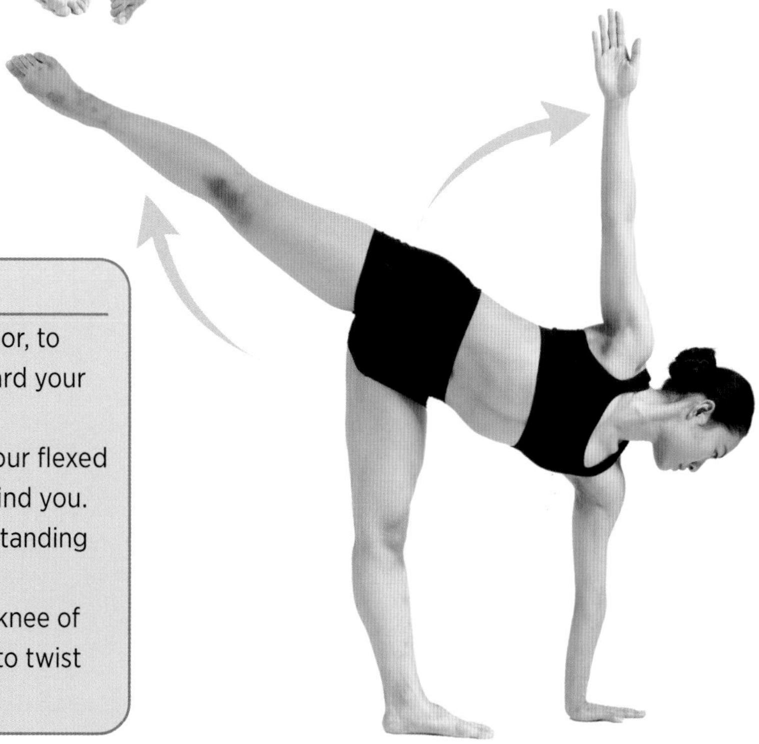

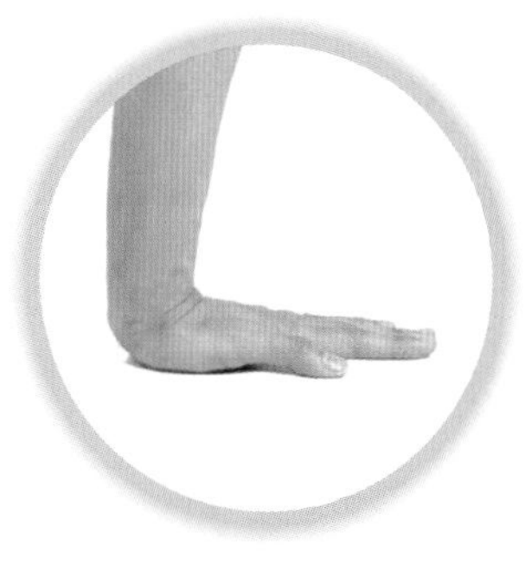

DO IT RIGHT

- Gaze toward the floor, to the side, or up toward your raised hand.
- Imagine pressing your flexed foot into a wall behind you.
- Avoid letting your standing foot turn in.
- Avoid allowing the knee of your standing foot to twist out of alignment.

FACT FILE

SANSKRIT
- Ardha Chandrasana

TARGET
- Spine
- Hip adductors
- Hamstrings
- Rib cage
- Chest
- Shoulders

TYPE
- Dynamic

BENEFITS
- Stretches hip, groin, torso, arms, and spine
- Strengthens thighs and ankles
- Stimulates digestion and elimination
- Improves balance

CAUTIONS
- Knee issues
- Shoulder issues
- Diarrhea
- Headache
- High or low blood pressure
- Neck issues

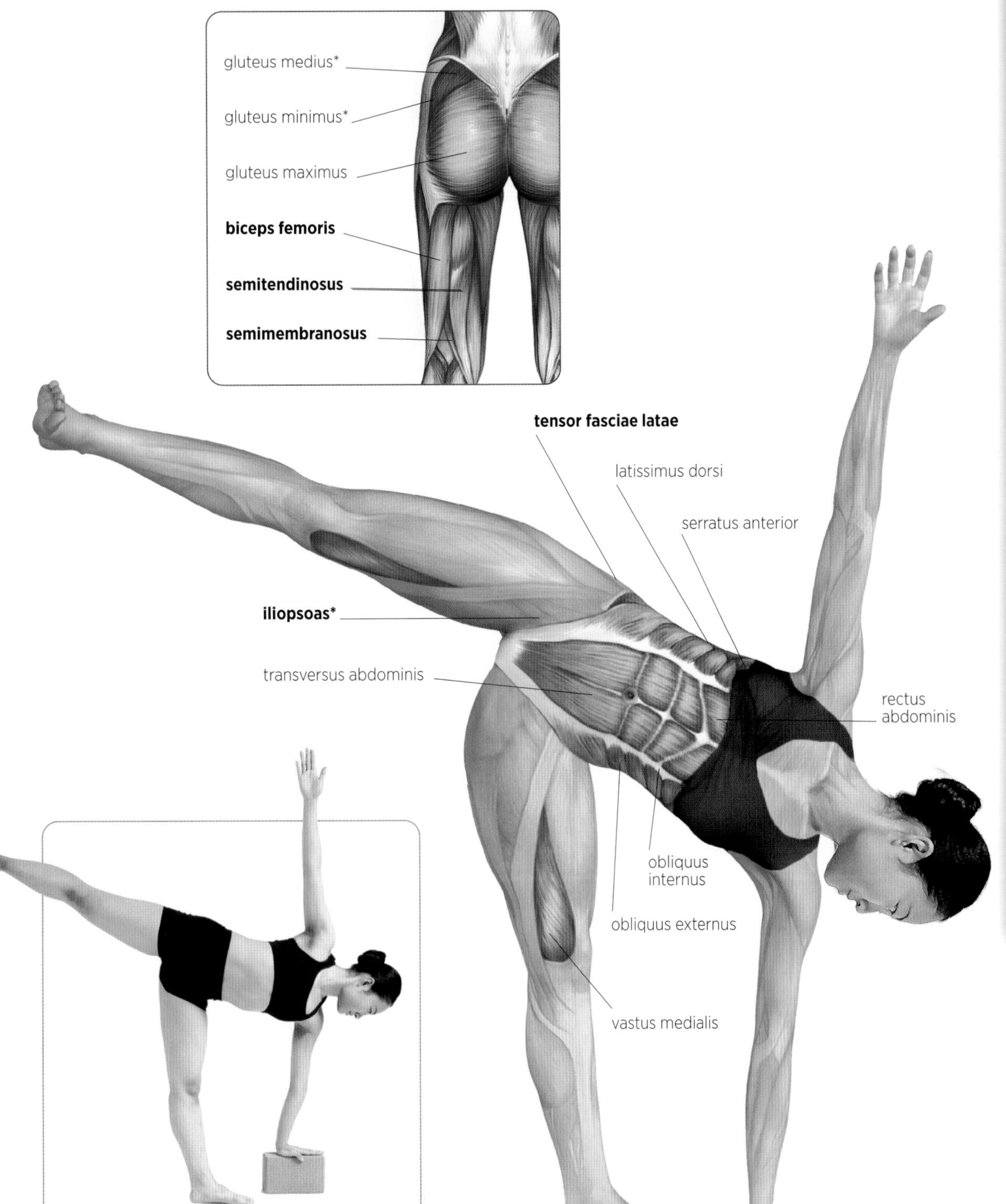

MODIFICATION

EASIER: Rest your hand on a block if it is challenging for you to straighten your standing leg. If needed, increase the height of the block by resting it on its side.

Annotation Key
Bold text indicates target muscles
Light text indicates other working muscles
* indicates deep muscles

Side Angle Pose

Mastering Side Angle Pose is the first step in achieving the strength and flexibility necessary to move on to the more difficult standing postures. On its own, it's a great side stretch and core strengthener.

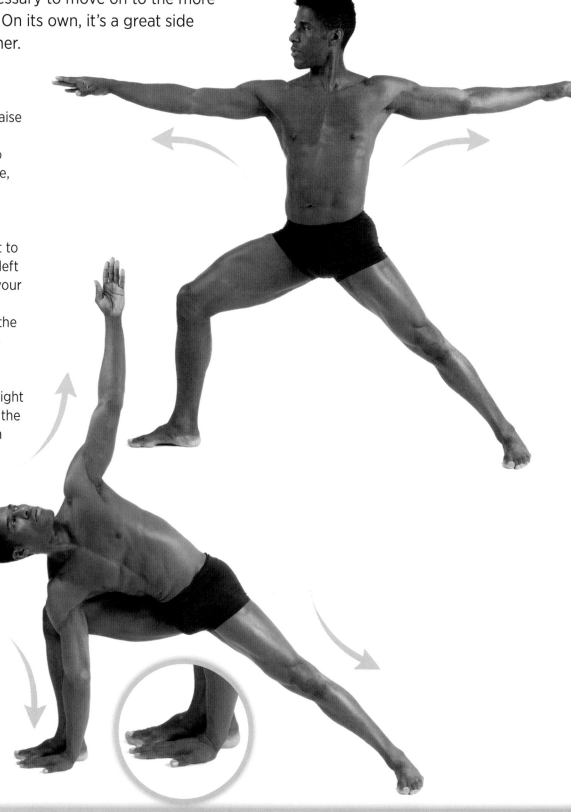

HOW TO DO IT

- Leading with your right foot, raise your arms parallel to the floor and reach them actively out to the sides, shoulder blades wide, palms down.
- Turn your right foot slightly to the right and your left foot out to the left 90 degrees. Align the left heel with the right heel. Firm your thighs and turn your left thigh outward so that the center of the left knee cap is in line with the center of the left ankle.
- Bend your torso toward your right knee, reaching your fingers to the floor as you raise your left arm straight toward the ceiling.
- Hold for the recommended breaths, and then repeat on the other side.

FACT FILE

SANSKRIT
- Parsvakonasana

TARGETS
- Core
- Hips

TYPE
- Dynamic

BENEFITS
- Strengthens core
- Opens hips
- Stretches leg from hip to ankle
- Stretches shoulders, chest, and spine
- Relieves the symptoms of menopause

CAUTIONS
- High or low blood pressure
- Neck issues

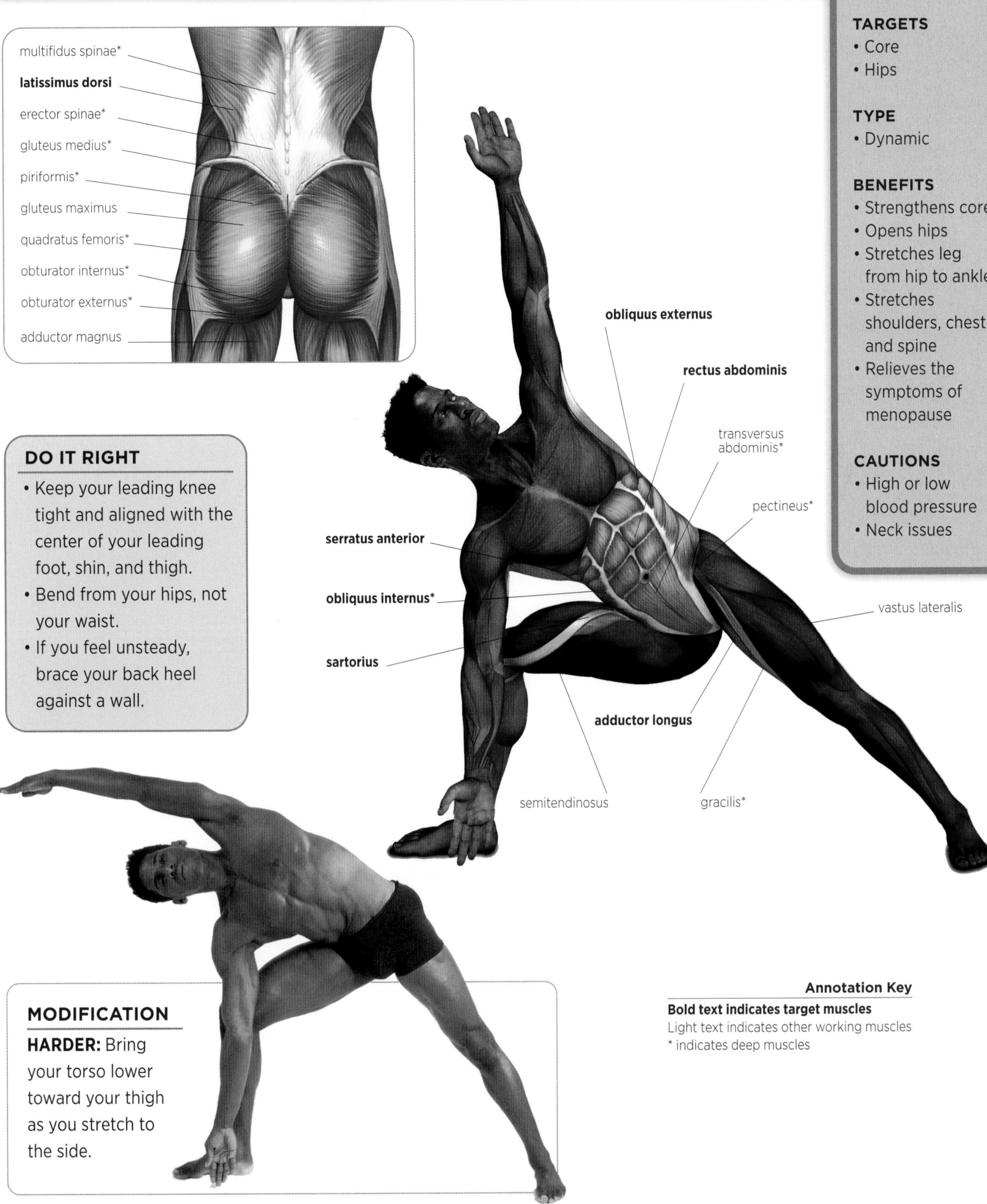

DO IT RIGHT

- Keep your leading knee tight and aligned with the center of your leading foot, shin, and thigh.
- Bend from your hips, not your waist.
- If you feel unsteady, brace your back heel against a wall.

MODIFICATION

HARDER: Bring your torso lower toward your thigh as you stretch to the side.

Annotation Key
Bold text indicates target muscles
Light text indicates other working muscles
* indicates deep muscles

Crossed-Foot Forward Bend

This Crossed-Foot Forward Bend improves flexibility and loosens tight leg muscles and glutes. The foot position also engages your iliotibial band, the fibrous tissue that runs along your outer thigh and stabilizes your hip and knee joints.

HOW TO DO IT

- Stand with your arms relaxed at your sides. Cross one foot over the other so that the outer edges of your soles are aligned.

- Bend at your waist, and gradually reach toward the floor with your hands.

- Press your palms to the floor, and hold for the recommended breaths. Release, slowly roll up, and repeat on the other side.

DO IT RIGHT

- Keep your knees straight, yet soft, throughout the exercise.
- Let your head drop.
- Avoid bending or locking your knees.
- Avoid twisting your neck, shoulders, or torso to either side.

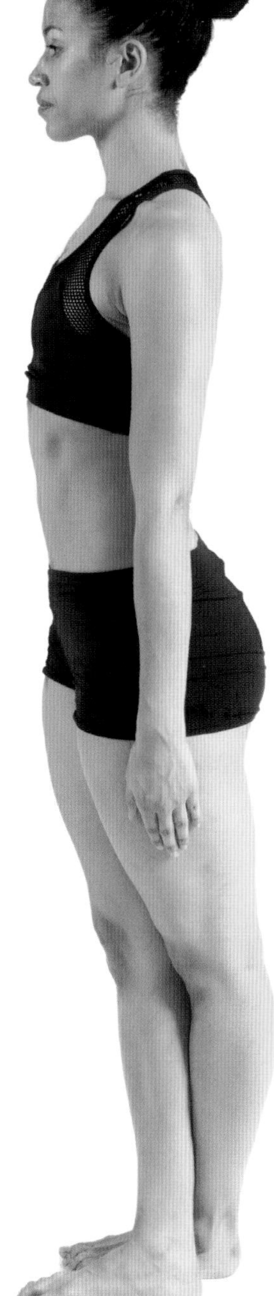

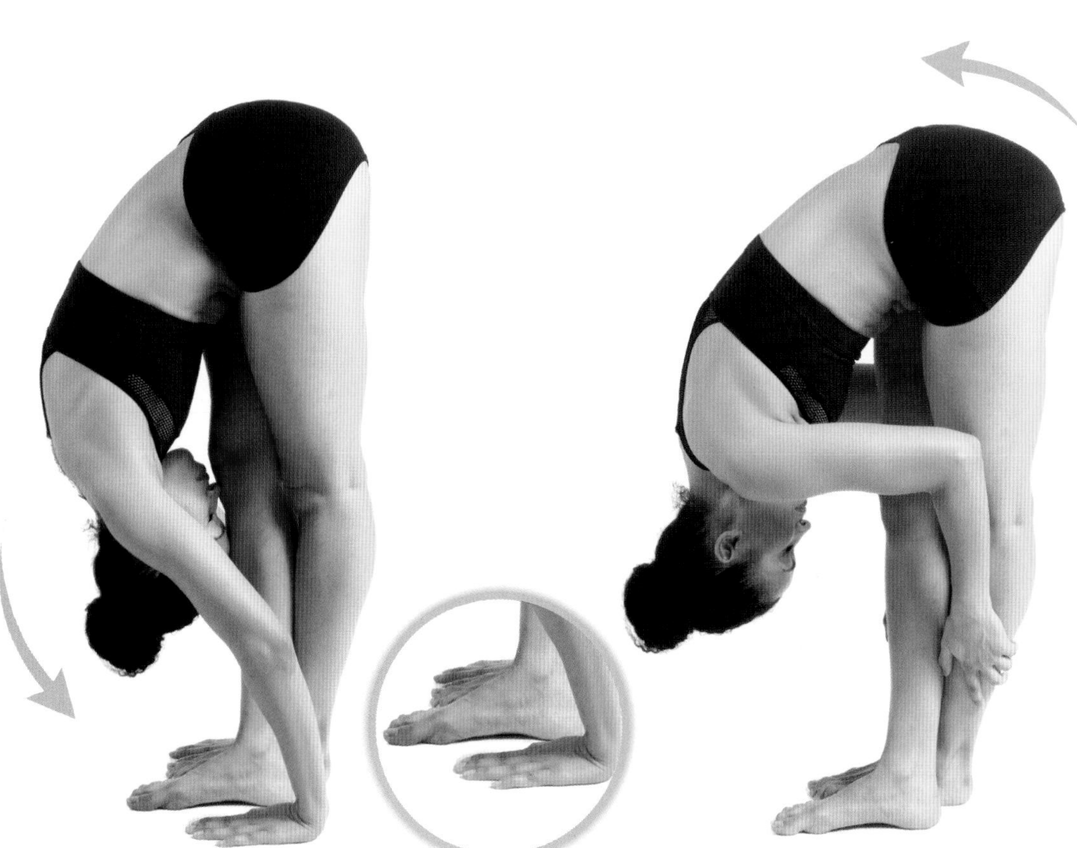

FACT FILE

SANSKRIT
- None

TARGETS
- Hamstrings
- Upper back
- Lower back
- Calves
- Iliotibial band

TYPE
- Static

BENEFITS
- Stretches iliotibial band
- Counteracts effects of wearing high heels

CAUTIONS
- Hip injury

MODIFICATION

EASIER: If you find it difficult to reach your hands to the floor while maintaining your form, reach only to the point where you are comfortable. Try to extend your hands slightly lower each time you stretch.

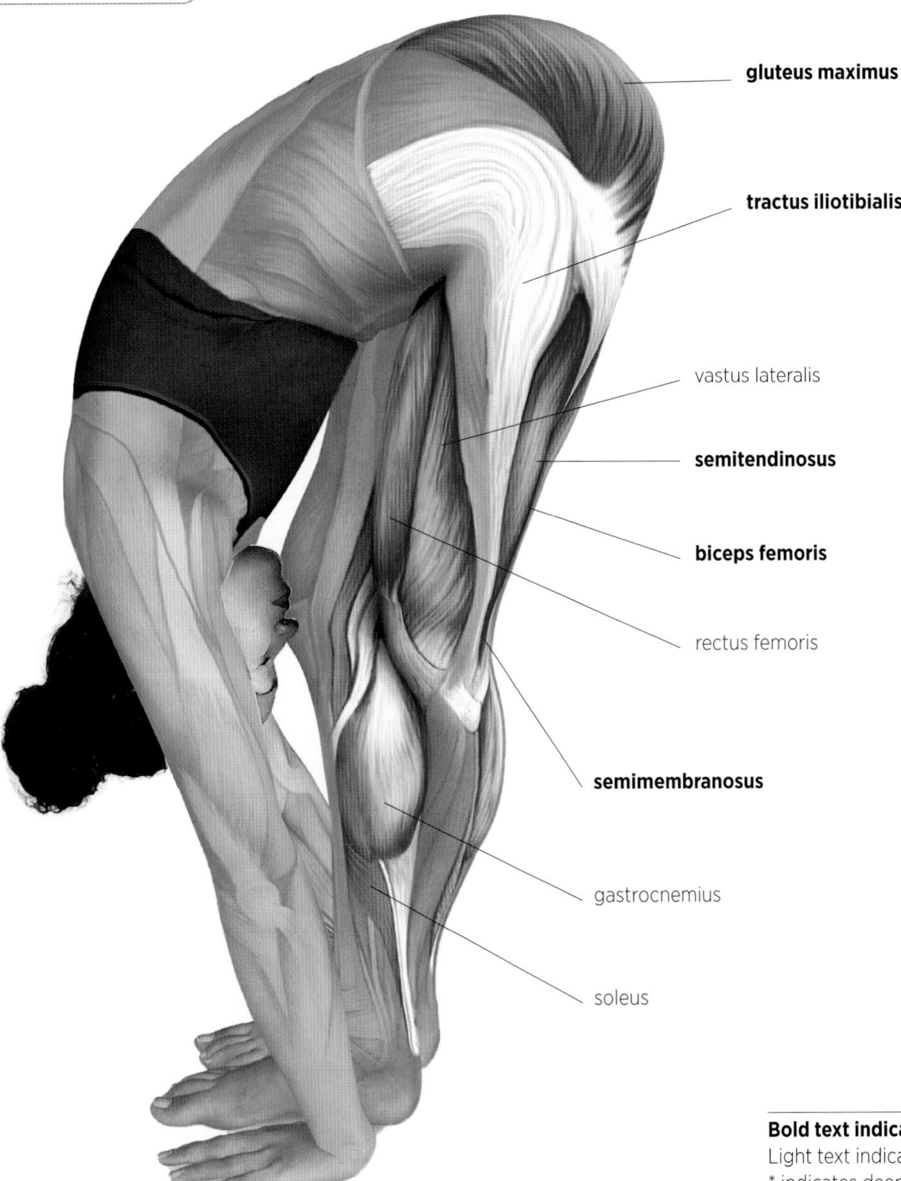

Annotation Key
Bold text indicates target muscles
Light text indicates other working muscles
* indicates deep muscles

Wide-Legged Forward Bend

Wide-Legged Forward Bend is one of the most effective ways to stretch your hamstrings and spine. Dancers frequently use it to relieve stress before a performance. This forward bend is also technically an inversion pose because your head is positioned below your heart.

HOW TO DO IT

- Stand with your legs and feet parallel and generously more than shoulder-width apart. Bend your knees slightly, and tuck your pelvis forward. Press your shoulder blades together and downward.

- Inhale and lengthen your spine. Lift your chest, and find a slight bend in your upper back, bringing your gaze up to the ceiling.

- Exhale and hinge forward from your hips with your back flat. Reach your palms to the floor, with your fingers facing forward. Bring the crown of your head toward the floor, lifting your shoulders toward your ears to make space for your neck.

- Firm your thighs, and lift your kneecaps. Let your sit bones move toward the ceiling as your tailbone draws down toward the floor.

- Hold for the recommended breaths.

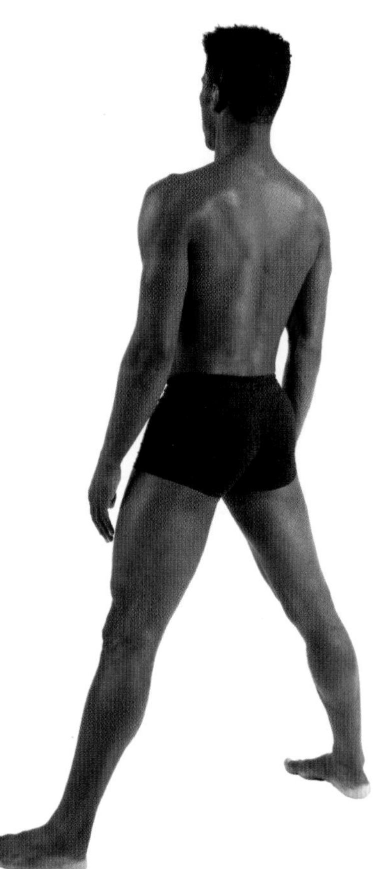

DO IT RIGHT

- Keep your knees soft.
- Hinge forward with your chest open and your back flat.
- Bend only as far forward as you can go while keeping your back flat.
- Keep your hips lined up above your heels.
- Avoid rounding your back to cheat your hands to the floor.
- Avoid locking your knees.

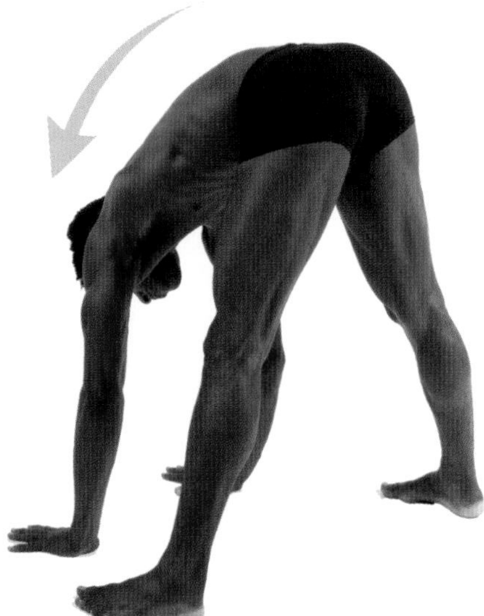

MODIFICATION

EASIER: If you find it difficult to reach the floor with your hands, place some blocks on the floor and reach for them instead.

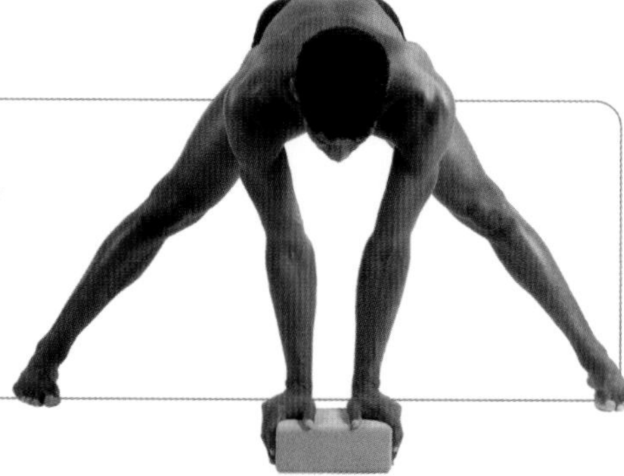

FACT FILE

SANSKRIT
- Prasarita Padottanasana

TARGETS
- Hamstrings
- Lower back
- Glutes
- Calves

TYPE
- Static

BENEFITS
- Strengthens spine
- Stretches inner and outer hips
- Releases groin
- Calms mind and body

CAUTIONS
- Back issues
- Hamstring issues

MODIFICATION

ADVANCED: Walk your hands in between your legs, bend your elbows, and gently rest your forehead on the floor. Your hands should be available, if necessary, to keep your balance.

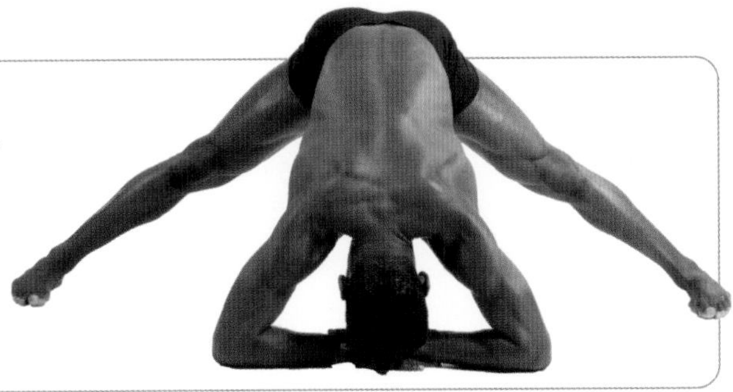

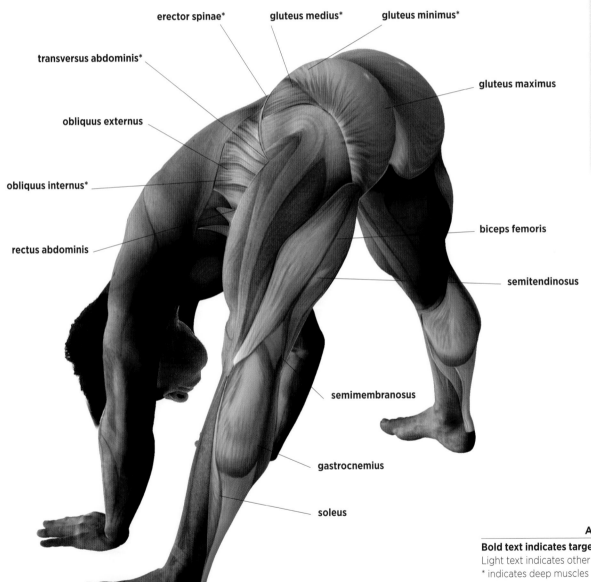

Annotation Key
Bold text indicates target muscles
Light text indicates other working muscles
* indicates deep muscles

One-Legged Bridge

This Bridge Pose stretches your chest, spine, and thighs while strengthening your core and buttocks. It also eases stress by relieving tension in your back and shoulders.

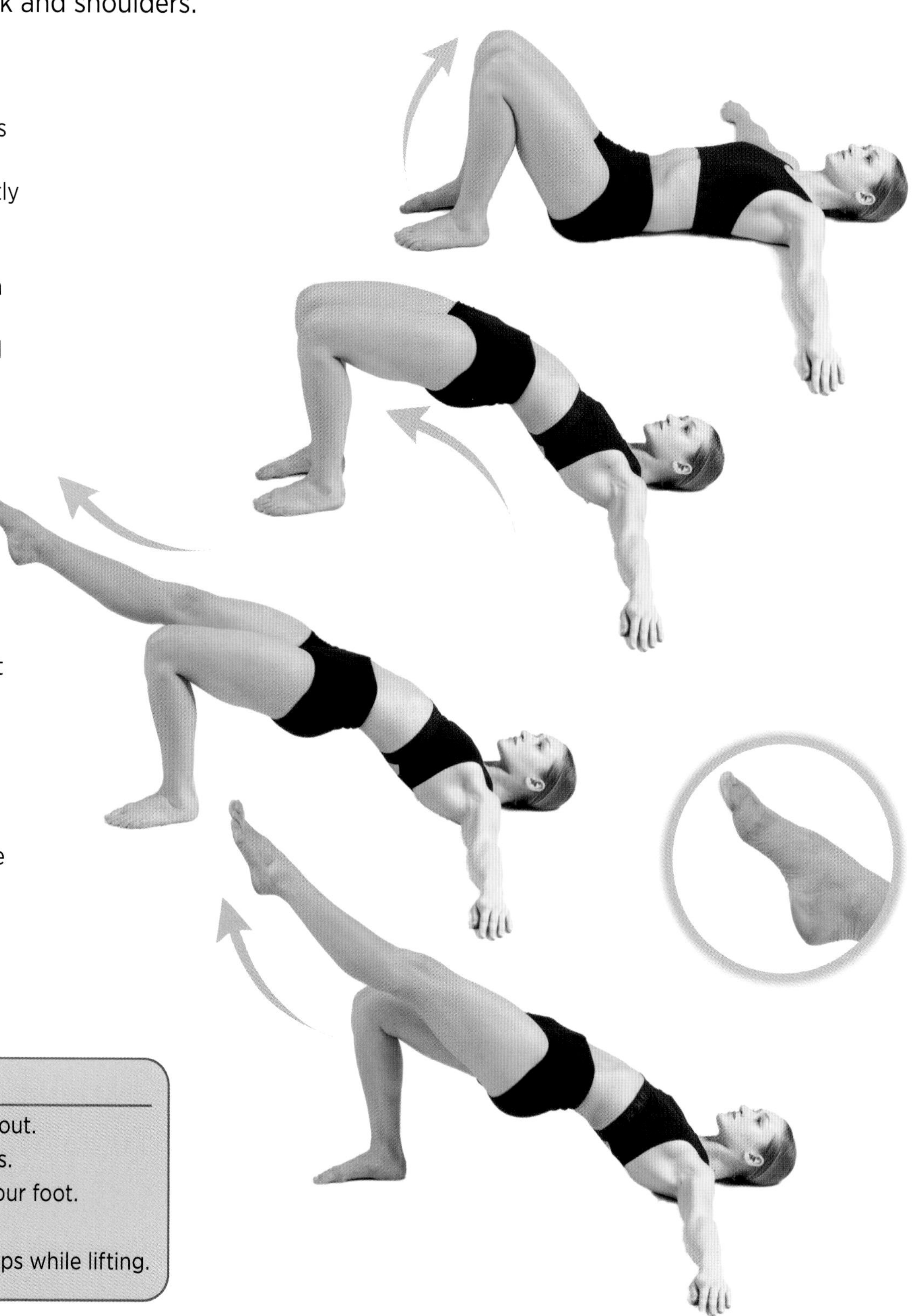

HOW TO DO IT

- Lie on your back with your arms out to your sides. Bend your knees and align your feet directly under your knees.
- Exhale and press down through your feet to lift your buttocks off the floor. With your feet and thighs parallel, push your arms into the floor while extending through your fingertips.
- Lengthen your neck away from your shoulders. Lift your hips higher so that your torso rises from the floor.
- Straighten your right leg so that it is fully extended, forming a straight line from hip to toe.
- Hold for the recommended breaths, return to the starting position, and then repeat on the opposite side.

DO IT RIGHT

- Engage your buttocks throughout.
- Keep your hips level at all times.
- Extend your leg out through your foot.
- Avoid arching your back.
- Avoid twisting or tilting your hips while lifting.

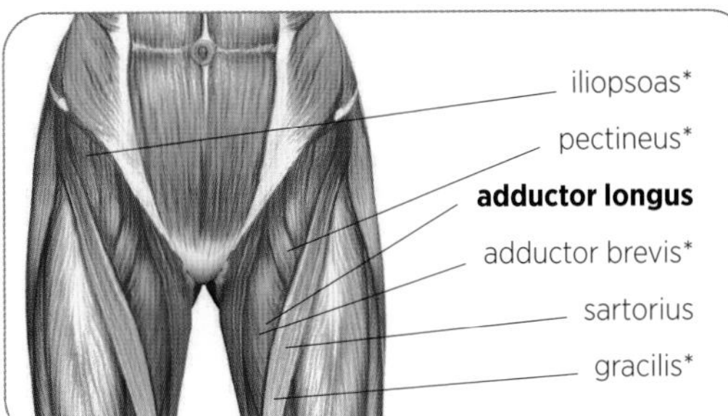

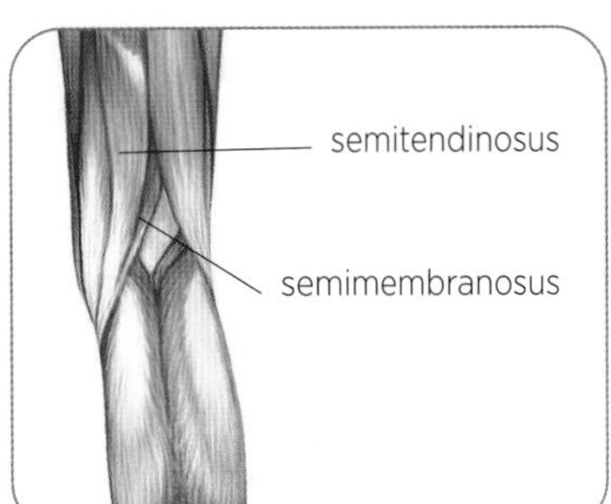

MODIFICATION

HARDER: Follow the first four steps and then draw your hands together above your chest, keeping your elbows straight. Hold for the recommended breaths, and then repeat on the opposite side.

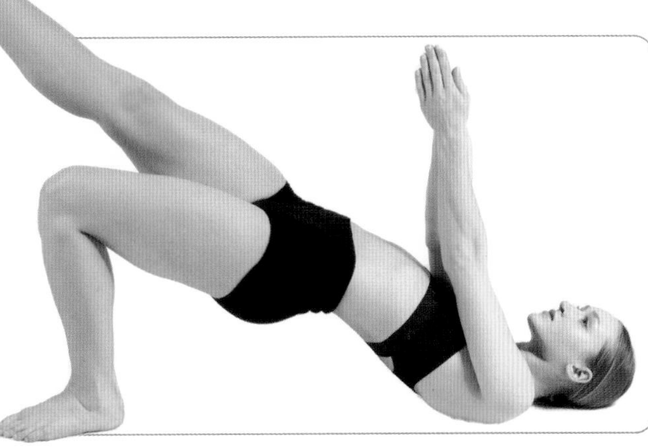

Annotation Key

Bold text indicates target muscles
Light text indicates other working muscles
* indicates deep muscles

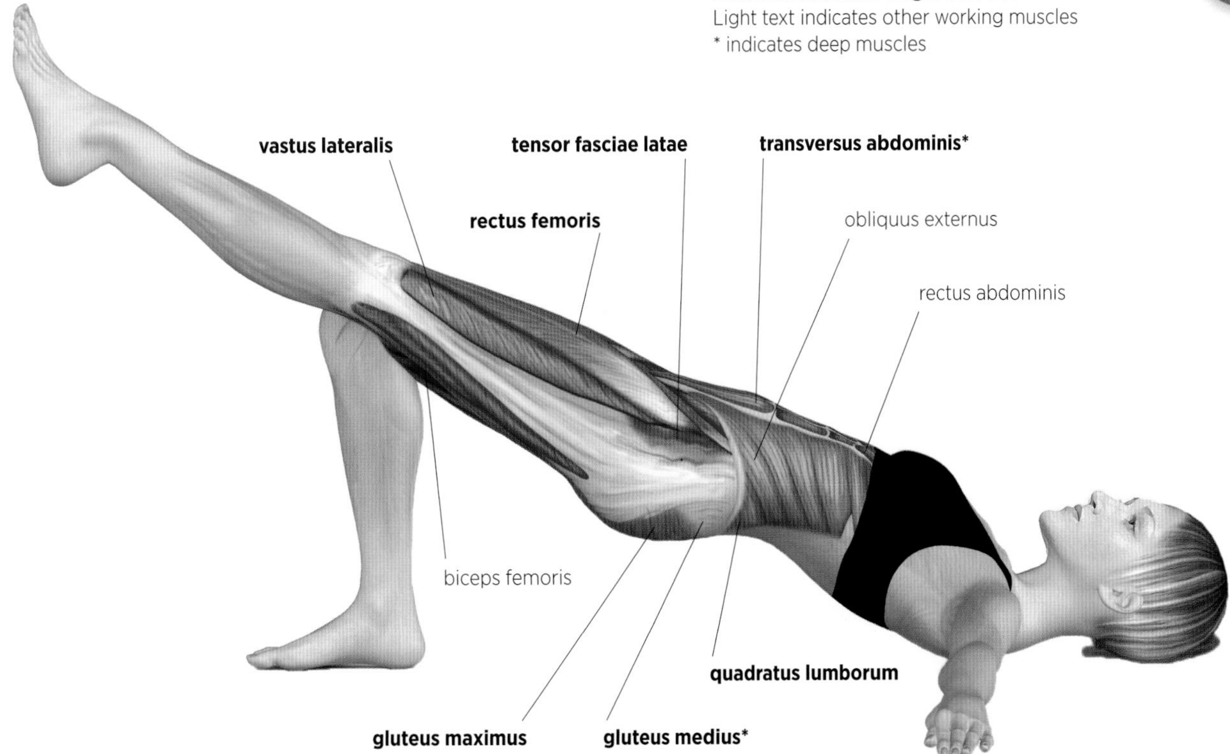

FACT FILE

SANSKRIT
- Setu Bandha Sarvangasana

TARGETS
- Spine
- Abdominals
- Thighs
- Glutes

TYPE
- Static

BENEFITS
- Stretches chest and spine
- Strengthens thighs and buttocks
- Stimulates digestion
- Stimulates thyroid
- Reduces stress

CAUTIONS
- Shoulder issues
- Back issues
- Neck issues
- Lower-back issues

Lord of the Dance Pose

The Sanskrit name of this pose, Natarajasana, refers to the Hindu god Shiva, who is known as the Lord of the Dance. This pose requires a strong sense of balance and is very effective at opening your hips and shoulders.

HOW TO DO IT

- Begin standing in Mountain Pose (pages 74–75). Bend your right knee, and draw your right heel toward your buttocks. Contract the muscles of your left thigh. Keep both hips open.
- Turn your right palm outward, reach behind your back, and grasp the inside of your right foot. Lift through your spine, from your tailbone to the top of your neck.
- Raise your right foot toward the ceiling, and push back against your right hand. At the same time, lift your left arm up toward the ceiling, and bring your left thumb and index finger together in Gyan Mudra, a gesture of unity.
- Lift your chest and arm to help you stand upright and increase your flexibility, rather than tilting your torso forward as you raise your back leg.
- Hold for the recommended breaths. Release your foot, and repeat on the opposite side.

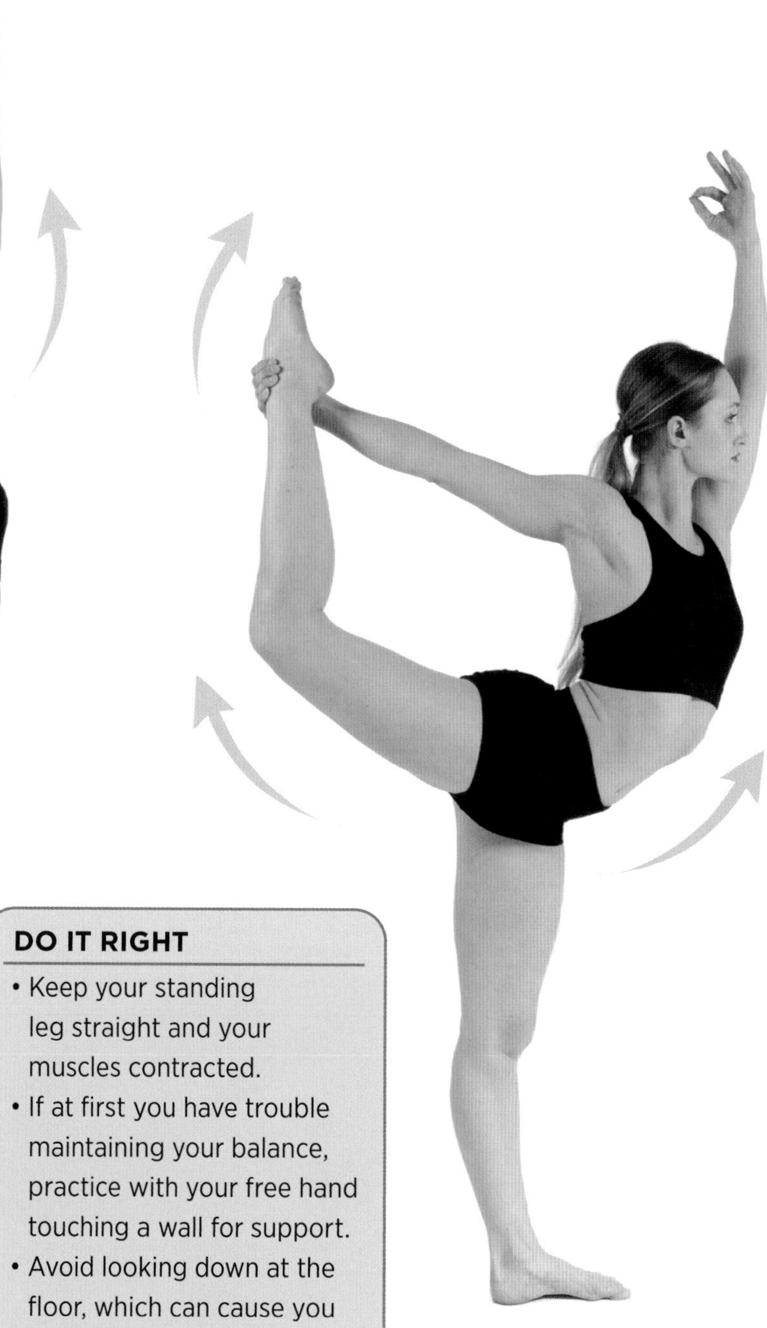

DO IT RIGHT

- Keep your standing leg straight and your muscles contracted.
- If at first you have trouble maintaining your balance, practice with your free hand touching a wall for support.
- Avoid looking down at the floor, which can cause you to lose your balance.
- Avoid compressing your lower back.

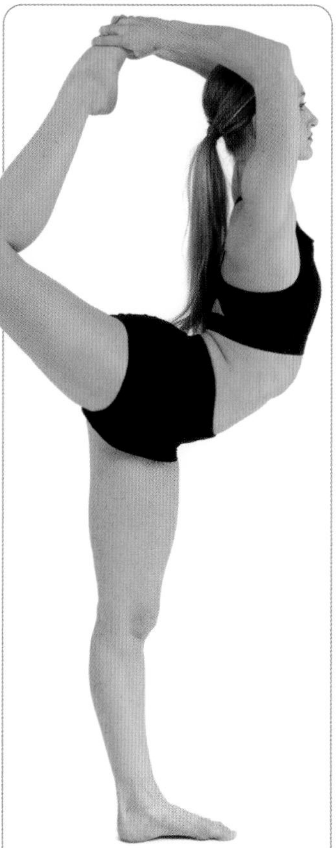

MODIFICATION

HARDER: Follow the first step. Turn your right palm outward, but instead of grasping the inside of your right foot, reach for the outside of your foot. Rotate your shoulder so that your right elbow points up toward the ceiling. Lift your leg and open your chest. Reach over your head with your left arm, bending your elbow, and grasp the top of your raised foot. Slowly walk your fingers back until both hands are holding your toes.

Annotation Key
Bold text indicates target muscles
Light text indicates other working muscles
* indicates deep muscles

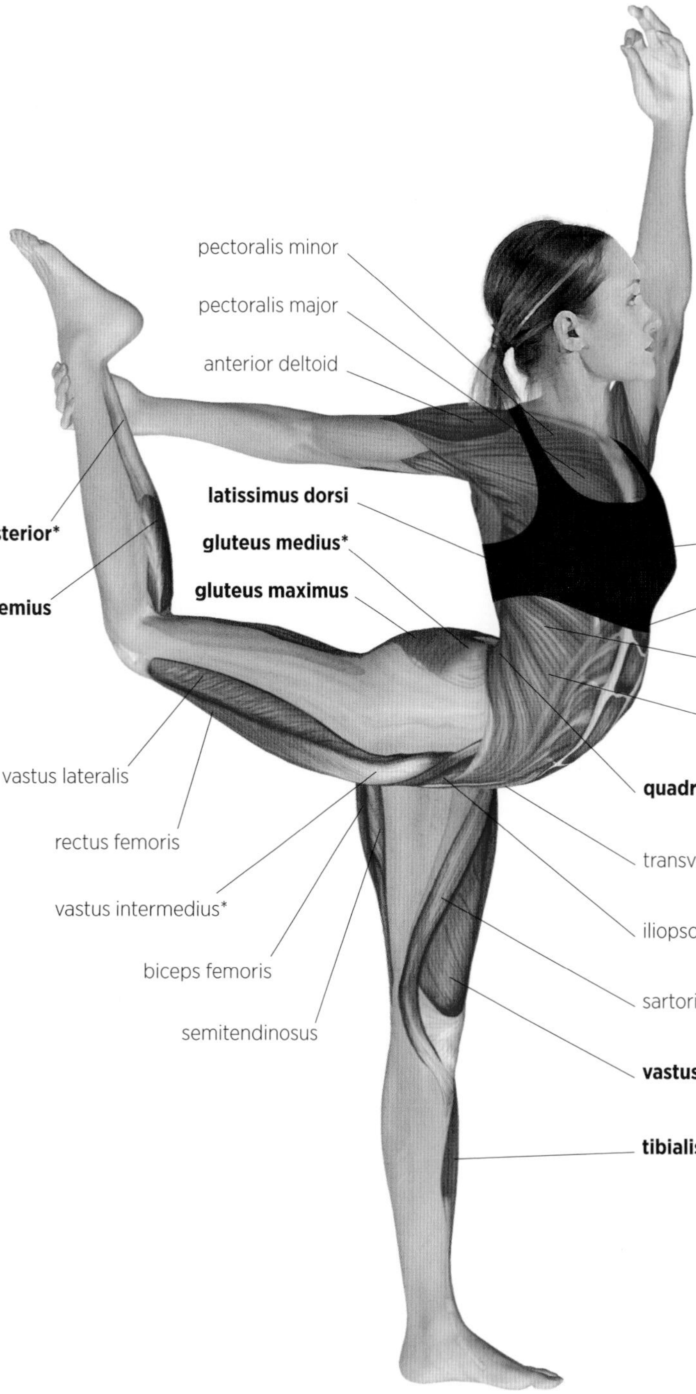

pectoralis minor
pectoralis major
anterior deltoid
latissimus dorsi
gluteus medius*
gluteus maximus
tibialis posterior*
gastrocnemius
vastus lateralis
rectus femoris
vastus intermedius*
biceps femoris
semitendinosus
serratus anterior
rectus abdominis
obliquus externus
obliquus internus*
quadratus lumborum
transversus abdominis*
iliopsoas*
sartorius
vastus medialis
tibialis anterior

FACT FILE

SANSKRIT
- Natarajasana

TARGETS
- Thighs
- Groin
- Chest
- Shoulders

TYPE
- Static

BENEFITS
- Stretches thighs, groin, abdomen, shoulders, and chest
- Strengthens spine, thighs, hips, and ankles
- Improves balance

CAUTIONS
- Back injury
- Low blood pressure

CHAPTER THREE

CARDIO EXERCISES

Aerobic exercise is essential for good health; it gets your heart rate up, making your blood pump faster, and in doing so delivers more oxygen throughout your body, which in turn keeps your heart and lungs healthy; in fact, cardiovascular exercise plays a vital role in how effective our workout routines are. Regular cardio exercise can also help you lose weight, get better sleep, and decrease the risk of chronic disease. And if you can't get outside for a daily jog or run, there are still plenty of cardio exercises you can do at home.

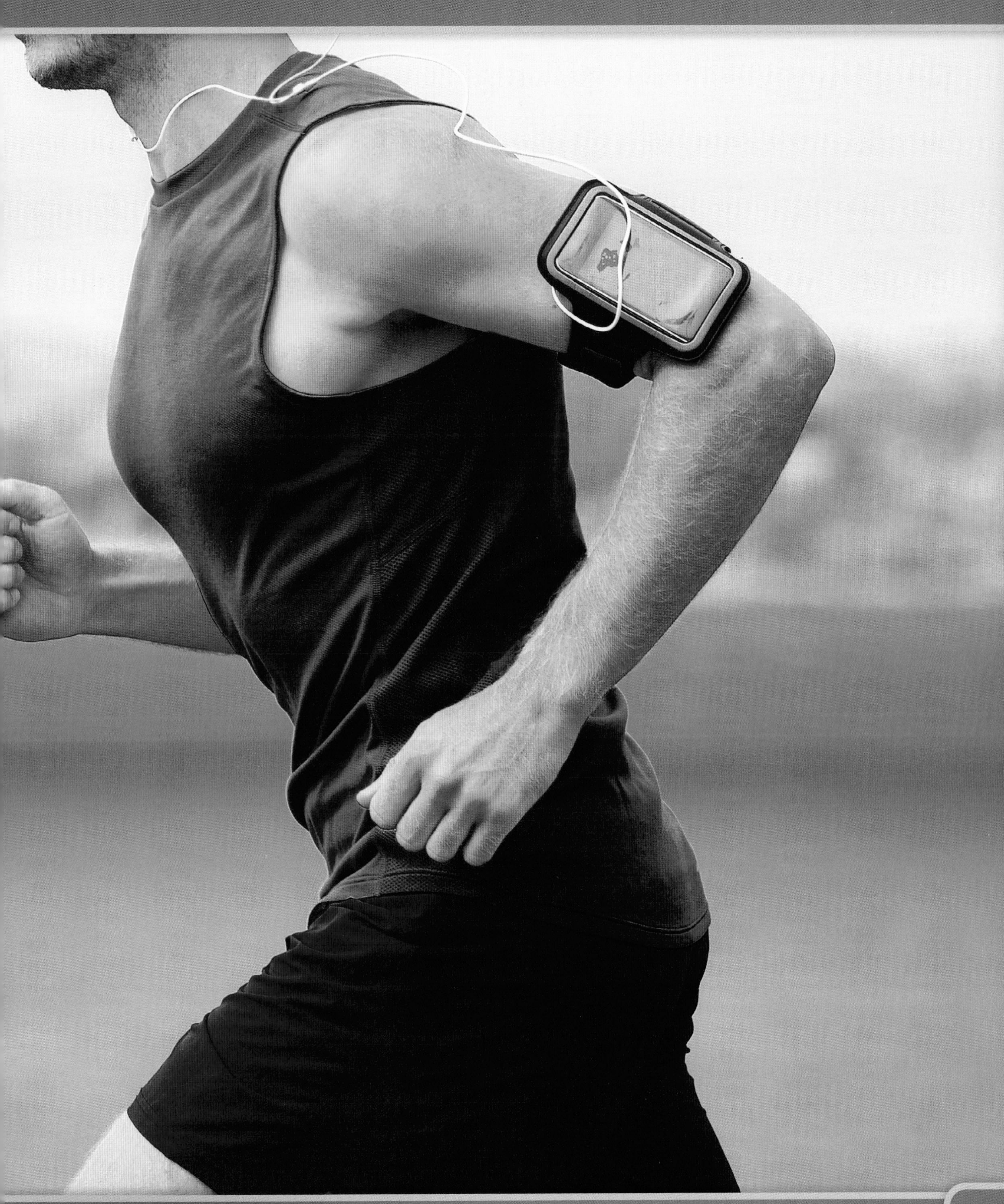

Burpee

The Burpee, a plyometric powerhouse of an exercise, combines the strength-training benefits of a squat or push-up move with high-intensity cardio. Challenge yourself with one of this versatile exercise's many variations; for example, you can add different kinds of jumps or perform it on one leg.

HOW TO DO IT

- Stand with your feet together and your arms above your head.
- Drop into a squat, placing your hands on the floor in front of you.
- In one quick, explosive motion, kick your feet back to assume a high plank position.
- Lower your chest to the floor to perform a push-up.
- In another quick motion, jump your feet back into a squat, and then jump into the air.
- Return to the starting position. Continue performing for the desired time or repetitions.

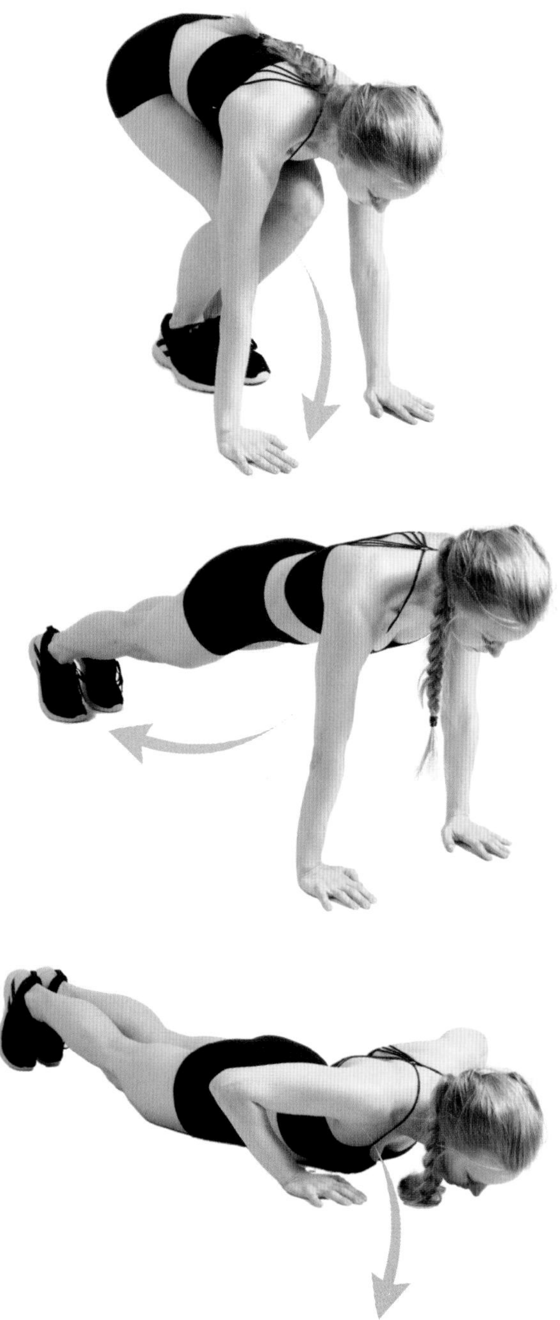

DO IT RIGHT

- Make sure your chest touches the floor during the push-up.
- Jump as high as you can as you rise from the squat.
- Avoid moving with floppy or jerky motions—your movement should be smooth and controlled.

FACT FILE

TARGETS
- Triceps
- Deltoids
- Abdominals
- Back
- Hip flexors
- Quadriceps
- Hamstrings
- Glutes

TYPE
- Dynamic

BENEFITS
- Increases cardiovascular endurance
- Increases agility and speed
- Strengthens entire body

CAUTIONS
- Shortness of breath
- Shoulder issues
- Wrist issues
- Lower-back pain

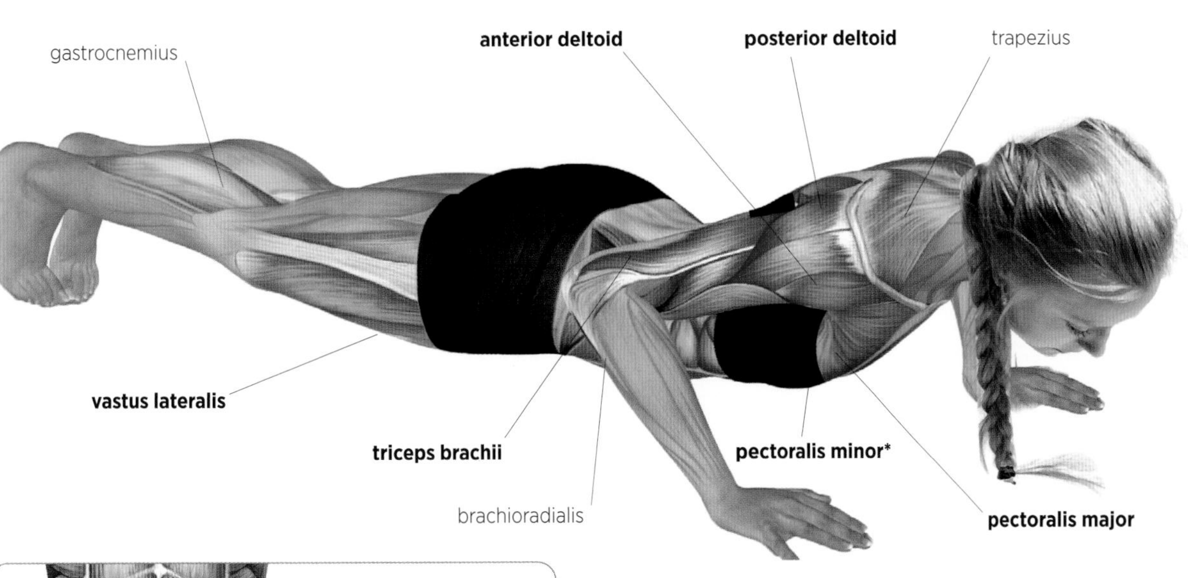

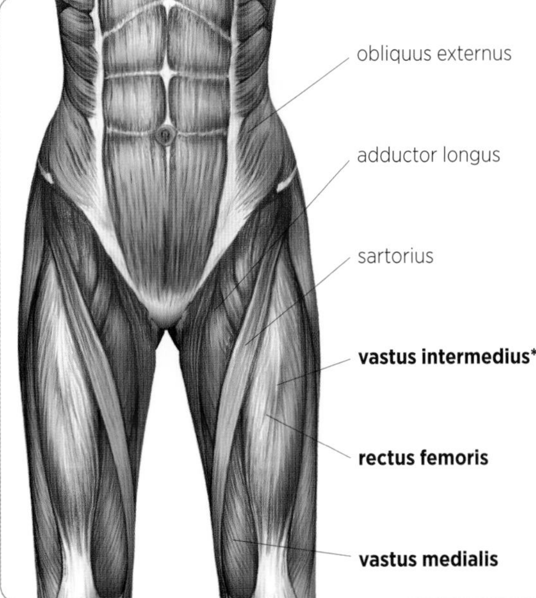

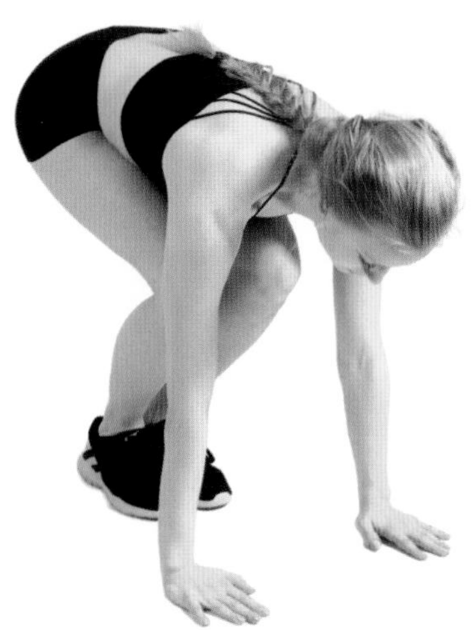

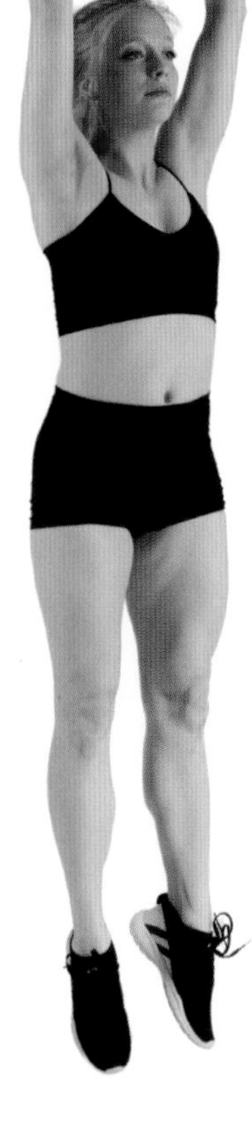

Annotation Key
Bold text indicates target muscles
Light text indicates other working muscles
* indicates deep muscles

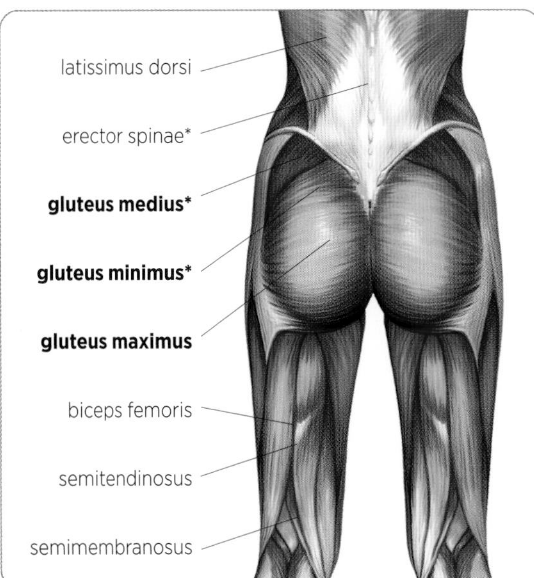

Butt Kick

Butt Kicks will work as a stand-alone strength exercise or as a great warm-up move, especially for your quadriceps. It also gets your blood pumping as it burns calories.

HOW TO DO IT

- Begin in a standing position, and then jog in place.
- Kick your heels up high toward your glutes.
- Continue jogging in place, lifting your heels high and increasing your speed as you go. Perform for the recommended time.

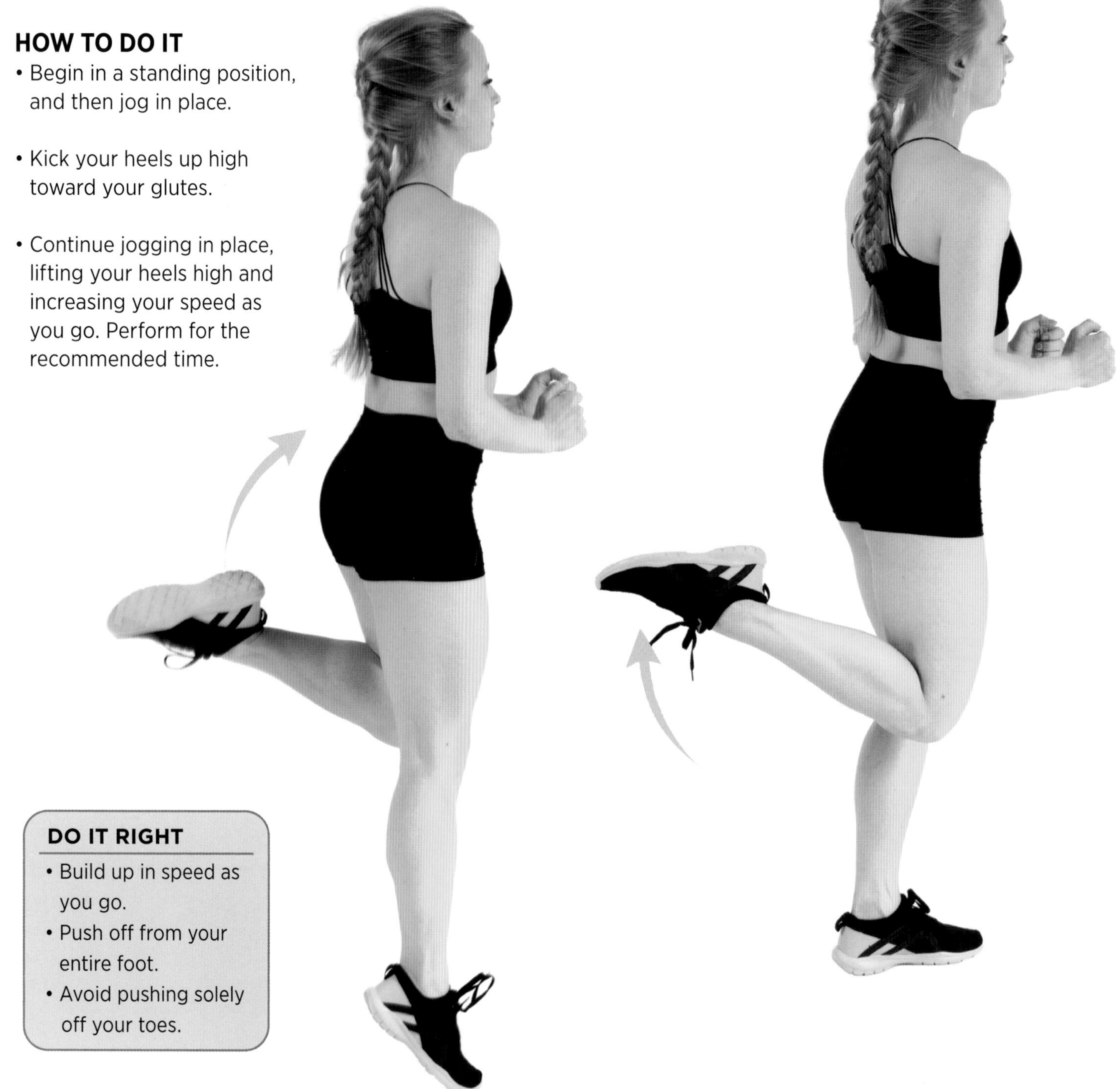

DO IT RIGHT

- Build up in speed as you go.
- Push off from your entire foot.
- Avoid pushing solely off your toes.

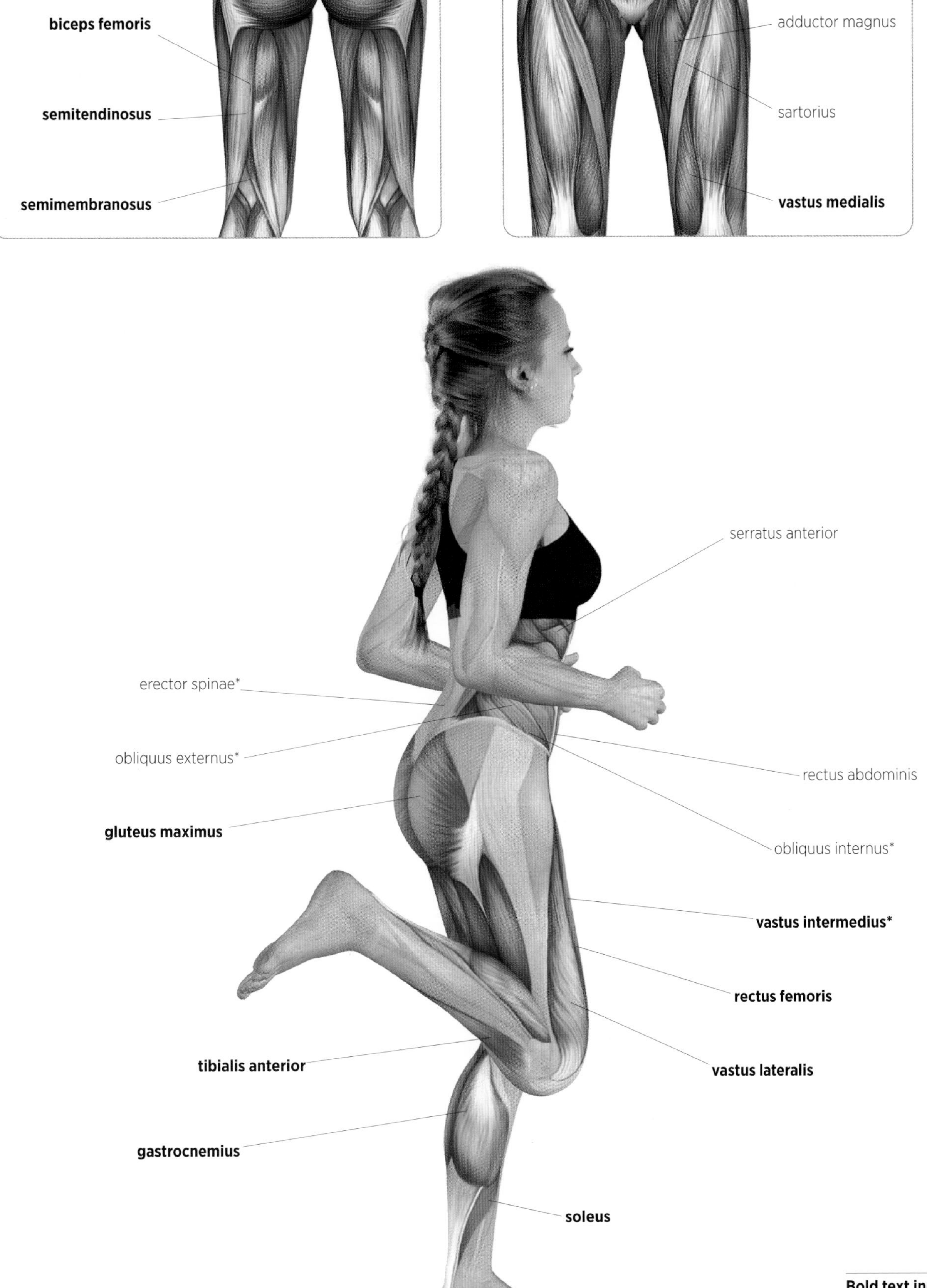

FACT FILE

TARGETS
- Glutes
- Quadriceps
- Hamstrings
- Calves

TYPE
- Dynamic

BENEFITS
- Strengthens lower body
- Serves as a warm-up for other exercises
- Builds endurance

CAUTIONS
- Knee issues
- Ankle pain

Annotation Key

Bold text indicates target muscles
Light text indicates other working muscles
* indicates deep muscles

Warm-Up Obstacle Course

The Warm-Up Obstacle Course exercise will get your heart pumping and test your agility and coordination. This fun exercise prepares you for complicated Weight-Free workouts.

HOW TO DO IT

- Set up seven small objects on the floor to form a triangle and a square.
- Taking small, quick steps, step around all of the objects in the triangle.
- Stand in front of the square, and jump forward to land in the middle of the square. Complete a Jumping Jack (see box on opposite page).
- Jump forward to land outside the square. Jog back to the beginning of the course, and repeat for the recommended time or repetitions.

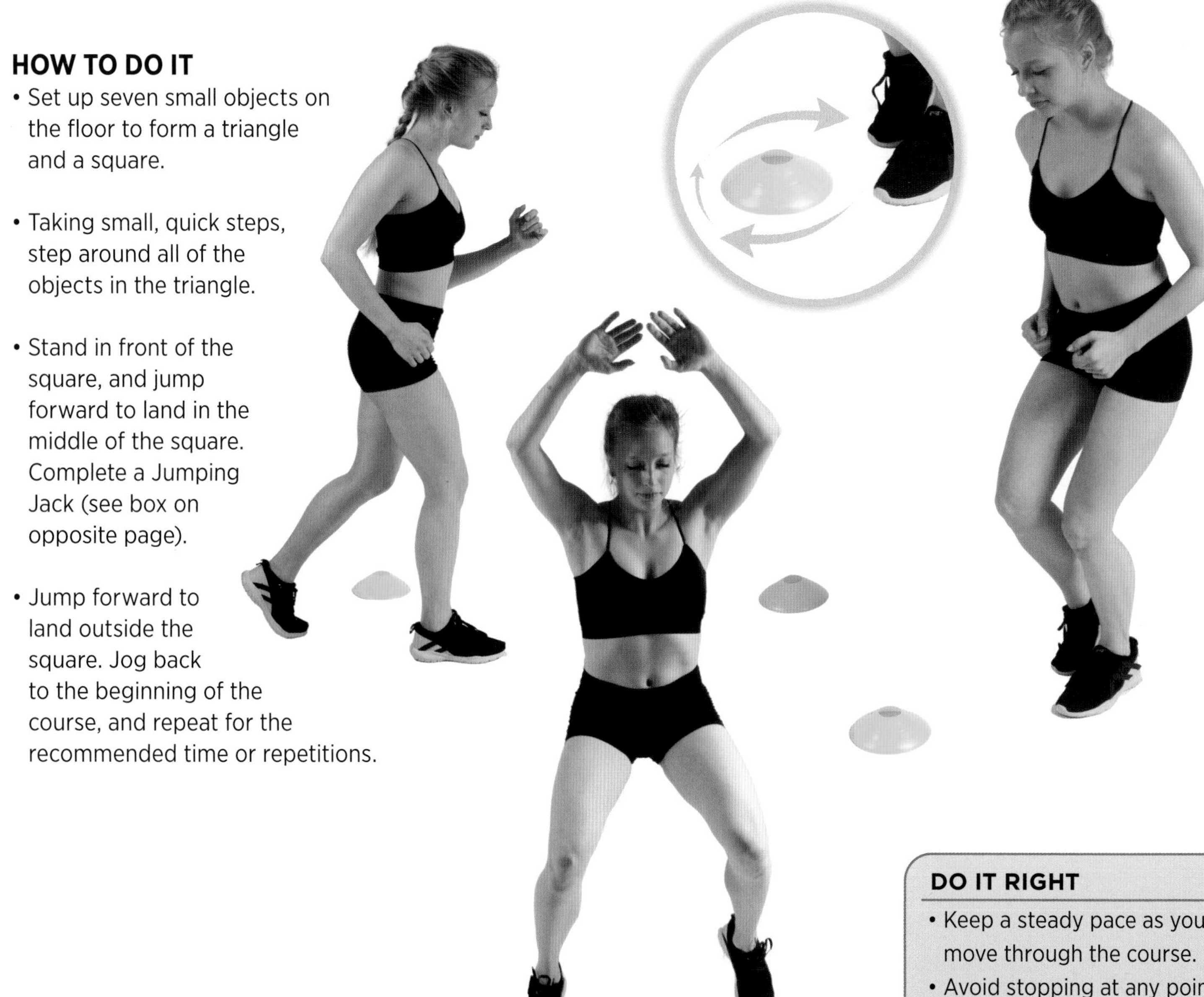

DO IT RIGHT

- Keep a steady pace as you move through the course.
- Avoid stopping at any point.
- Avoid moving too quickly throughout the course.
- Take small steps, focusing on coordination.
- Stand upright.
- Keep your abdominal muscles engaged.

FACT FILE

TARGETS
- Abdominals
- Glutes
- Hamstrings
- Quadriceps

TYPE
- Dynamic

BENEFITS
- Warms up muscles
- Improves agility

CAUTIONS
- Knee issues

EQUIPMENT
- Small cones

multifidus spinae*
gluteus minimus*
vastus lateralis
biceps femoris
semitendinosus
semimembranosus

MODIFICATION

EASIER: To perform a Jumping Jack, stand with your arms at your sides and with your feet together and knees slightly bent. Keeping your knees bent, jump up, spreading your legs and bringing your arms up to touch overhead. Return to the starting position.

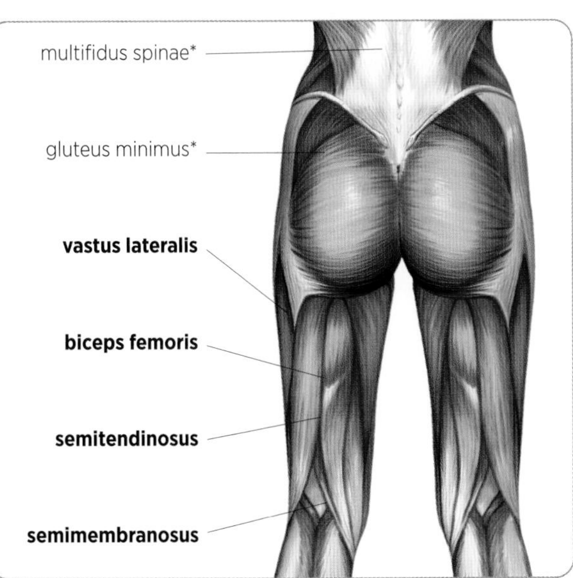

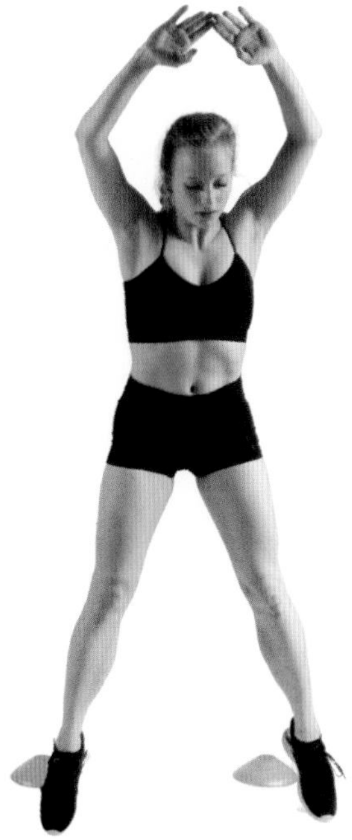

rectus abdominis
vastus intermedius*
rectus femoris
vastus medialis
gluteus medius*
tensor fasciae latae
biceps femoris
gastrocnemius

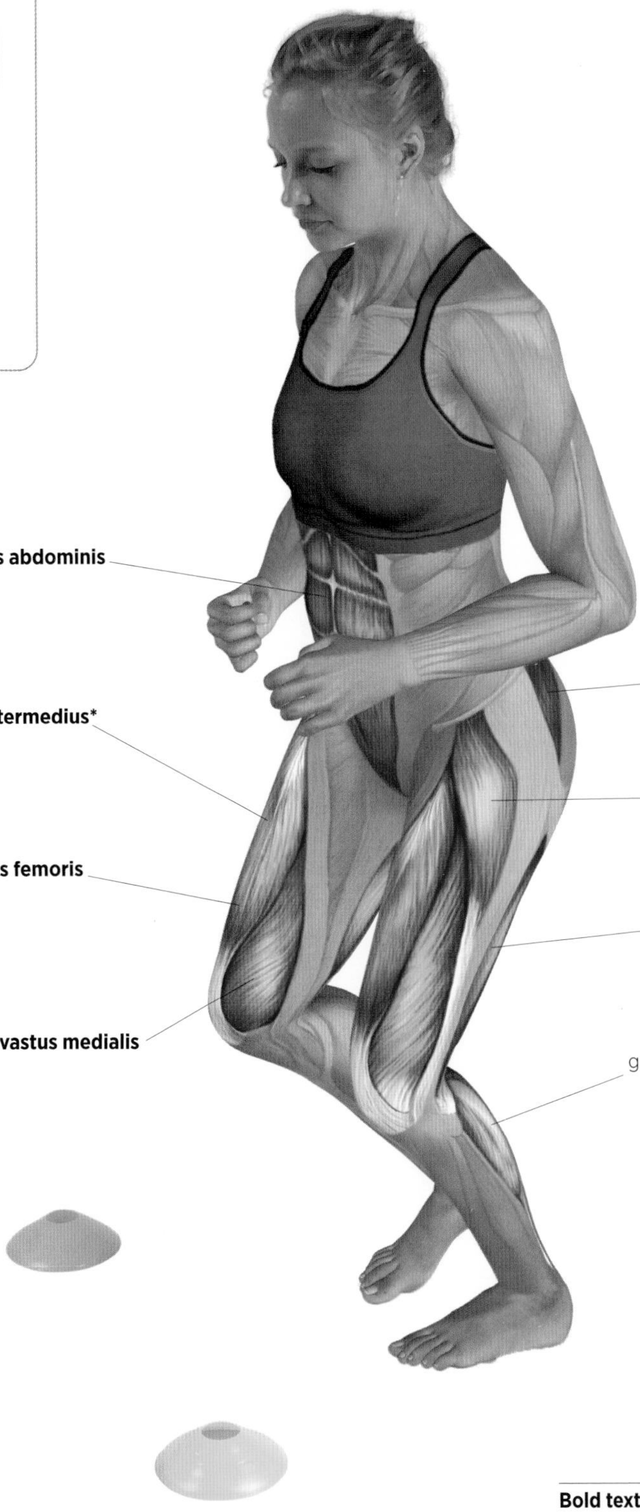

Annotation Key
Bold text indicates target muscles
Light text indicates other working muscles
* indicates deep muscles

Twisting Knee Raise

Work your abdominals—especially your obliques—while developing leg strength and endurance with Twisting Knee Raise. It will also burn calories as you prepare for a rigorous Weight-Free workout.

HOW TO DO IT

- Stand with your feet hip-width apart and your arms at your sides. Raise both arms and bend your elbows so that each arm forms a right angle, palms facing forward.
- Raise your left knee toward your abdomen. At the same time, bring your right elbow toward the knee. Aim for your knee and elbow to touch.
- Return to starting position. Repeat on the opposite side, alternating sides for the recommended repetitions.

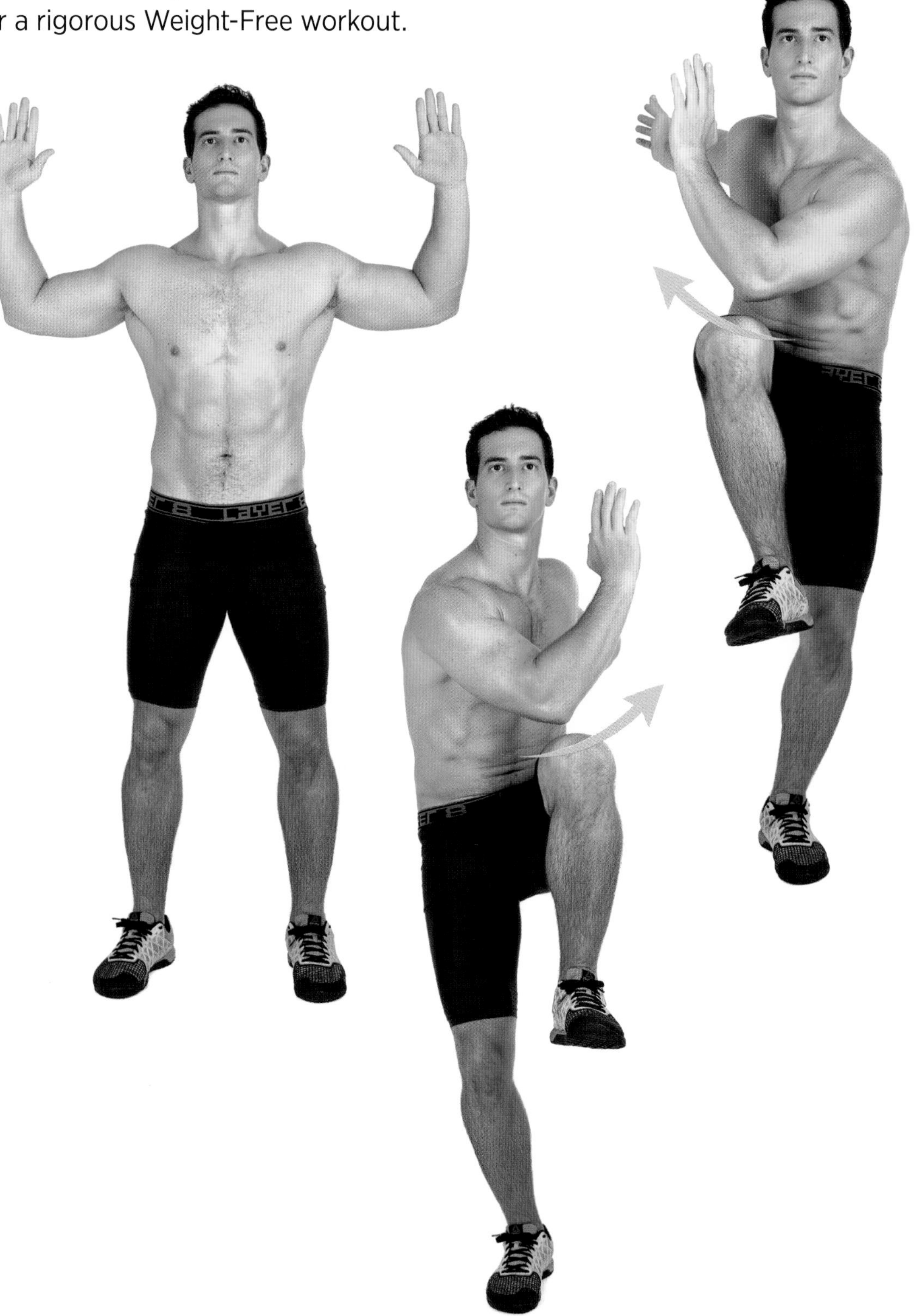

DO IT RIGHT

- Keep your abs engaged and contracted.
- Maintain a quick, consistent pace.
- Face forward as you perform the twist.
- Avoid hyperextending your back.
- Don't excessively twist your hips.

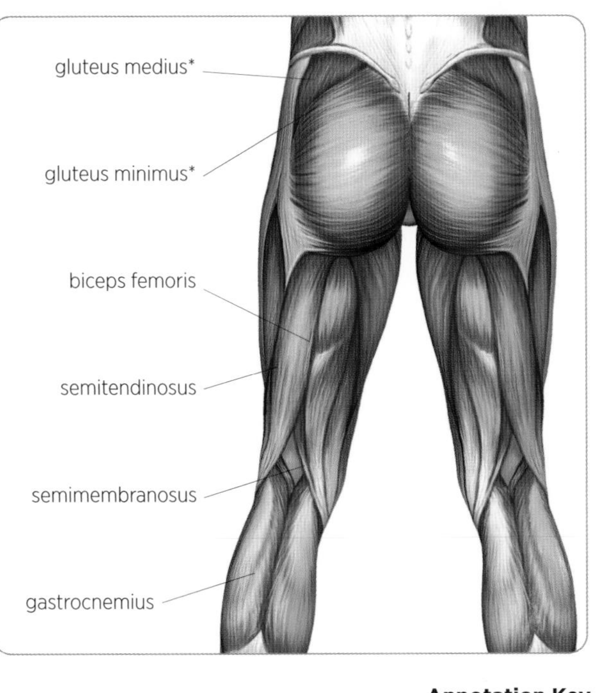

Annotation Key

Bold text indicates target muscles
Light text indicates other working muscles
* indicates deep muscles

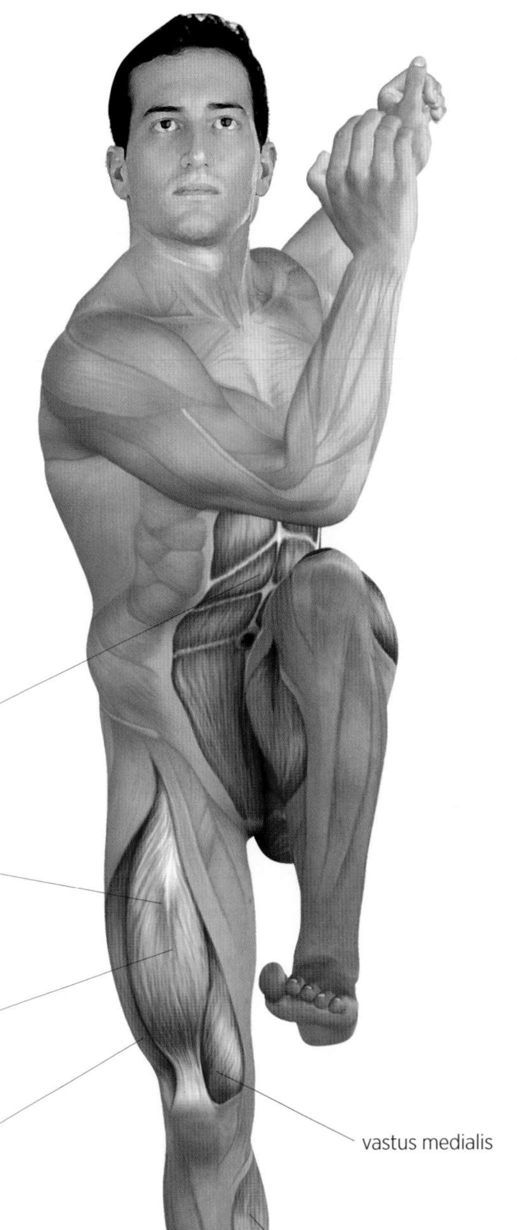

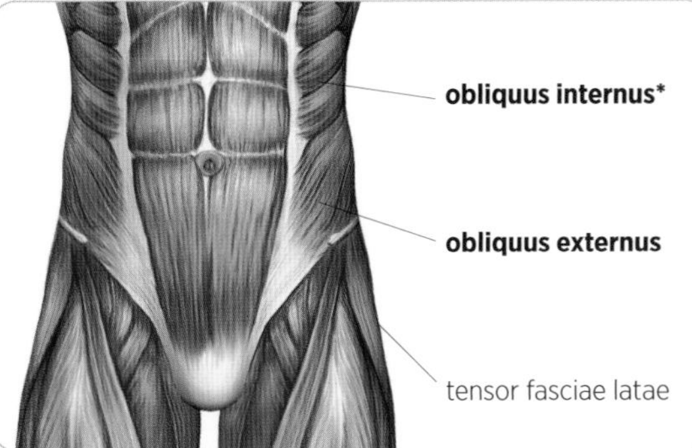

FACT FILE

TARGETS
- Abdominals
- Legs

TYPE
- Dynamic

BENEFITS
- Improves balance and coordination
- Improves agility and power
- Burn calories
- Elevates heart rate
- Strengthens and tones core muscles and calves

CAUTIONS
- Lower-back issues
- Knee issues

Star Jump

The Star Jump exercise helps develop leg strength and cardio endurance. It is not easy as it looks—you must be able to jump high enough to simultaneously extend your legs and arms outward.

HOW TO DO IT

- Stand with your feet together, and then squat down, keeping your knees in line with your toes.
- In one explosive movement, jump as high as possible while spreading your arms and legs as wide as you can. Your body will make a star shape in the fully extended point of the jump.
- Bend your knees slightly as you land in the standing position. Sink back to a squat, and repeat. Each jump equals one repetition. Repeat for the recommended repetitions.

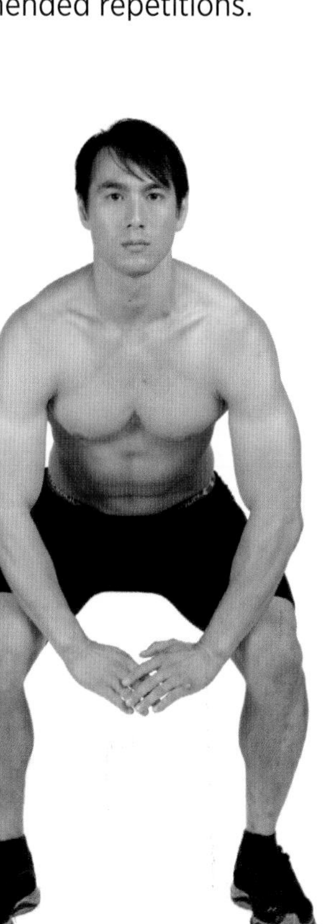

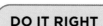

DO IT RIGHT

- Perform these on a soft surface, such as an exercise mat or padded carpeting, to reduce the impact of your landing.
- Flare out your legs as far as possible.
- Avoid twisting in the jump; landing in an awkward position could cause a torque injury.

gluteus medius*
gluteus minimus*
obturator externus
adductor magnus
biceps femoris
semitendinosus
semimembranosus

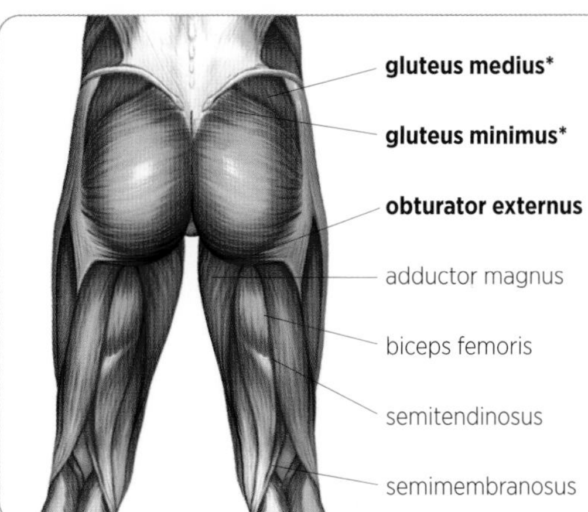

Annotation Key

Bold text indicates target muscles
Light text indicates other working muscles
* indicates deep muscles

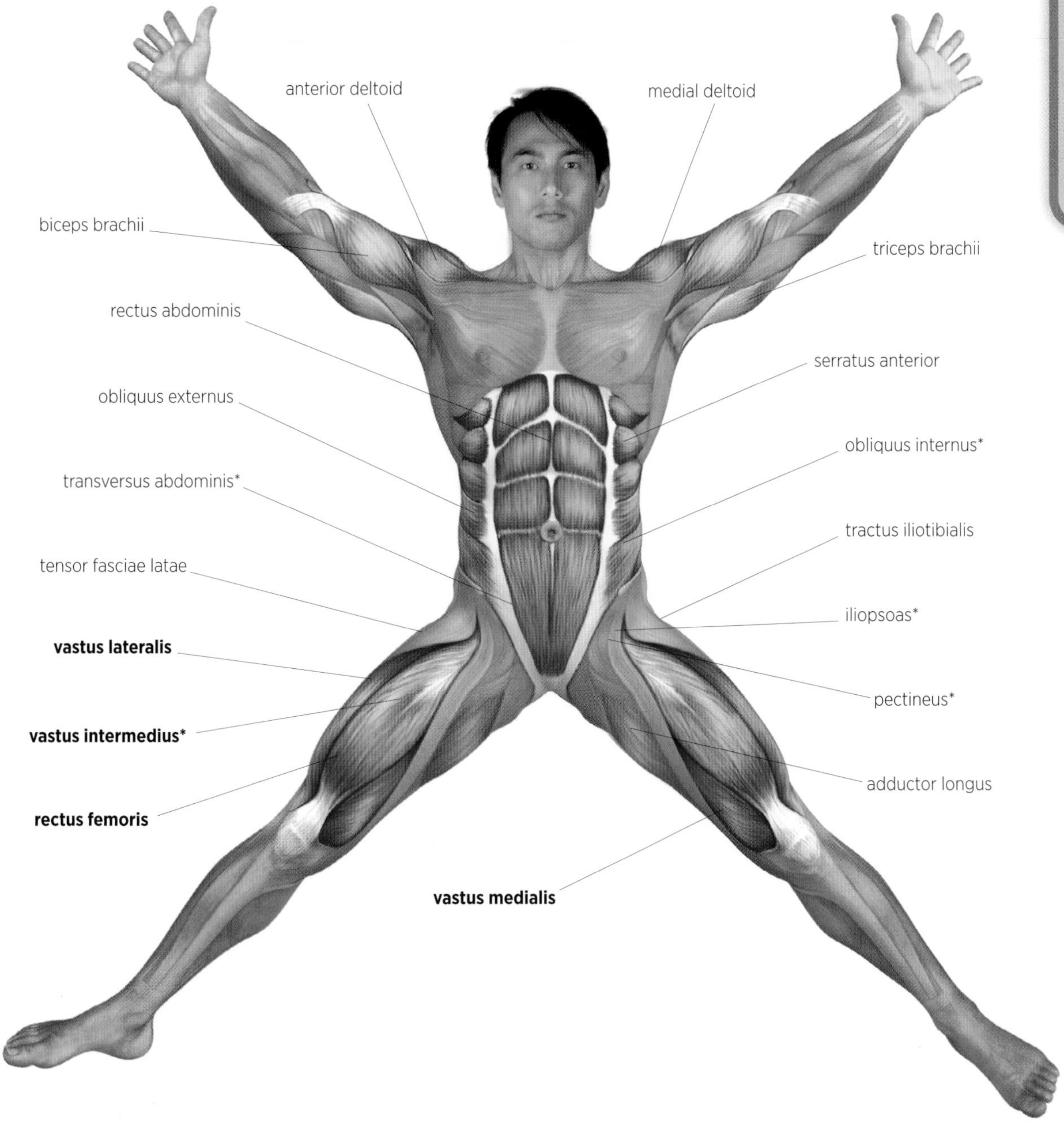

anterior deltoid
medial deltoid
biceps brachii
triceps brachii
rectus abdominis
serratus anterior
obliquus externus
obliquus internus*
transversus abdominis*
tractus iliotibialis
tensor fasciae latae
iliopsoas*
vastus lateralis
pectineus*
vastus intermedius*
adductor longus
rectus femoris
vastus medialis

FACT FILE

TARGETS
- Shoulders
- Abdominals
- Quadriceps
- Hamstrings
- Glutes

TYPE
- Dynamic

BENEFITS
- Strengthens upper and lower body
- Increases agility
- Improves coordination
- Increases cardiovascular endurance

CAUTIONS
- Ankle issues

Abdominal Kick

This intense exercise strengthens and stabilizes your abdominals, particularly your lower abs. Perform the Abdominal Kick at a steady, controlled pace for the best results.

HOW TO DO IT

- Lie faceup with your legs straight and your head raised off the floor.
- Pull your right knee toward your chest, and straighten your left leg, raising it about 45 degrees from the floor. Place your left hand on the inside of your right ankle and your right hand on your bent knee.
- Switch your legs two times, switching your hand placement simultaneously.
- Switch your legs two more times, keeping your hands in their proper placement. Continue alternating sides for the recommended repetitions.

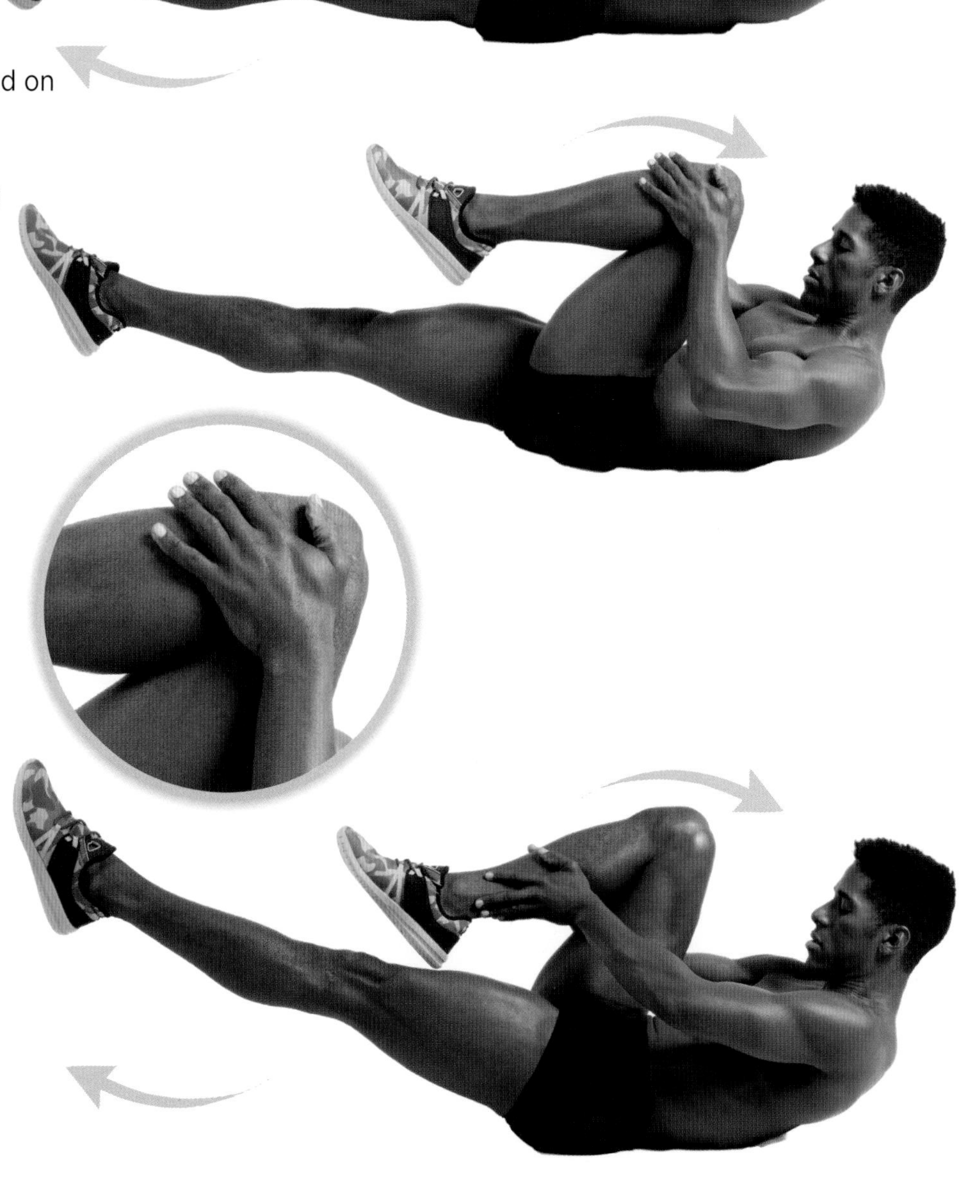

DO IT RIGHT

- Place your hand on the ankle of your bent leg and your inside hand on your bent knee.
- Lift the top of your sternum forward.
- Avoid allowing your lower back to rise up off the floor; use your abdominals to stabilize core while switching legs.

FACT FILE

TARGETS
- Abdominals

TYPE
- Dynamic

BENEFITS
- Strengthens abdominals
- Stabilizes core while extremities are in motion

CAUTIONS
- Neck issues
- Lower-back pain

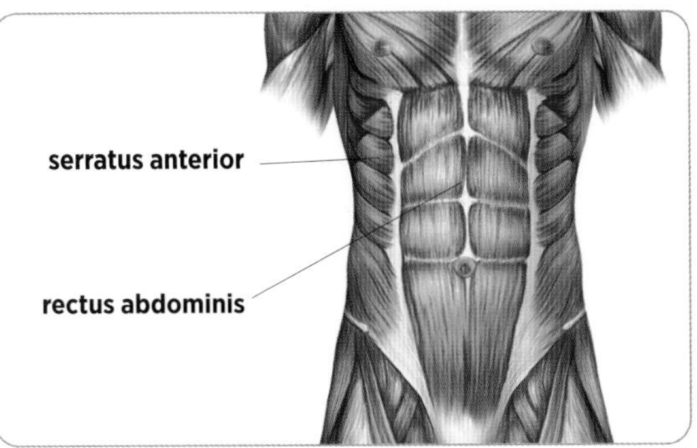

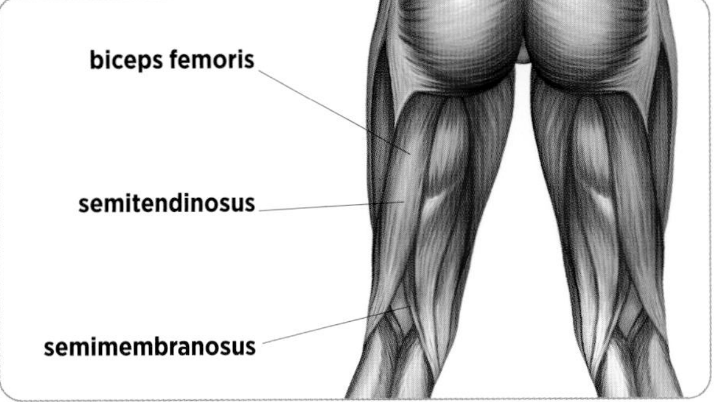

Annotation Key

Bold text indicates target muscles
Light text indicates other working muscles
* indicates deep muscles

gastrocnemius

rectus femoris

triceps brachii

tibialis anterior

tensor fasciae latae

deltoideus anterior

deltoideus posterior

vastus lateralis

gluteus maximus

obliquus internus*

transversus abdominis *

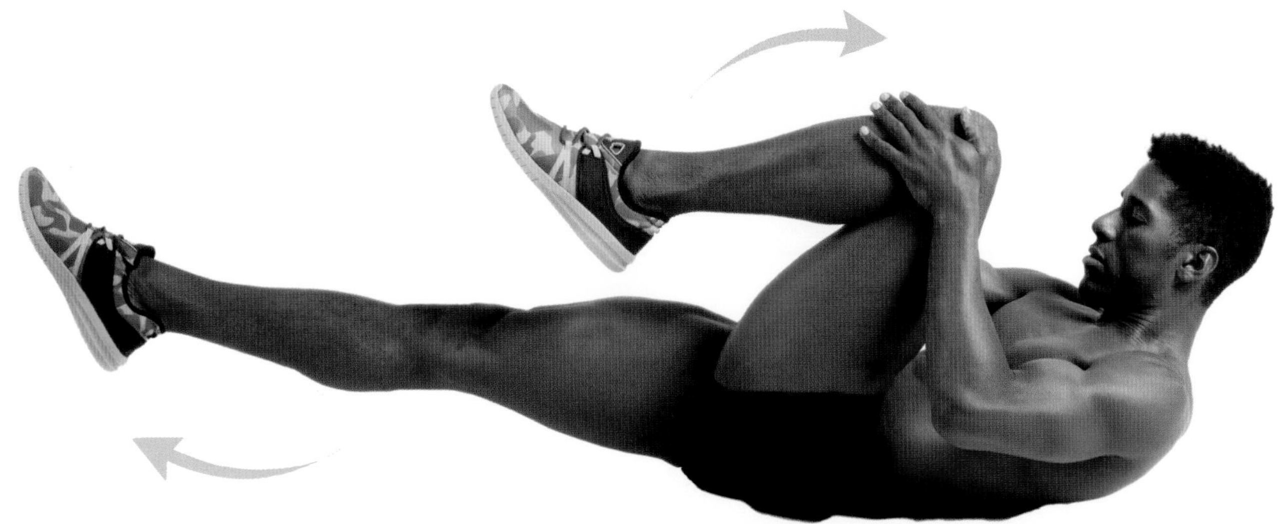

Speed Skater

The Speed Skater helps you stabilize your knee and hip joints by targeting their supporting muscles, including your iliotibial bands, hip adductors, and hip abductors. Be sure to perform this exercise on a smooth, friction-free surface to bring out your inner skater.

HOW TO DO IT

- Stand in a half-squat position, and place your left leg behind your right.
- Jump to your left as far as possible while swinging your arms toward the left. Land in a half-squat position with your right leg behind your left.
- Immediately jump back toward the right as far as possible, as if you were skating in long strides. Switching back and forth equals one repetition. Repeat for the recommended repetitions.

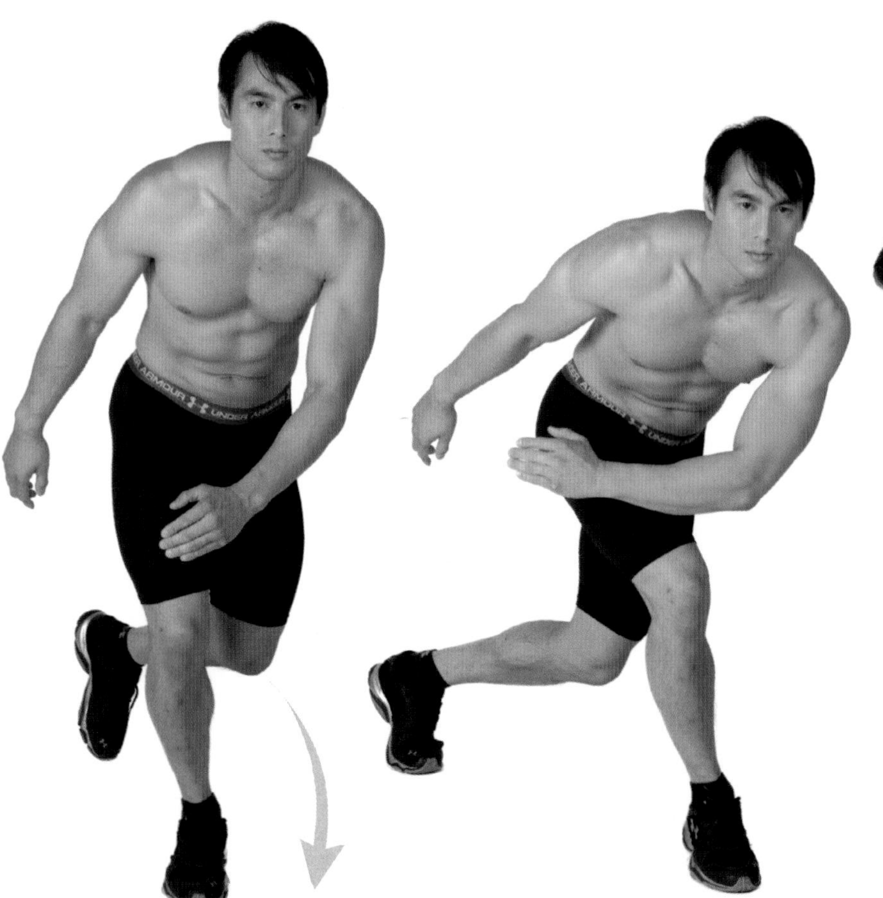

DO IT RIGHT

- Swing your arms together in the direction of the jump.
- Avoid moving your arms in any direction other than the direction of the jump.

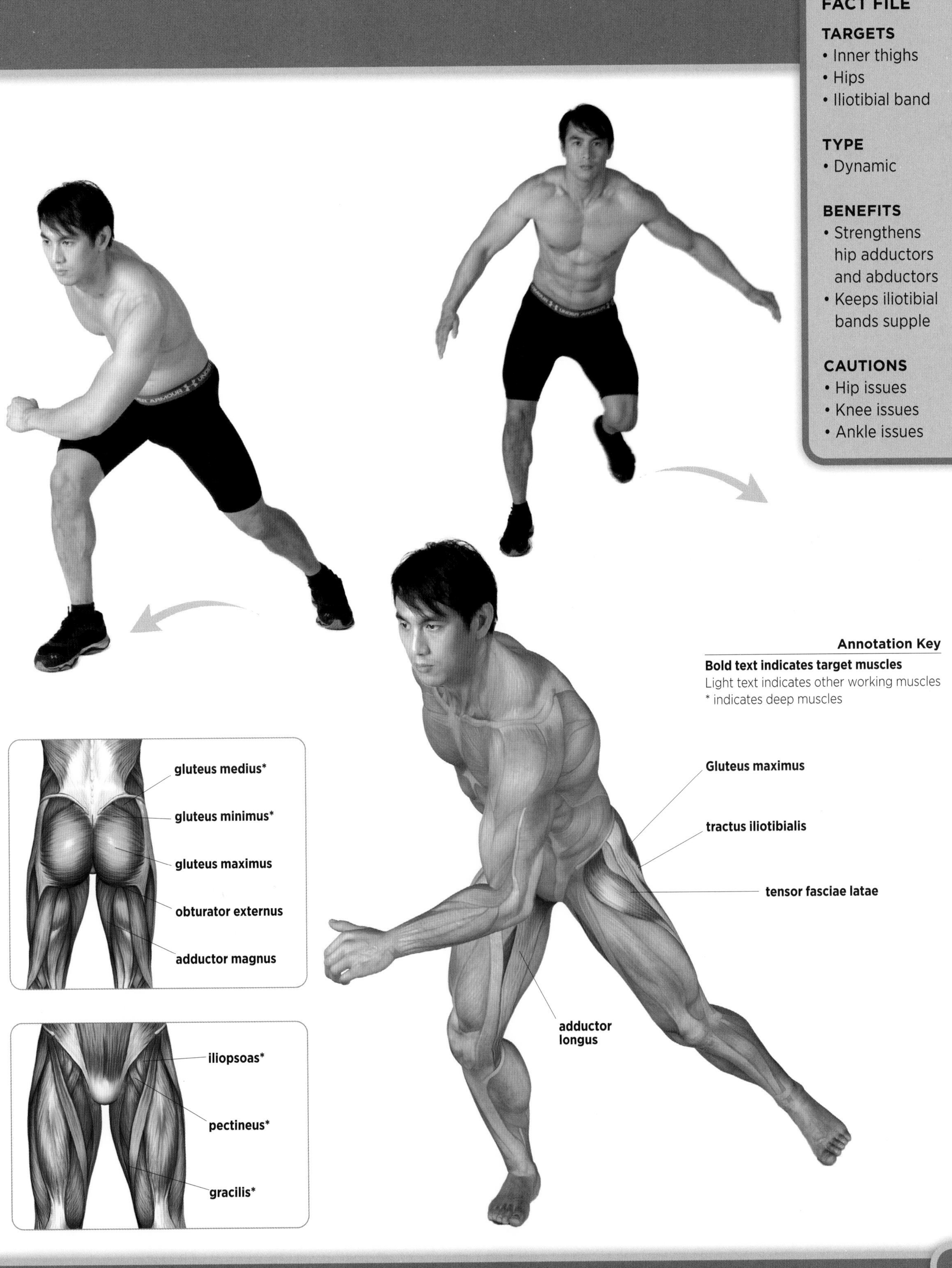

FACT FILE

TARGETS
- Inner thighs
- Hips
- Iliotibial band

TYPE
- Dynamic

BENEFITS
- Strengthens hip adductors and abductors
- Keeps iliotibial bands supple

CAUTIONS
- Hip issues
- Knee issues
- Ankle issues

Plyo Knee Drive

This dynamic exercise uses the form of the standardized lunge combined with the benefits of plyometric training. Focusing on your quadriceps, glutes, calves, and hip flexors, the Plyo Knee Drive will undoubtedly hit nearly every part of your legs.

HOW TO DO IT

- Begin in a staggered stance with your right leg placed forward and your feet approximately hip-width apart.
- Bend both knees to drop the knee of your left leg toward the floor.
- With one explosive motion, extend both legs, launching yourself into the air while drawing your left leg in toward your torso, driving your knee forward.
- Before returning to the floor, return your left leg back behind you, landing in the starting position.
- Repeat on the opposite side. Continue alternating sides for the recommended repetitions.

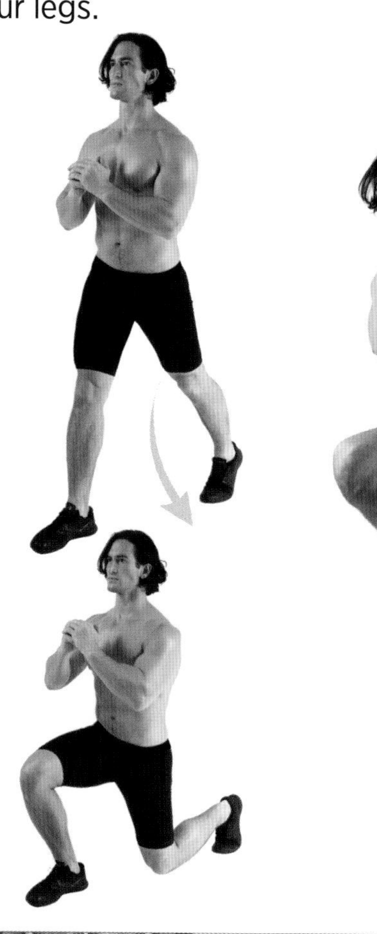

FACT FILE

TARGETS
- Abdominals
- Hip flexors
- Quadriceps
- Glutes

TYPE
- Dynamic

BENEFITS
- Strengthens and tones abdominals and legs
- Increases cardiovascular endurance
- Improves coordination

CAUTIONS
- Lower-back issues

DO IT RIGHT

- Keep your motions quick and powerful.
- Avoid small motions; drive your lifted knee high and outward with exaggerated movements.

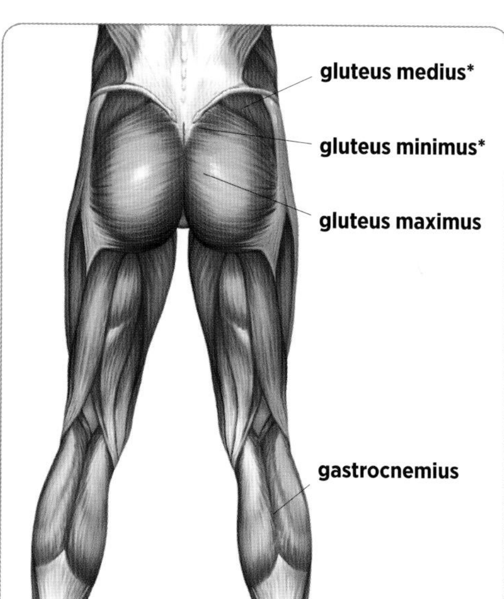

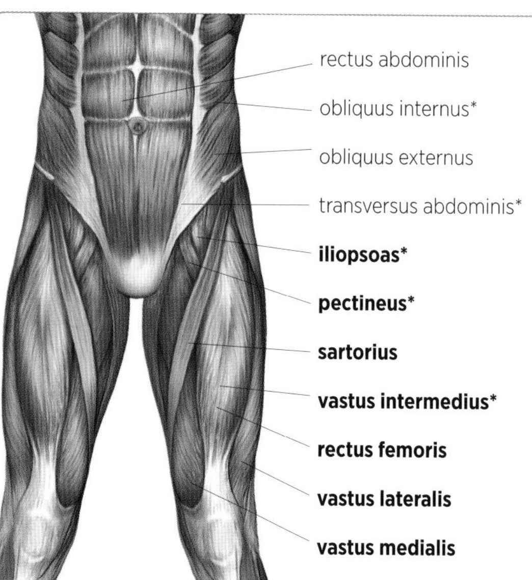

Annotation Key
Bold text indicates target muscles
Light text indicates other working muscles
* indicates deep muscles

Pistol

Essentially a single-leg squat, Pistols provide all the lower-body and core benefits of a basic squat, but doubles the intensity. As with any exercise that requires a single-leg stance, they will tax your midline stability, balance, and coordination.

HOW TO DO IT

- Stand on your left leg with it centered underneath your center of gravity. Raise your arms straight in front of you at shoulder height, palms facing downward.
- Shift your weight backward, and extend your right leg straight out, flexing at your hip, knee, and ankle as you lower into a squat until the top of your right thigh is parallel with the floor.
- Drive your left foot into the floor, extending your leg and hips to return to the starting position.
- Repeat on the opposite side. Continue alternating sides for the recommended repetitions.

FACT FILE

TARGETS
- Quadriceps
- Glutes
- Back

TYPE
- Dynamic

BENEFITS
- Strengthens and tones back and legs
- Improves balance

CAUTIONS
- Knee issues

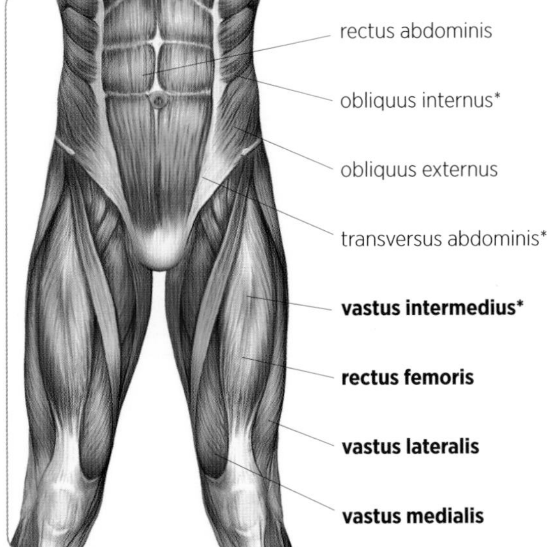

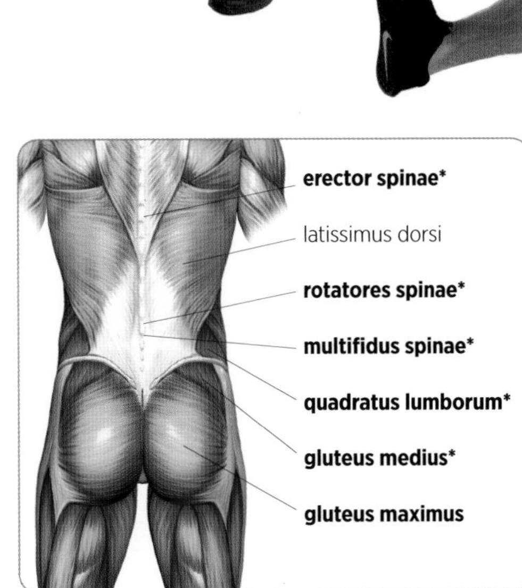

Annotation Key

Bold text indicates target muscles
Light text indicates other working muscles
* indicates deep muscles

DO IT RIGHT

- Keep your back as upright as possible.
- Keep your weight shifted back and through your heel of your supporting foot.

Kneeling Squat Jump

Body-weight leg exercise . . . check. Explosive . . . check. Sweat-inducing . . . check! This advanced, dynamic plyometric exercise targets your quadriceps, glutes, calves, abdominals, and last, but not least, your endurance! A great one to go all out on, this explosive movement demands a lot, but gives even more!

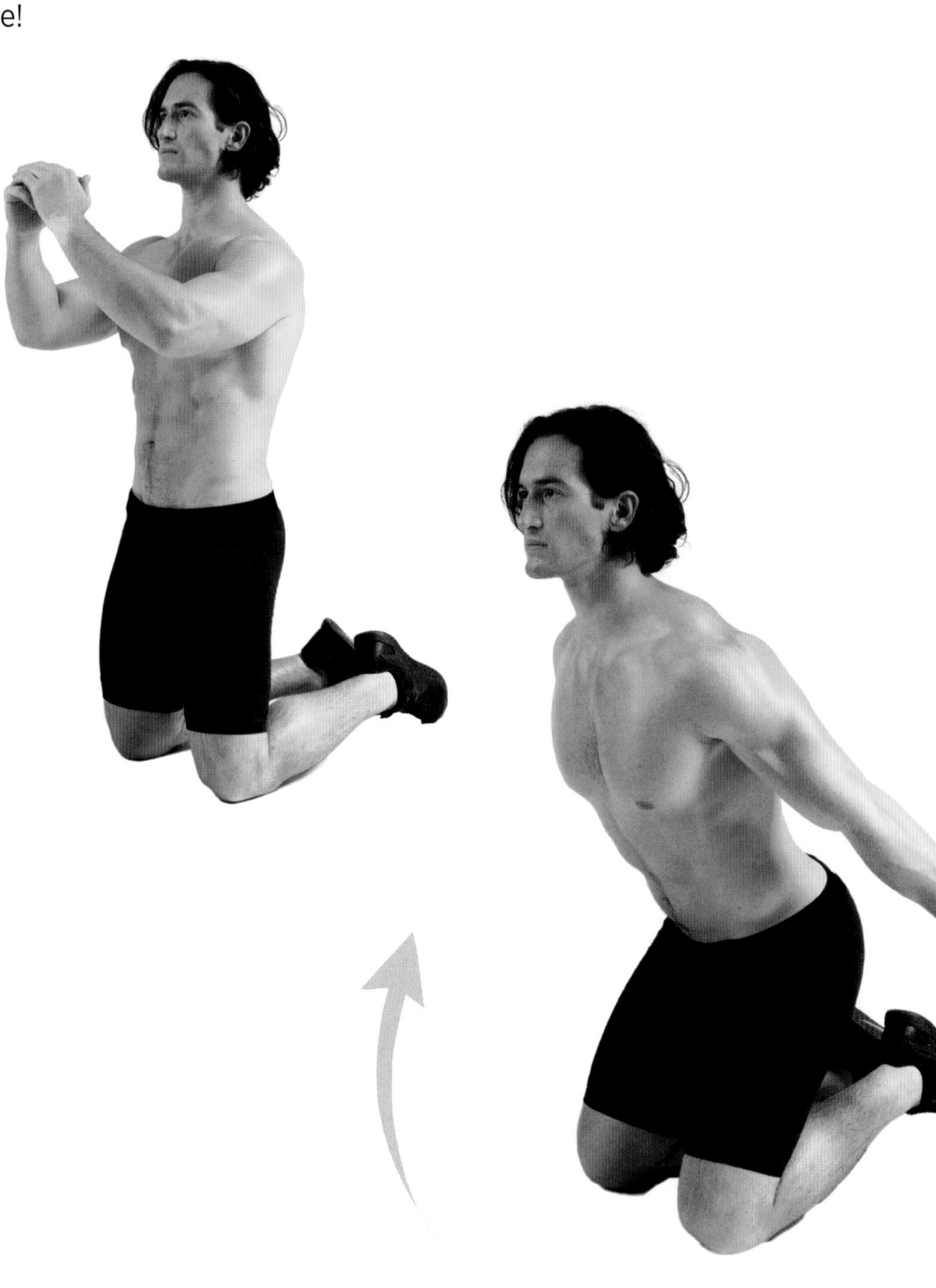

HOW TO DO IT

- Kneel on the floor with your legs bent and tucked underneath you.
- Drop your hips back, bending at your knees and hips, and swing your arms back and behind you.
- In one explosive motion, swing your arms forward while thrusting your hips forward and extending your legs to power off the floor before pulling your feet underneath you to catch yourself in a squat.
- Come to a standing position by extending your legs and hips.
- Lower yourself back down to the starting position, and then repeat for the recommended repetitions.

DO IT RIGHT

- When catching yourself in the squat, make sure to have your feet positioned beneath you, tracking your knees over toes.
- Imagine pressing into the floor as you rise from the squat, creating your body's own resistance in your leg muscles.

TARGETS
- Hip flexors
- Quadriceps
- Glutes
- Abdominals

TYPE
- Dynamic

BENEFITS
- Strengthens and tones abdominals and legs
- Improves coordination
- Increases cardiovascular endurance
- Increases lower-extremity power

CAUTIONS
- Hip issues
- Knee issues

Annotation Key
Bold text indicates target muscles
Light text indicates other working muscles
* indicates deep muscles

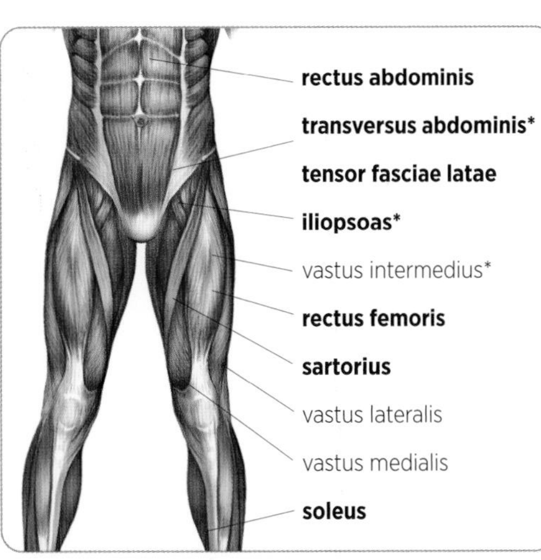

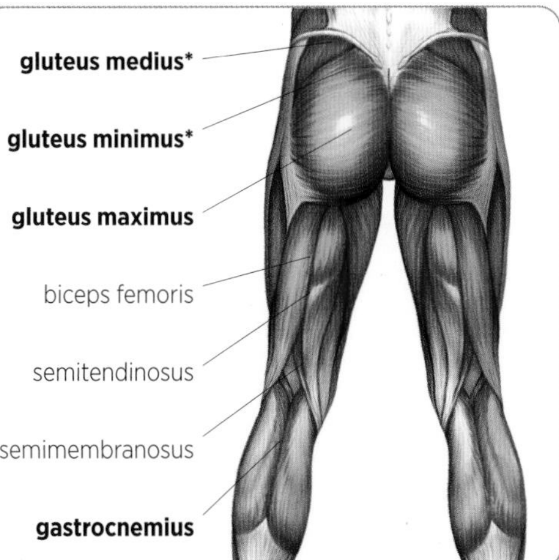

Sphinx Push-Up

Inspired by the statuesque Egyptian figure, this exercise will give you rock-hard muscles that will stand the test of time. With a focus on the triceps, this intermediate exercise combines the best benefits of planks and push-ups into one high-intensity movement.

FACT FILE

TARGETS
- Triceps
- Pectorals
- Abdominals

TYPE
- Dynamic

BENEFITS
- Strengthens and tones arms, abdominals, and chest
- Improves core stability

CAUTIONS
- Wrist issues

HOW TO DO IT

- Assume a low plank position with your forearms positioned directly under your shoulders, your palms facing downward, your legs extended behind you, and your feet firmly planted.
- While engaging your core, press into the floor with both hands, extending at your elbows to lift your body away from the floor until your arms are straight and you are in a high plank position.
- Bend your elbows until you are again resting on your forearms to return to the starting position.

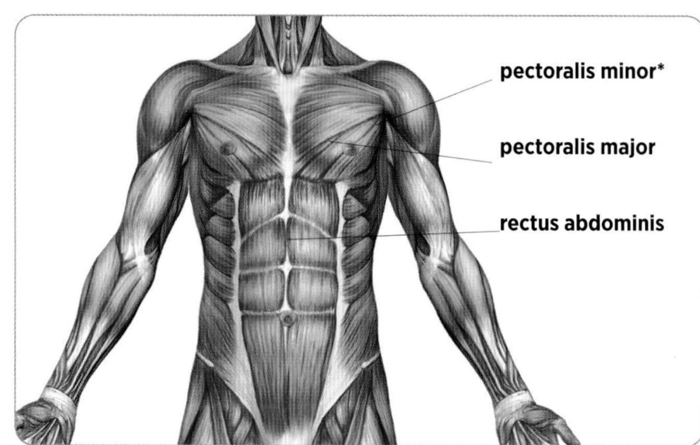

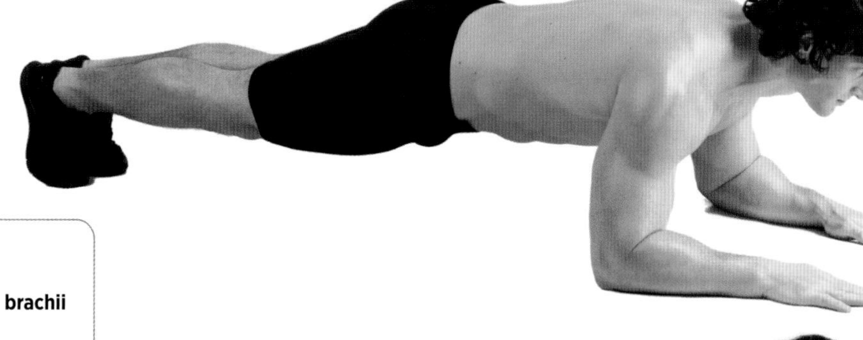

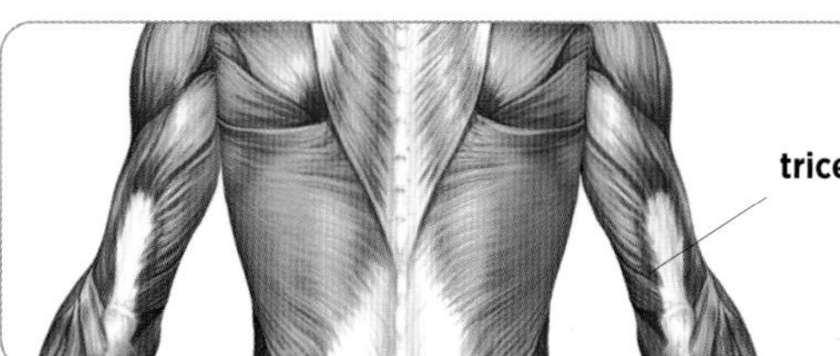

Annotation Key
Bold text indicates target muscles
Light text indicates other working muscles
* indicates deep muscles

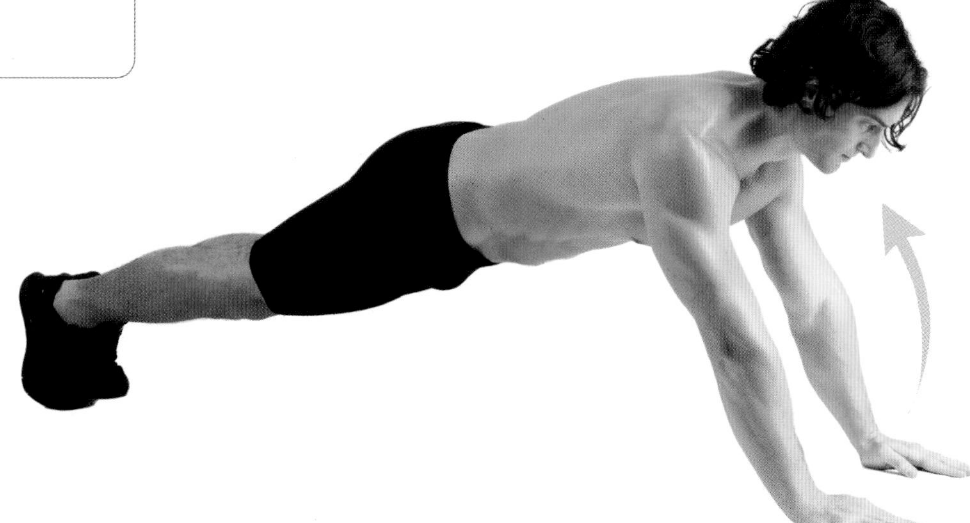

DO IT RIGHT

- Keep your back straight.
- Keep your hands in line with your shoulders.
- Avoid excessive arching of your spine.

Star Push-Up

This stellar exercise says goodbye to the earthly confines of the basic push-up and will launch your workout to a higher level. The Star Push-Up places high stress on the pectorals, as well as the serratus anterior, core, quadriceps, and many other muscles.

HOW TO DO IT

- Lie facedown with your arms and legs extended, creating a star shape with your body.
- Keeping your core engaged, simultaneously press your hands and feet into the floor to lift your body. Keep your arms and legs as straight as possible.
- Return to the starting position, and then repeat for the recommended repetitions.

DO IT RIGHT

- Keep your back straight.
- Keep your abdominals engaged.
- Avoid bending your arms or legs.

FACT FILE

TARGETS
- Biceps
- Pectorals
- Abdominals
- Hip flexors
- Quadriceps

TYPE
- Dynamic

BENEFITS
- Strengthens and tones abdominal, chest, arms, and legs
- Improves core stability

CAUTIONS
- Lower-back issues

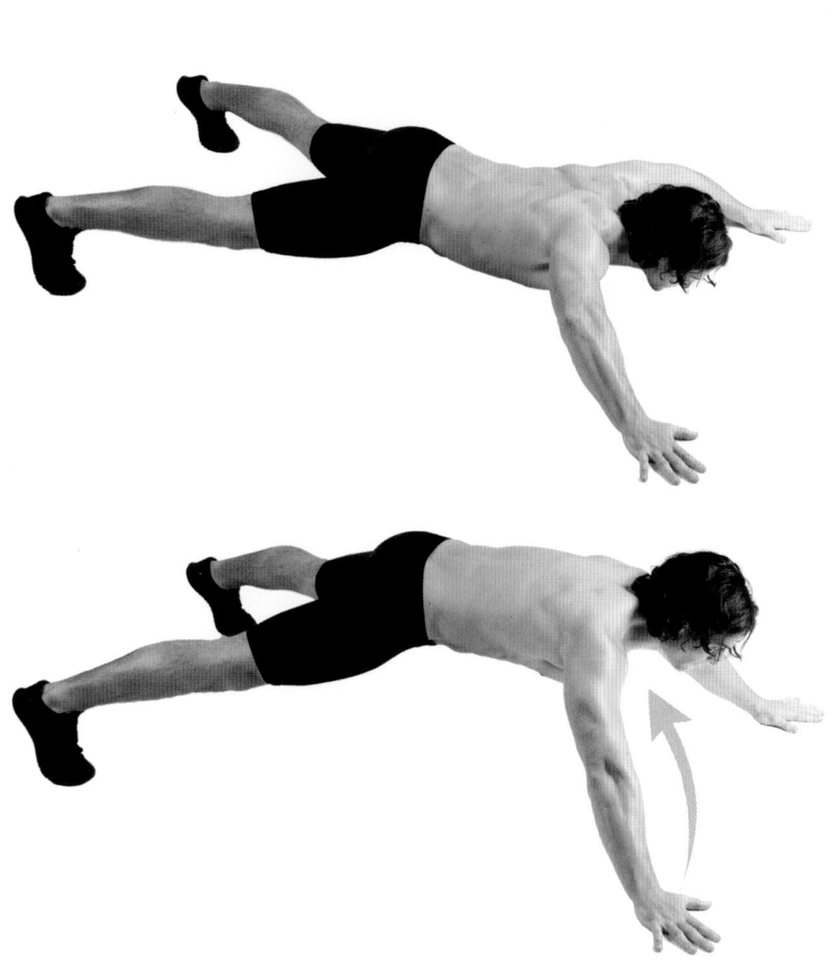

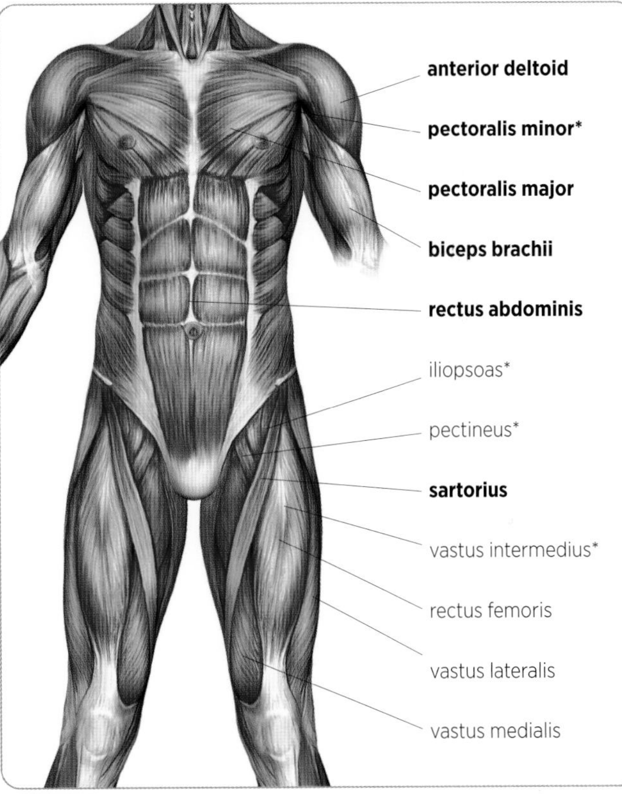

Annotation Key

Bold text indicates target muscles
Light text indicates other working muscles
* indicates deep muscles

High Knees

This simple exercise offers a high-intensity, calorie-burning cardiovascular workout that also strengthens your abdominals, thighs, calves, and glutes. You can perform High Knees while jogging over a distance or just running in place.

HOW TO DO IT

- Stand tall with your hands either on your hips or down by your sides.
- Raise your left knee as high as you are able, and then return to the starting position.
- Alternate legs while increasing your speed as you jog over distance or run in place. Continue for the recommended time or repetitions.

DO IT RIGHT

- Build up in speed as you go.
- Push off from your entire foot.
- Avoid pushing solely off your toes.

FACT FILE

TARGETS
- Abdominals
- Glutes
- Quadriceps
- Hamstrings
- Calves

TYPE
- Dynamic

BENEFITS
- Strengthens lower body
- Serves as a warm-up for other exercise
- Builds endurance

CAUTIONS
- Knee issues
- Ankle pain

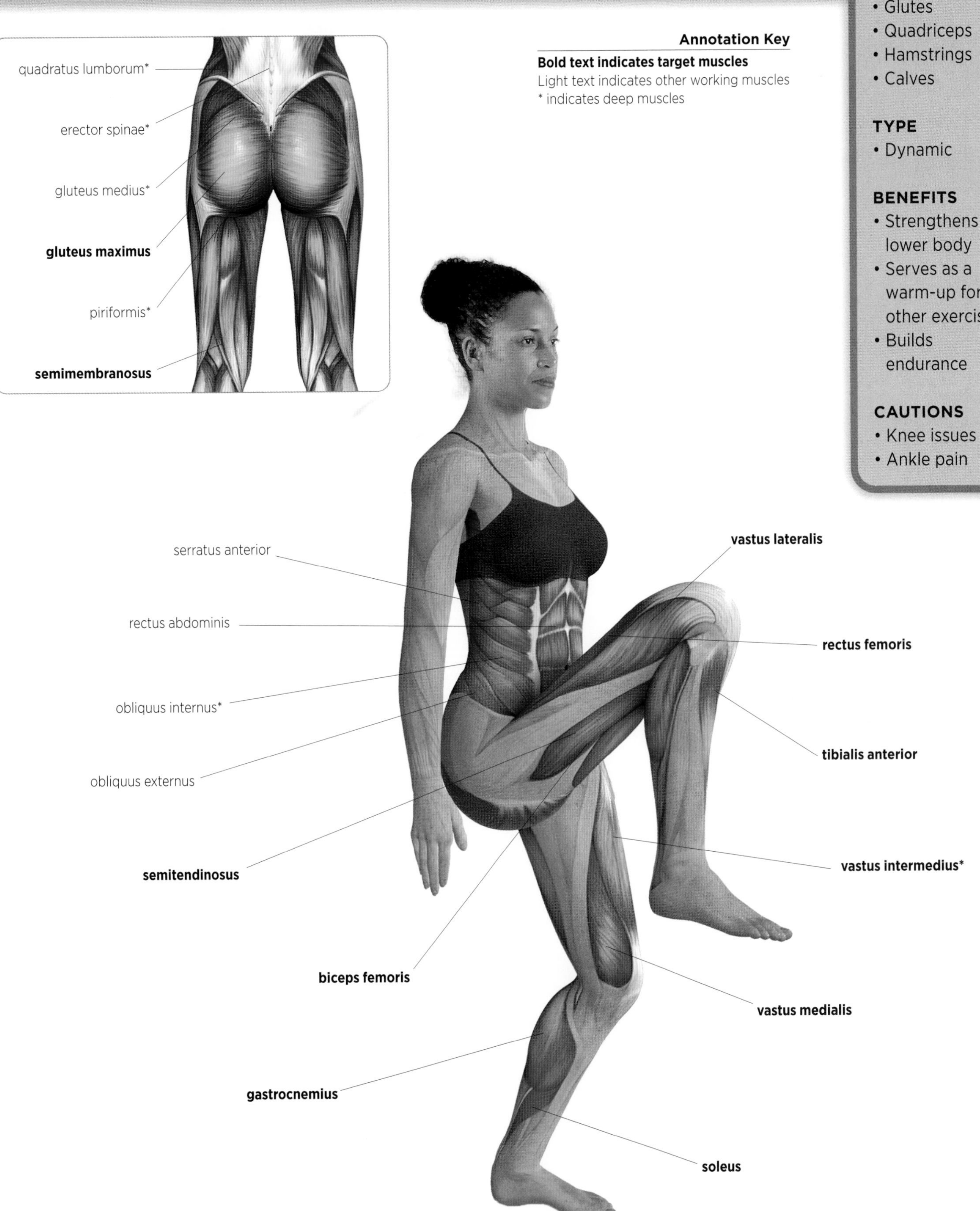

Switch Lunge

The dynamic Switch Lunge takes a basic lunge a step further, calling for you to jump upward to switch legs. It will stabilize your hips, knees, and ankles; stretch your hip flexors; and strengthen your hamstrings, quadriceps, and glutes.

HOW TO DO IT

- Stand with your left leg stepped out in front of your body. Keep a slight bend in your left knee.
- Drop your right knee, touching it lightly on the floor.
- Jump up, switching your legs in the air.
- Land with your right leg forward, and drop your left knee. Lunging and jumping once on each leg equals one repetition. Continue alternating sides for the recommended repetitions.

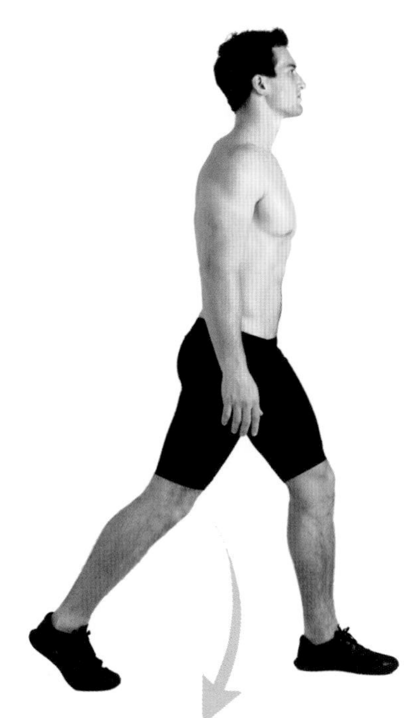

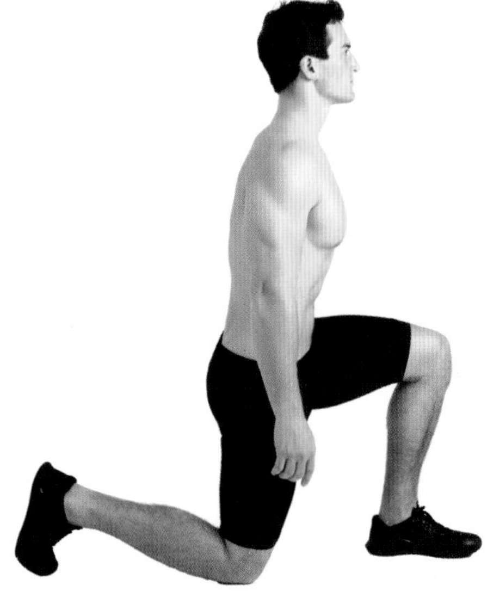

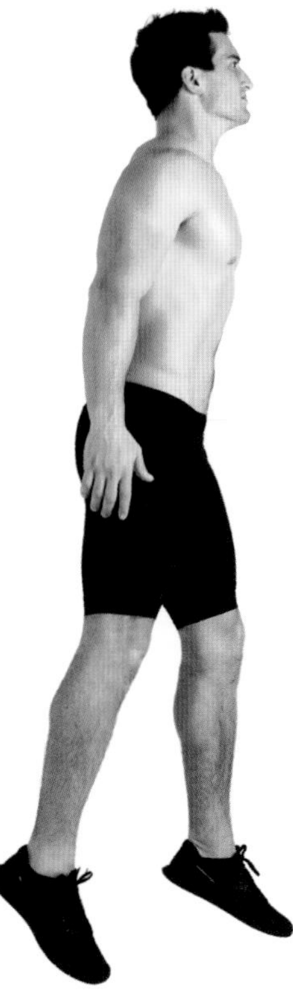

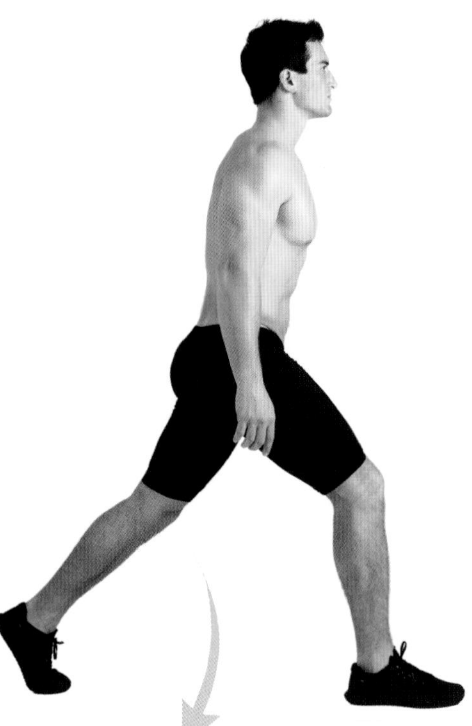

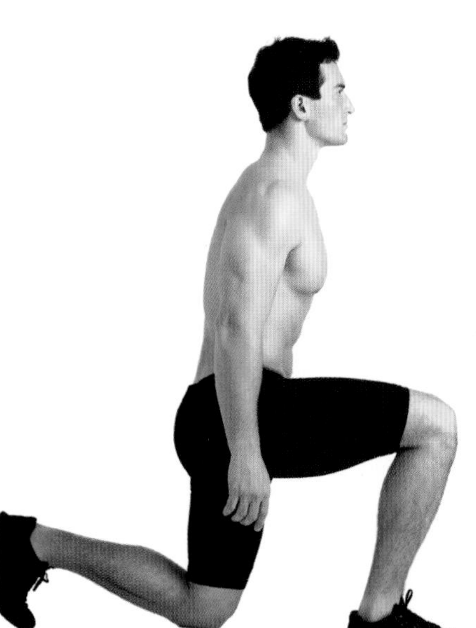

FACT FILE

TARGETS
- Quadriceps
- Hamstrings
- Glutes
- Calves

TYPE
- Dynamic

BENEFITS
- Strengthens quadriceps, hamstrings, glutes, and calves
- Stabilizes hips
- Increases cardiovascular endurance

CAUTIONS
- Knee issues
- Ankle pain

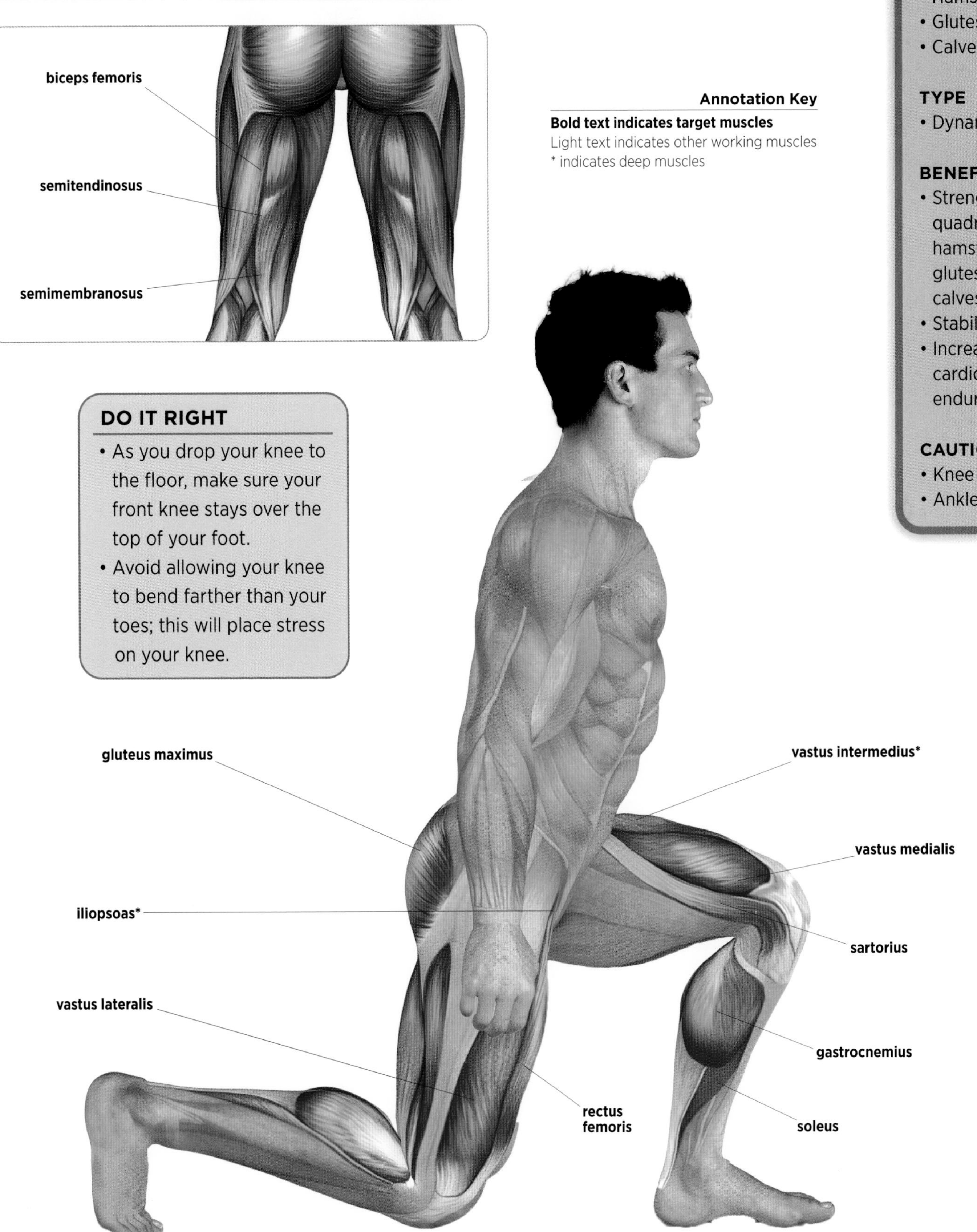

Annotation Key

Bold text indicates target muscles

Light text indicates other working muscles

* indicates deep muscles

DO IT RIGHT
- As you drop your knee to the floor, make sure your front knee stays over the top of your foot.
- Avoid allowing your knee to bend farther than your toes; this will place stress on your knee.

High Plank Kick-Through

The High Plank Kick-Through is a high-intensity exercise that engages your upper body, core, and lower body. A great conditioning exercise, it provides a high-rep sweat maker.

HOW TO DO IT

- Begin in a high plank position with your hands shoulder-width apart, your palms on the floor, your feet together, and your back straight.
- Bring your right leg in toward your body and underneath it while twisting your torso so that your leg crosses your midline toward your left side.
- Without touching the floor with your right leg, draw back underneath your body to return to the high plank position.
- Repeat on the opposite side. Continue alternating sides for the recommended repetitions.

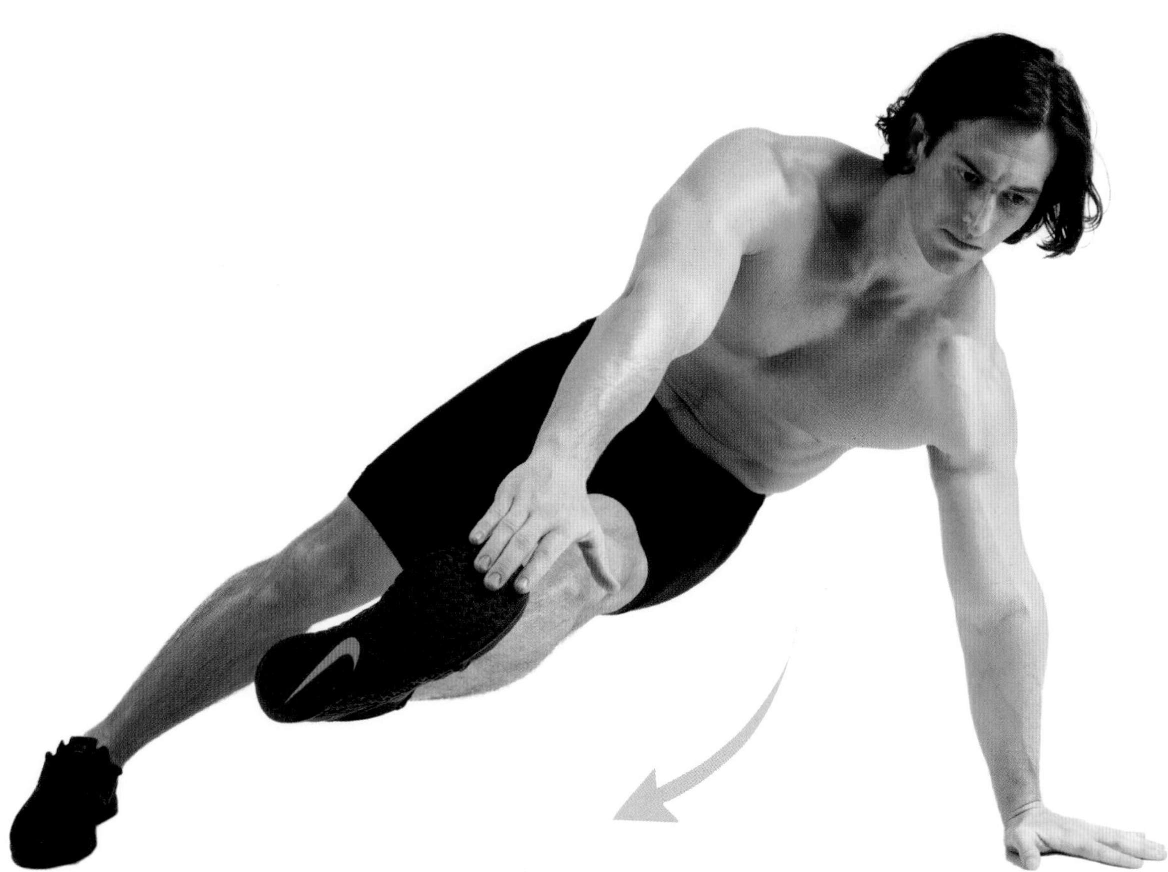

FACT FILE

TARGETS
- Pectorals
- Triceps
- Deltoids
- Abdominals
- Back
- Hip flexors
- Quadriceps
- Glutes

TYPE
- Dynamic

BENEFITS
- Develops core stability
- Improves coordination
- Strengthens and tones abdominals, chest, arms, and legs

CAUTIONS
- Wrist issues
- Lower-back issues

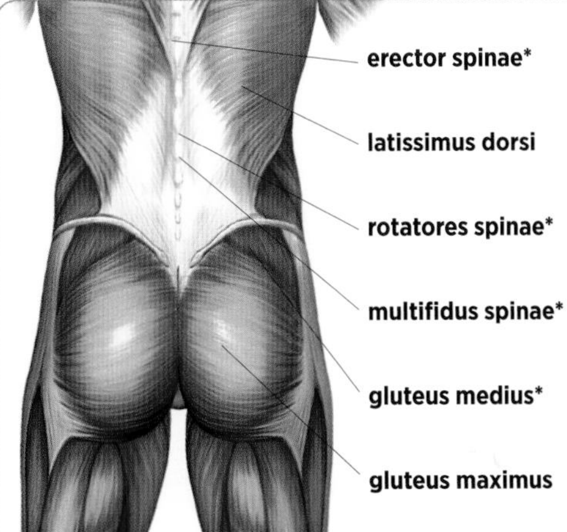

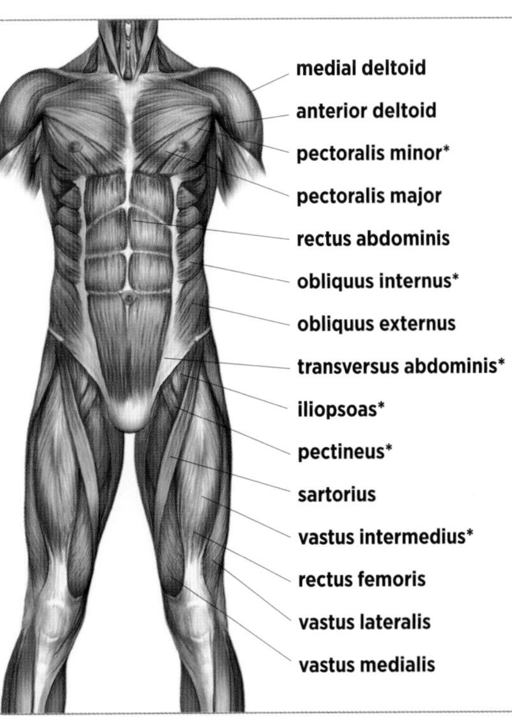

Annotation Key
Bold text indicates target muscles
Light text indicates other working muscles
* indicates deep muscles

DO IT RIGHT
- Keep your back straight.
- Bend your elbows when performing the twist.
- Keep your moving leg as straight as possible.

Two-Level Push-Up

The explosive Two-Level Push-Up takes your fitness to another level. This plyometric exercise uses a higher power movement to target your chest in a way that will improve power, strength, and coordination.

HOW TO DO IT

- Place two aerobics steps or low boxes on the floor. Position your palms shoulder-width apart between the steps, and assume a high plank position, balancing on your toes with your feet together and your back in a neutral position.
- Keeping your torso rigid and your legs straight, bend your elbows to lower your chest toward the floor to perform a push-up.
- In one explosive movement, press up from the floor, extending your arms dynamically to elevate your body with enough velocity to allow yourself to place your hands on the steps on either side of your torso.
- In a high plank position on the steps, repeat the steps above, performing a push-up on the steps, and then catching yourself once again on the floor between the equipment. Repeat for the recommended repetitions.

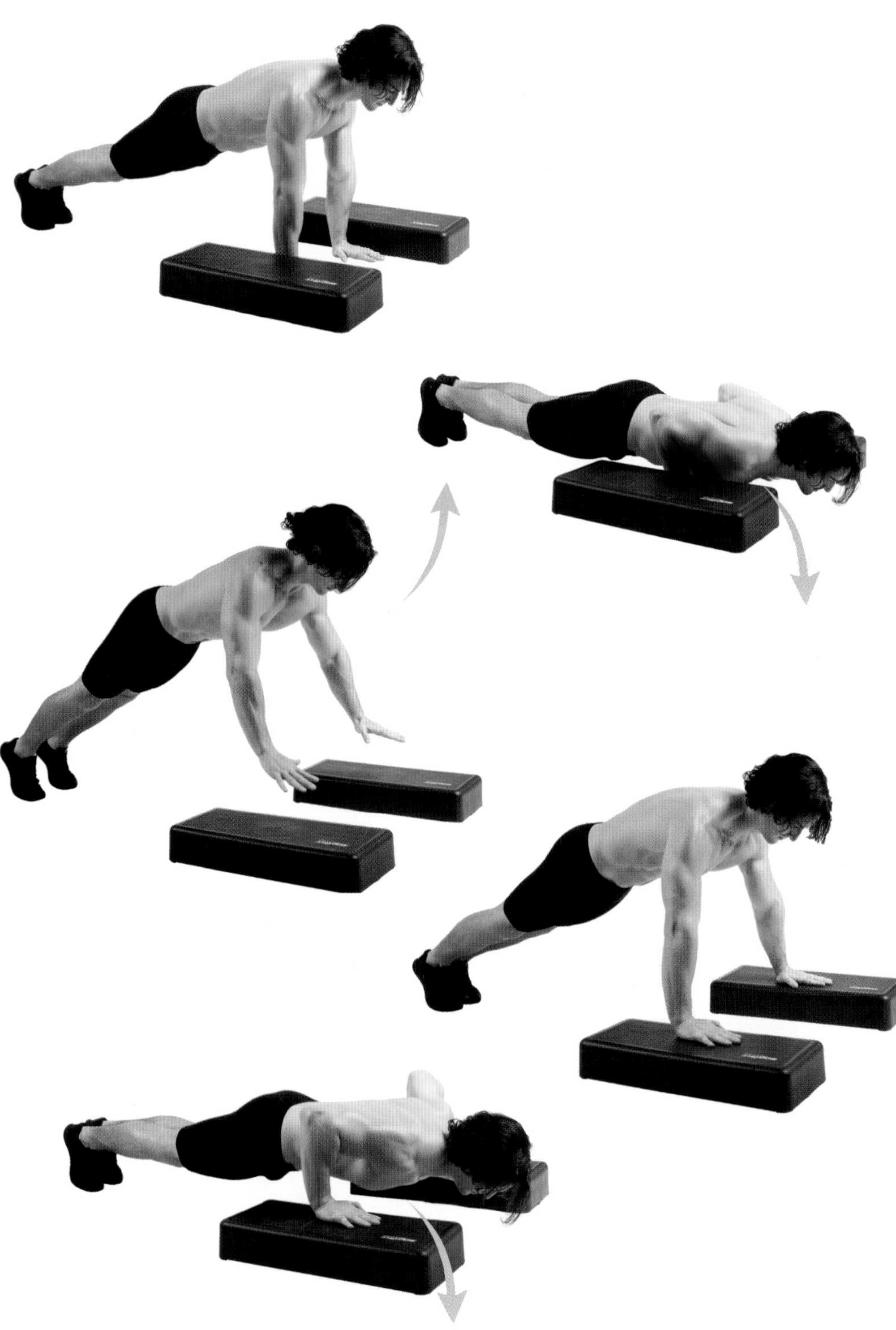

DO IT RIGHT

- Keep your back straight.
- Avoid any excessive arching in the spine.
- Bend your elbows to absorb the shock of landing.

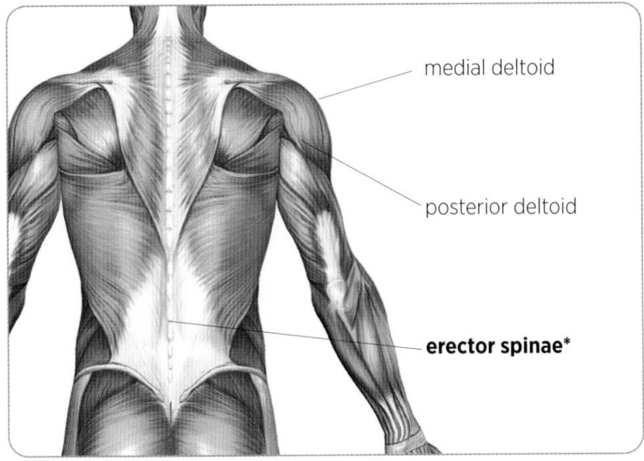

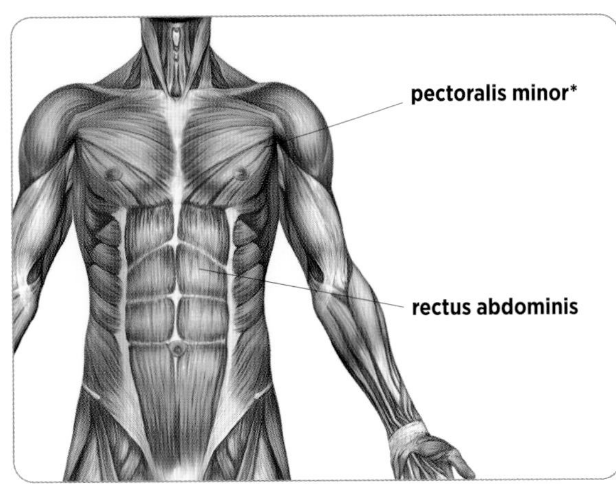

latissimus dorsi

obliquus externus

obliquus internus*

anterior deltoid

pectoralis major

biceps brachii

triceps brachii

rectus femoris

Annotation Key

Bold text indicates target muscles
Light text indicates other working muscles
* indicates deep muscles

FACT FILE

TARGETS
- Pectorals
- Deltoids
- Abdominals
- Triceps

TYPE
- Dynamic

BENEFITS
- Strengthens and tones abdominals, chest, and arms
- Increases cardiovascular endurance
- Improves coordination

CAUTIONS
- Shoulder issues
- Wrist issues
- Elbow issues

EQUIPMENT
- Boxes or steps

Jump Rope

Channel your inner child and perform this school-yard favorite. Jump Rope, also called Skip Rope, is a great cardio and strength exercise. This calorie burner works mainly on your calf muscles, while strengthening your bones and improving your balance and coordination. Perform as a rest between other exercise sets to recover your heart rate.

HOW TO DO IT

- Stand holding a rope in your hands, letting it hang behind your feet.

- Swing the rope around your body and jump over it. Keep your arms as straight as you can during the movement, and land with both feet together on the floor. Perform for recommended time.

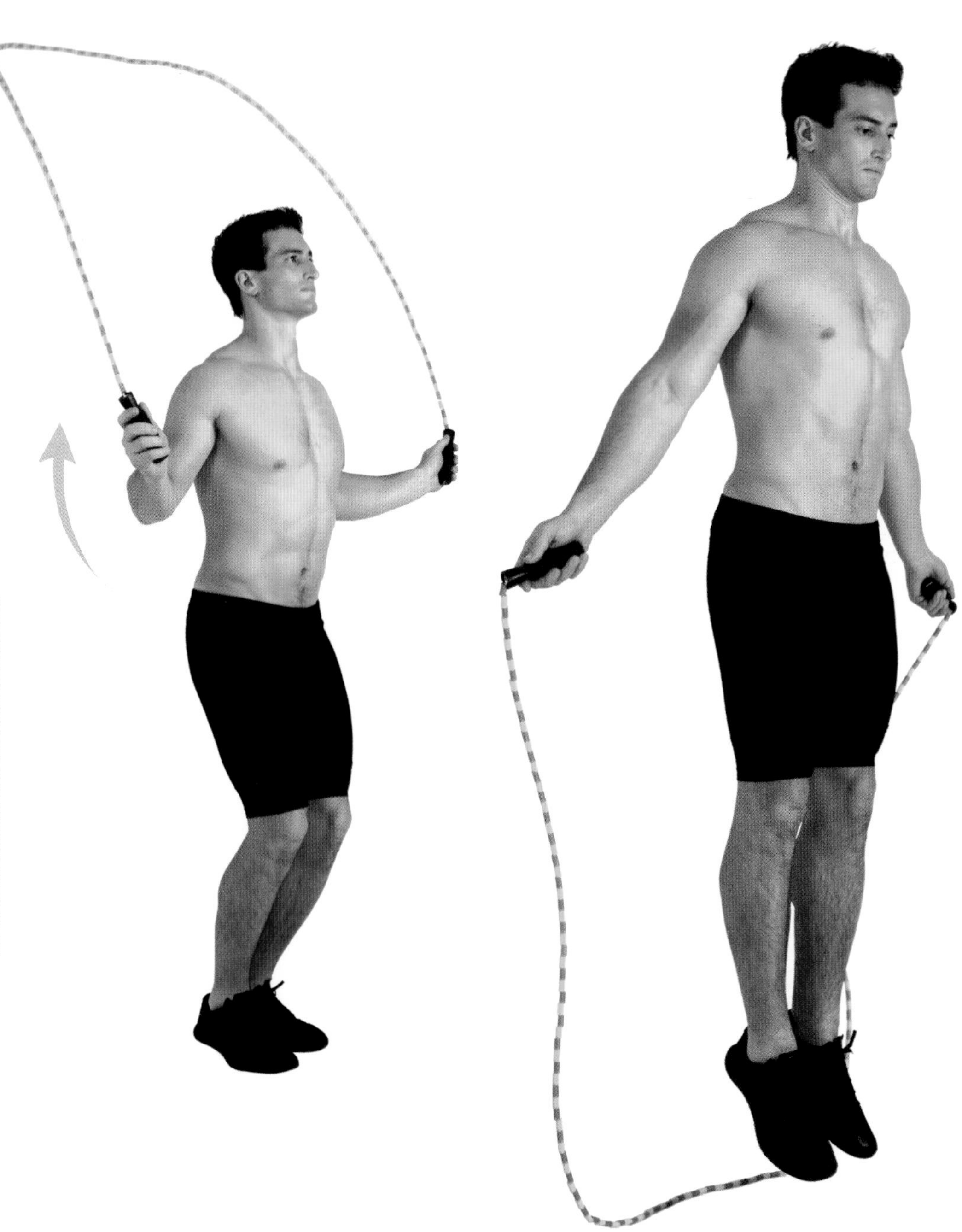

DO IT RIGHT

- Land on the balls of your feet; landing flat on your feet can compact your knees.
- To check if a jump rope is the right size for you, place one foot in the center of the rope, and then lift the handles—they shouldn't reach higher than your armpits.

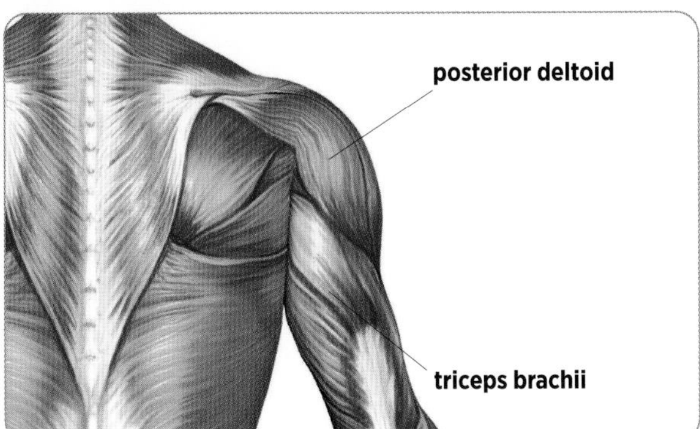

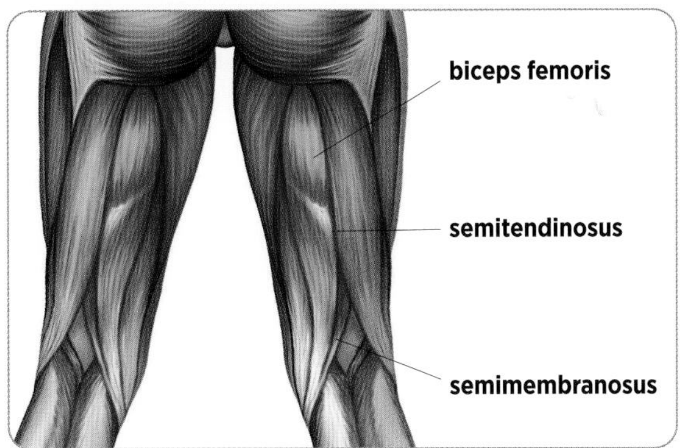

FACT FILE

TARGETS
- Legs
- Arms
- Shoulders
- Back

TYPE
- Dynamic

BENEFITS
- Strengthens arms, legs, back, and shoulders
- Increases cardiovascular endurance

CAUTIONS
- Wrist issues
- Ankle issues
- Knee pain

EQUIPMENT
- Jump rope

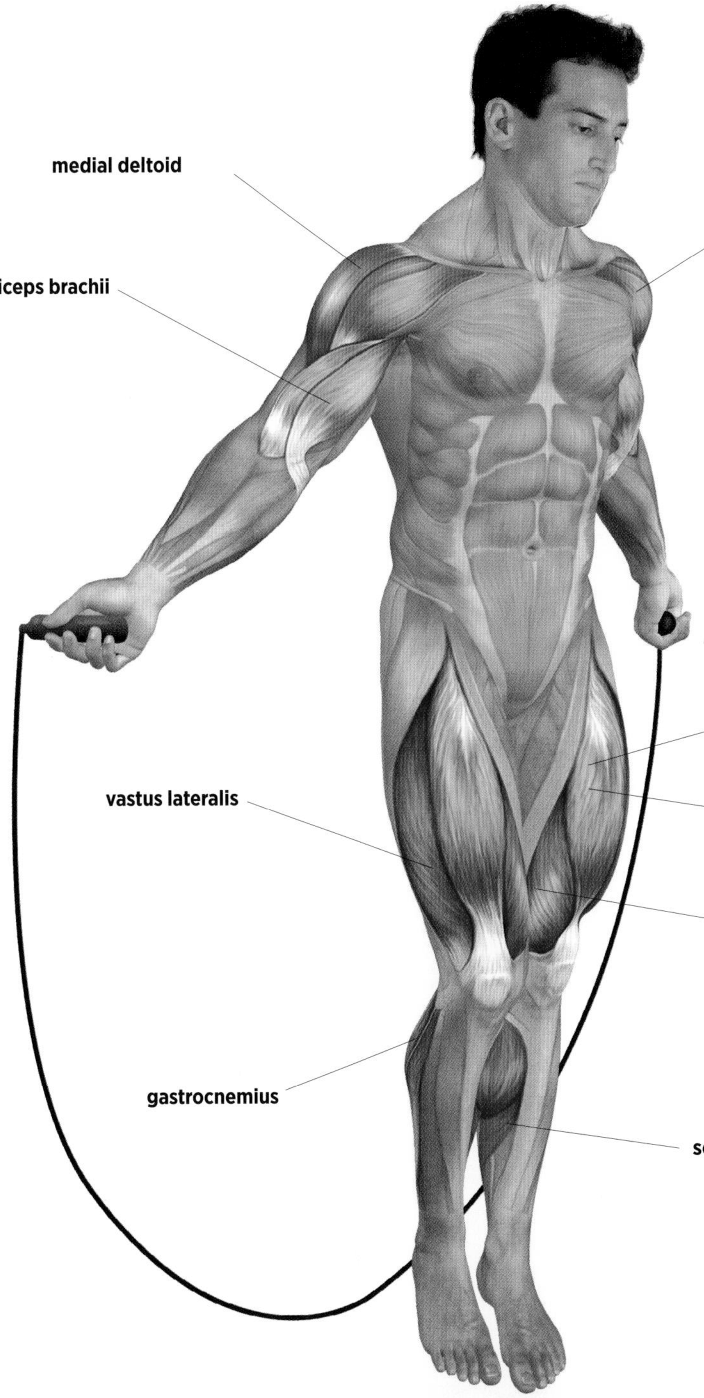

Annotation Key

Bold text indicates target muscles

Light text indicates other working muscles

* indicates deep muscles

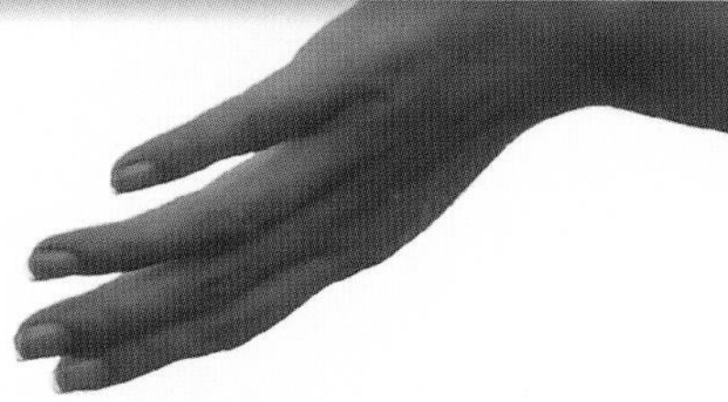

CHAPTER FOUR

BACK EXERCISES

Strengthening your back muscles can help prevent injuries and ensure that your entire body works smoothly during daily movement. It is very important to train your back muscles for posture because most of us sit all day long at work, often letting our shoulders roll forward. Your upper back muscles and lats are one of the largest muscular areas of the upper body and, as such, are essential in fat-loss workouts as well as hypertrophy workouts. That said, the back is one of the most difficult body parts to exercise because it is so energy draining when trained properly, so take your time and persevere.

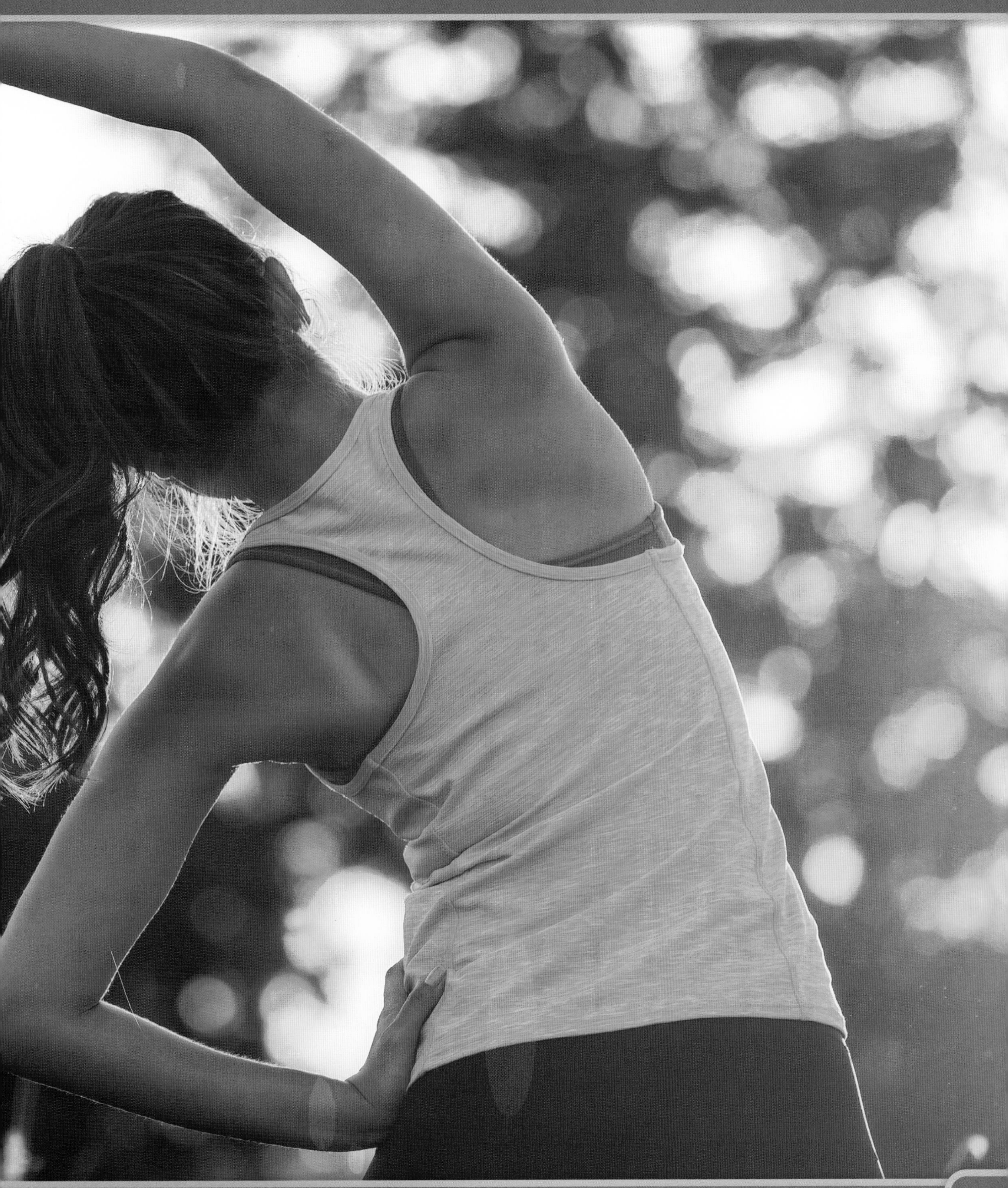

Thread the Needle

This spine-strengthener is popular in all kinds of training regimens. Thread the Needle gives your body a thorough rotation, with the arm movement building your core stability.

HOW TO DO IT

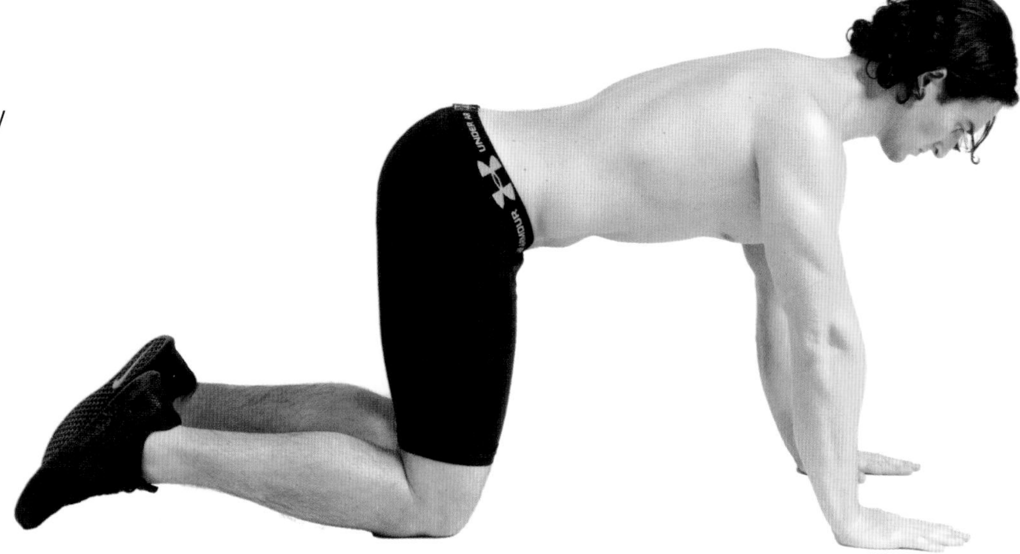

- Begin on all fours with your back flat and palms downward, directly below your shoulders.
- Turn your left hand over, so the back of your hand is now on the floor. Slide this hand behind your right arm and out to your right side, keeping the back of your hand on the floor. Bend your supporting arm as you slide your left hand out farther.
- Continue sliding until your left shoulder rests on the floor and your supporting arm is bent perpendicular. The side of your head should be resting on the floor with your gaze to the right.

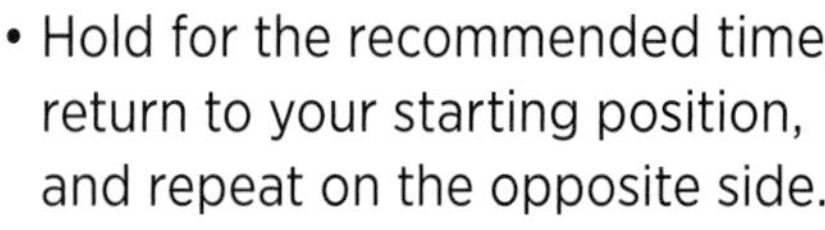

- Hold for the recommended time, return to your starting position, and repeat on the opposite side.

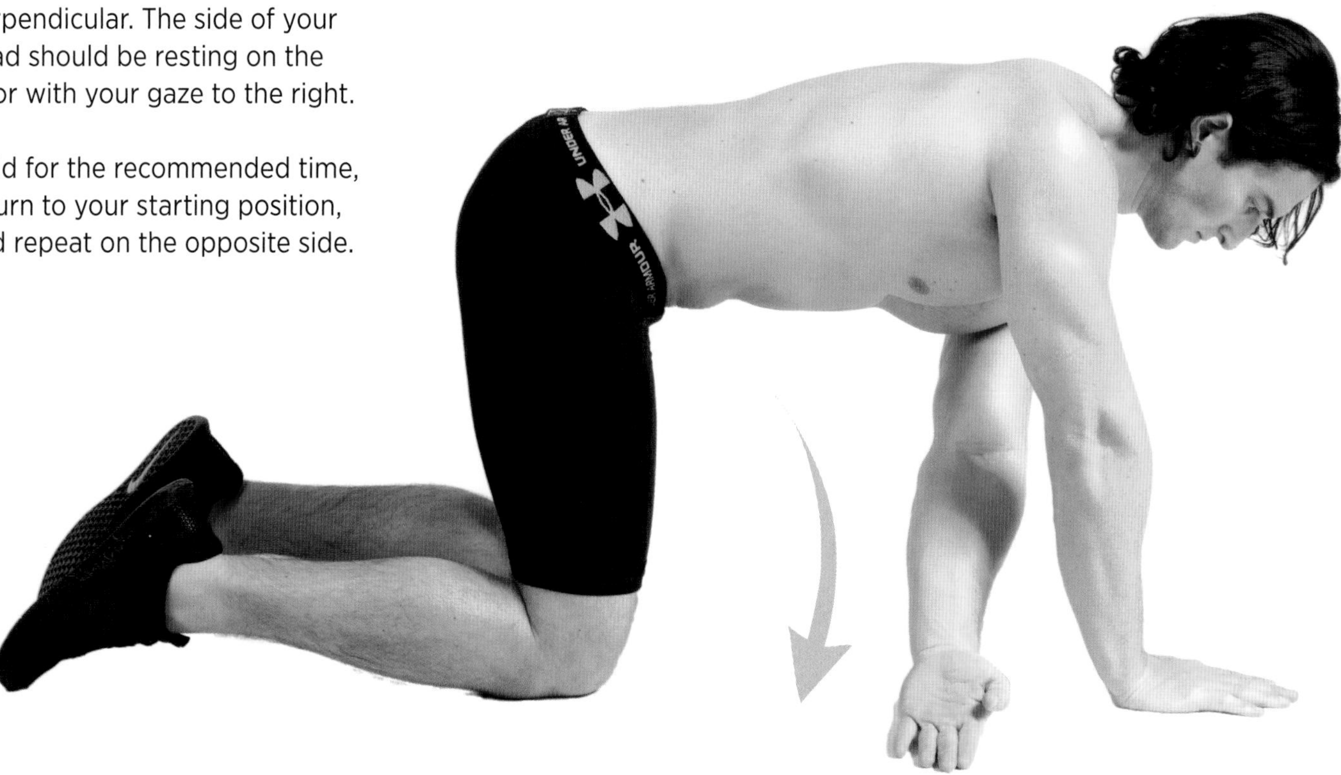

FACT FILE

TARGETS
- Back

TYPE
- Dynamic

BENEFITS
- Improves back and shoulder mobility
- Increases spinal flexibility

CAUTIONS
- Lower-back pain
- Wrist or elbow pain
- Shoulder issues

DO IT RIGHT

- Rotate evenly throughout.
- Move slowly through the exercise to complete the full range of motion.
- Keep your supporting arm engaged to maintain balance.

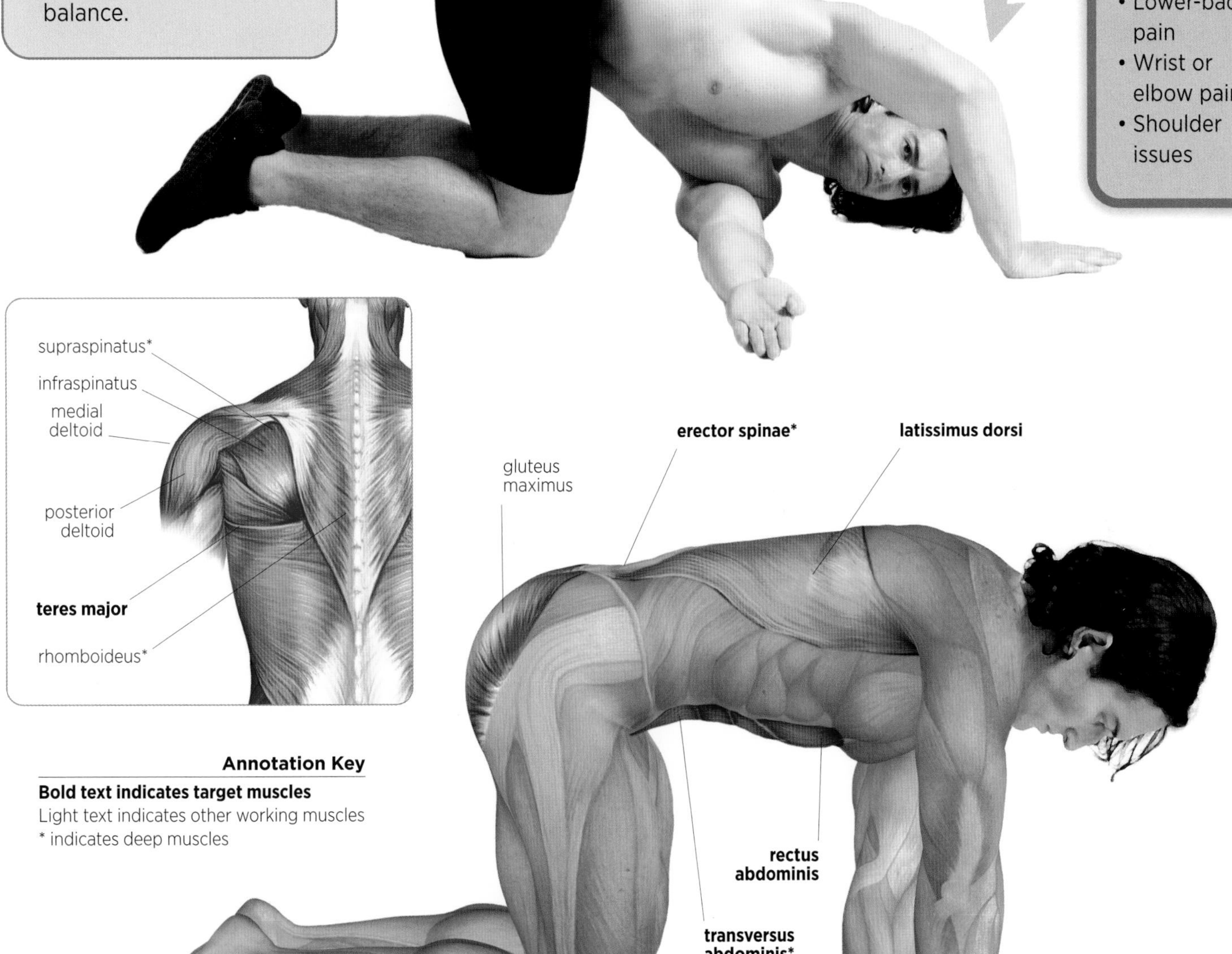

Annotation Key
Bold text indicates target muscles
Light text indicates other working muscles
* indicates deep muscles

Hip Crossover

The Hip Crossover effectively consolidates your core. As with many core exercises, aim for controlled movements. You want your muscles—not momentum—to move you.

HOW TO DO IT

- Lie on your back with your arms lengthened away from your body and your legs bent at a 90-degree angle and lifted off the floor.
- Brace your abs, and lower your knees to your right side, dropping them as close to the floor as possible without lifting your shoulders off the floor.
- Return to the starting position, hold for the recommended time, and repeat on the opposite side.

DO IT RIGHT

- Keep your core centered.
- Move carefully and with control.
- Avoid swinging your legs excessively.

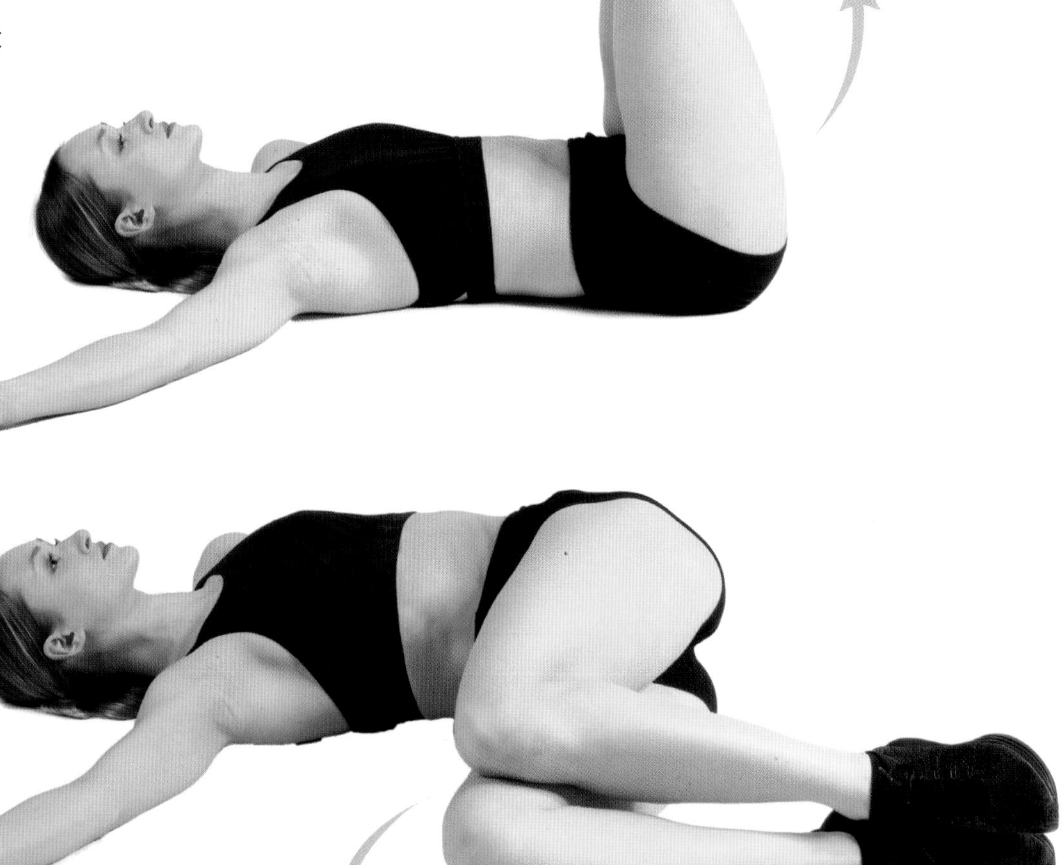

FACT FILE

TARGETS
- Lower back
- Obliques

TYPE
- Dynamic

BENEFITS
- Tones abdominals
- Stabilizes core

CAUTIONS
- Lower-back issues

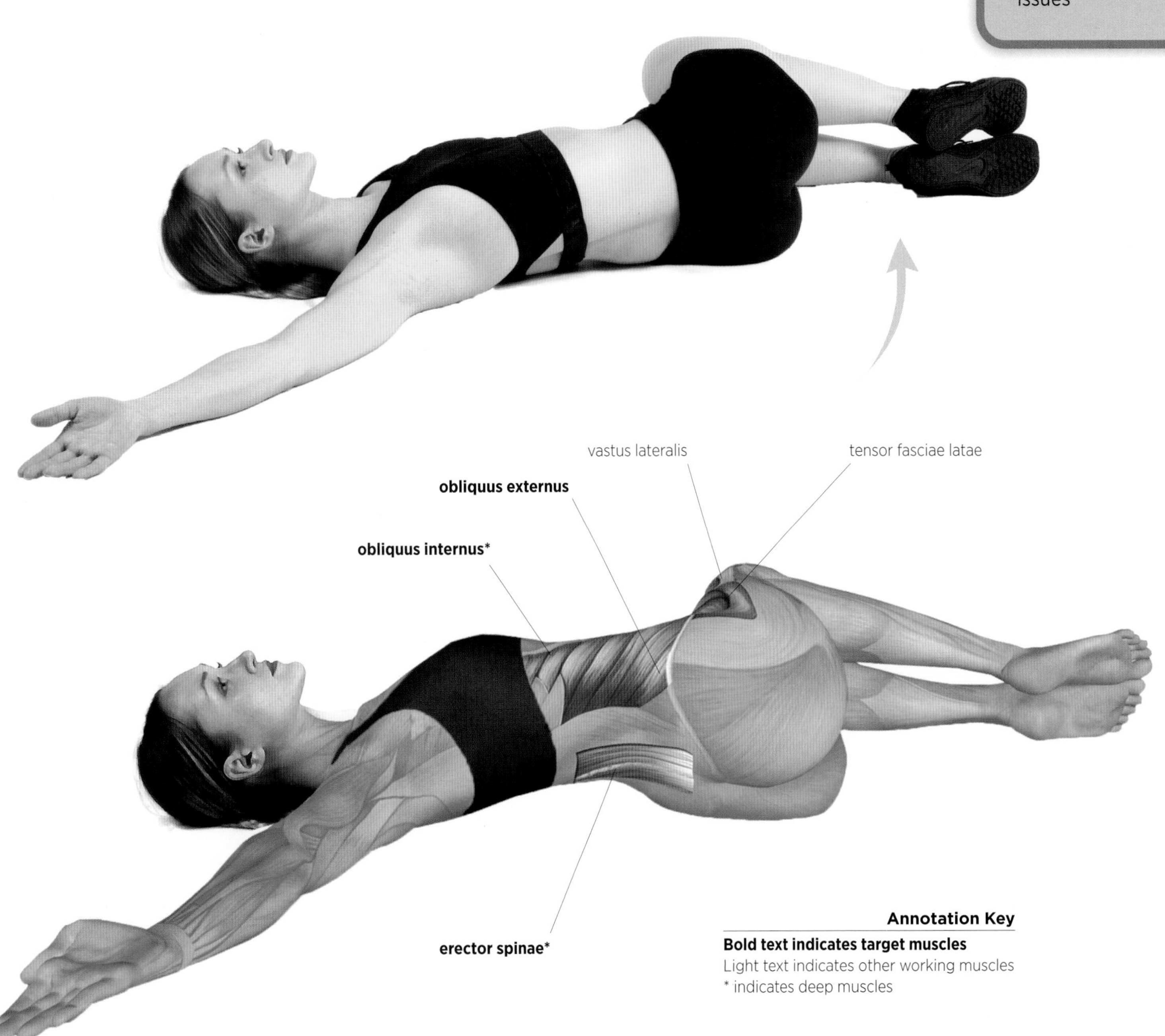

Annotation Key

Bold text indicates target muscles

Light text indicates other working muscles

* indicates deep muscles

Swimmer

The Swimmer engages pretty much every muscle in your body, but it is especially effective at strengthening both your hip extensors and the muscles that support your spine.

HOW TO DO IT

- Lie facedown with your legs hip-width apart. Stretch your arms beside your ears on the floor. Engage your pelvic floor, and draw your navel into your spine.
- Extend through your upper back as you lift your left arm and right leg simultaneously. Lift your head and shoulders off the floor.
- Lower your arm and leg to the starting position, maintaining a stretch in your limbs throughout.
- Extend your opposite arm and leg off the floor, lengthening and lifting your head and shoulders.
- Elongate your limbs as you return to the starting position. Repeat, alternating sides for the recommended repetitions.

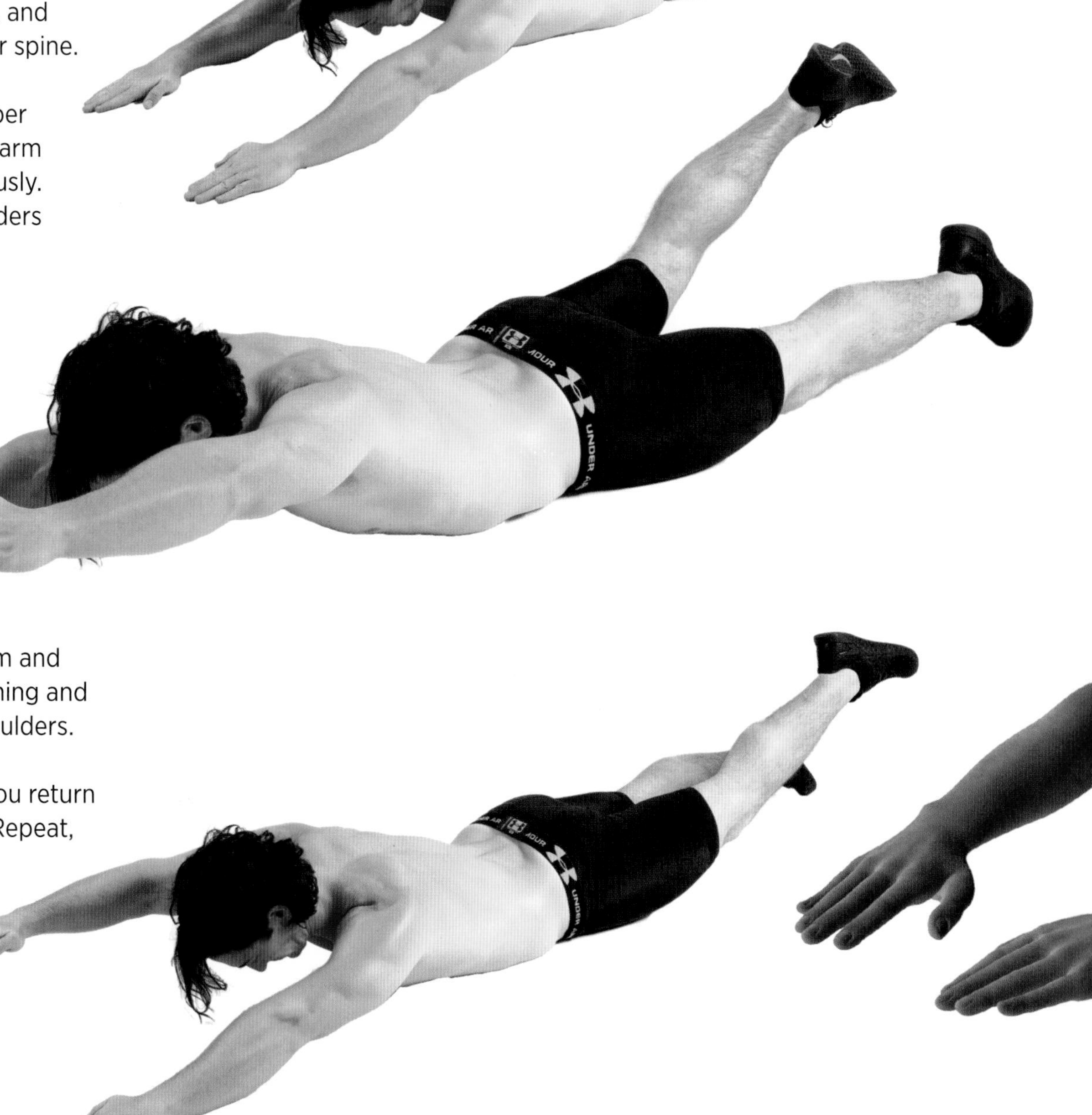

MODIFICATION

HARDER: Instead of lifting the opposite leg and arm, lift both arms and legs simultaneously, continuing to draw your navel into your spine. This version of the exercise is known as the Superman.

FACT FILE

TARGETS
- Hips
- Spine

TYPE
- Dynamic

BENEFITS
- Strengthens hip and spine extensors
- Challenges stabilization of the spine against rotation

CAUTIONS
- Lower-back pain
- Extreme curvature of upper spine
- Curvature of lower spine

Annotation Key

Bold text indicates target muscles

Light text indicates other working muscles

* indicates deep muscles

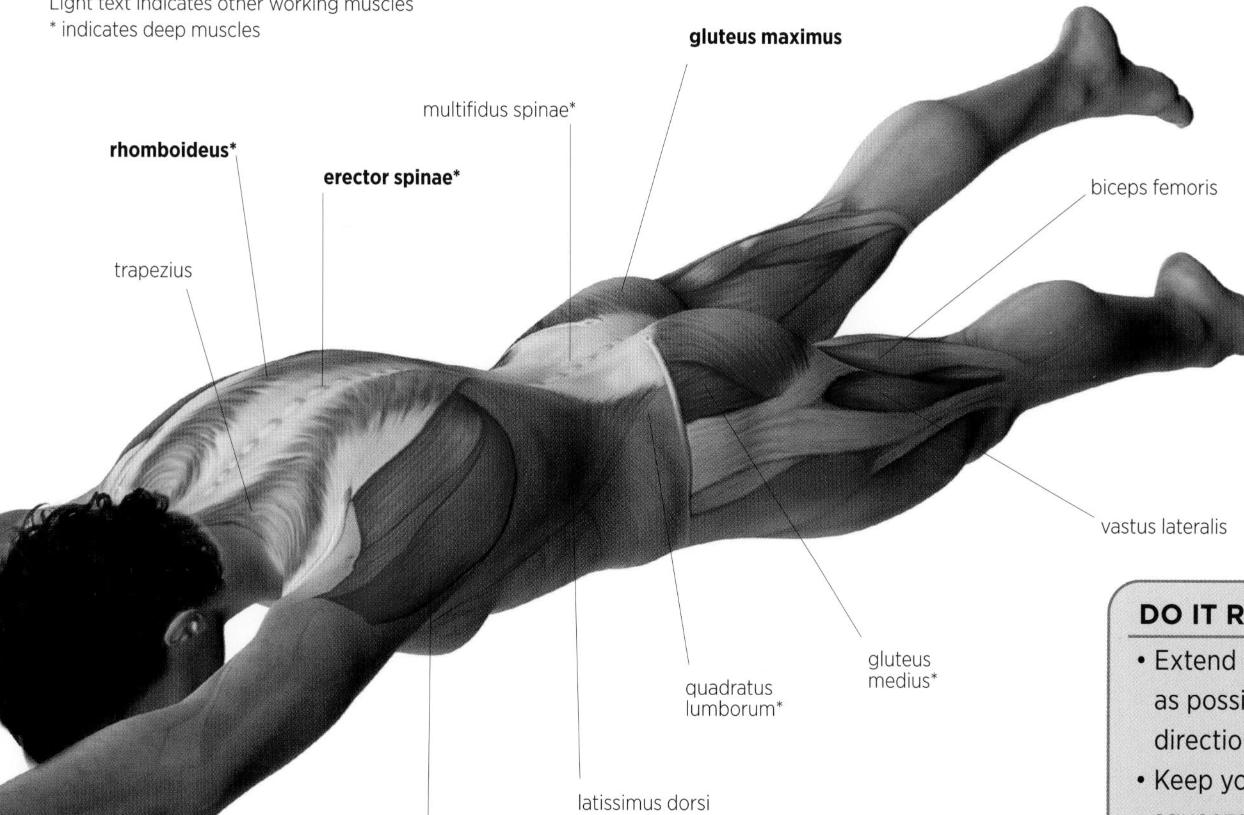

DO IT RIGHT

- Extend your limbs as long as possible in opposite directions.
- Keep your glutes tightly squeezed and your navel drawn in.
- Keep your neck long and relaxed.
- Avoid allowing your shoulders to lift toward your ears.

Alligator Crawl

In the fun but challenging Alligator Crawl, you imitate an alligator stalking its prey. The movements work your chest, shoulders, back, and arms.

HOW TO DO IT

- Begin in a high plank position with your palms on the floor and your back straight.
- Lower into a half push-up position, keeping your back straight.
- Keeping your body low to the floor, bring your right knee to your right elbow while walking your left hand forward.
- Repeat on the opposite side by walking your right hand forward and bringing your left knee to your left elbow.
- Continue moving forward, alternating your hand and knee positions. Perform for the recommended time.

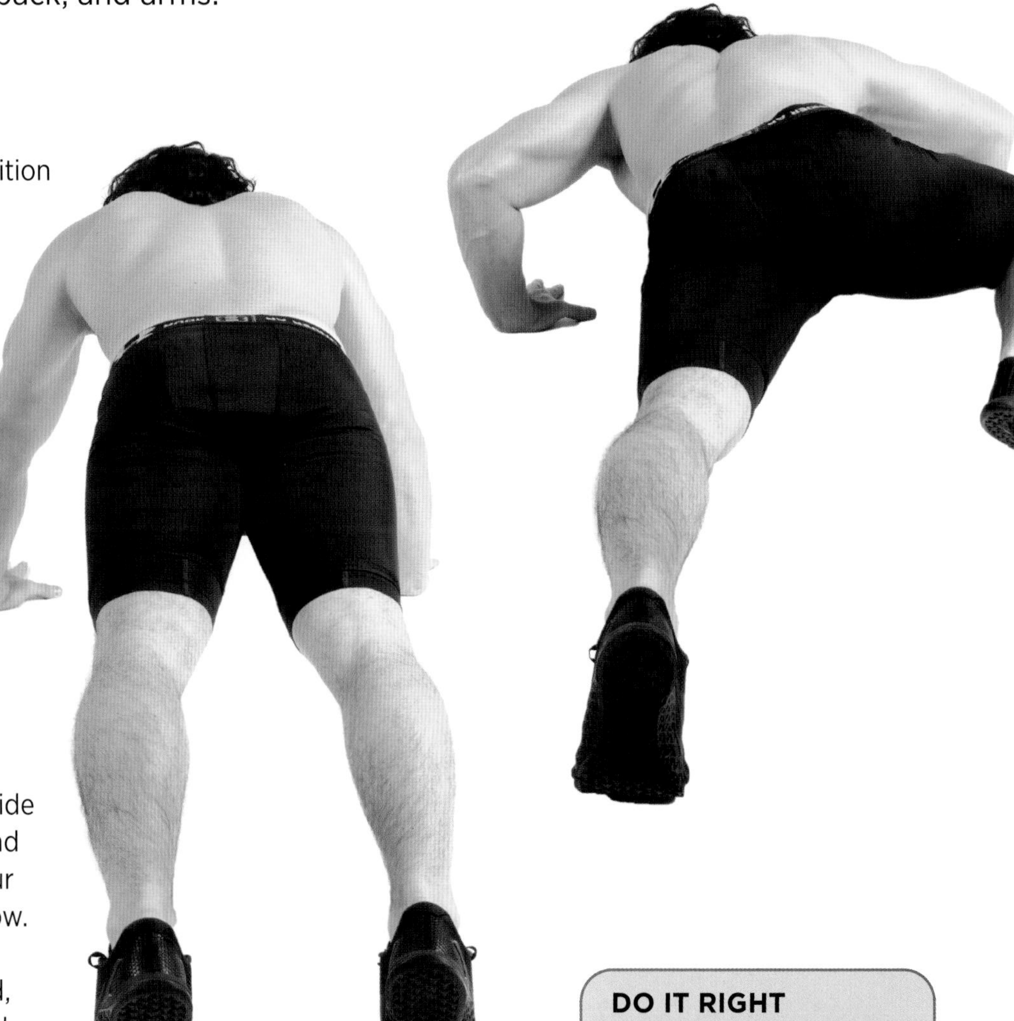

DO IT RIGHT

- Keep your body in a hover position close to the floor, with your elbows at 90 degrees during the entire exercise.
- Avoid allowing your hips to rise.
- Avoid straightening your arms.

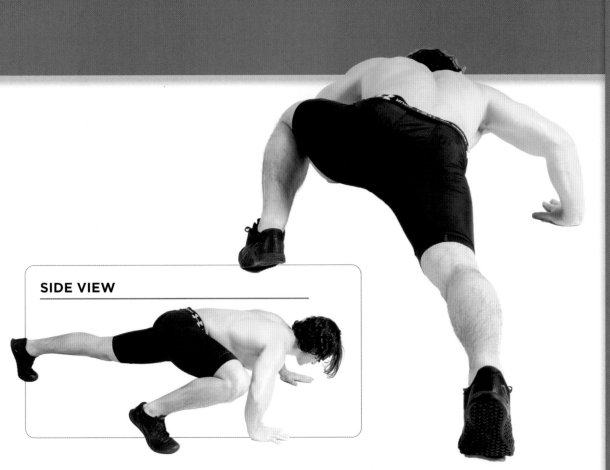

FACT FILE

TARGETS
- Pectorals
- Deltoids
- Back
- Biceps
- Triceps

TYPE
- Dynamic

BENEFITS
- Strengthens upper body
- Increases agility
- Improves coordination

CAUTIONS
- Shoulder issues
- Wrist issues
- Lower-back issues

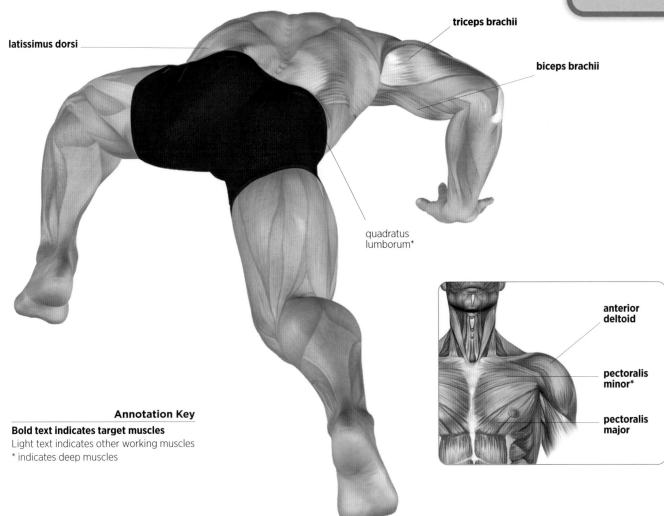

latissimus dorsi

triceps brachii

biceps brachii

quadratus lumborum*

anterior deltoid

pectoralis minor*

pectoralis major

Annotation Key

Bold text indicates target muscles

Light text indicates other working muscles

* indicates deep muscles

Back Burner

The Back Burner strengthens your lower back as well as all of your abdominal muscles. With regular practice, you'll build a strong core while enhancing your posture.

HOW TO DO IT

- Lie on your stomach with your arms extended in front of you. Your legs should be weighted into the floor with feet pointed. Press your navel to your spine and your shoulders down your back.

- Lift your extended arms off the floor and pulse them up and down for the recommended repetitions.

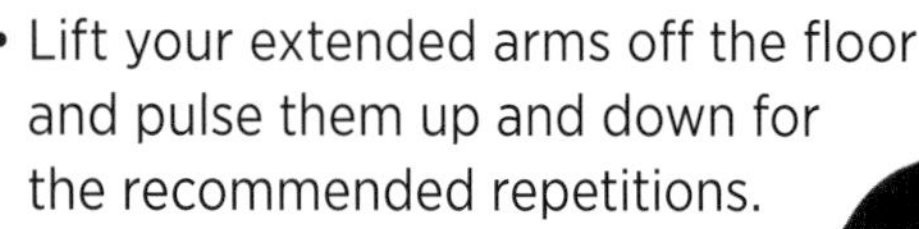

- Reposition your arms so that they are at 10:00 and 2:00 on an imaginary clock. Perform a further recommended number of pulses from this position.

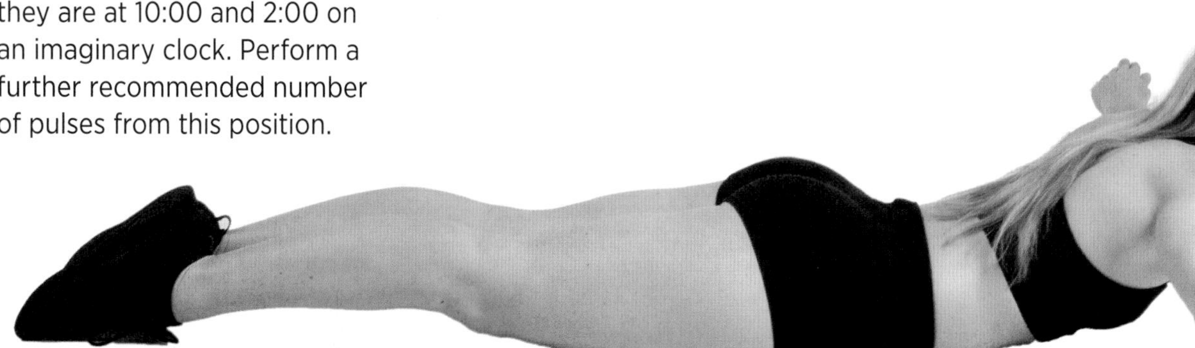

- Keeping your shoulders down, move your arms to the 3:00 and 9:00 position. Perform a further recommended number of pulses from this position.

- Bring both arms behind you, angled slightly with palms inward. With the action originating from your shoulders, perform a further recommended number of pulses from this position.

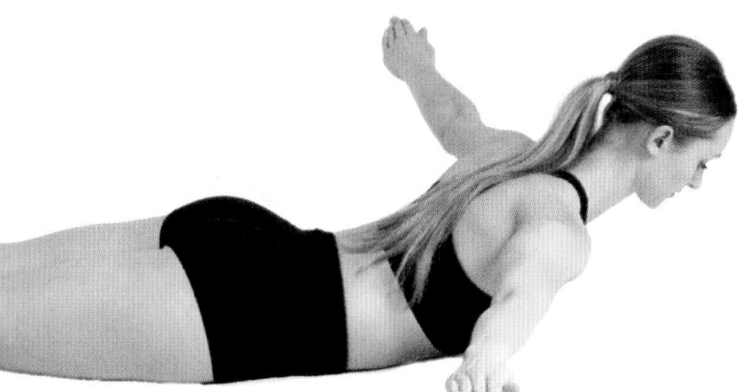

FACT FILE

TARGETS
- Lower back
- Abdominals
- Glutes

TYPE
- Dynamic

BENEFITS
- Strengthens lower-back muscles
- Strengthens abdominals
- Improves posture

CAUTIONS
- Lower-back issues
- Other back issues
- Shoulder issues

DO IT RIGHT

- Keep your abdominals strong and your hips stable.
- Look toward the floor to elongate your neck.
- Keep your torso and legs still throughout.
- Move your arms from under your shoulder blades.
- Avoid hunching your shoulders.
- Avoid lifting your feet off the floor.

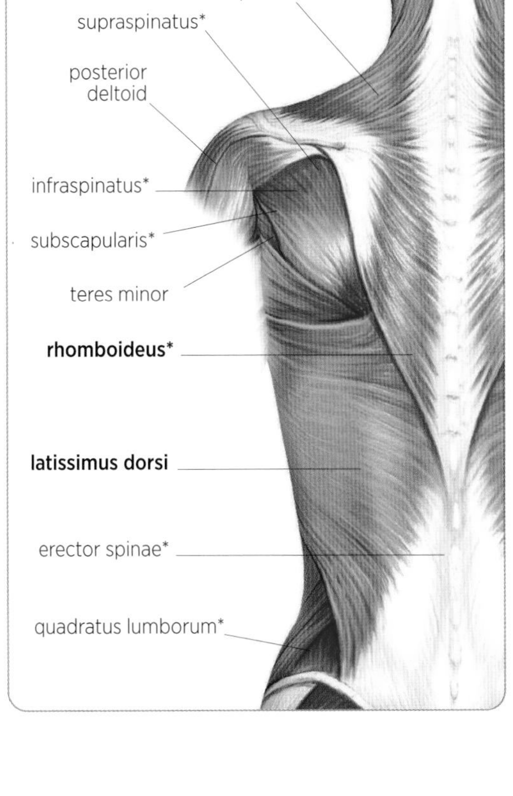

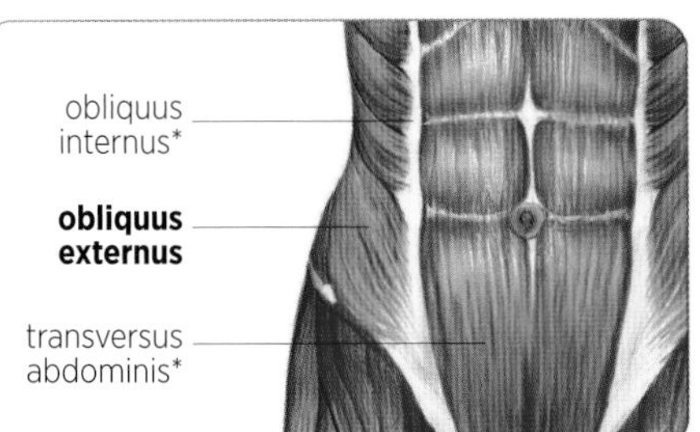

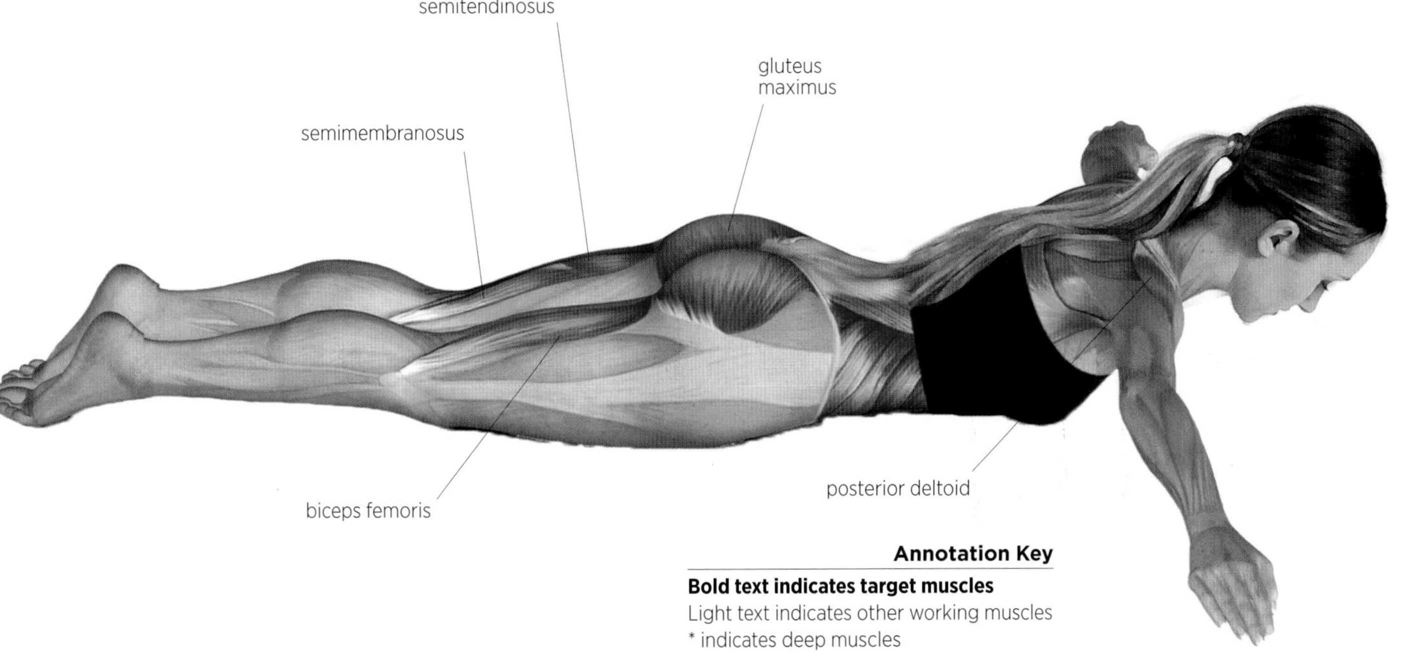

Annotation Key

Bold text indicates target muscles

Light text indicates other working muscles

* indicates deep muscles

Arm Hauler

A go-to exercise of special forces teams, the Arm Hauler builds upper-back and rear-shoulder strength. It is also an effective stabilizing exercise that can help prevent shoulder injuries.

HOW TO DO IT

- Lie facedown, and spread your arms wide, keeping them level with your shoulders.
- Lift your head, keeping your chin up while arching your lower back. Bring your arms off the floor, and reach as far behind you as possible.
- Without letting your hands touch the floor, bring your arms forward in front of you, touching your fingers together.
- Bring your hands back to the starting position, and repeat for the recommended repetitions.

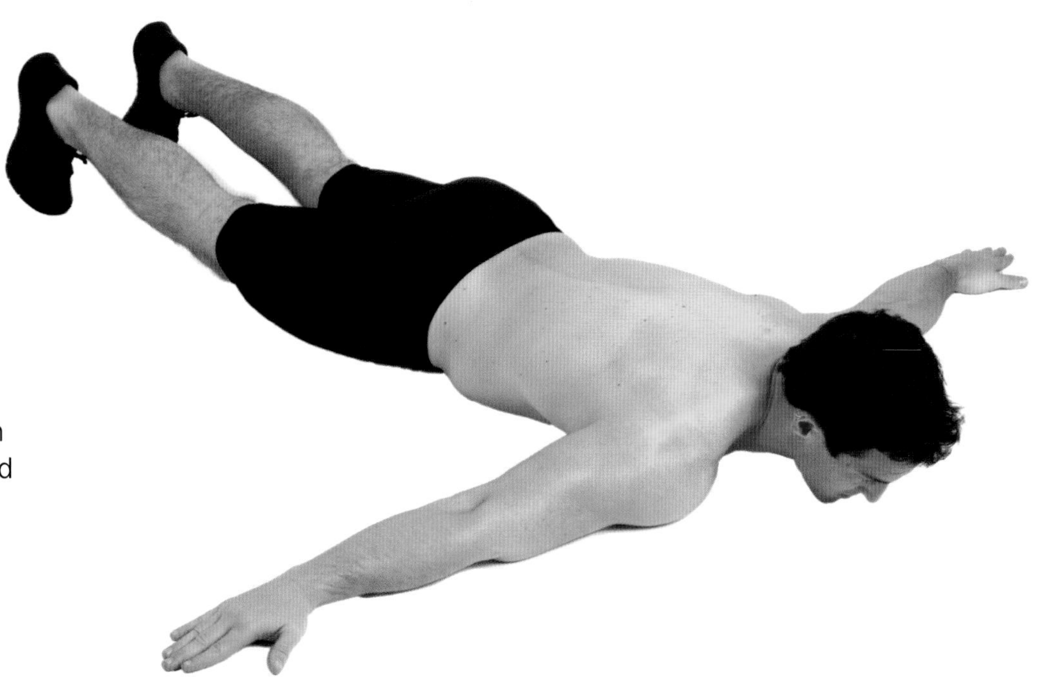

DO IT RIGHT

- Keep your chin up.
- Keep your lower back arched.
- Avoid dropping your head so that your chin touches the floor.

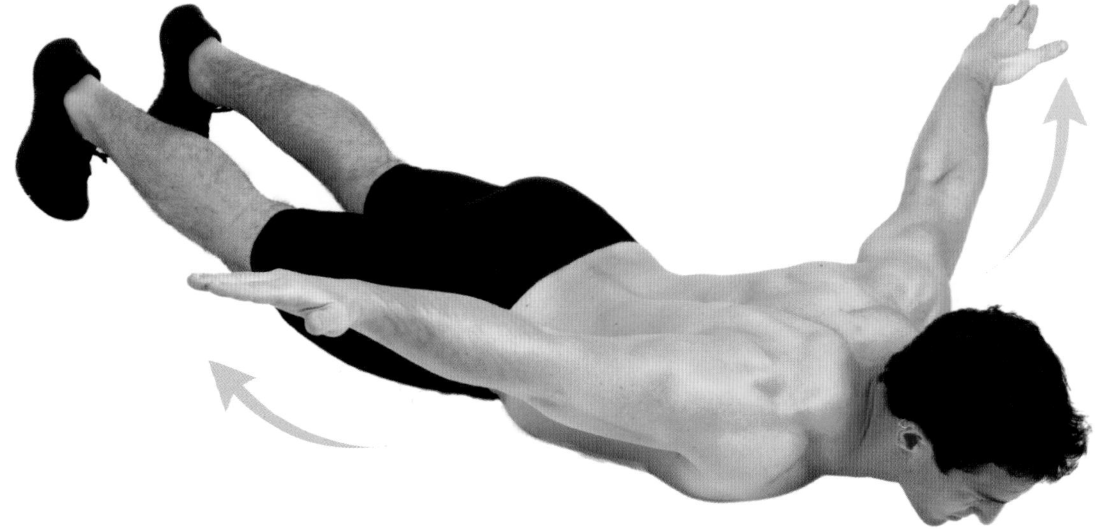

FACT FILE

TARGETS
- Upper back
- Shoulders

TYPE
- Dynamic

BENEFITS
- Strengthens and stabilizes back and shoulders

CAUTIONS
- Shoulder issues

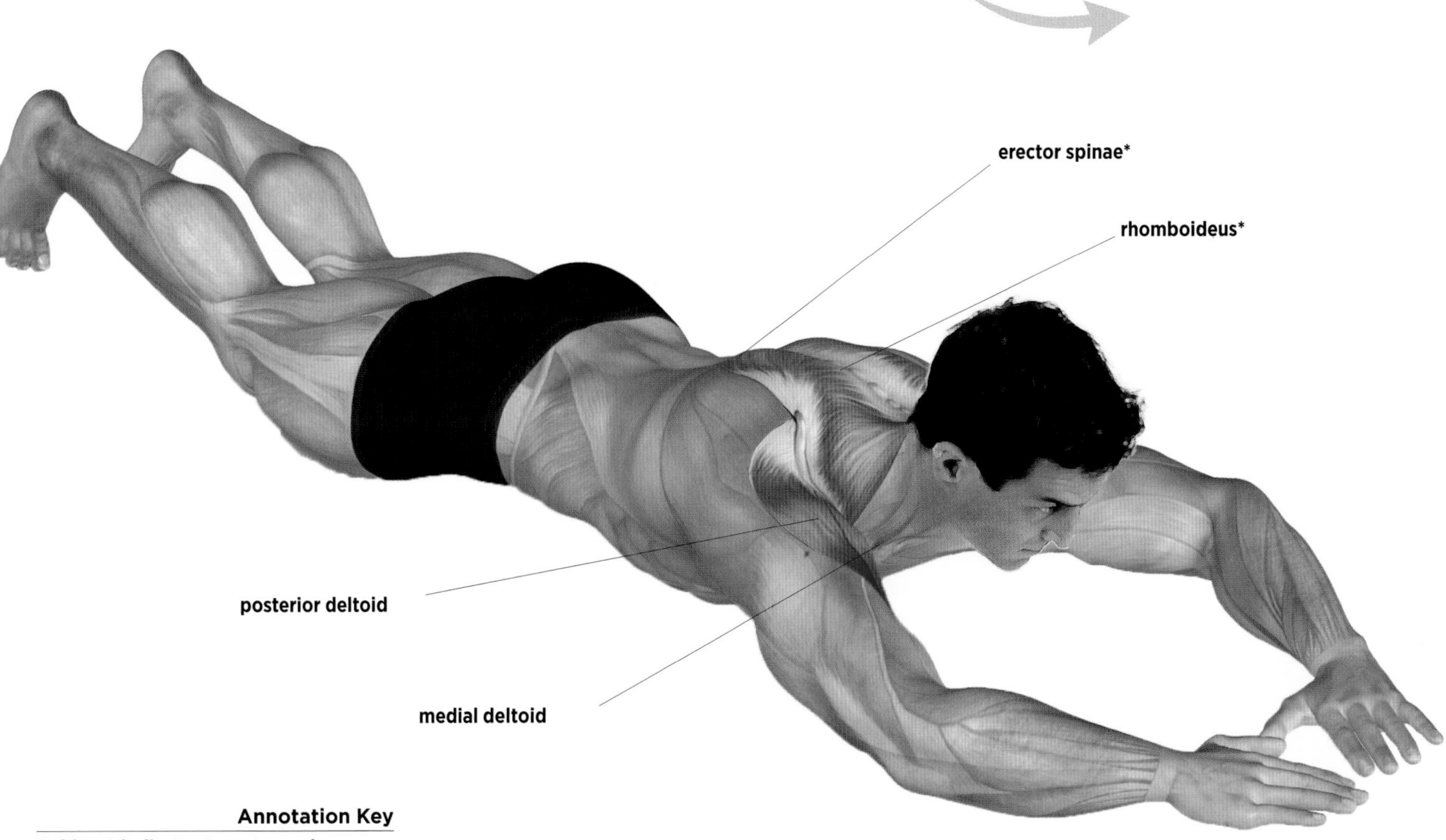

Annotation Key

Bold text indicates target muscles
Light text indicates other working muscles
* indicates deep muscles

Advanced Superman

The Advanced Superman builds on the Swimmer (pages 158–59), creating a medium-intensity exercise that strengthens your core and lower-back muscles.

HOW TO DO IT

- Lie facedown, and bend your elbows, placing your hands behind your ears. Extend your legs, and press down into the floor with your thighs and the tops of your feet.
- Lift your chest and legs off the floor. Hold for a few moments, and then lower yourself to the floor. Repeat for the recommended repetitions.

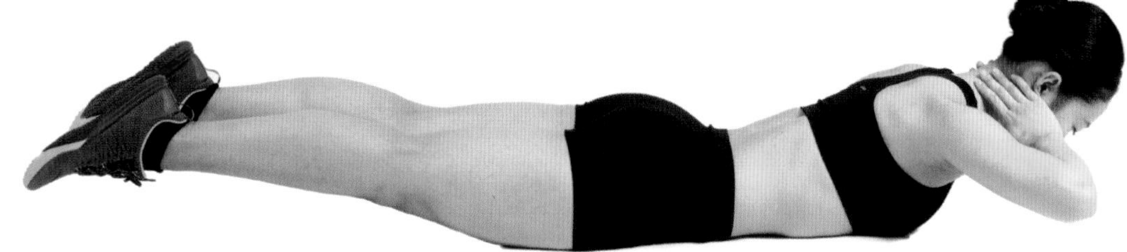

DO IT RIGHT

- Keep your body in a straight line.
- Avoid bending your knees.
- Avoid overarching your back.

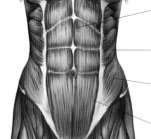

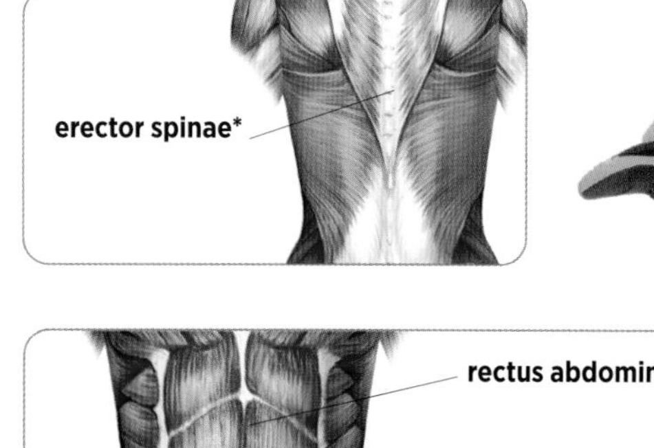

FACT FILE

TARGETS
- Core
- Lower back

TYPE
- Dynamic

BENEFITS
- Strengthens core and lower back

CAUTIONS
- Wrist pain
- Shoulder issues
- Lower-back pain

The Y

Named for the shape your body takes while performing it, The Y is a great body-weight exercise that develops your postural muscles. If you want a healthier back, this strengthener is one of the essentials you'll need to keep in your toolbox.

HOW TO DO IT

- Lie facedown on the floor with arms extended front and above you, placing your body in the shape of a Y.
- Keeping your lower body and torso planted on the floor, lift both arms. Lead with your thumbs and reach as high as possible.
- Return your arms to the floor, and repeat for the recommended repetitions.

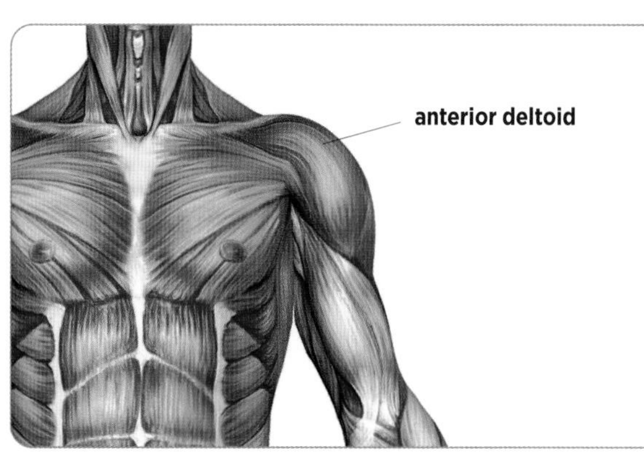

FACT FILE

TARGETS
- Deltoids
- Middle back

TYPE
- Dynamic

BENEFITS
- Warms up muscles
- Promotes proper scapular-humeral movement
- Strengthens and tones midscapular muscles

CAUTIONS
- Lower-back pain
- Extreme curvature of upper spine
- Curvature of lower spine

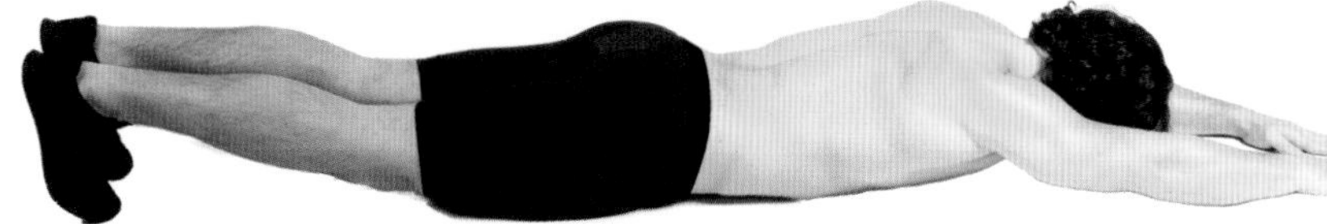

DO IT RIGHT

- Keep your torso on the floor.
- Avoid excessive trunk movement during exercise.
- Flare your hands out to ease shoulder stress.

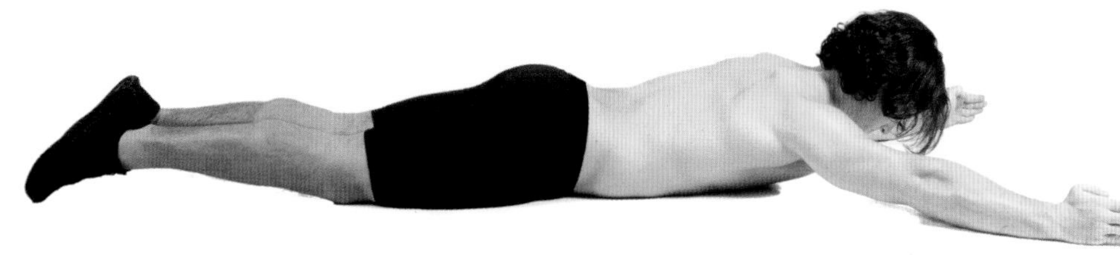

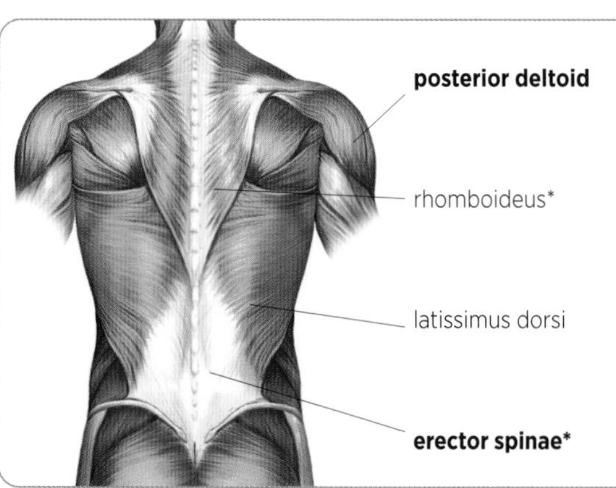

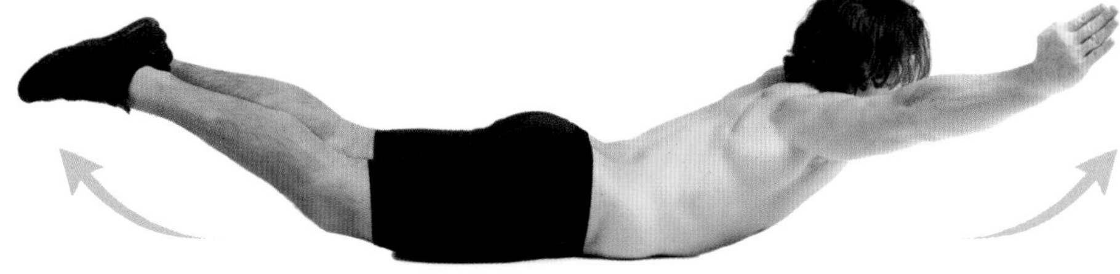

Annotation Key
Bold text indicates target muscles
Light text indicates other working muscles
* indicates deep muscles

Rotated Back Extension

The Rotated Back Extension, performed on a Swiss ball, gives your back and sides a significant stretch. It requires an engaged core, making it a strengthening exercise as well.

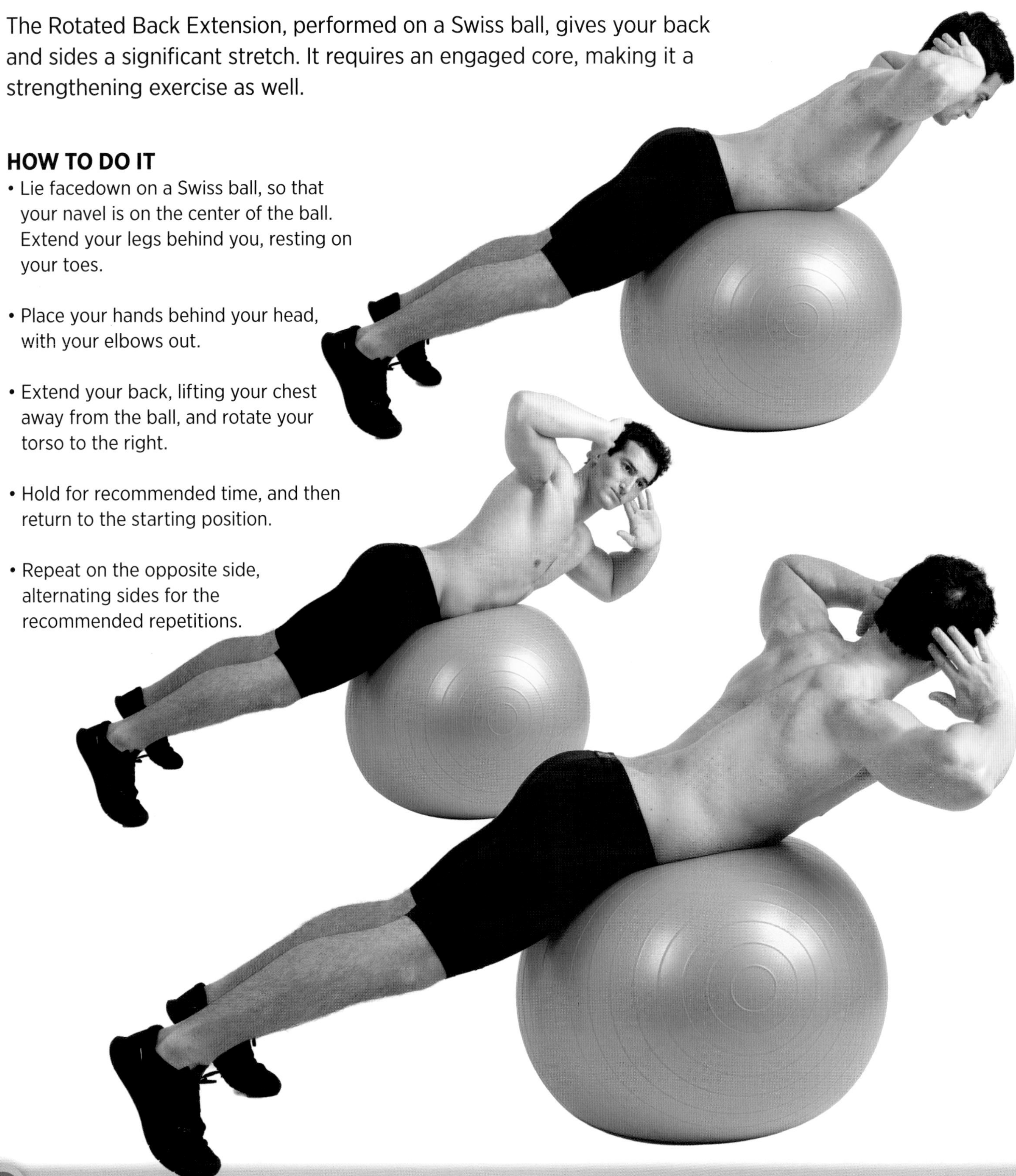

HOW TO DO IT

- Lie facedown on a Swiss ball, so that your navel is on the center of the ball. Extend your legs behind you, resting on your toes.
- Place your hands behind your head, with your elbows out.
- Extend your back, lifting your chest away from the ball, and rotate your torso to the right.
- Hold for recommended time, and then return to the starting position.
- Repeat on the opposite side, alternating sides for the recommended repetitions.

Annotation Key

Bold text indicates target muscles

Light text indicates other working muscles

* indicates deep muscles

pectoralis major
obliquus externus
transversus abdominis*
iliacus*
sartorius
anterior deltoid
rectus abdominis
serratus anterior
obliquus internus*
iliopsoas*

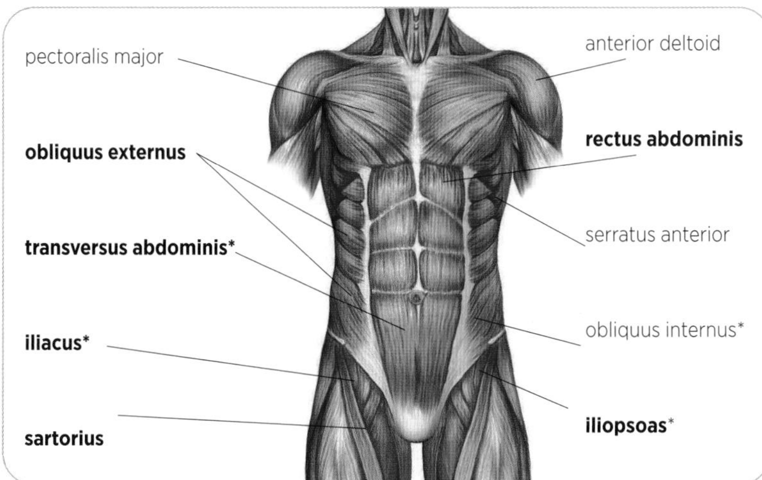

DO IT RIGHT

- Keep your toes firmly planted on the floor.
- Keep your arms out at a 90-degree angle to your body with your elbows bent.
- Widen your feet for increased stability.
- Avoid shifting your hips as you rotate—hold them square to the ball throughout the movement.

FACT FILE

TARGETS
- Middle back
- Lower-back
- Obliques

TYPE
- Dynamic

BENEFITS
- Stretches lower-back and obliques
- Strengthens core and back

CAUTIONS
- Neck issues
- Lower-back pain

EQUIPMENT
- Swiss ball

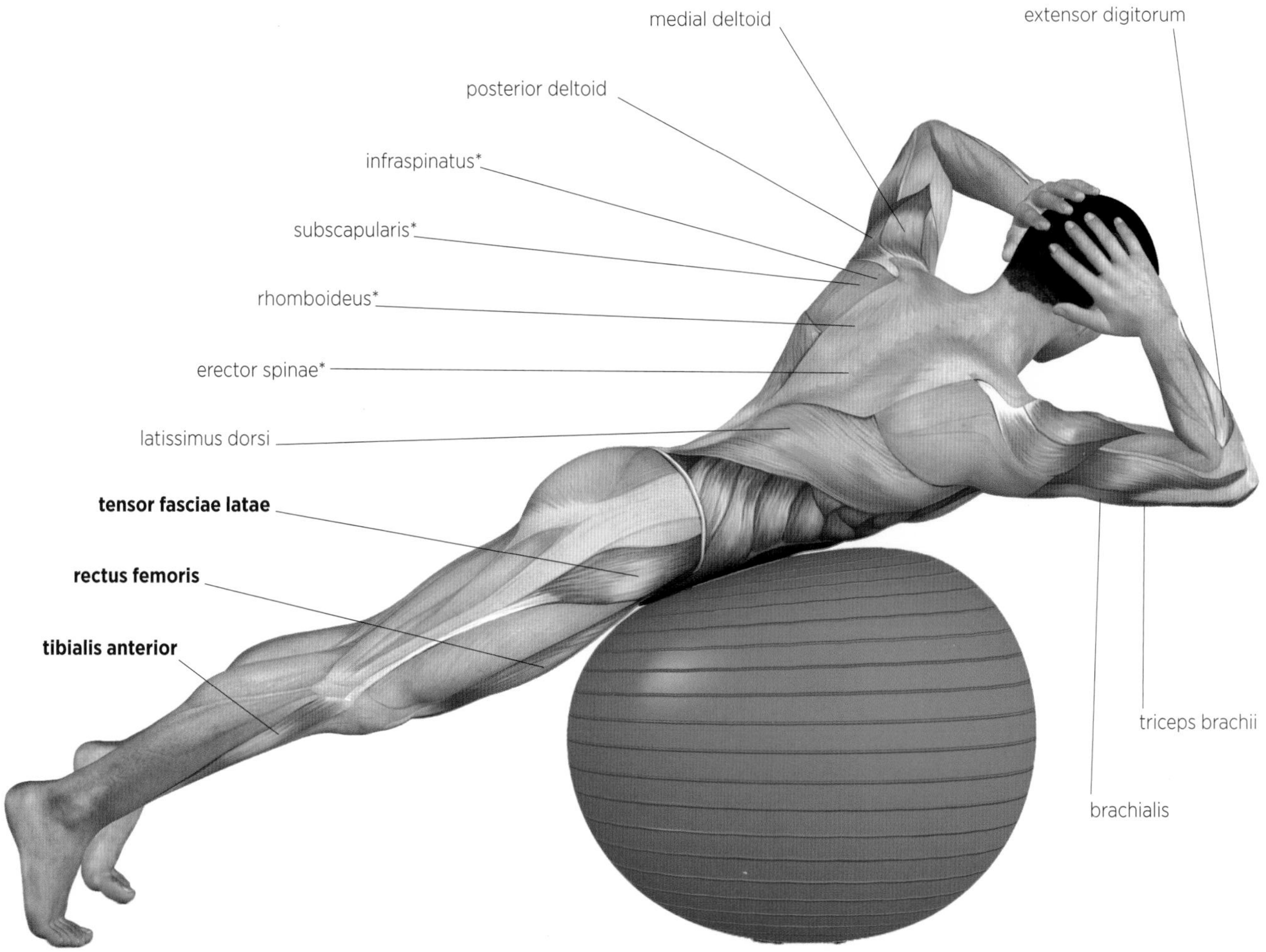

medial deltoid
extensor digitorum
posterior deltoid
infraspinatus*
subscapularis*
rhomboideus*
erector spinae*
latissimus dorsi
tensor fasciae latae
rectus femoris
tibialis anterior
triceps brachii
brachialis

Good Morning Bow

Good Morning Bows are a healthy back essential to keep in your toolbox. This simple exercise specifically focuses on your erector spinae, a bundle of deep muscles also known as your lumbar extensors. By strengthening these muscles, you can avoid lower back pain.

HOW TO DO IT

- Stand with your feet hips-width apart, arms positioned behind your head.
- Keeping your lower back in a neutral position and your legs straight, hinge at the hip to 90 degrees, or as far down as flexibility will allow.
- Return to upright position, by engaging your hip extensors, pushing your hips forward until you have assumed the starting position.

FACT FILE

TARGETS
- Lumbar extensors
- Hamstrings
- Glutes
- Core

TYPE
- Static

BENEFITS
- Warms up muscles
- Strengthens back, core, legs, and glutes

CAUTIONS
- Severe lower-back pain

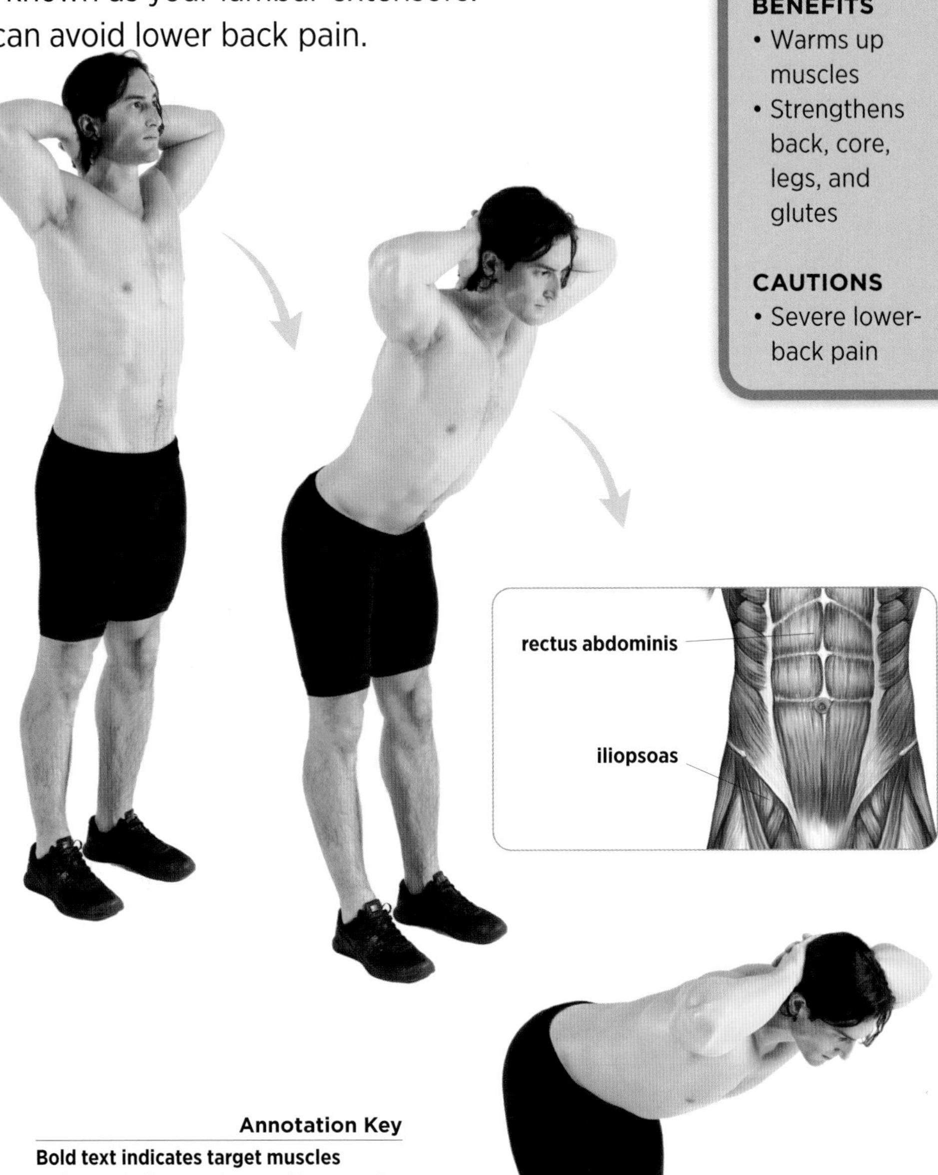

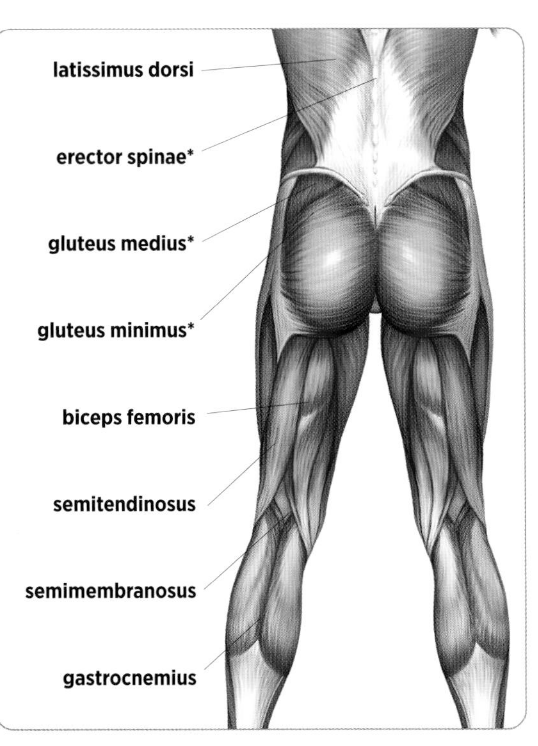

Annotation Key

Bold text indicates target muscles
Light text indicates other working muscles
* indicates deep muscles

DO IT RIGHT

- Keep your back and legs straight.
- Keep your shoulder blades pulled back and down.
- Avoid slumping.

Layout Push-Up

The Layout Push-Up is an advanced movement requiring intense effort from your back and core musculature. Don't let the "push-up" name fool you because this is not your average gym class exercise—rather than your pectorals, it mainly focuses on your triceps and lats.

HOW TO DO IT

- Lie facedown with your feet together. Stretch your arms upward beside your ears on the floor. Engage your pelvic floor, and draw your navel into your spine.

- While keeping your core engaged, lift your body up and away from the floor.

- Lower yourself back to the starting position, and repeat for the recommended repetitions.

DO IT RIGHT

- Keep your core engaged.
- Avoid excessive arching of your spine.

Annotation Key

Bold text indicates target muscles
Light text indicates other working muscles
* indicates deep muscles

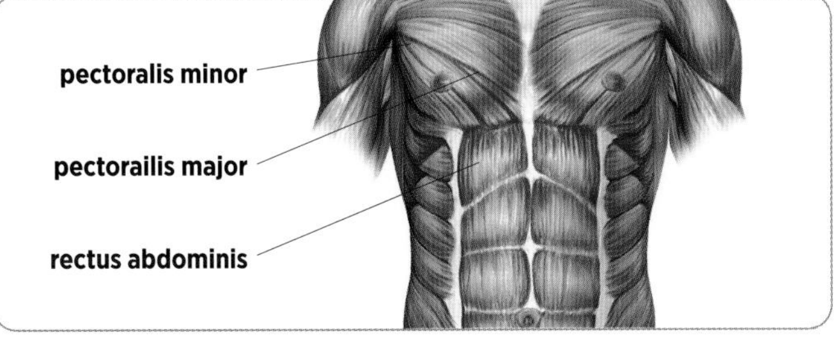

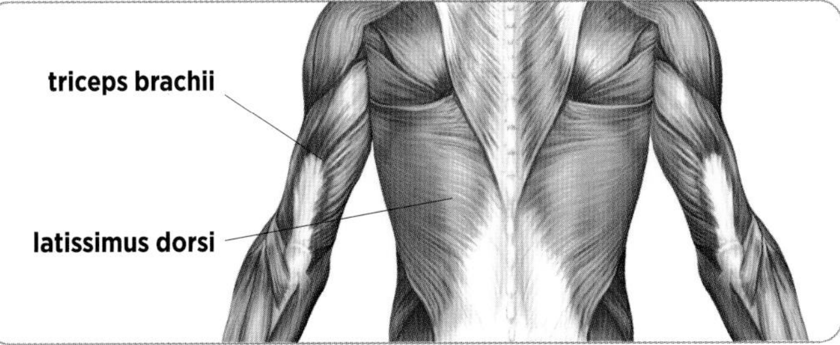

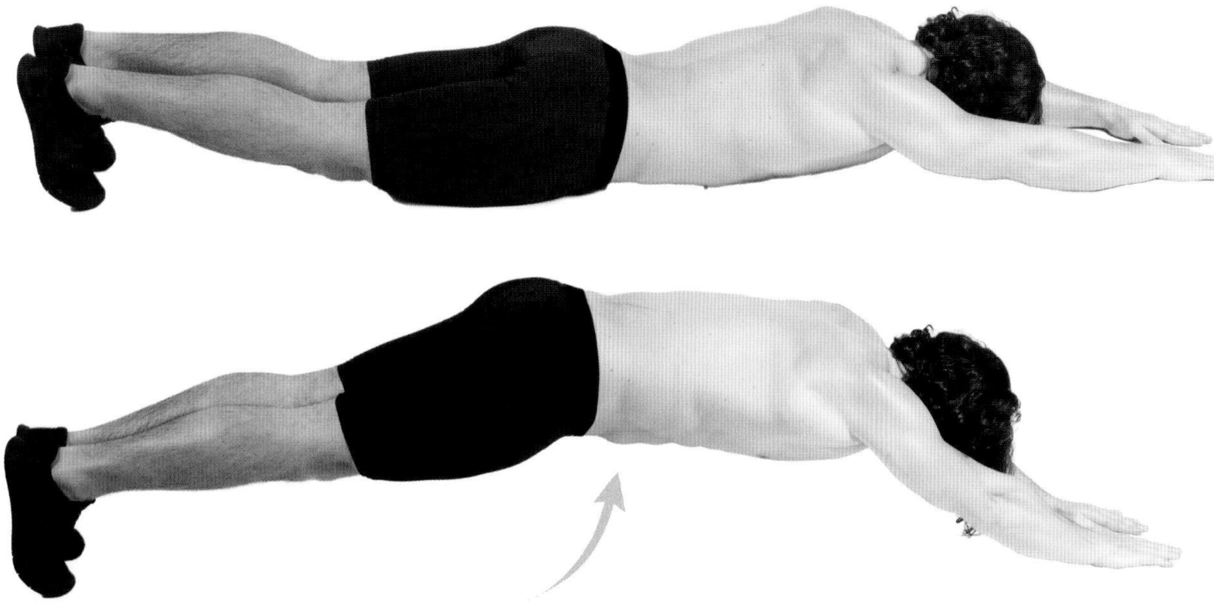

FACT FILE

TARGETS
- Latissimus dorsi
- Triceps
- Pectorals
- Abdominals

TYPE
- Dynamic

BENEFITS
- Strengthens triceps, lats, abdominals, and pectorals
- Increases core stability

CAUTIONS
- Shoulder or rotator cuff issues

Camel Yoga Stretch

The yoga-inspired Camel exercise stretches nearly all the major muscles of your body, particularly your shoulders and lower back. It also tones your chest, abdomen, and thighs.

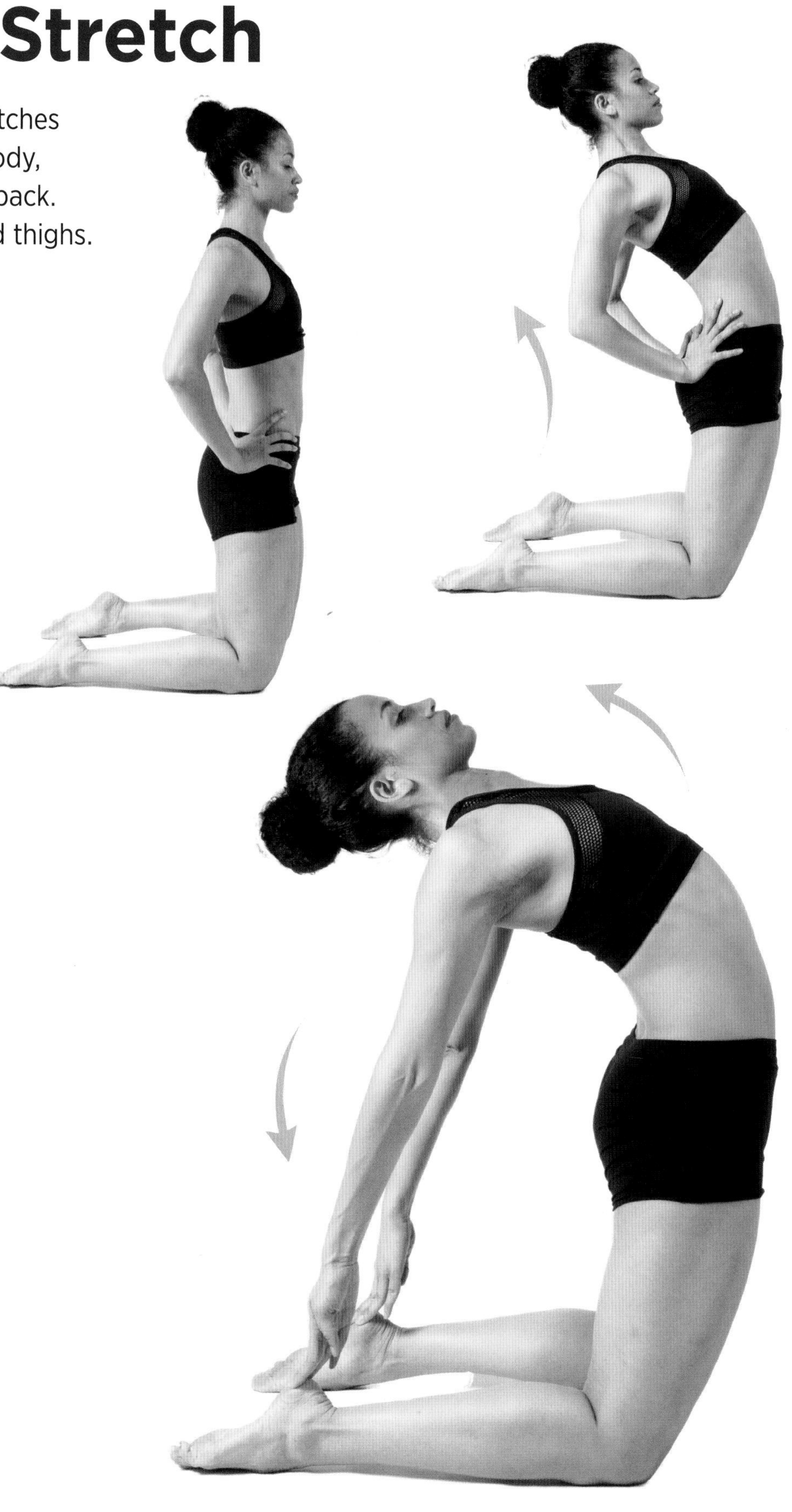

HOW TO DO IT

- Kneel on the floor, with your knees hip-width apart and your shins and feet aligned behind your knees. The tops of your feet should rest on the floor, with your toes pointing straight back.
- Bend your elbows, and bring your hands to your lower back, fingers pointing upward. Draw your elbows together, opening your chest.
- Bend from your upper back, and straighten your arms as you reach behind you to grasp your heels. Keep your hips directly above your knees; if your hips shift backward as you reach for your toes, keep your hands on your lower back instead.
- Broaden your collarbones and press your shoulder blades together to open your chest and shoulders. Allow your head to drop back. Hold for the recommended time.

Annotation Key

Bold text indicates target muscles
Light text indicates other working muscles
* indicates deep muscles

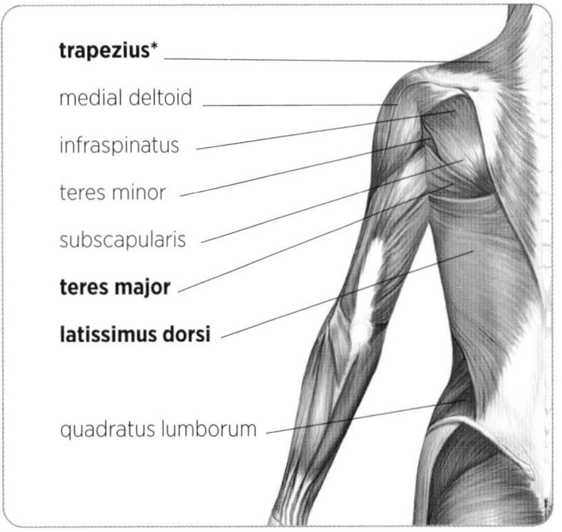

scalenus*
pectoralis minor*
pectoralis major
rectus abdominis
transversus abdominis*
levator scapulae*
trapezius
gluteus medius*
gluteus maximus
anterior deltoid
iliopsoas*
biceps femoris
rectus femoris

FACT FILE

TARGETS
- Lower Back
- Chest
- Shoulders
- Abdominals
- Thighs

TYPE
- Dynamic

BENEFITS
- Stretches hip flexors, thighs, and abdominals
- Opens shoulders and chest
- Improves posture

CAUTIONS
- Knee issues
- Lower-back issues
- Neck issues

DO IT RIGHT
- While bending backward, keep your thighs perpendicular to the floor.
- If your neck feels strained when you drop your head backward, keep your head lifted instead and gaze forward.
- Avoid bending from your hips.

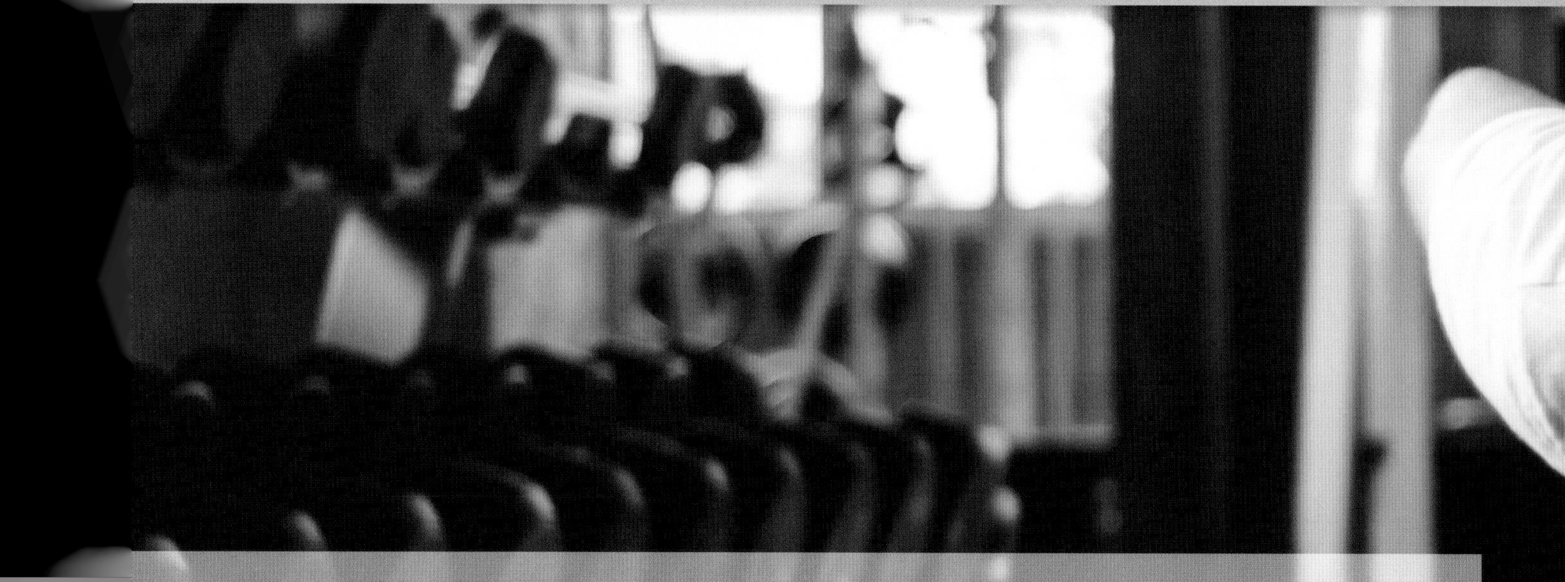

CHAPTER FIVE

ARM AND SHOULDER EXERCISES

These muscles are essential in pushing, pulling and lifting, and are therefore used in most everyday activity. Exercising the shoulders can improve the range of motion. It is understandable to think that successful runners only need strong legs, and therefore should focus on leg and glute exercises, but exercizing your arms can actually boost your speed and endurance. Arm workouts can also strengthen your bones, building bone density—especially important in later life. Arm exercises should form an integral part of any healthy workout plan.

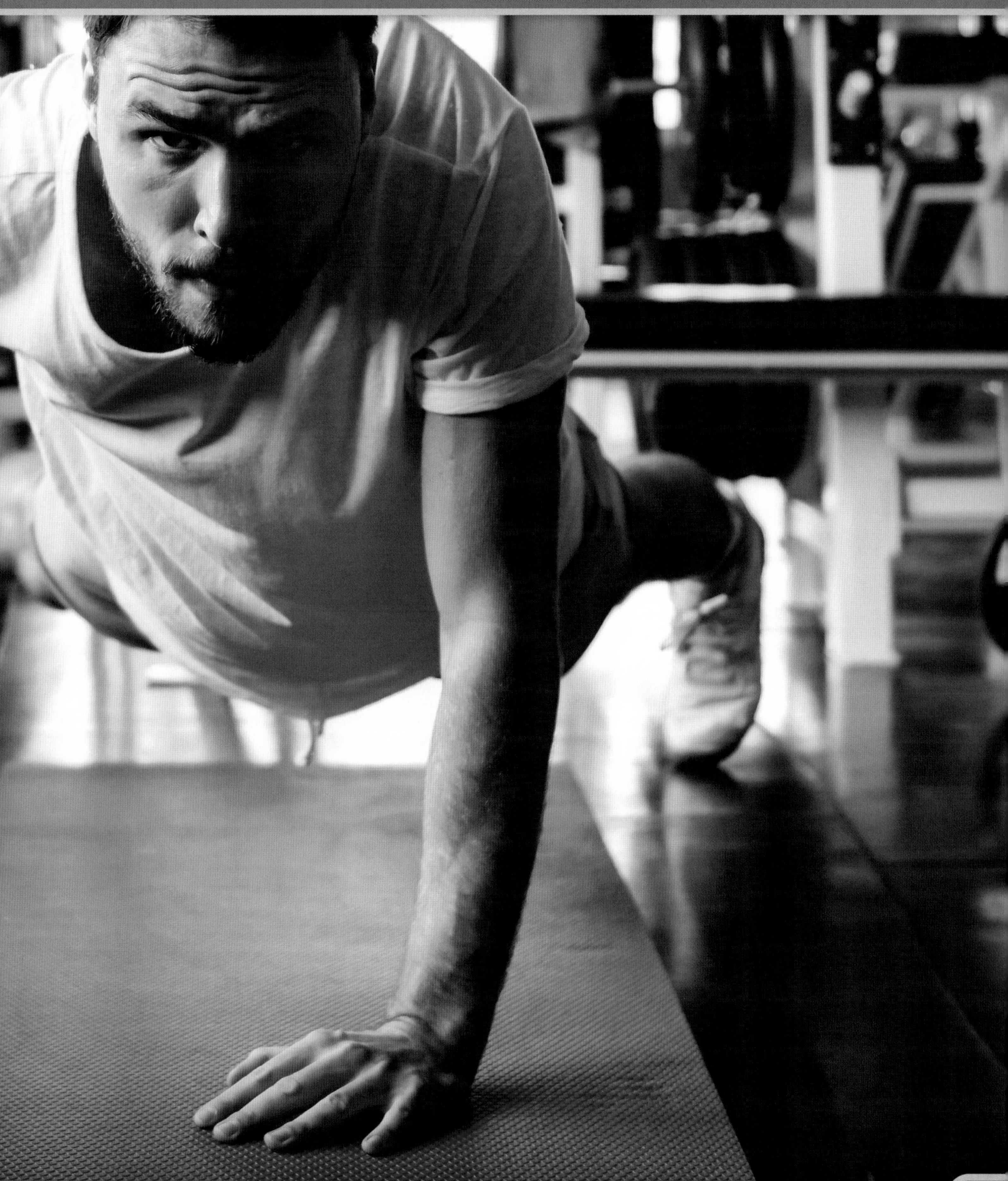

Bench Dip

The Bench Dip is a classic body-weight exercise that targets your hard-to-isolate triceps. This version replaces a weight bench with an ordinary chair.

HOW TO DO IT

- Sit up tall near the front of a sturdy chair. Place your hands beside your hips, wrapping your fingers over the front edge of the chair.
- Extend your legs in front of you slightly, and place your feet flat on the floor. Scoot off the edge of the chair until your knees align directly above your feet and your torso will be able to clear the chair as you dip down.
- Bend your elbows directly behind you without splaying them out to the sides, and lower your torso until your elbows make a 90-degree angle.
- Press into the chair, raising your body back to the starting position. Repeat for the recommended repetitions.

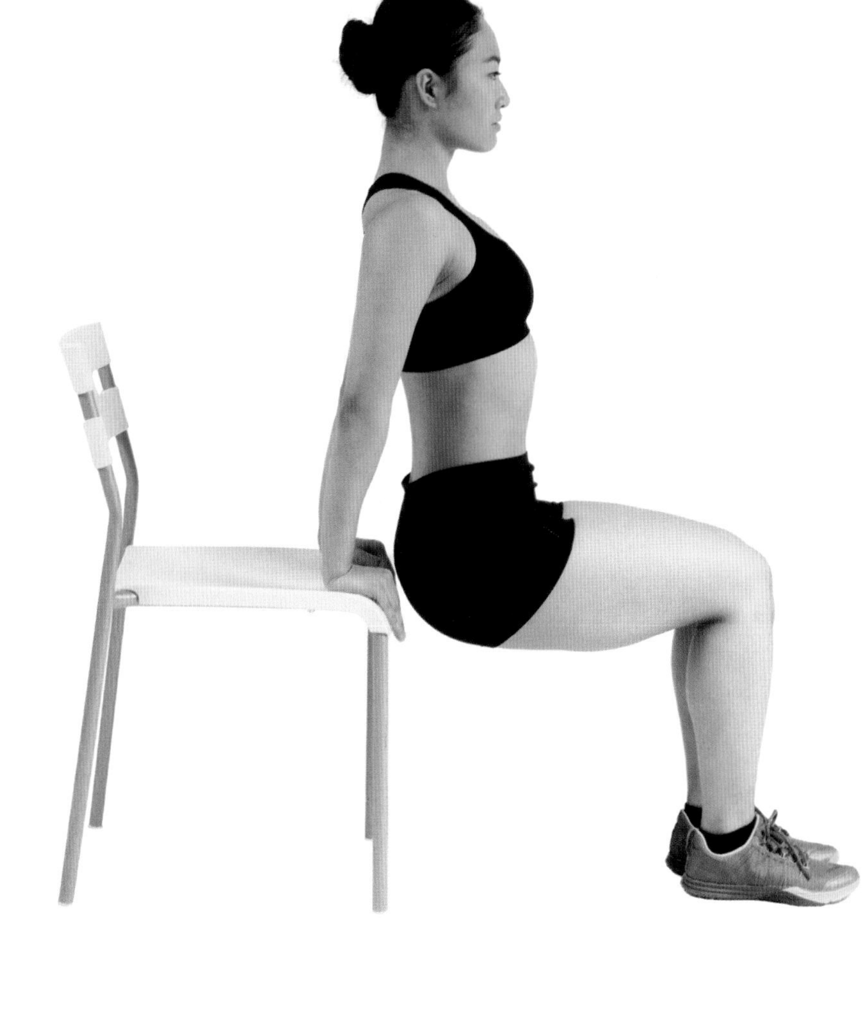

DO IT RIGHT

- Keep your body close to the chair.
- Keep your spine in a neutral position.
- Avoid allowing your shoulders to lift toward your ears.
- Avoid moving your feet.
- Avoid rounding your back as you lower your hips.
- Avoid pushing up solely with your feet. Instead use your arm strength.

FACT FILE

TARGETS
- Triceps
- Shoulders
- Core

TYPE
- Dynamic

BENEFITS
- Tones triceps
- Strengthens shoulder girdle

CAUTIONS
- Shoulder issues
- Wrist issues

EQUIPMENT
- Bench or chair

MODIFICATION

HARDER: Perform the exerise with one leg raised and stretched out in front, continuing to draw your navel into your spine. Repeat with the other leg.

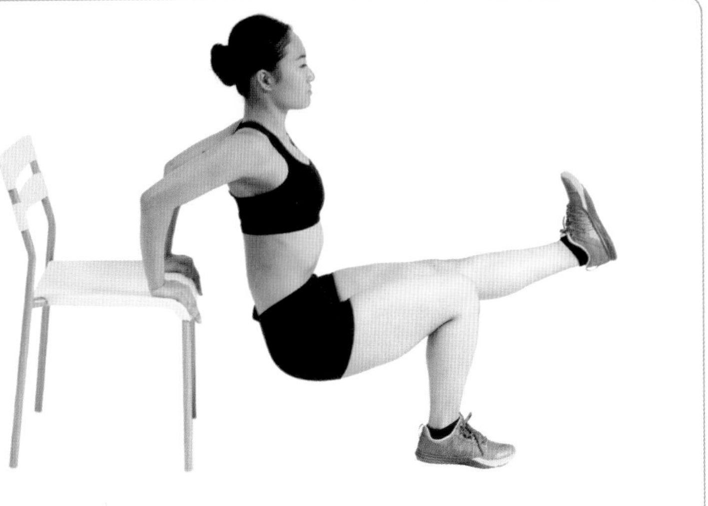

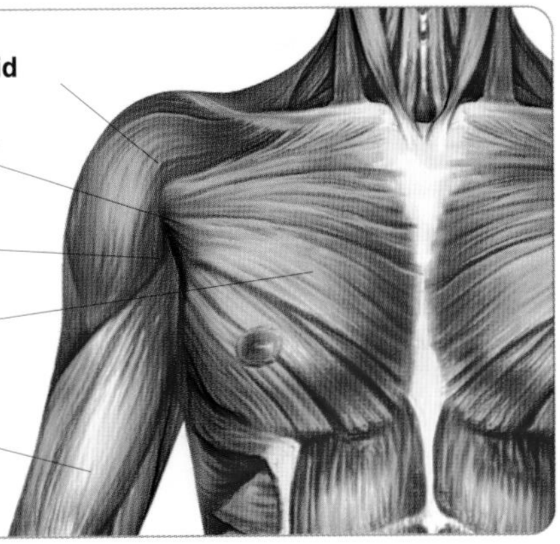

anterior deltoid

pectoralis minor*

coracobrachialis

pectoralis major

biceps brachii

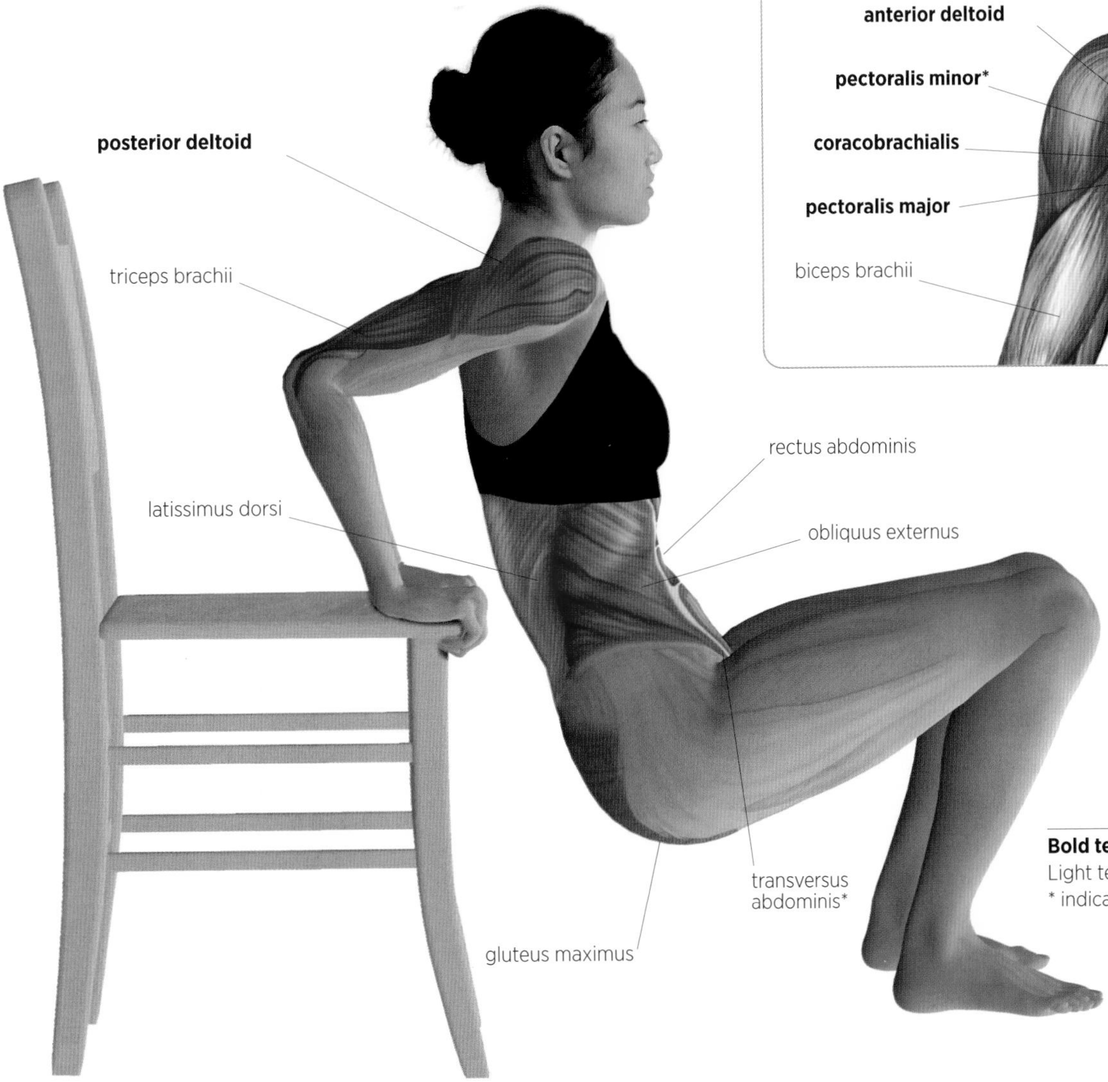

posterior deltoid

triceps brachii

latissimus dorsi

rectus abdominis

obliquus externus

transversus abdominis*

gluteus maximus

Annotation Key

Bold text indicates target muscles

Light text indicates other working muscles

* indicates deep muscles

Triceps Push-Up

Hand position has a significant impact on which muscles work hardest. In a basic push-up, your pectorals are the primary movers. In this version, you plant your hands closer together to place greater emphasis on your shoulders and triceps.

HOW TO DO IT

- With your hands close together, place your palms on the floor and assume a plank position with your weight on the balls on your feet. Your wrists should be directly beneath your shoulders, with your arms straight and your fingers pointing forward.
- Bend your arms, and lower your torso until your chest touches the floor.
- Straighten your arms to rise back to the starting position. Repeat for the recommended repetitions.

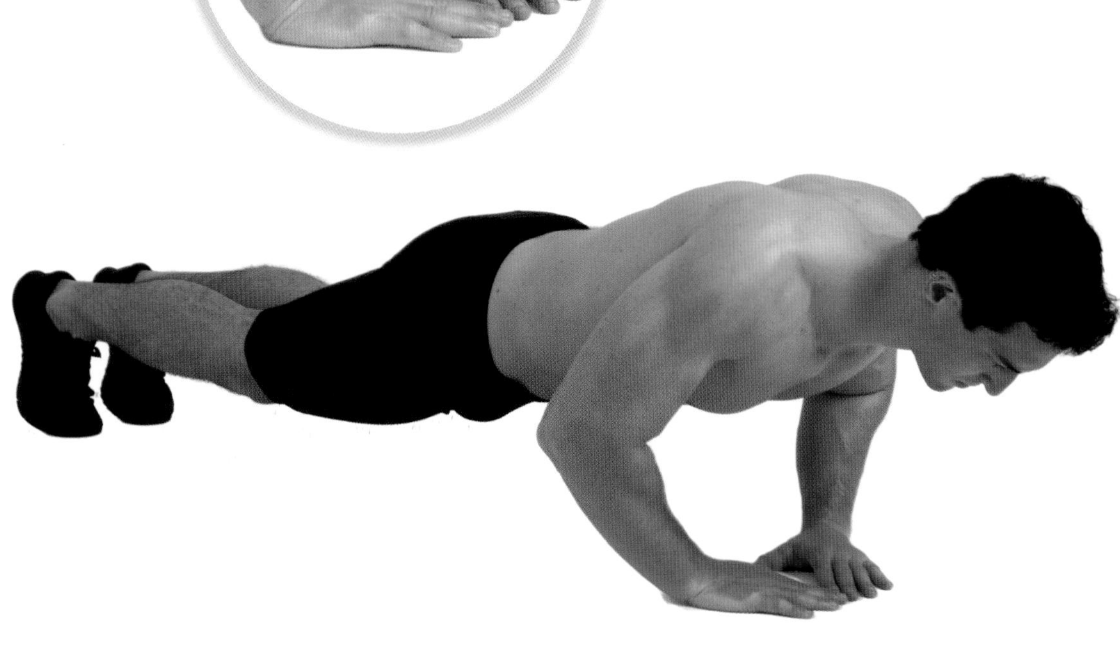

DO IT RIGHT

- Keep your elbows close to your rib cage as you lower your chest to the floor.
- Avoid pushing your hips into the air.
- Avoid pointing your elbows to the side during the down movement; this places undue stress on your front deltoids.

FACT FILE

TARGETS
- Triceps
- Shoulders
- Core

TYPE
- Dynamic

BENEFITS
- Tones triceps
- Strengthens upper body and abdominals
- Stabilizes core

CAUTIONS
- Shoulder issues
- Wrist issues
- Lower-back pain

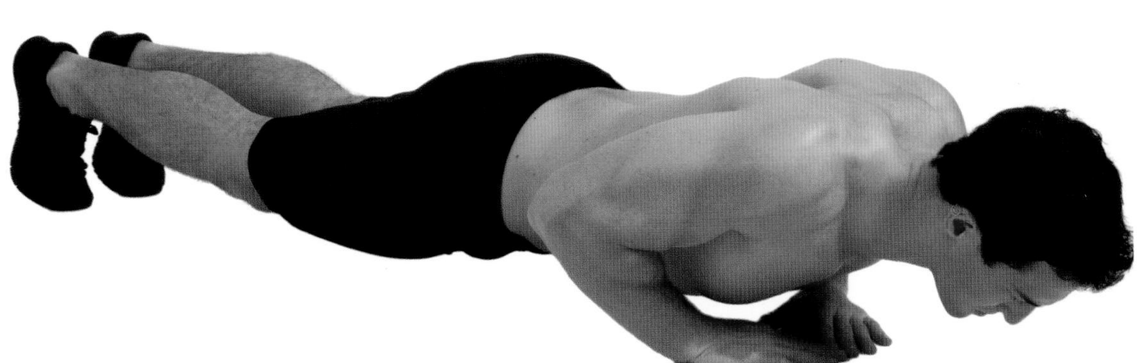

Annotation Key

Bold text indicates target muscles
Light text indicates other working muscles
* indicates deep muscles

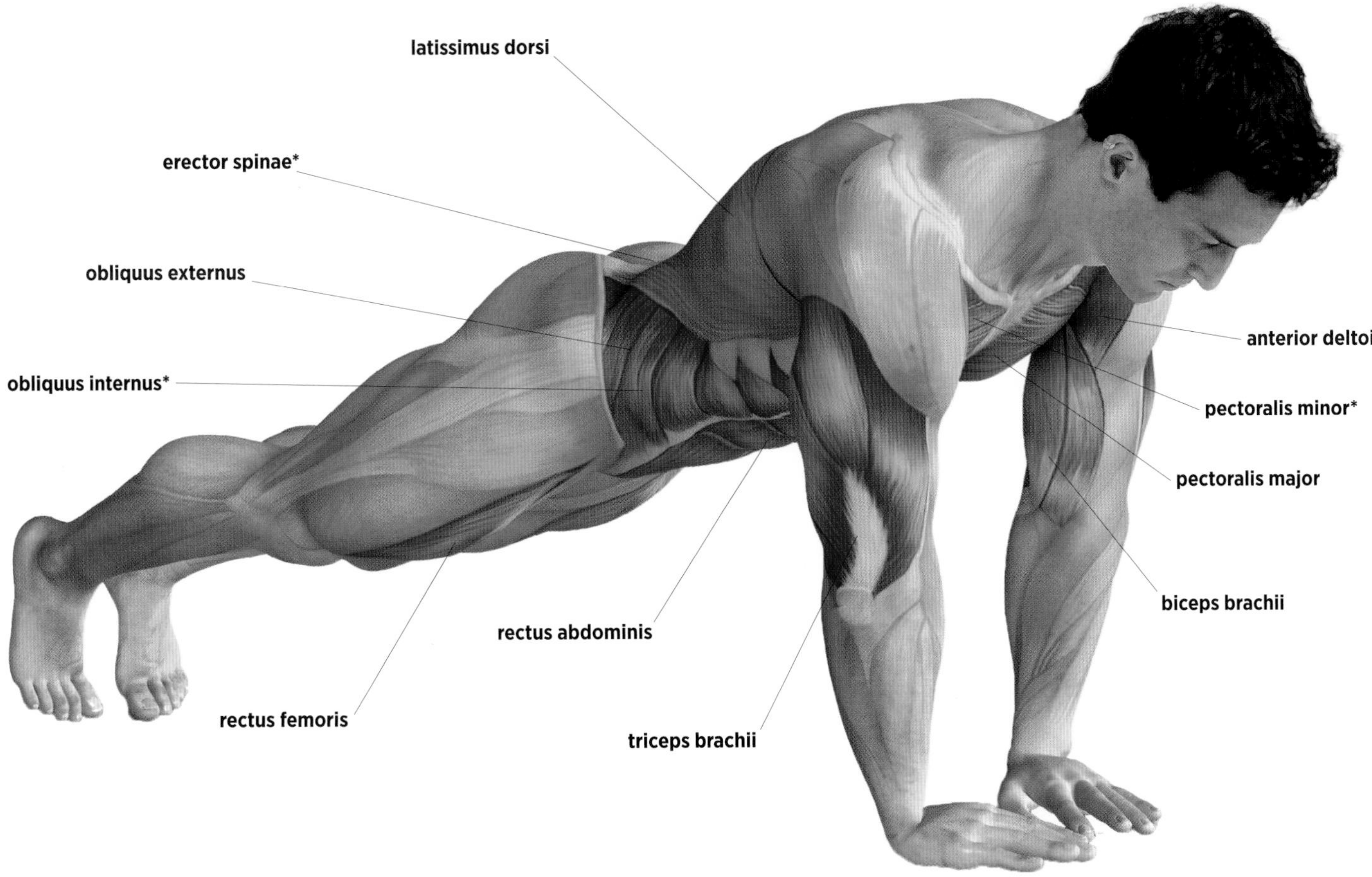

latissimus dorsi
erector spinae*
obliquus externus
obliquus internus*
anterior deltoid
pectoralis minor*
pectoralis major
biceps brachii
rectus abdominis
rectus femoris
triceps brachii

Plank-Up

Plank-Up is an effective exercise to strengthen your abdominals and arms. Focus on your form, keeping your core fully engaged as you move from low to high and back again.

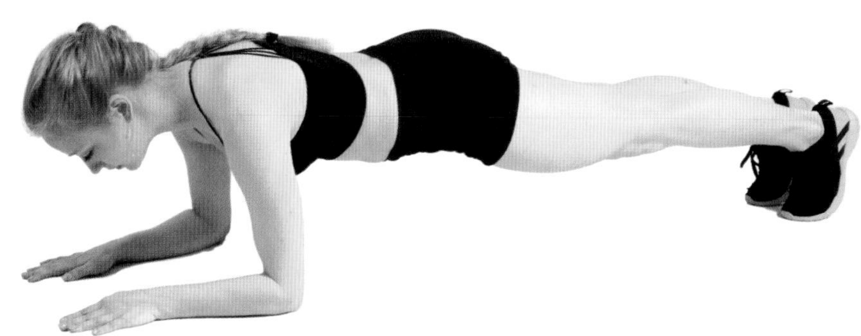

HOW TO DO IT

- Begin in a forearm plank position with your weight evenly distributed on your forearms and the balls of your feet. Take a moment to stabilize your hips and fully engage your abdominals.
- Reposition your left arm and then the right so that your hands are planted beneath your shoulders, lifting your body into a high plank position.
- Return to the forearm plank, repositioning your left arm and then the right.
- Repeat for the recommended repetitions, alternating leading with one arm and then the other.

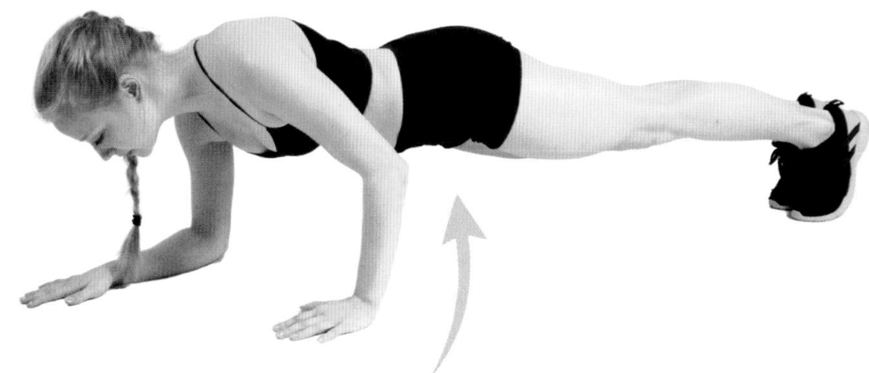

DO IT RIGHT

- Pull your navel in toward your spine to engage your abdominals.
- Avoid letting your stomach or ribcage sag.
- Avoid lifting your shoulders up or forward.
- Avoid shifting your weight when you change levels.

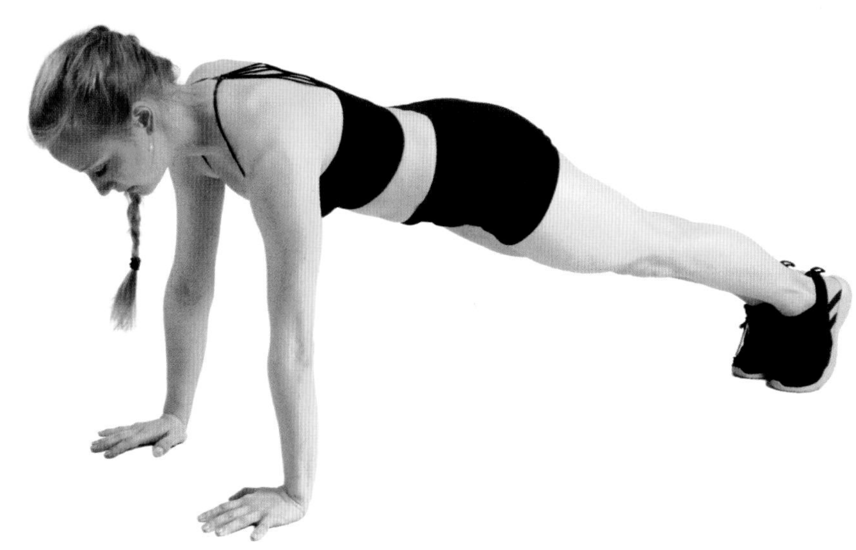

FACT FILE

TARGETS
- Triceps
- Abdominals

TYPE
- Static

BENEFITS
- Stabilizes core
- Strengthens abdominals
- Strengthens triceps

CAUTIONS
- Shoulder issues
- Back issues
- Wrist issues

Annotation Key

Bold text indicates target muscles
Light text indicates other working muscles
* indicates deep muscles

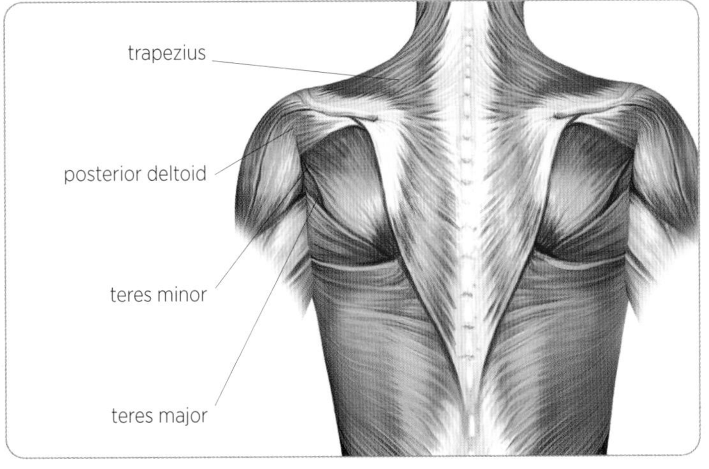

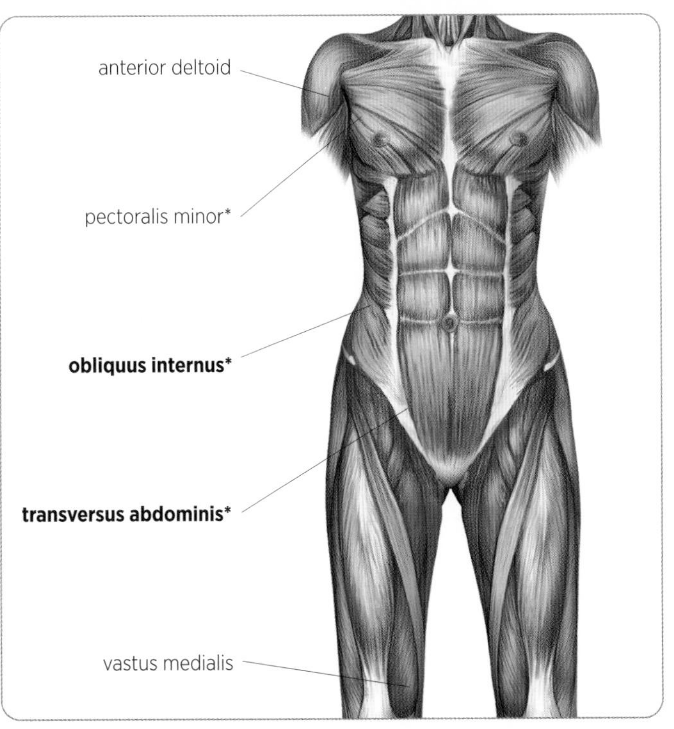

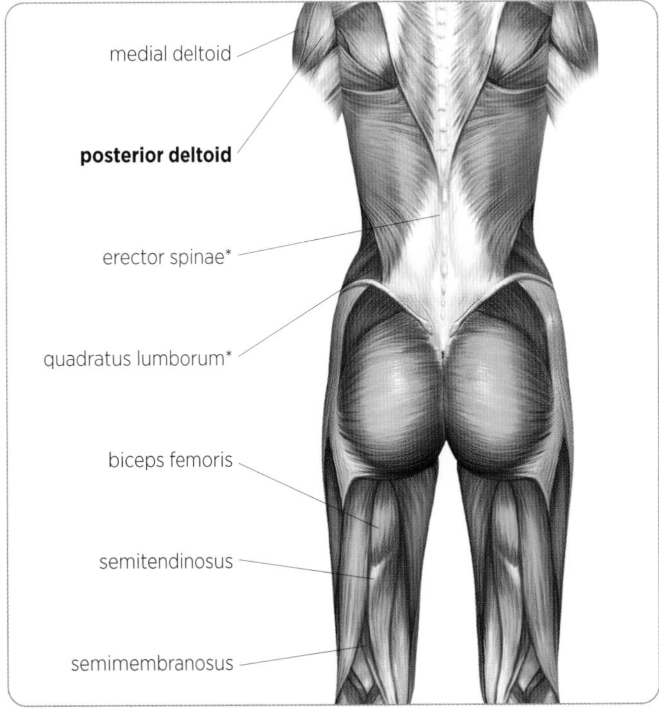

Power Punch

The Power Punch gives you a great upper-body workout, strengthening and toning big muscles, such as the deltoids. It works as a cardio exercise, helping to raise your heart rate and burn calories.

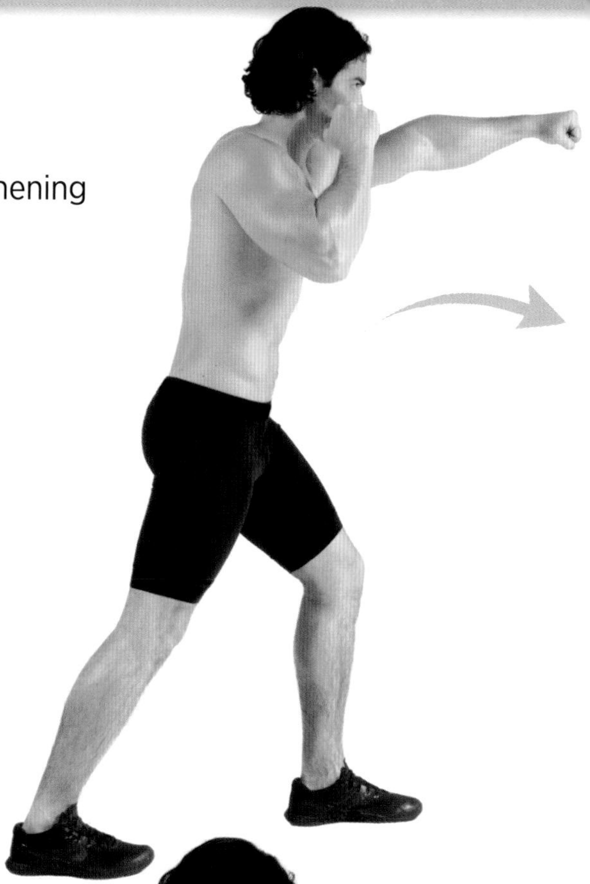

HOW TO DO IT

- Stand with your feet shoulder-width apart and your left leg placed slightly in front of the other, putting most of your weight on your back leg. Keep your elbows in, and raise your fists up.

- Transferring your weight to your front leg, punch straight in front of you with your right fist as you turn your torso in to lend power to the punch.

- Punch for the recommended repetitions, and then switch arms and legs to repeat on the opposite side. Continue alternating sides for the recommended repetitions.

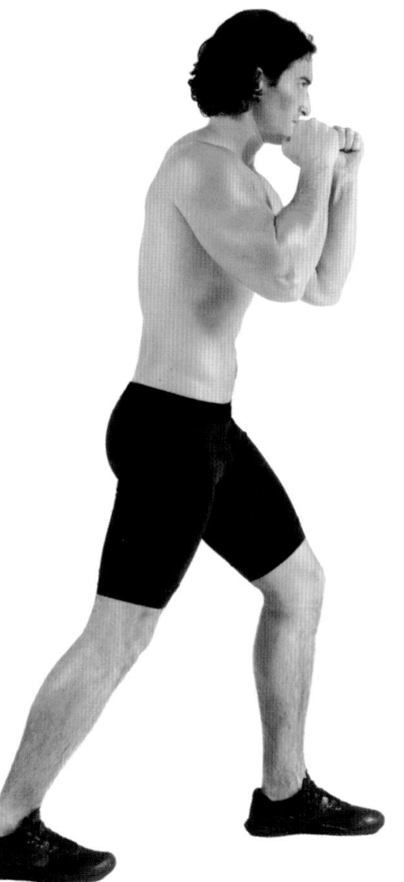

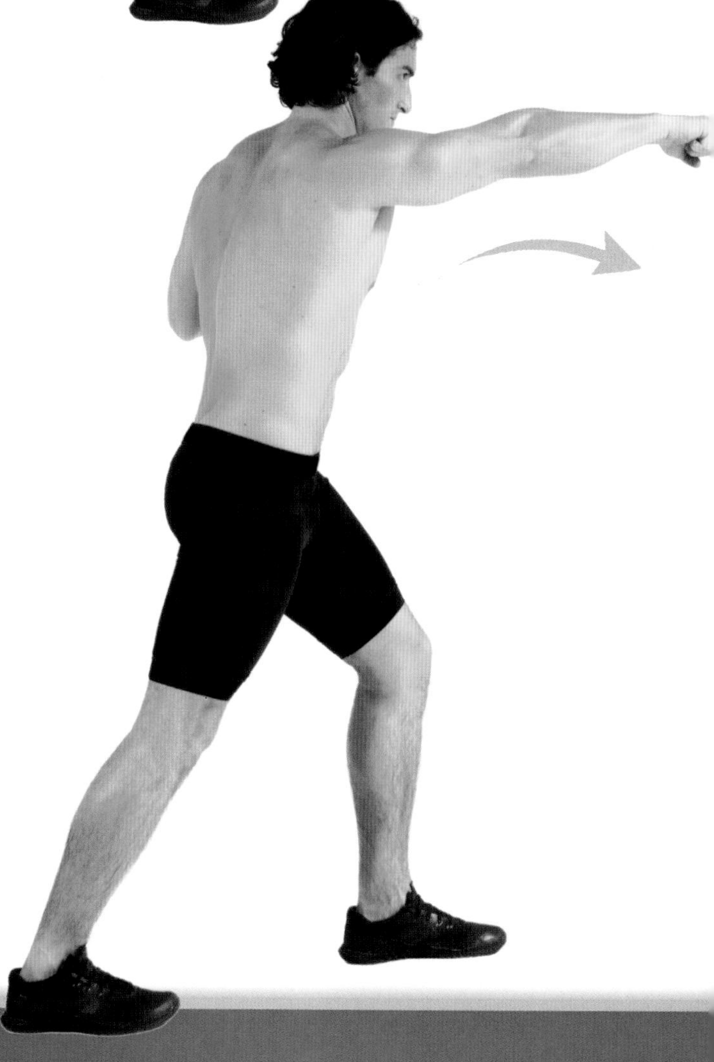

DO IT RIGHT

- Maintain a steady, even—but modest—pace.
- Rotate your torso to drive the movement.
- Keep your fists up.
- Avoid excessive speed.
- Avoid sloppy form.

FACT FILE

TARGETS
- Back
- Shoulders
- Abdominals

TYPE
- Dynamic

BENEFITS
- Strengthens back and shoulders
- Builds endurance

CAUTIONS
- Shoulder issues

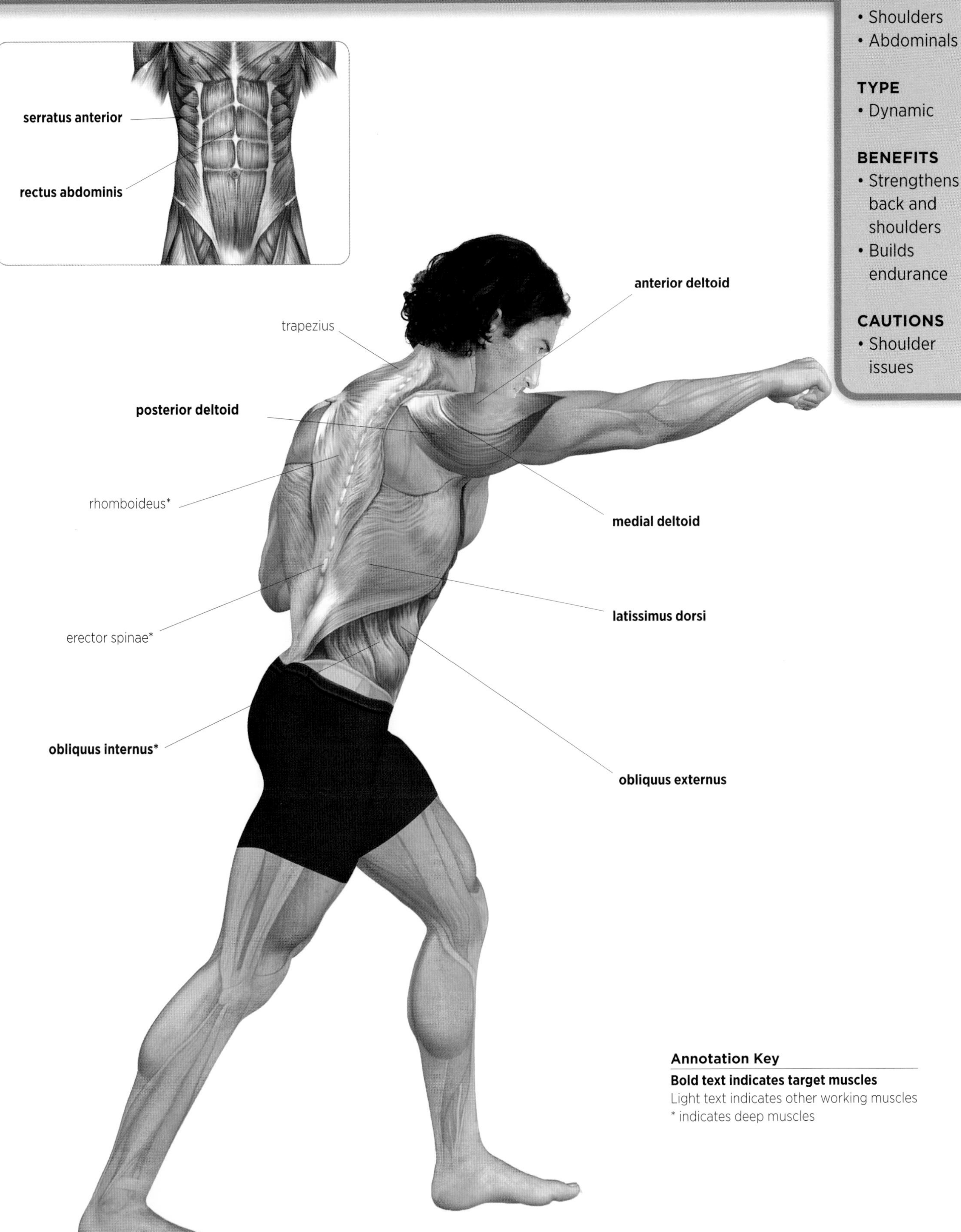

Annotation Key

Bold text indicates target muscles

Light text indicates other working muscles

* indicates deep muscles

Uppercut

This exercise builds upper-body strength, especially in your shoulders. It also lightly works your feet and legs, which are engaged in the upward drive.

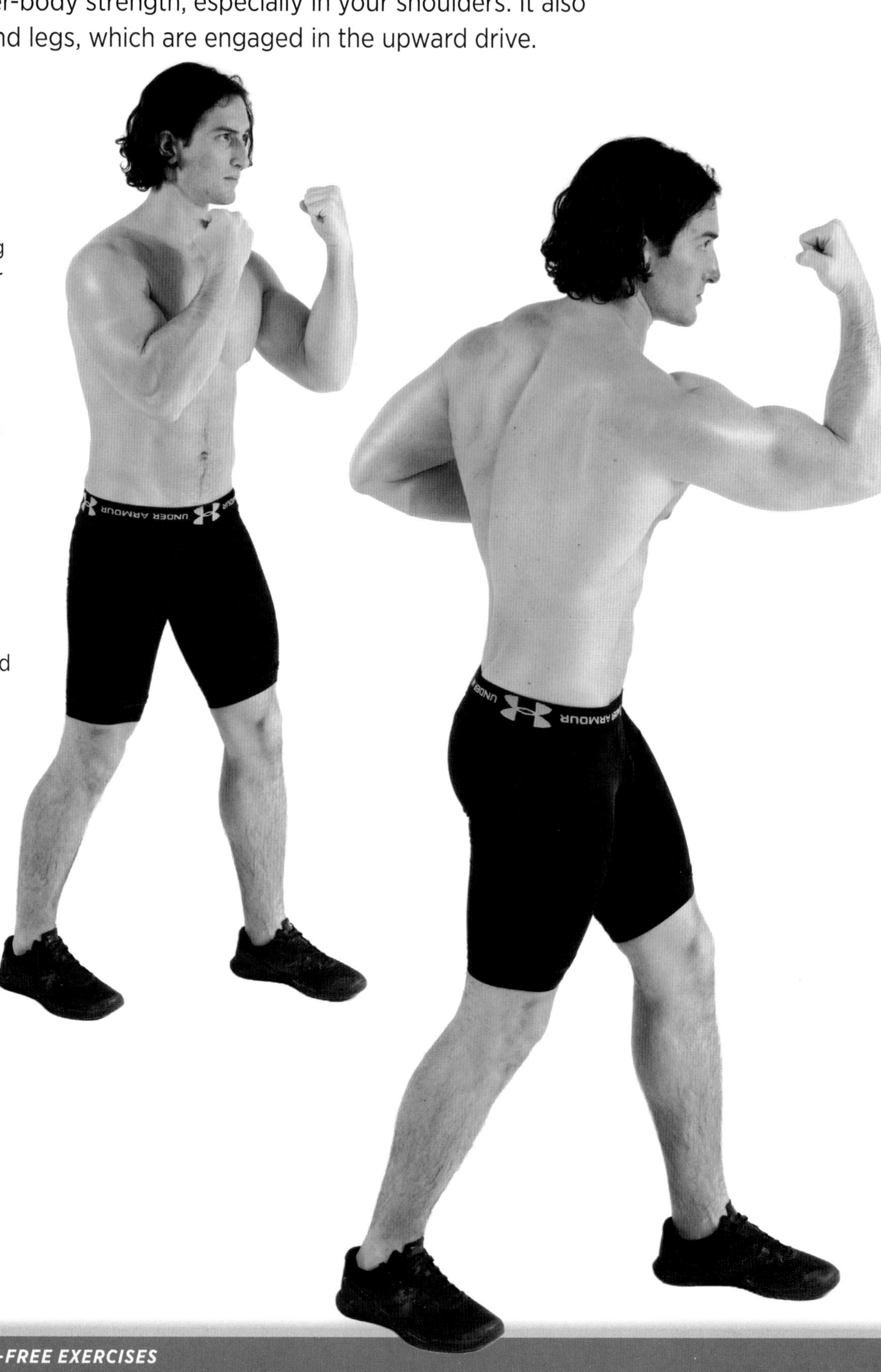

HOW TO DO IT

- Stand with your feet shoulder-width apart and your left leg placed slightly in front of your right, putting most of your weight on your back leg. Keep your elbows in, and raise both fists.
- Keeping your elbows in and your fists raised, punch upward toward the sky with your right fist as you rotate your torso slightly toward the left and transfer most of your weight to your front foot.
- Punch for the recommended number of times, and then reverse sides, switching your legs and arm.

DO IT RIGHT

- Maintain a steady, even, but modest pace.
- Rotate your torso to drive the movement.
- Keep your fists up.
- Avoid excessive speed.
- Avoid sloppy form.

FACT FILE

TARGETS
- Back
- Shoulders
- Abdomen

TYPE
- Dynamic

BENEFITS
- Strengthens back and shoulder muscles
- Builds endurance

CAUTIONS
- Shoulder issues

Annotation Key
Bold text indicates target muscles
Light text indicates other working muscles
* indicates deep muscles

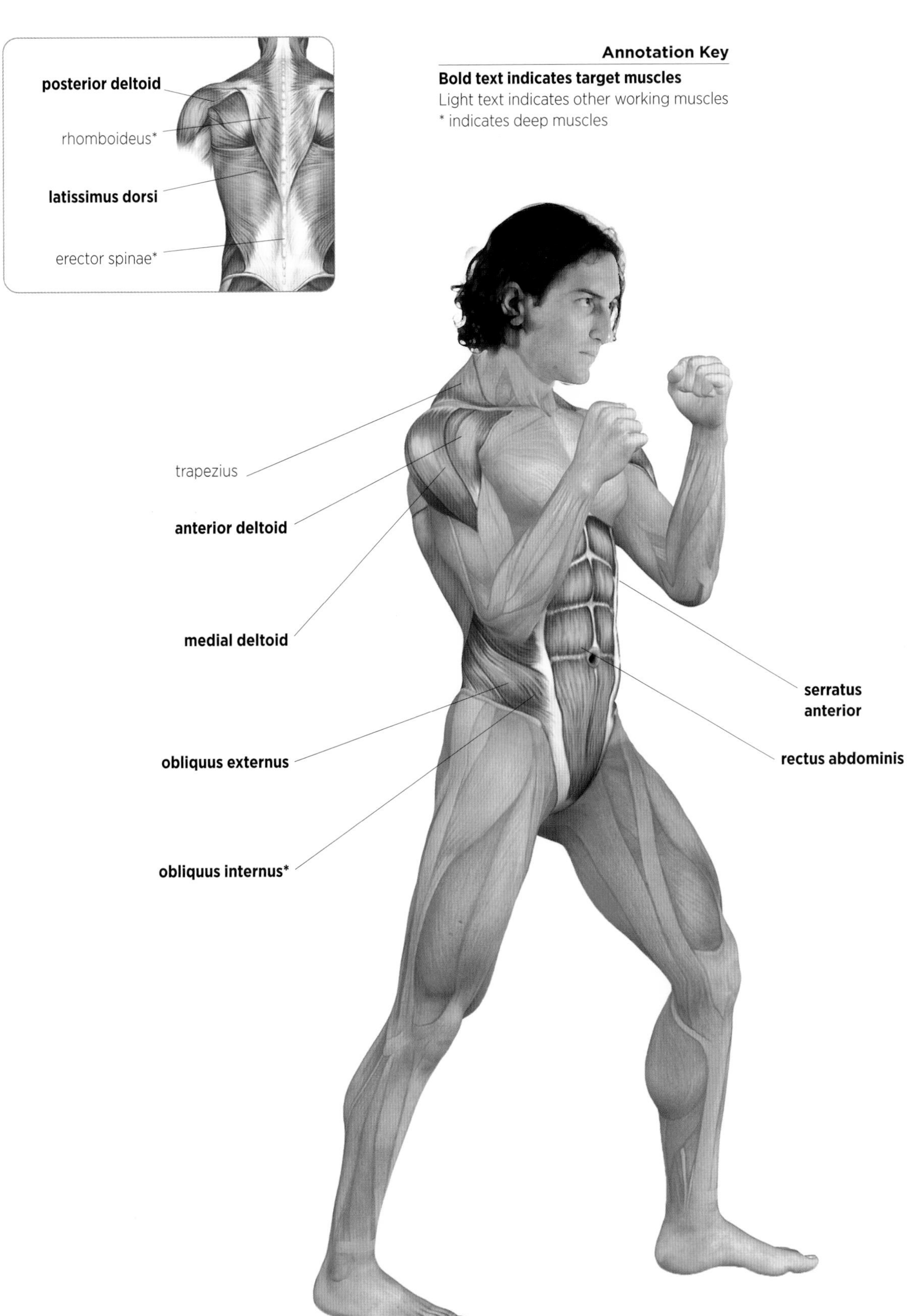

Inchworm

The Inchworm, also known as Monkey Walk, is a good gauge of overall fitness. It requires core and upper-body strength, and this full-body stretch really tests the limits of your flexibility.

HOW TO DO IT

- Stand tall, and then carefully bend forward toward the floor until your palms are flat on the floor in front of you.
- Slowly walk your hands out to a plank position with your wrists directly under your shoulders. Keep your body parallel to the floor, legs hip-width apart, navel pressing toward your spine and shoulders pressing down your back.
- Pop your hips upward, and push your weight back onto your heels. Your body should be in the shape of an upside-down V. Hold for a few moments before slowly walking your hands back toward your legs.
- Carefully rise back to a standing position. Pause, and then repeat for the recommended repetitions.

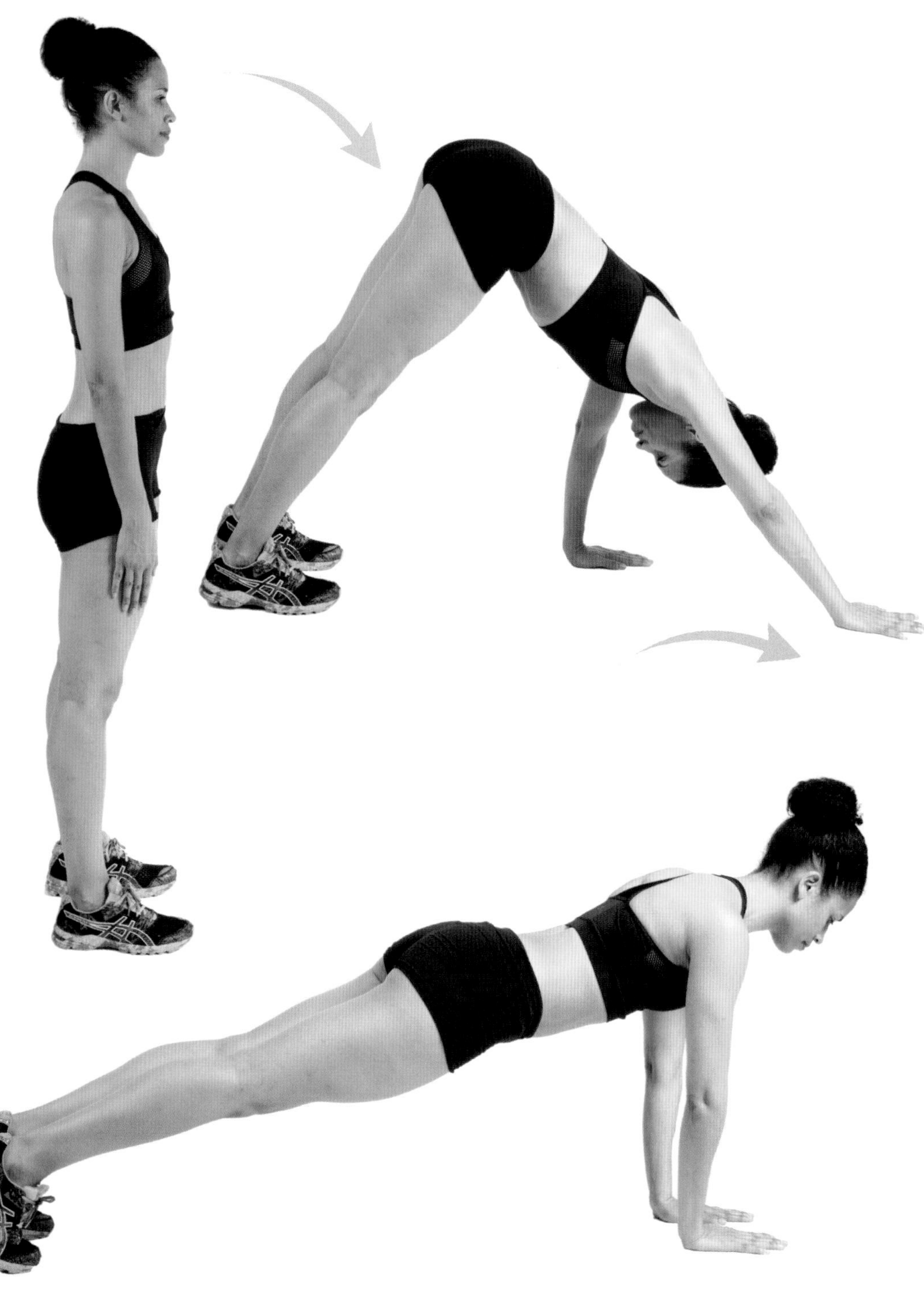

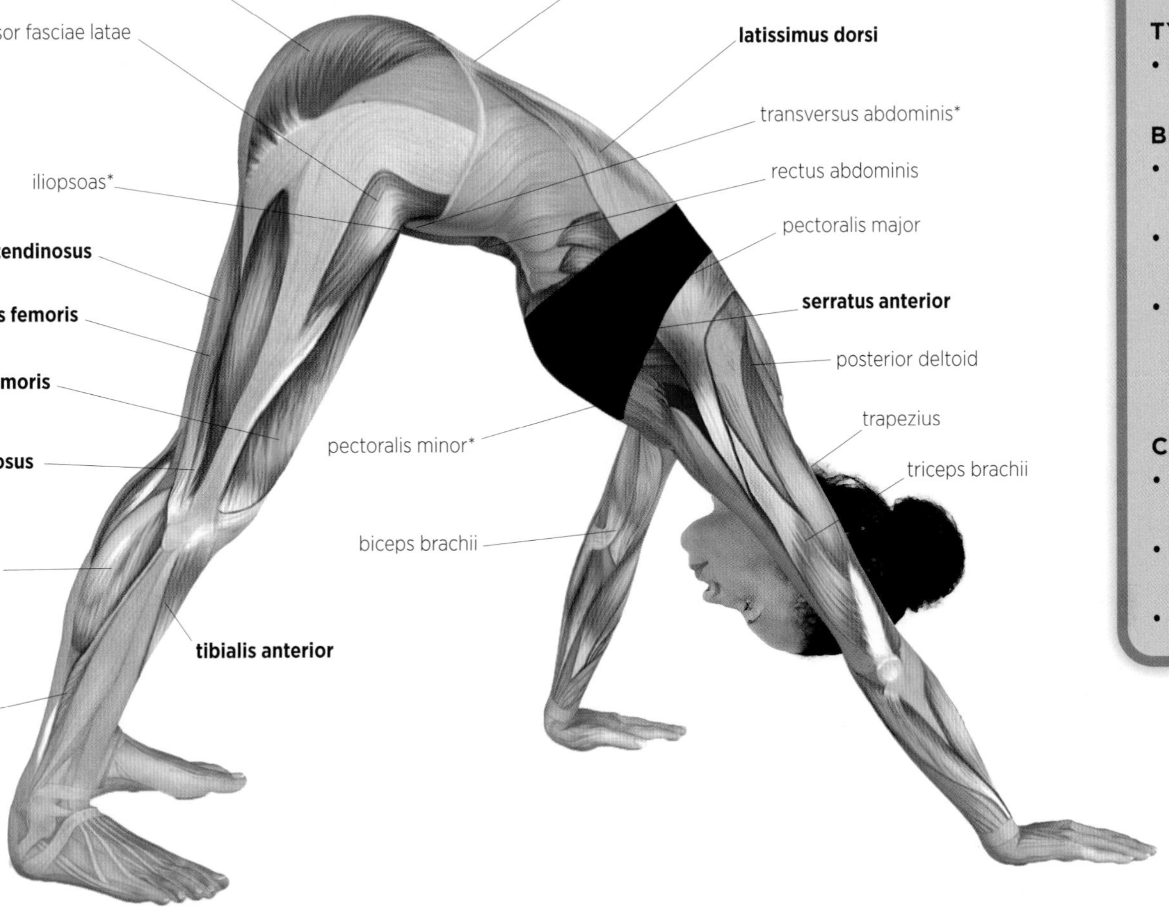

gluteus maximus
erector spinae*
tensor fasciae latae
latissimus dorsi
transversus abdominis*
iliopsoas*
rectus abdominis
pectoralis major
semitendinosus
biceps femoris
serratus anterior
rectus femoris
posterior deltoid
trapezius
pectoralis minor*
semimembranosus
triceps brachii
biceps brachii
gastrocnemius
tibialis anterior
soleus

FACT FILE

TARGETS
- Upper arms
- Back
- Legs
- Glutes

TYPE
- Dynamic

BENEFITS
- Warms up muscles
- Stretches back and legs
- Tones arms, glutes, and back

CAUTIONS
- Lower-back issues
- Shoulder issues
- Wrist issues

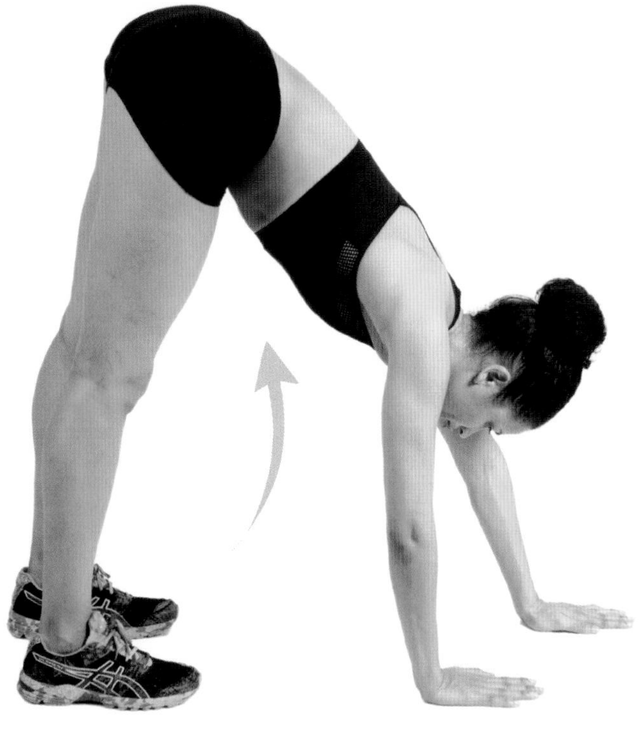

Annotation Key

Bold text indicates target muscles

Light text indicates other working muscles

* indicates deep muscles

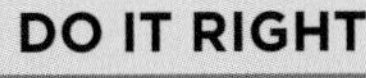

DO IT RIGHT
- Widen your stance if you have trouble reaching the floor with your hands.
- Keep your abdominals sleek and compact.
- Avoid rushing through the exercise.
- Avoid letting your stomach and spine sag while in the plank position.

Triceps Dip

You should really feel the Triceps Dip on the backs of your arms. Holding this body position works most of your other muscles, too.

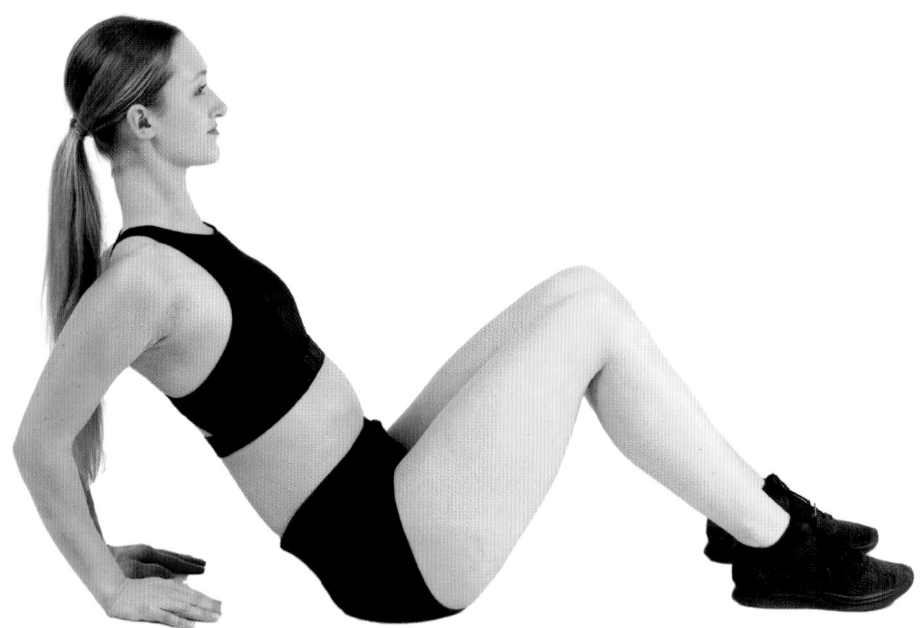

HOW TO DO IT

- Sit with your knees bent. Your arms should be behind you with your elbows bent and the palms of your hands pressing into the floor, fingers facing forward. Straighten your arms as you lift your hips a few inches off the floor.
- Shift your weight back toward your arms, and, keeping your heels pressed firmly into the floor, lift your toes. Keep your chest open and your gaze diagonally upward.
- Bending your elbows gradually, lower your body down slightly, but still above the floor. Then straighten your arms to raise your body up again, keeping your toes pointed upward the whole time. Repeat the up-and-down action for the recommended repetitions.
- Release back down to your starting position and repeat for the recommended repetitions.

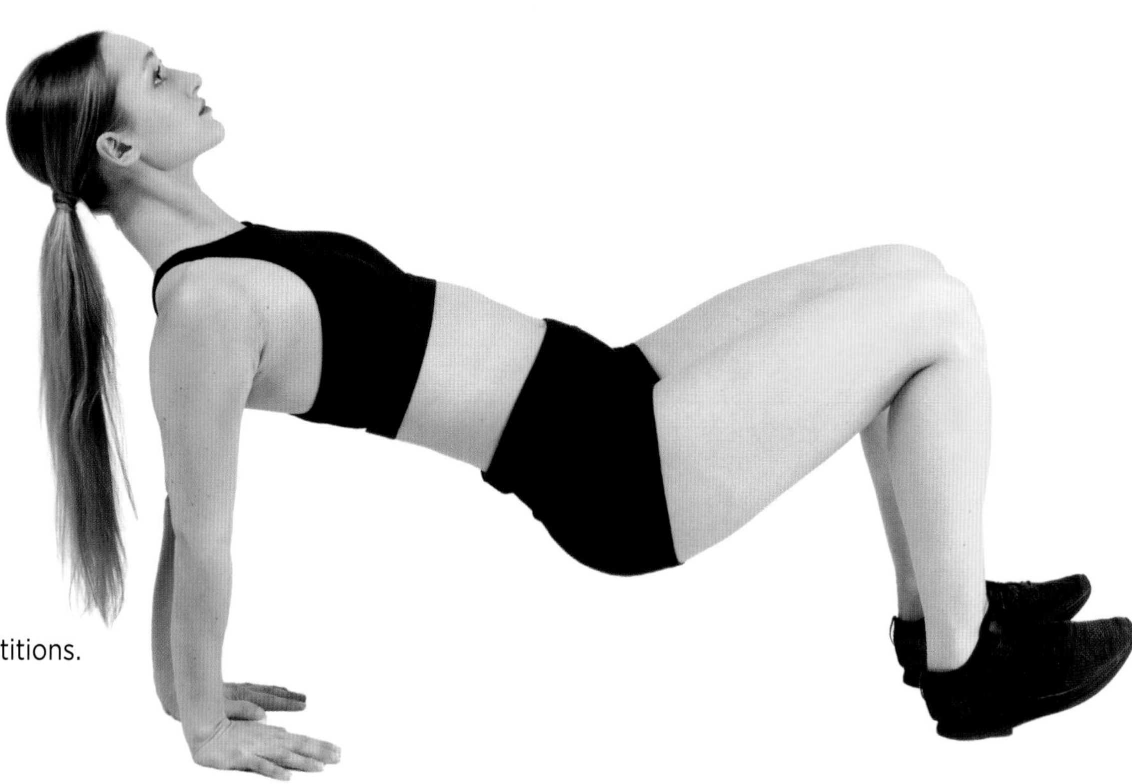

FACT FILE

TARGETS

- Triceps
- Deltoids
- Pectorals
- Lats

TYPE

- Dynamic

BENEFITS

- Strengthens triceps, shoulders, chest, back, and core
- Tones abdominals

CAUTIONS

- Back issues
- Shoulder issues

DO IT RIGHT

- Keep your chest lifted and open.
- Hold your shoulders down.
- Avoid arching your back.
- Avoid lifting your shoulders.
- Avoid rushing through the exercise.

Annotation Key

Bold text indicates target muscles
Light text indicates other working muscles
* indicates deep muscles

levator scapulae*
trapezius
posterior deltoid
teres minor
rhomboideus*
latissimus dorsi
erector spinae*

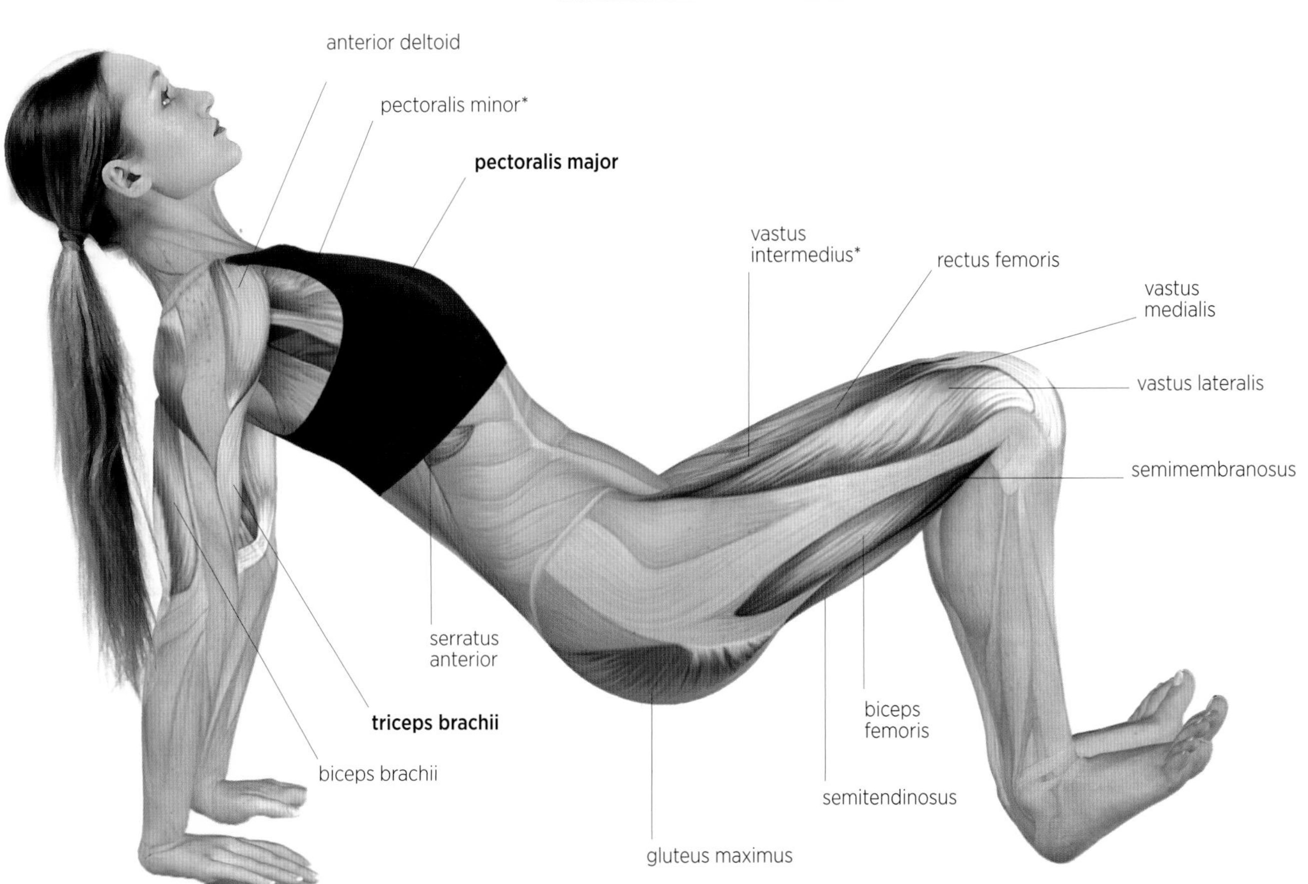

Bear Crawl

A Bear Crawl is an ideal way to build upper-body strength. This is an anaerobic exercise—meaning it is an intense strength promoter.

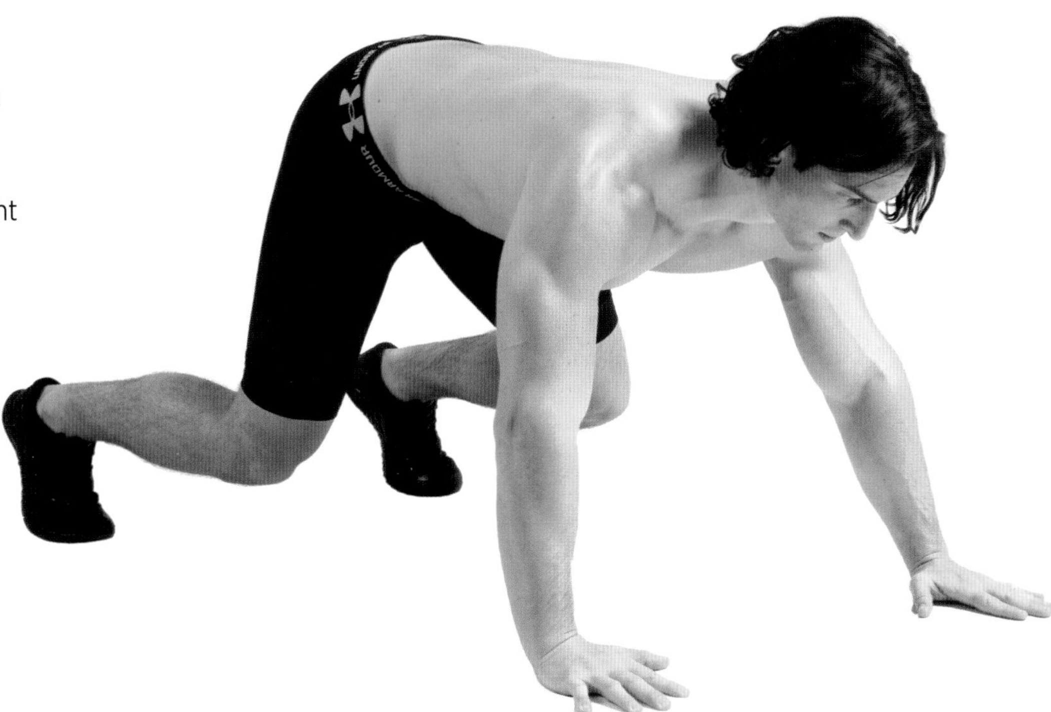

HOW TO DO IT

- To begin, place both hands and feet on the floor. Walk your left arm and right leg forward, and then your right arm and left leg.
- Now move backward in the same way.
- Keep moving forward and backward in this position, keeping your weight evenly distributed between your arms and legs. Perform for the recommended time.

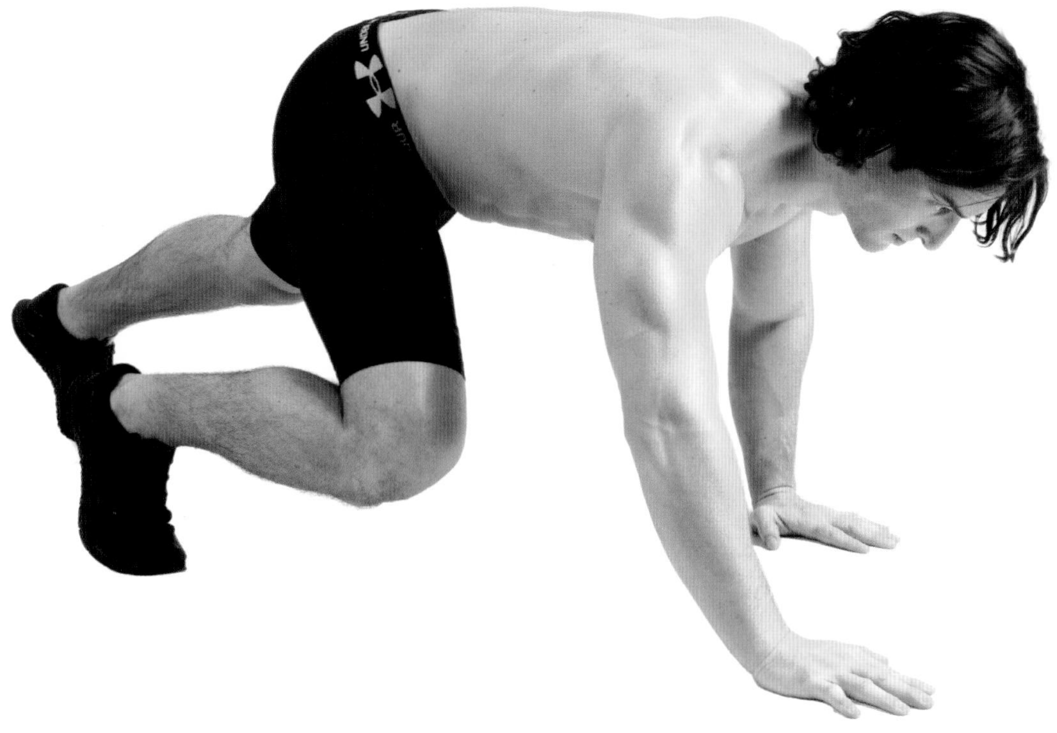

DO IT RIGHT

- Move steadily and smoothly.
- Avoid placing all of your weight on your arms and shoulders, which can stress your rotator cuffs.
- Avoid touching your knees to the floor.

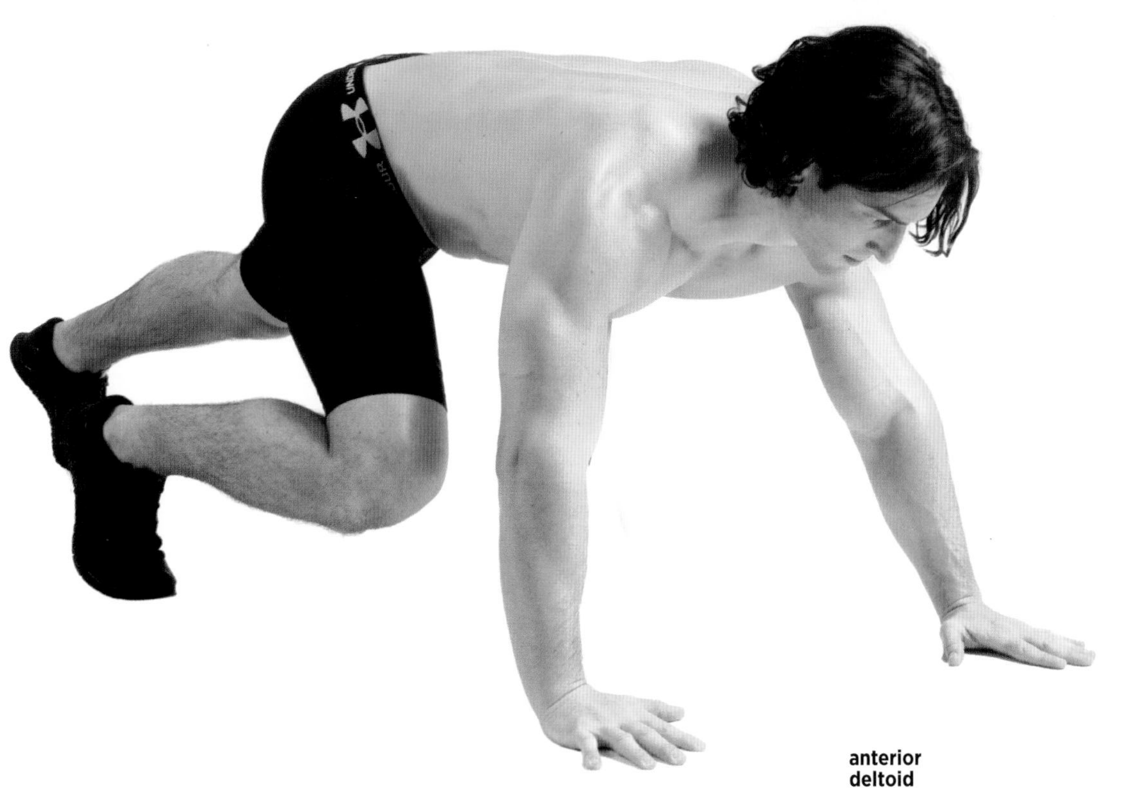

FACT FILE

TARGETS
- Pectorals
- Deltoids
- Biceps
- Triceps

TYPE
- Dynamic

BENEFITS
- Strengthens upper body
- Increases agility
- Improves coordination

CAUTIONS
- Back pain

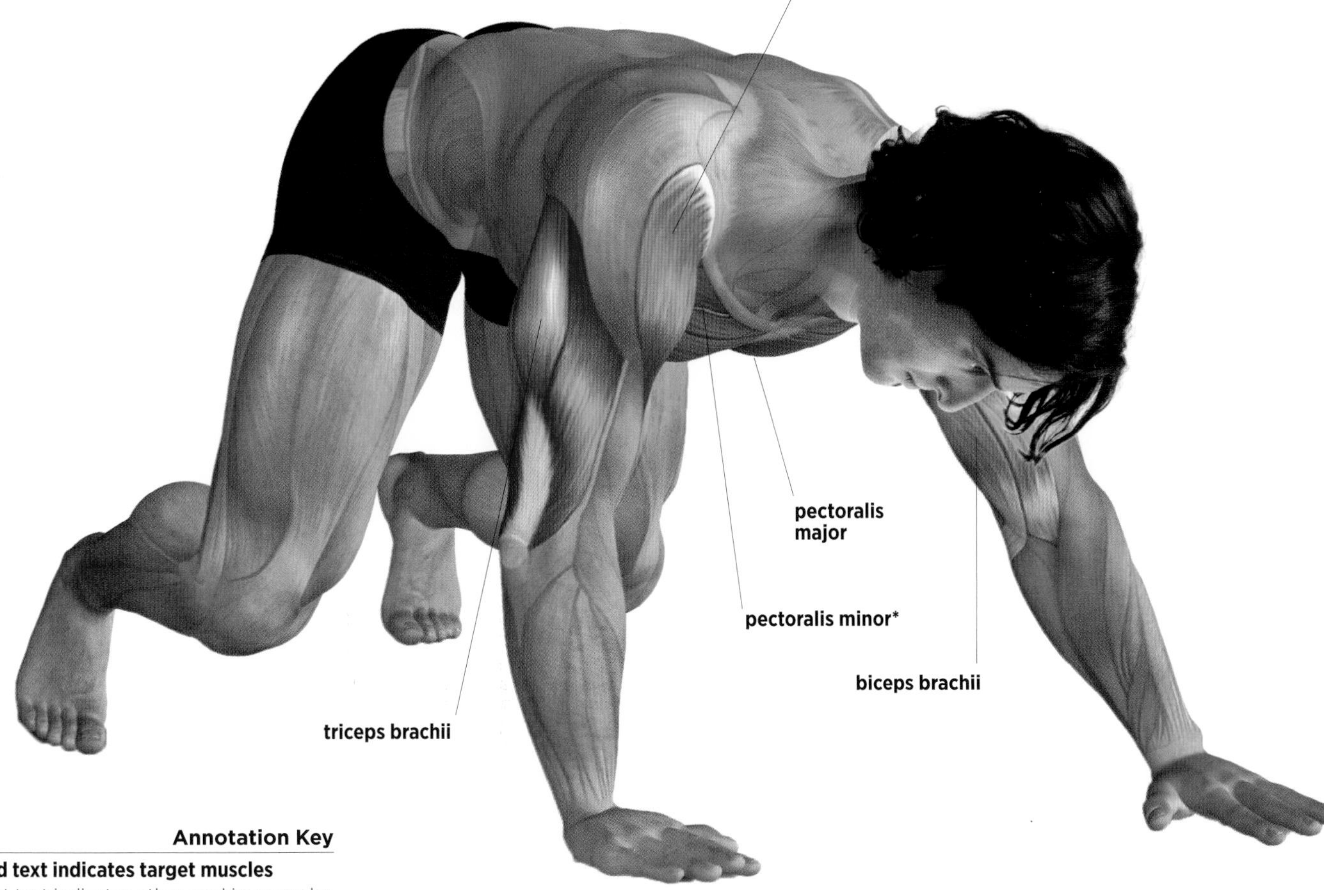

Annotation Key
Bold text indicates target muscles
Light text indicates other working muscles
* indicates deep muscles

Handstand Push-Up

The Handstand Push-Up is an advanced movement requiring an immense amount of upper-body strength, specifically from your shoulders and triceps, as well as midline stability from your core. Make sure you are strong and stable enough before attempting this exercise.

HOW TO DO IT

- Begin in a tripod position, with your head and hands on the floor, your head located between your hands and slightly forward making a triangle or tripod.
- Draw your legs above you, extending your hips and knees to stabilize your body in a single line, stacking your lower extremities above your trunk.
- Keeping your legs pointed toward the ceiling and your core engaged, press into the floor, extending your elbows, lifting your head and body up and away from the floor.
- Bending your elbows until your head makes contact with the mat. Repeat for the recommended repetitions.

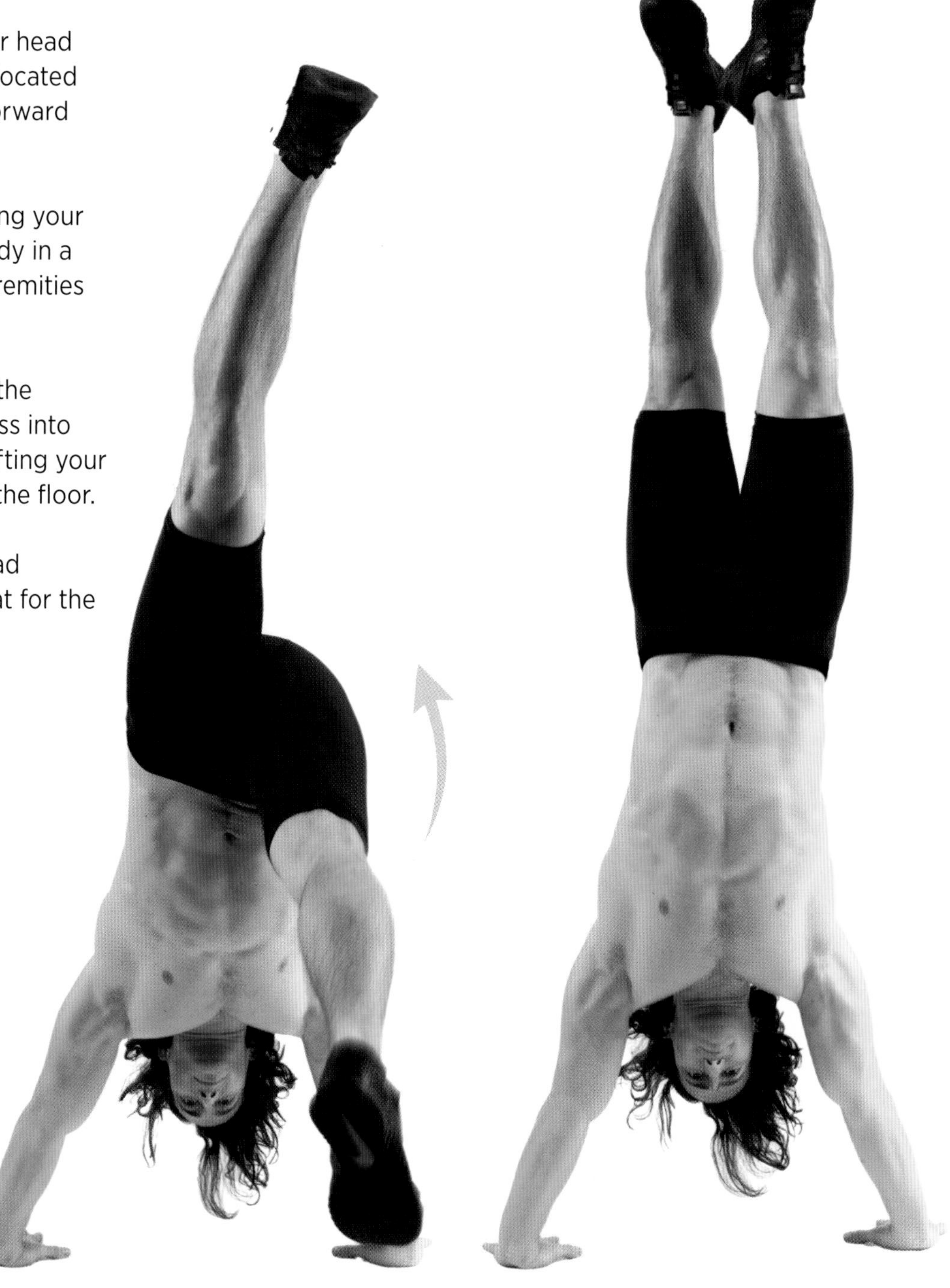

DO IT RIGHT

- Keep your back straight.
- Flare your hands out to ease stress on your wrists.
- Utilize a towel or pad underneath your head for safety and comfort.
- Avoid excessive trunk sway.
- As you master this exercise, perform it against a wall for added support.
- Use a spotter for safety.

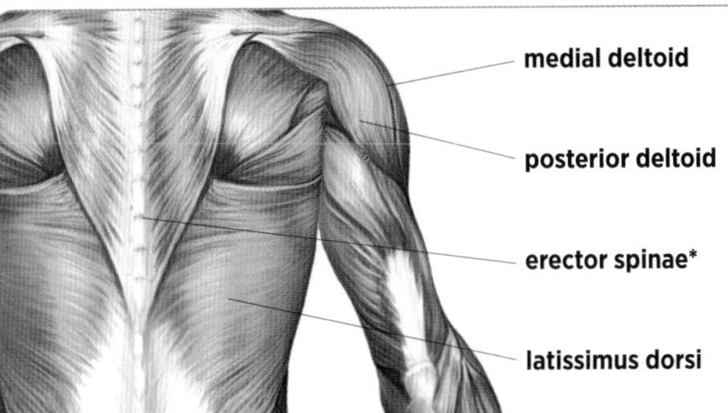

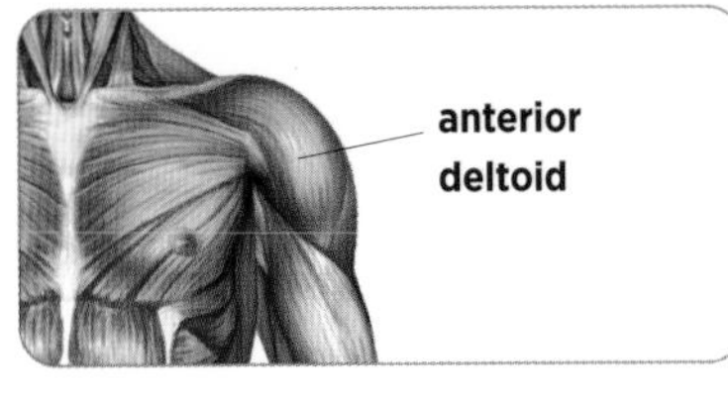

Annotation Key

Bold text indicates target muscles

Light text indicates other working muscles

* indicates deep muscles

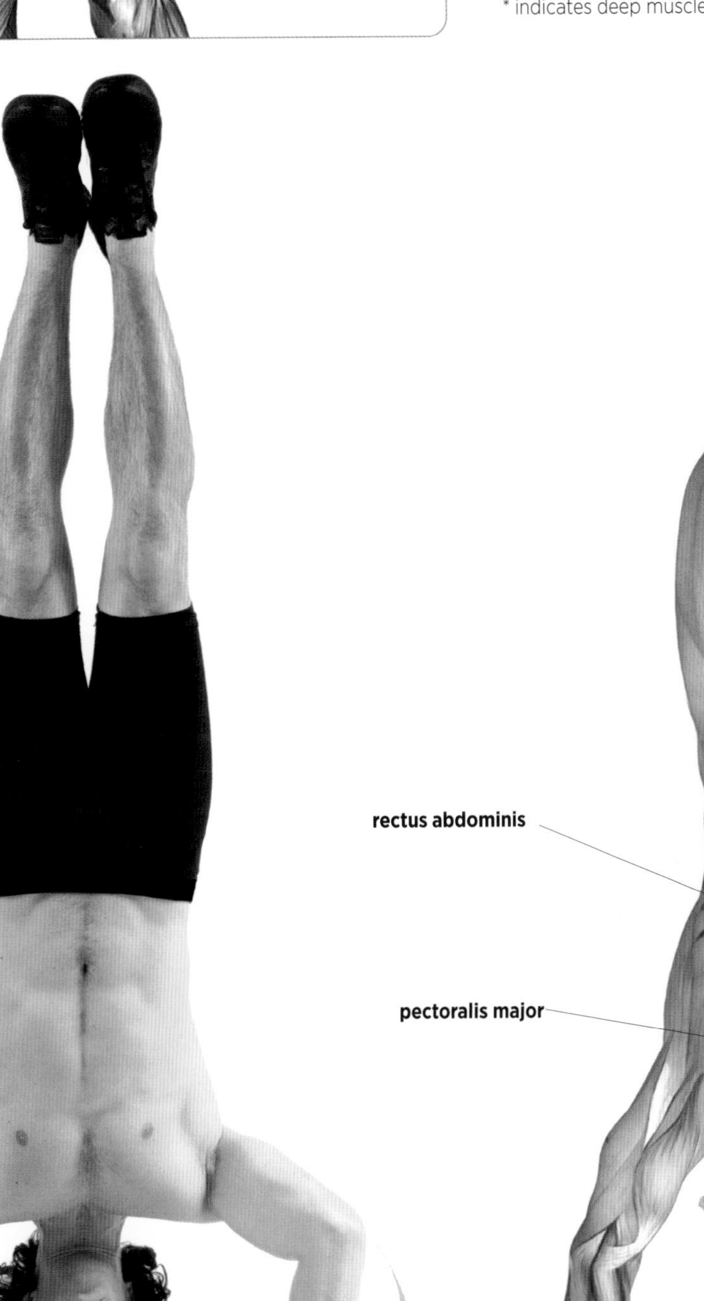

FACT FILE

TARGETS

- Triceps
- Deltoids
- Abdominals
- Back

TYPE

- Dynamic

BENEFITS

- Warms up muscles
- Improves coordination
- Strengthens and tones abdominals, chest, arms, and legs
- Increases cardiovascular endurance

CAUTIONS

- Wrist issues
- Shoulder issues

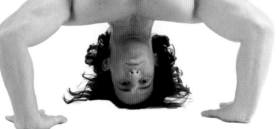

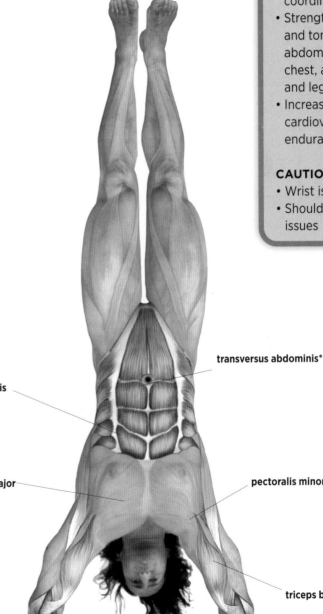

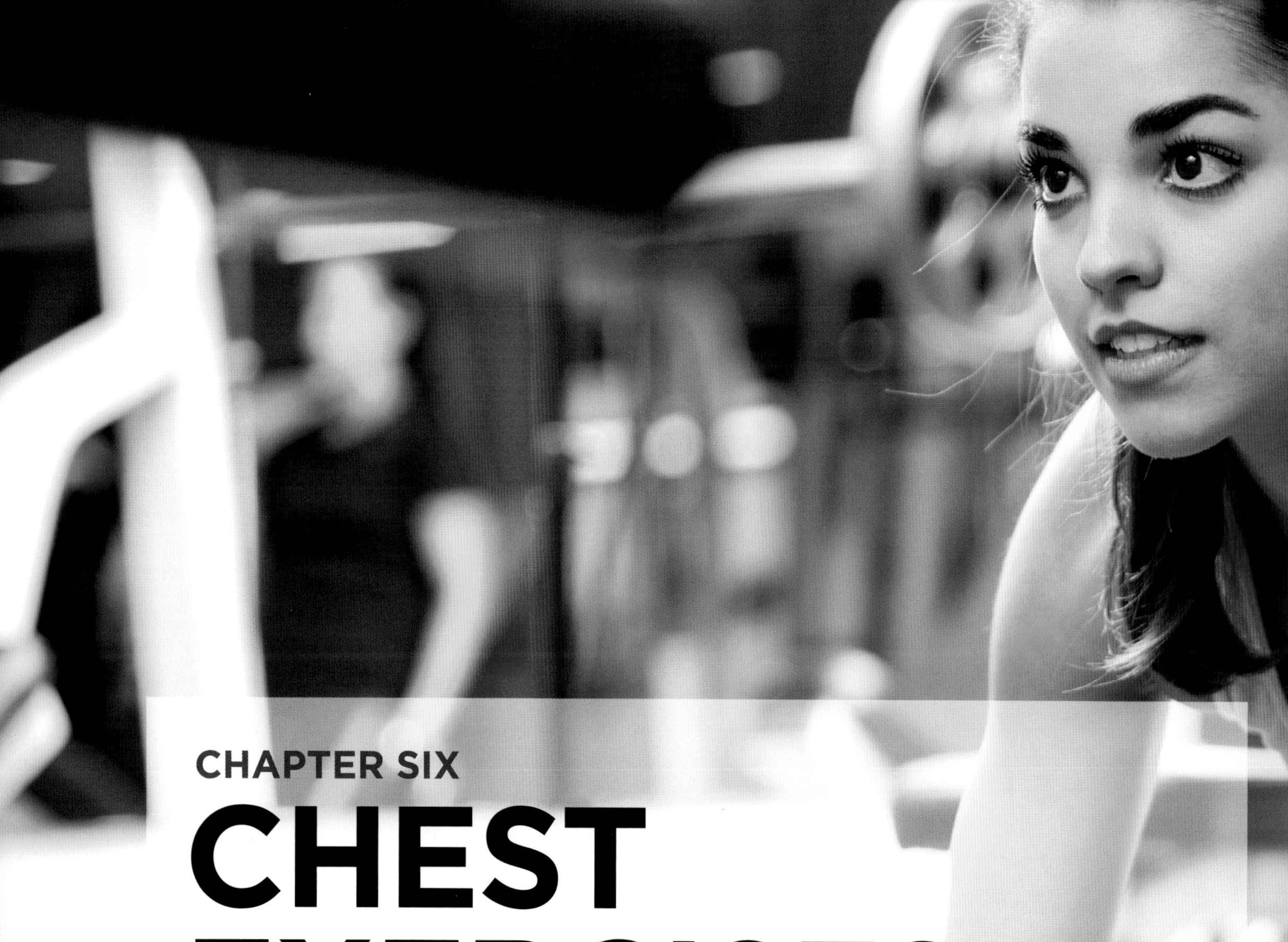

CHAPTER SIX

CHEST EXERCISES

Exercising your chest does more than improve your physique, the chest muscles are involved in essential functions. The chest muscles consist of the pectoralis major and, underneath that, the pectoralis minor, often referred to as the "pecs." The chest muscles are responsible for moving the arms across the body and up and down, as well as adduction, flexion, and rotation. The chest has some of the largest muscles in the body and you use them all day long—to open a door, pick up a parcel, or get up and down from the floor. It's important to keep these muscles strong!

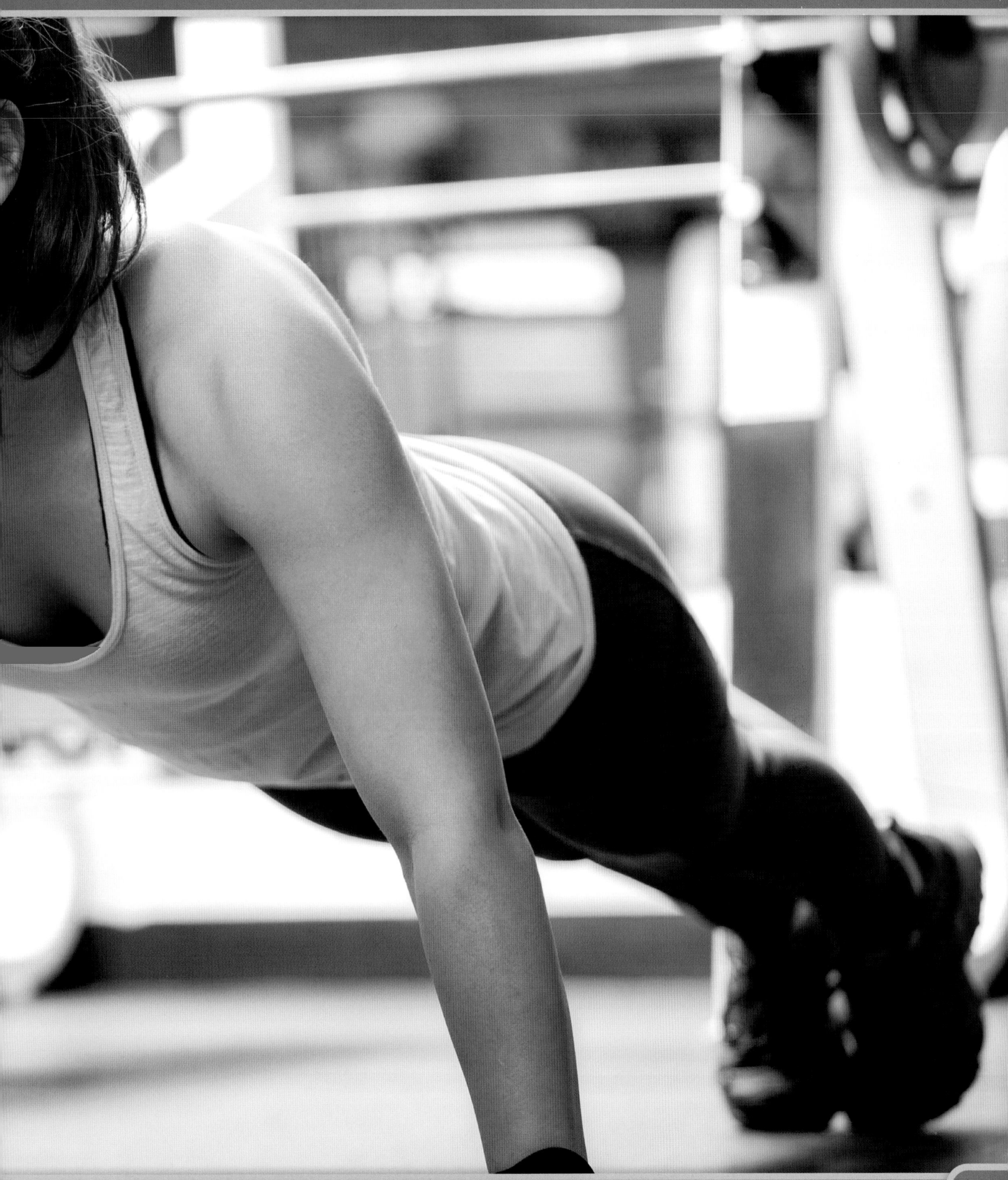

Push-Up

From military boot camps to high school gyms, you will find people performing the Push-Up. This proven calisthenics exercise works your chest, shoulders, arms, back, and core.

HOW TO DO IT

- Begin on your hands and knees, with your hands planted slightly wider than shoulder-width apart. Extend your legs back to come into a high plank position.
- With control, slowly lower the full length of your body toward the floor, bending your elbows.
- Straighten your elbows to return to the high plank position. Repeat for the recommended repetitions.

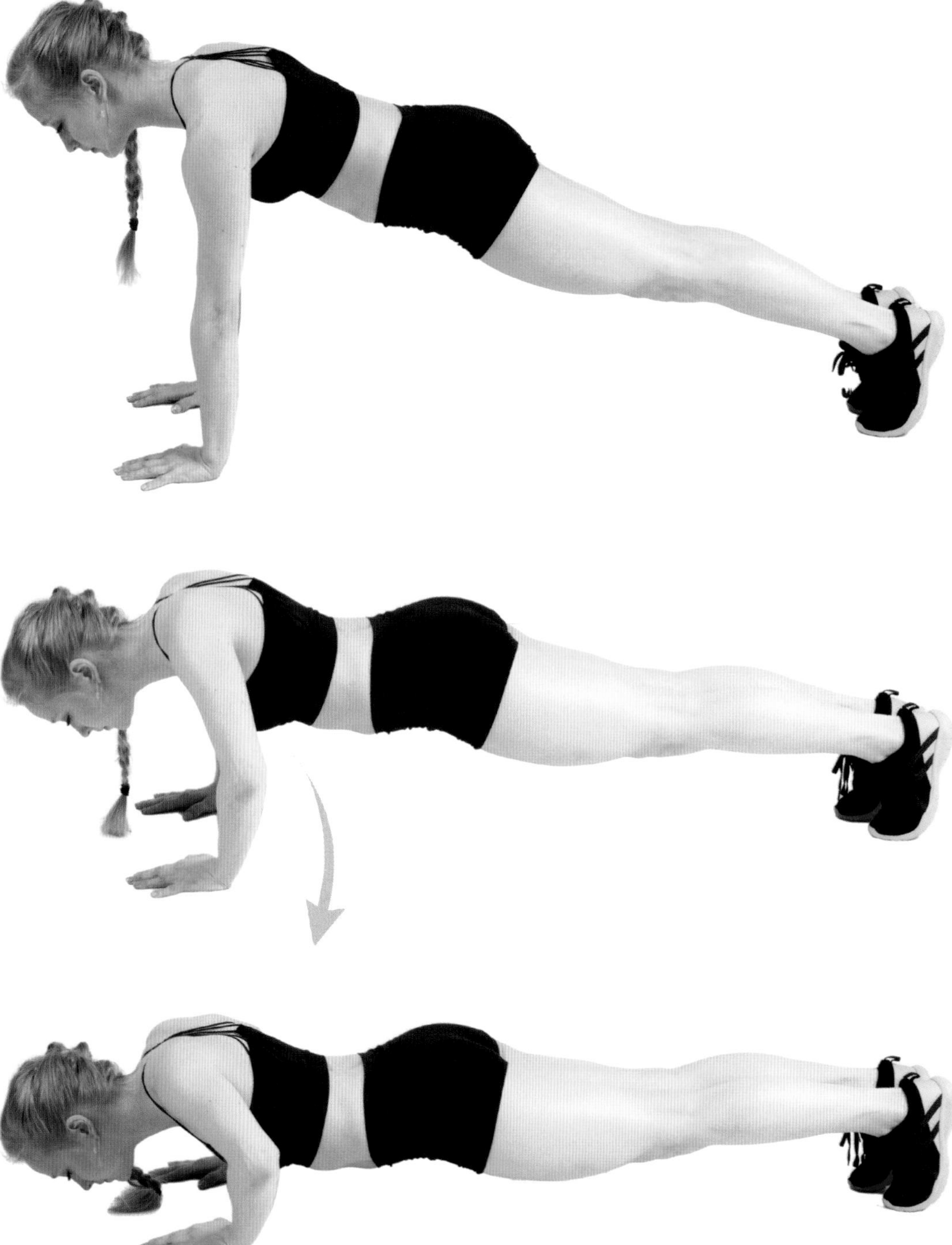

DO IT RIGHT

- Keep your shoulders pressed down your back.
- Imagine a straight line running from the top of your head to your heels.
- Avoid compromising the neutral alignment of your pelvis or spine.

FACT FILE

TARGETS
- Pectorals
- Biceps
- Deltoids
- Abdominals
- Back

TYPE
- Dynamic

BENEFITS
- Strengthens biceps, shoulders, chest, back, and core
- Tones abdominals

CAUTIONS
- Shoulder issues
- Wrist issues

MODIFICATION

EASIER: Kneel on all fours with your hands planted slightly wider than shoulder-width apart. Lift your feet toward your buttocks until your calves and thighs form a 90-degree angle. Perform as you would a basic push-up.

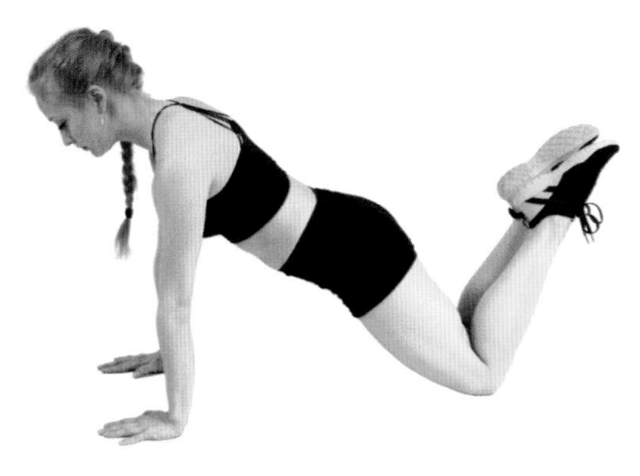

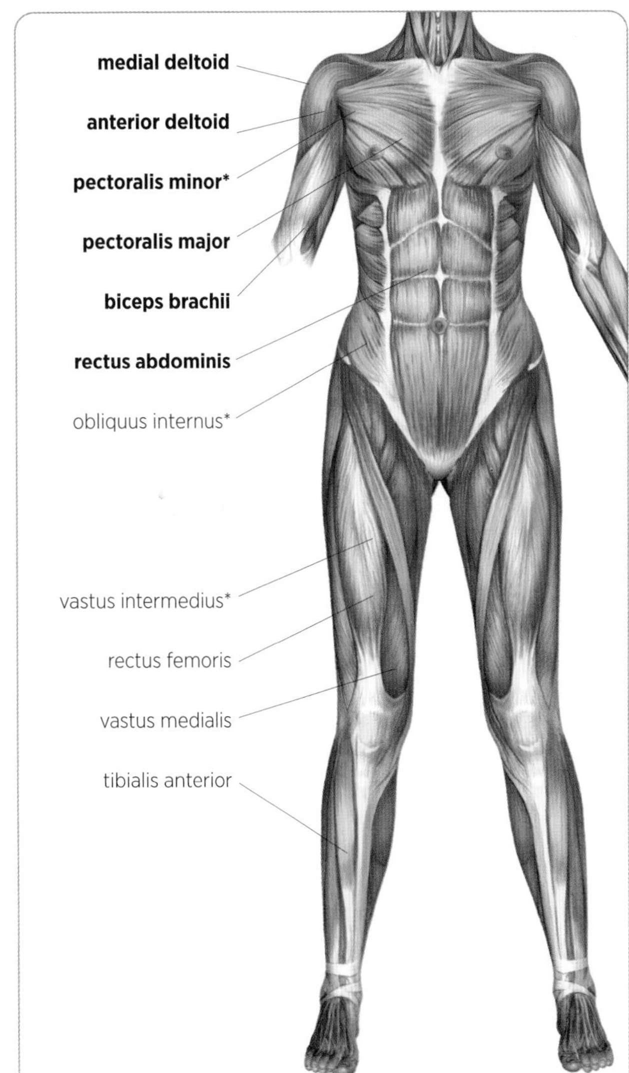

Annotation Key
Bold text indicates target muscles
Light text indicates other working muscles
* indicates deep muscles

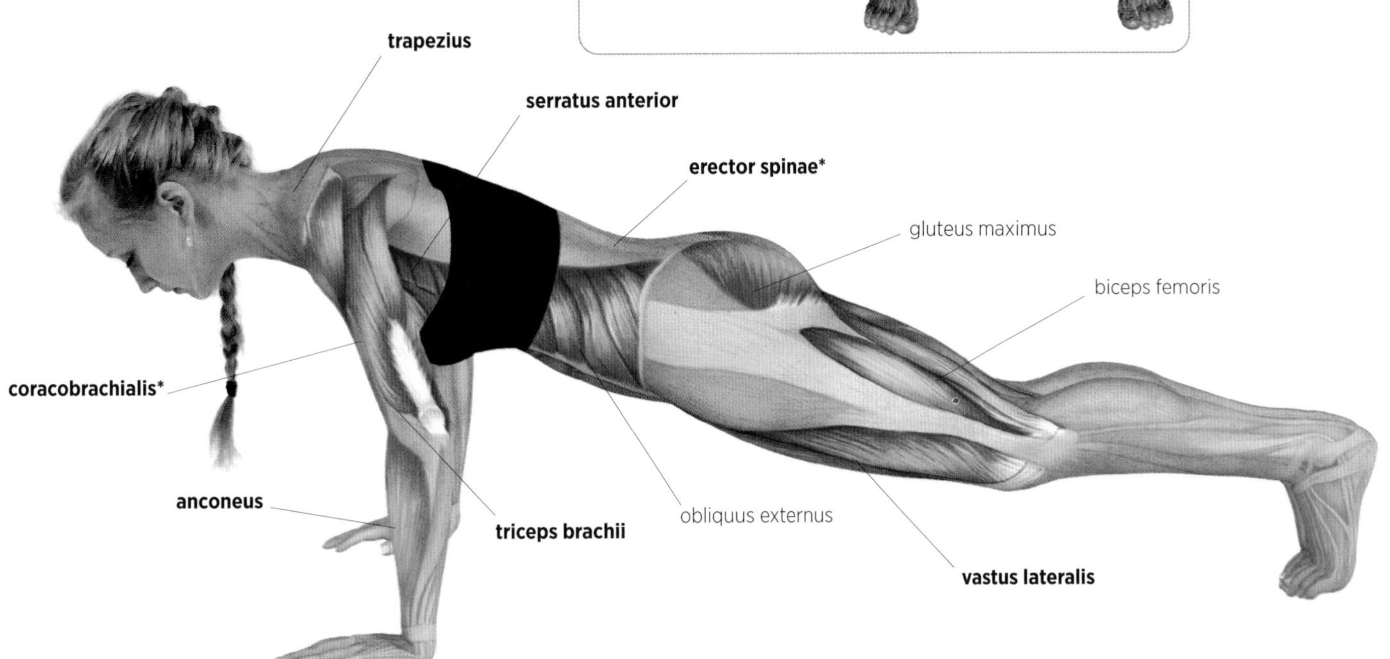

Alternating Single-Arm Push-Up

The Alternating Single-Arm Push-Up is an advanced, dynamically engaging chest exercise. It focuses on your pectorals, but it doesn't leave much untouched. With your triceps and deltoids engaged, as well as your core and legs providing a stable base, it will strengthen your entire body.

HOW TO DO IT

- Begin in a high plank position with your feet spread wider than hips-width apart and your hands planted beneath your shoulders.
- Place your right hand on the small of your back.
- Keeping your core engaged, bend your left elbow to bring your chest toward the floor.
- Press your left hand into the floor, and extend your elbow to return to the starting position.
- Repeat for the recommended repetitions, alternating arms with every rep.

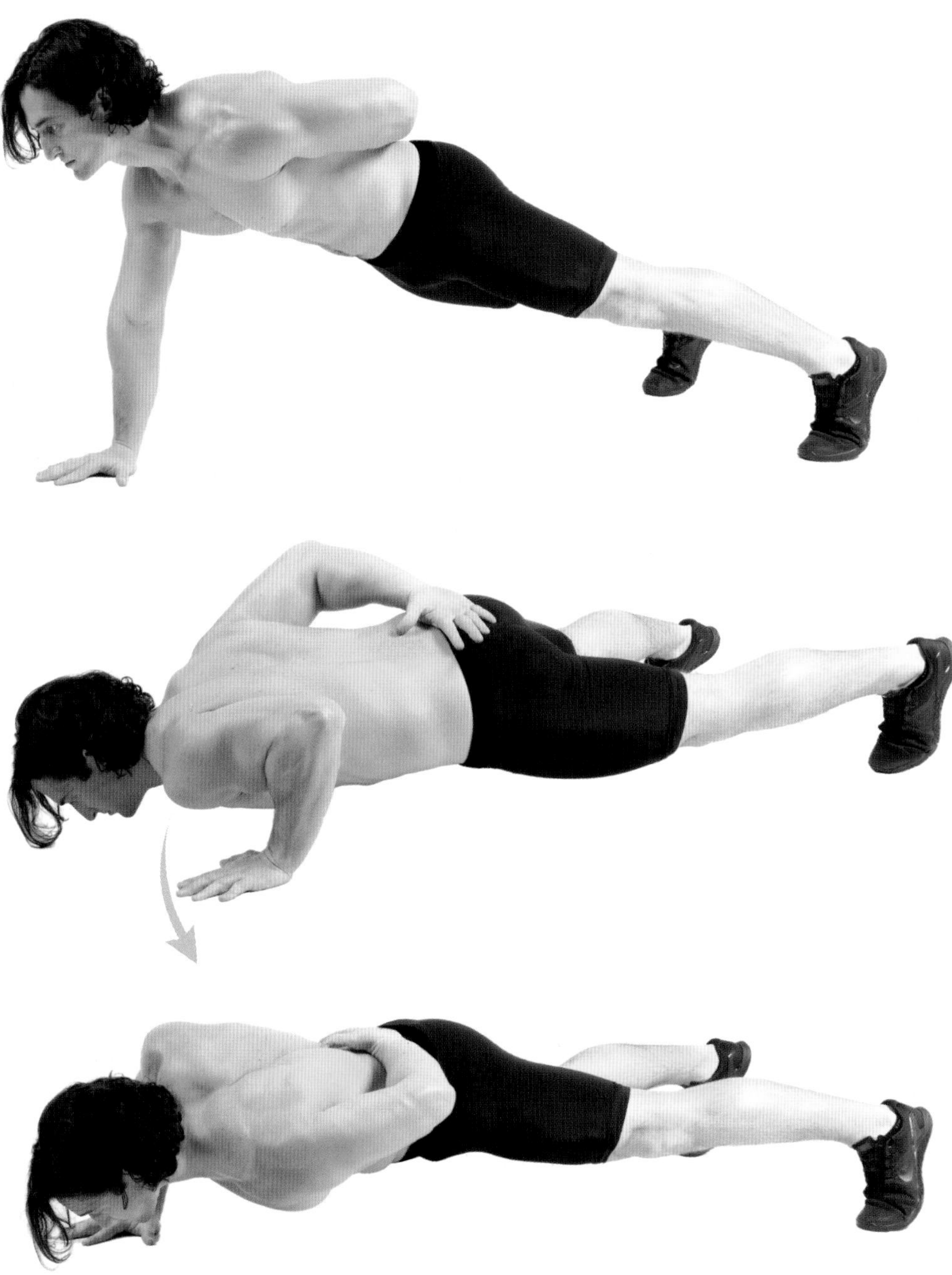

DO IT RIGHT

- Keep your back straight and hips square to the floor.
- Move with control.
- Avoid excessive arching of the spine.

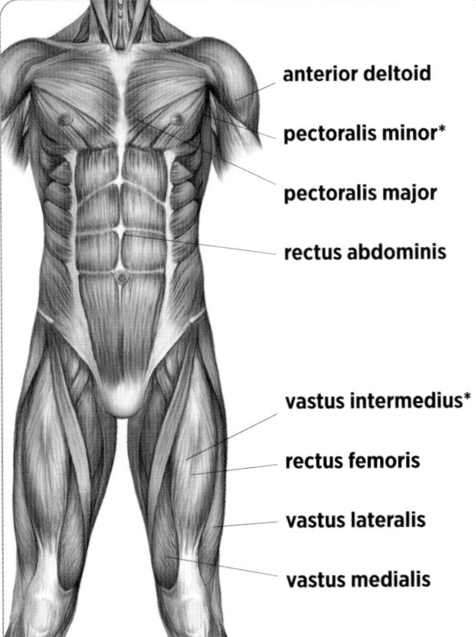

Annotation Key
Bold text indicates target muscles
Light text indicates other working muscles
* indicates deep muscles

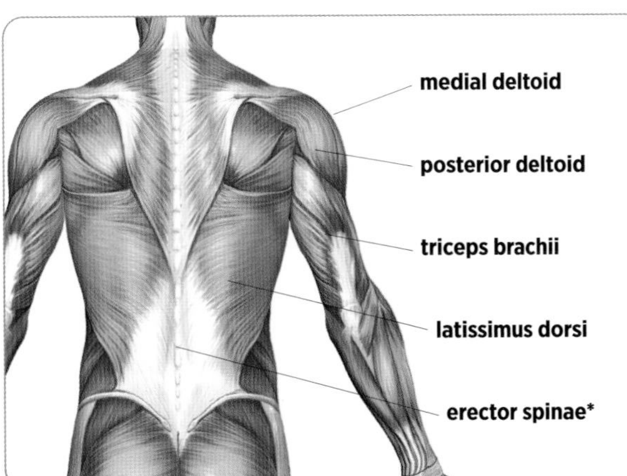

FACT FILE

TARGETS
- Pectorals
- Triceps
- Deltoids
- Abdominals
- Quadriceps

TYPE
- Dynamic

BENEFITS
- Improves balance
- Improves coordination
- Strengthens and tones chest, arms, abdominals, and legs

CAUTIONS
- Wrist issues
- Shoulder issues

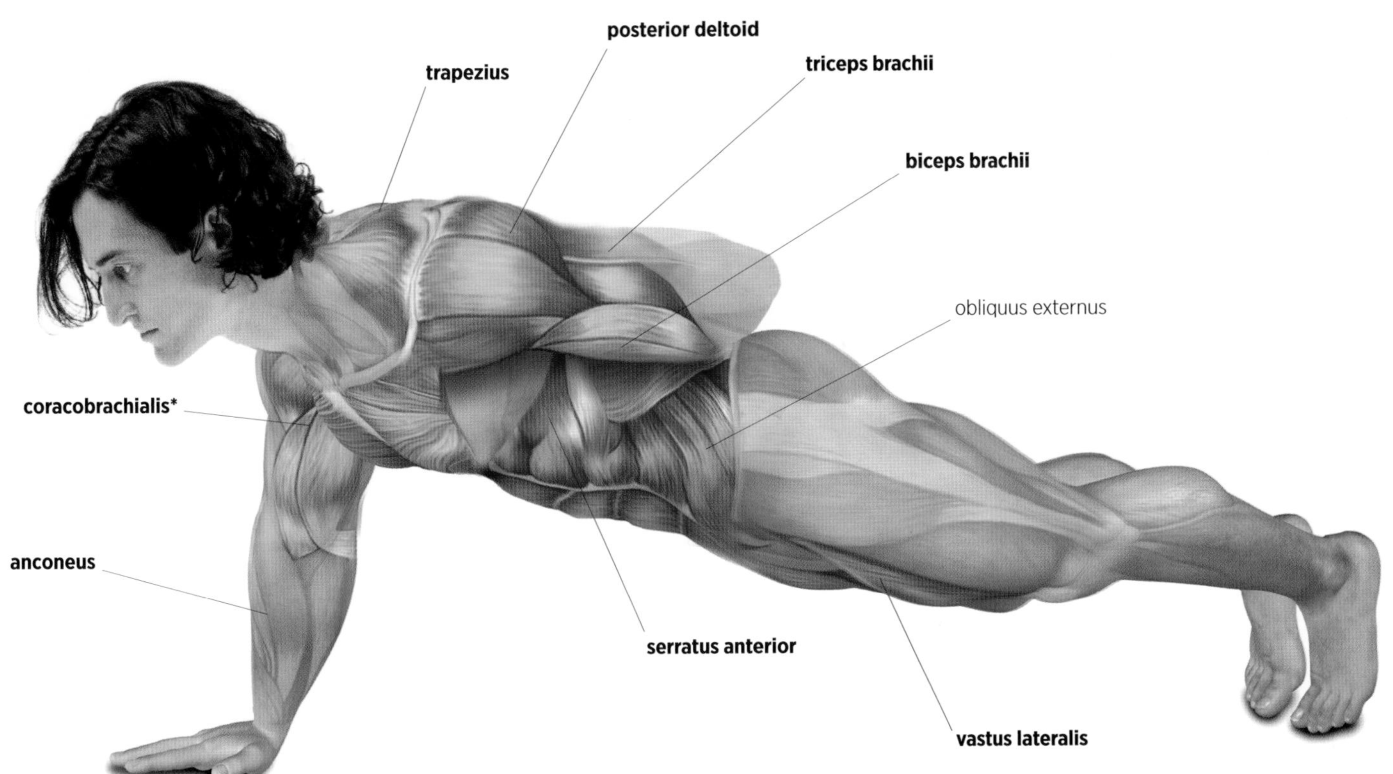

Towel Fly

The Towel Fly is a great addition to your chest workout. Its in-out movement not only engages your chest muscles but also recruits numerous other muscles, including those of the arms, back, hips, and abdomen, to keep your body stabilized.

HOW TO DO IT

- Place a towel on the floor in front of you. Assume a high plank position, with your elbows fully extended and the towel under your hands.
- Maintaining a rigid plank position and putting your weight into your heels, move your hands together. The towel should bunch together below your sternum.
- Straighten out the towel by pressing outward with your arms, returning to the starting position. Repeat for the recommended repetitions.

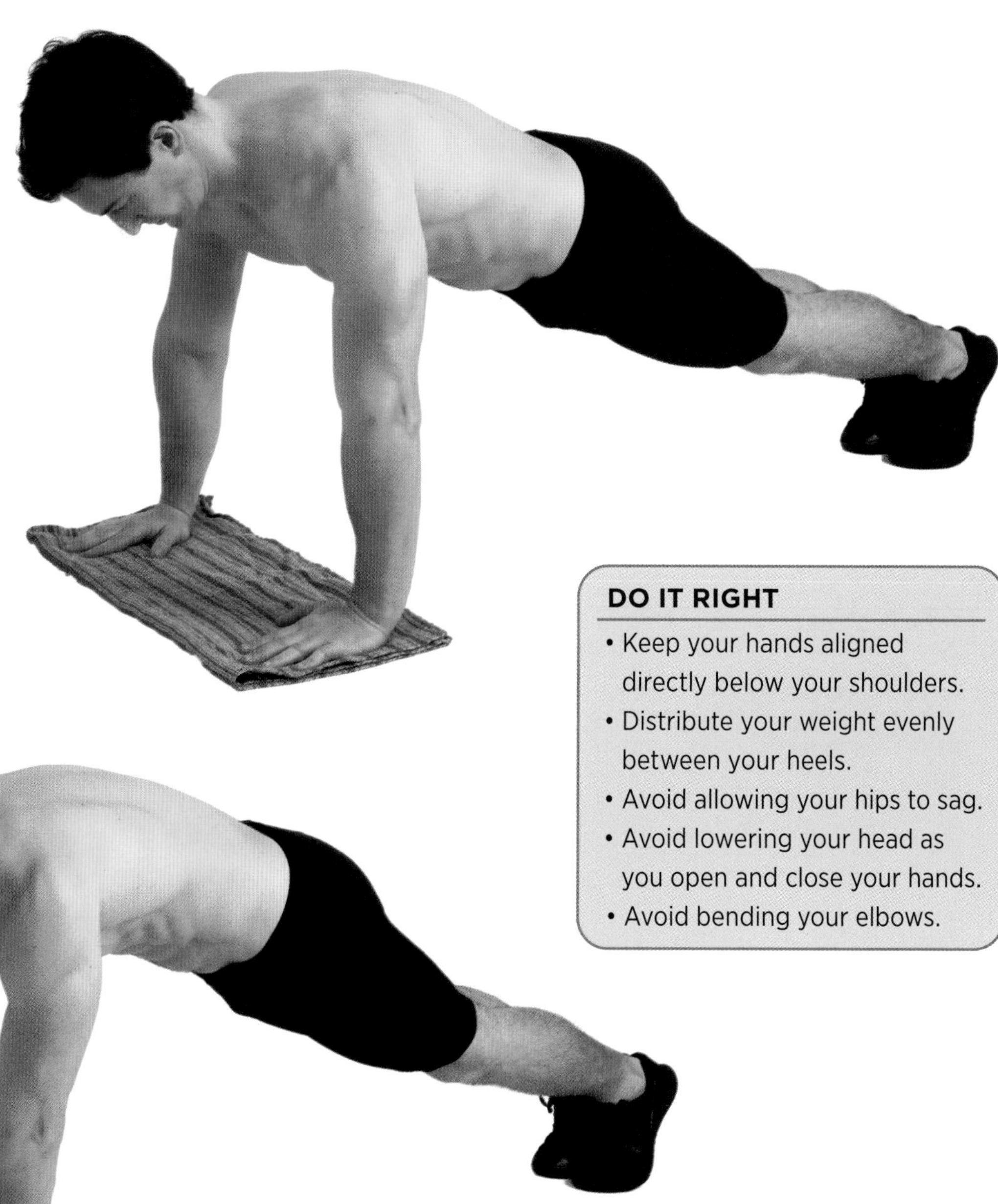

DO IT RIGHT

- Keep your hands aligned directly below your shoulders.
- Distribute your weight evenly between your heels.
- Avoid allowing your hips to sag.
- Avoid lowering your head as you open and close your hands.
- Avoid bending your elbows.

FACT FILE

TARGETS
- Pectorals
- Deltoids
- Hamstrings
- Back
- Abdominals

TYPE
- Dynamic

BENEFITS
- Strengthens chest and upper arm muscles
- Develops trunk and pelvic stability

CAUTIONS
- Shoulder issues
- Wrist issues
- Neck pain
- Lower-back pain

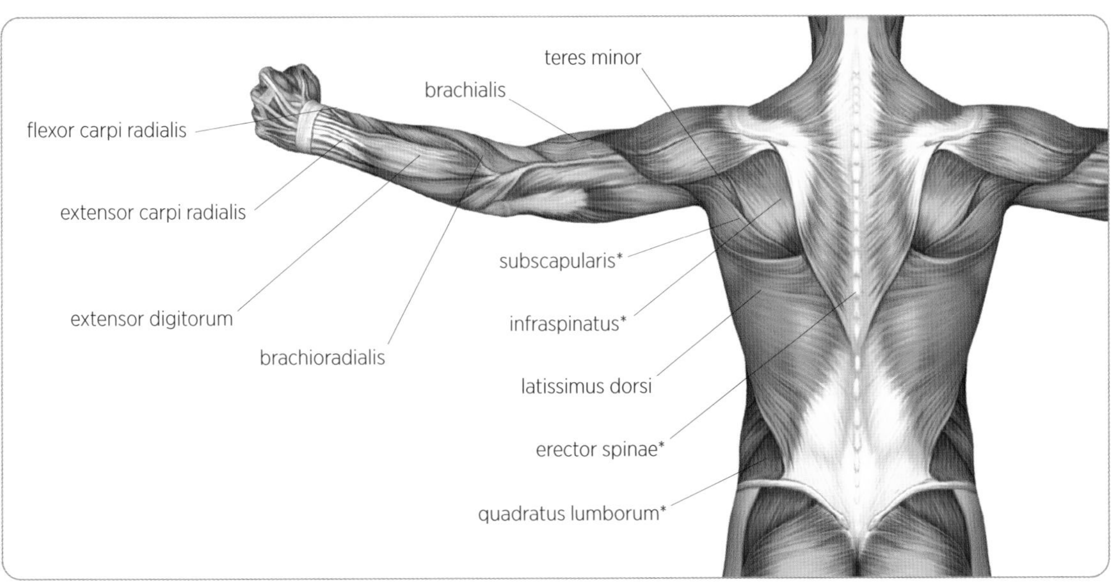

Annotation Key

Bold text indicates target muscles

Light text indicates other working muscles

* indicates deep muscles

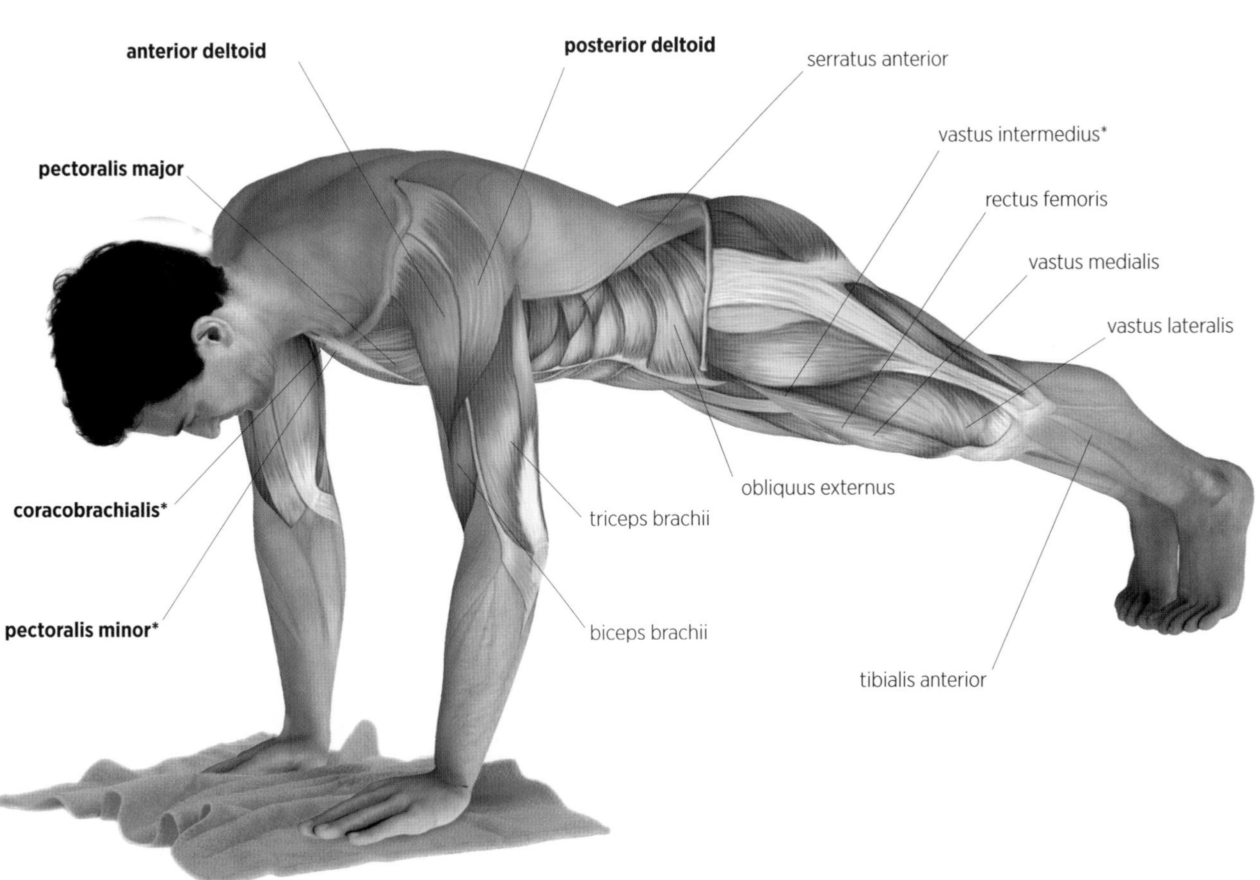

Sprawl Push-Up

Try the Sprawl Push-Up for a cardio-intensive version of the basic Push-Up. Perform this exercise as quickly as possible to increase the demand on your cardiovascular system.

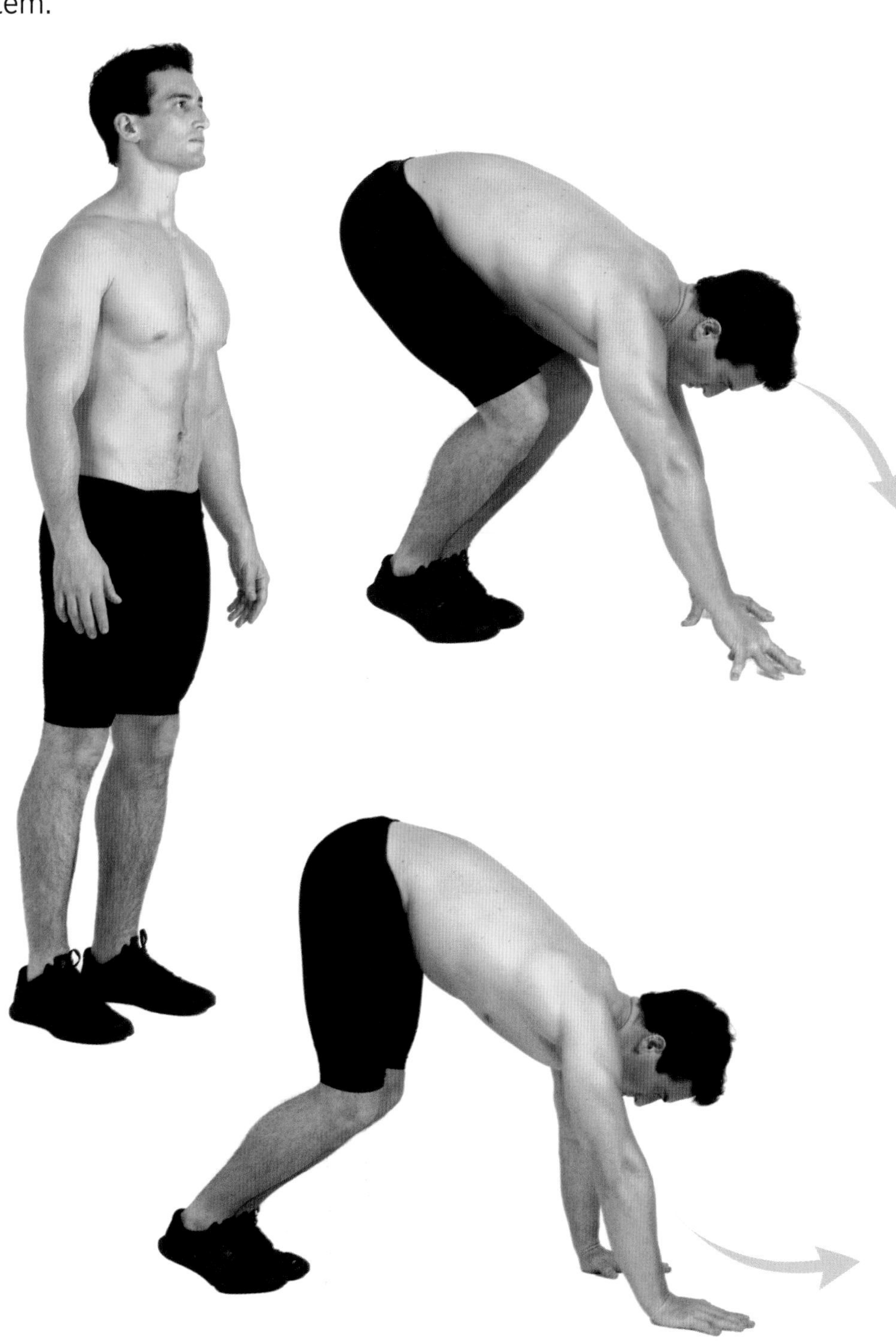

HOW TO DO IT

- Stand with your feet together.
- Bend forward from your hips, and place your hands on the floor, walking them forward.
- Continue walking your hands forward until you are in a flat Push-Up position.
- Raise your body to a high plank position with your feet spread wider than hips-width apart and your hands planted beneath your shoulders.
- Lower your chest back to floor. This is one repetition.
- Walk your hands back to your feet to return to a standing position. Perform as many repetitions as possible in the recommended time.

DO IT RIGHT

- Keep your legs and back straight during the push-up portion.
- Perform this exercise as quickly as possible to increase the demand on your cardiovascular system.
- Avoid pointing your elbows to the side during the down movement; this places undue stress on the anterior deltoids.

FACT FILE

TARGETS
- Pectorals
- Triceps
- Deltoids
- Abdominals
- Quadriceps

TYPE
- Dynamic

BENEFITS
- Strengthens upper and lower body
- Builds cardio and muscle endurance

CAUTIONS
- Shoulder issues
- Wrist issues
- Lower-back pain

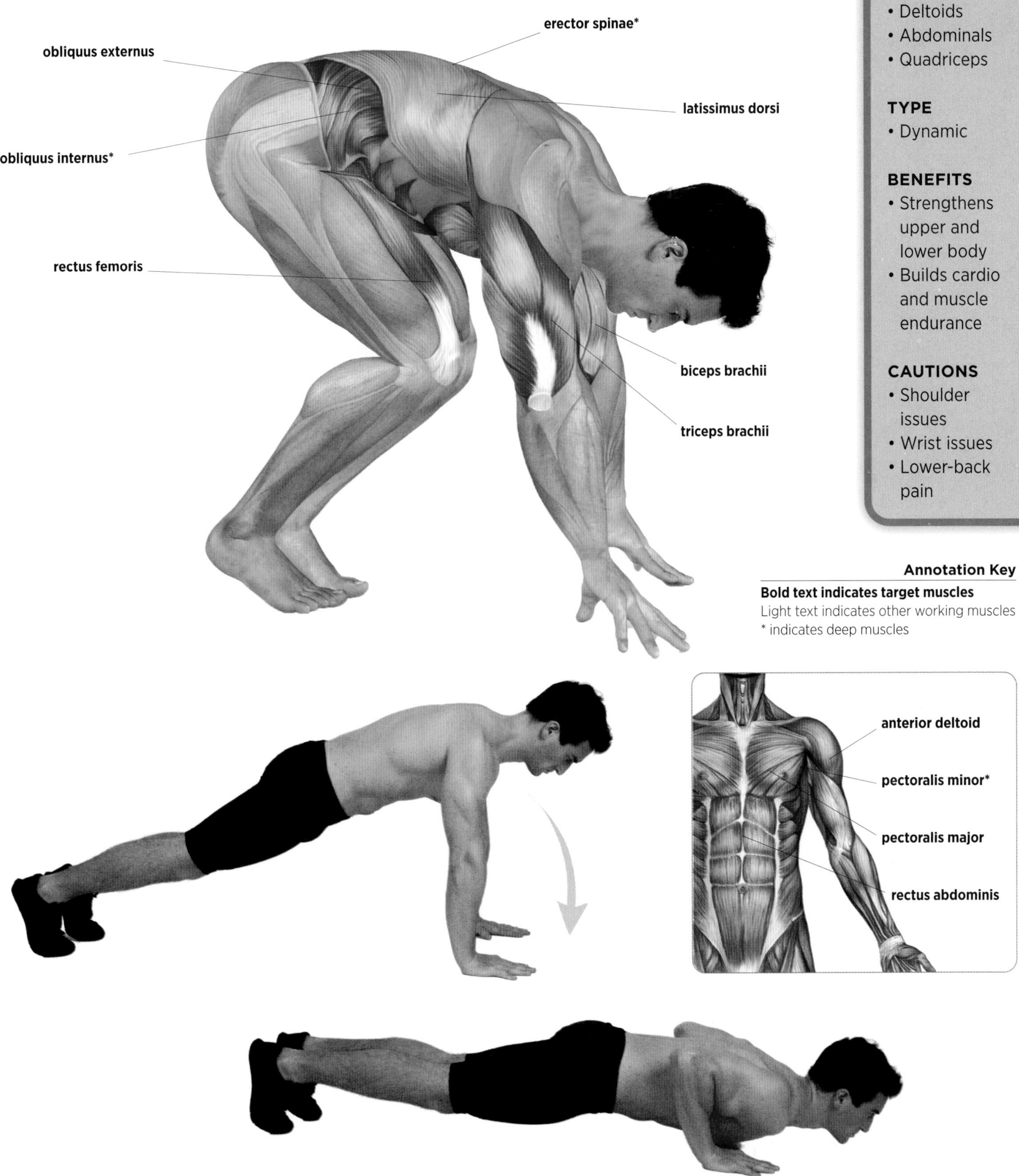

Annotation Key
Bold text indicates target muscles
Light text indicates other working muscles
* indicates deep muscles

Wide Push-Up

This Wide Push-Up emphasizes muscles differently than the basic Push-Up (pages 196–97). It especially strengthens the front of your shoulders and chest, with other—mostly upper-body—muscles helping out.

HOW TO DO IT

- Start on your hands and knees, with your hands much wider apart than shoulder-width.

- Push your body up so your arms are straight, with your legs extended backward, to come into a high plank position. Keep your palms on the floor, your feet together, your back straight, and your weight on the balls of your feet. This is your starting position.

- With control, slowly bend your arms, and lower your torso toward the floor. Lower as far as you can go comfortably—which may be until your chest touches the floor.

- Straighten your arms to rise back up to your starting plank position. Repeat for the recommended repetitions.

DO IT RIGHT

- Slightly flare your hands outward so your elbows go toward your hips as you lower yourself to the floor. This helps prevent shoulder tendonitis.
- If you cannot keep your back straight during the entire movement or you feel back pain, start this exercise on both knees and do a modified push-up.
- Avoid pushing your hips into the air.
- Avoid pointing your elbows to the side during the down movement. This places undue stress on the front of your shoulders.

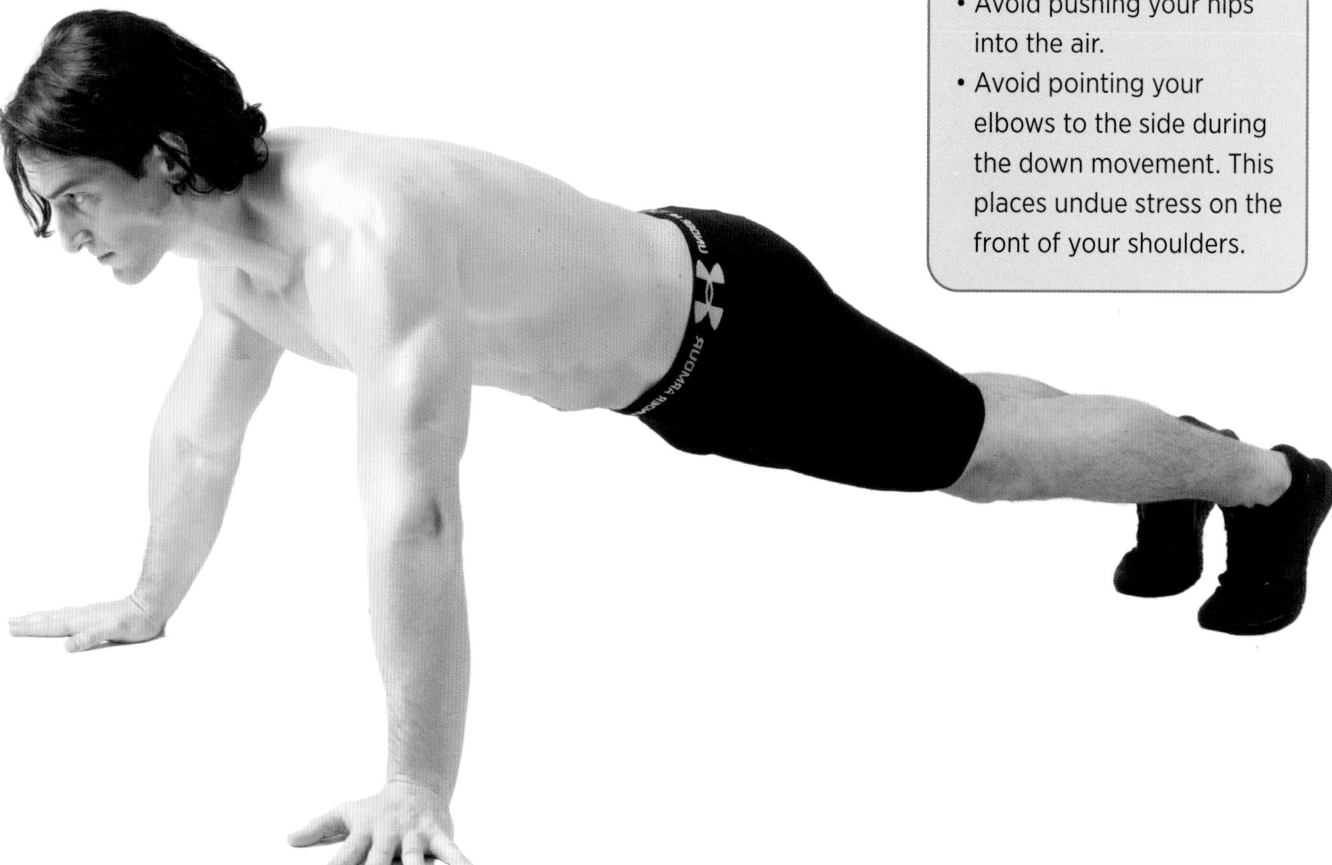

FACT FILE

TARGETS
- Chest
- Shoulders
- Abdominals
- Back
- Upper arms
- Front of thighs

TYPE
- Dynamic

BENEFITS
- Strengthens upper body
- Strengthens shoulders

CAUTIONS
- Shoulder issues
- Wrist issues
- Lower-back pain

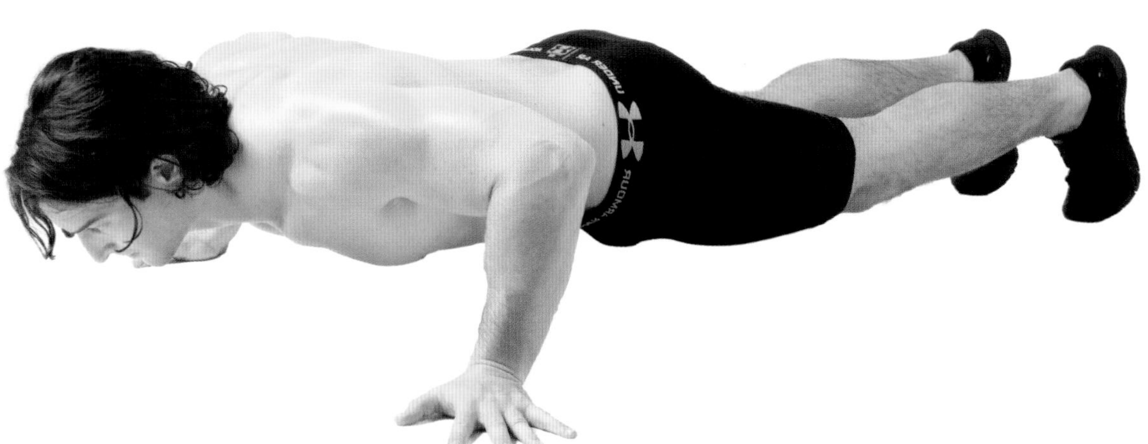

Annotation Key

Bold text indicates target muscles
Light text indicates other working muscles
* indicates deep muscles

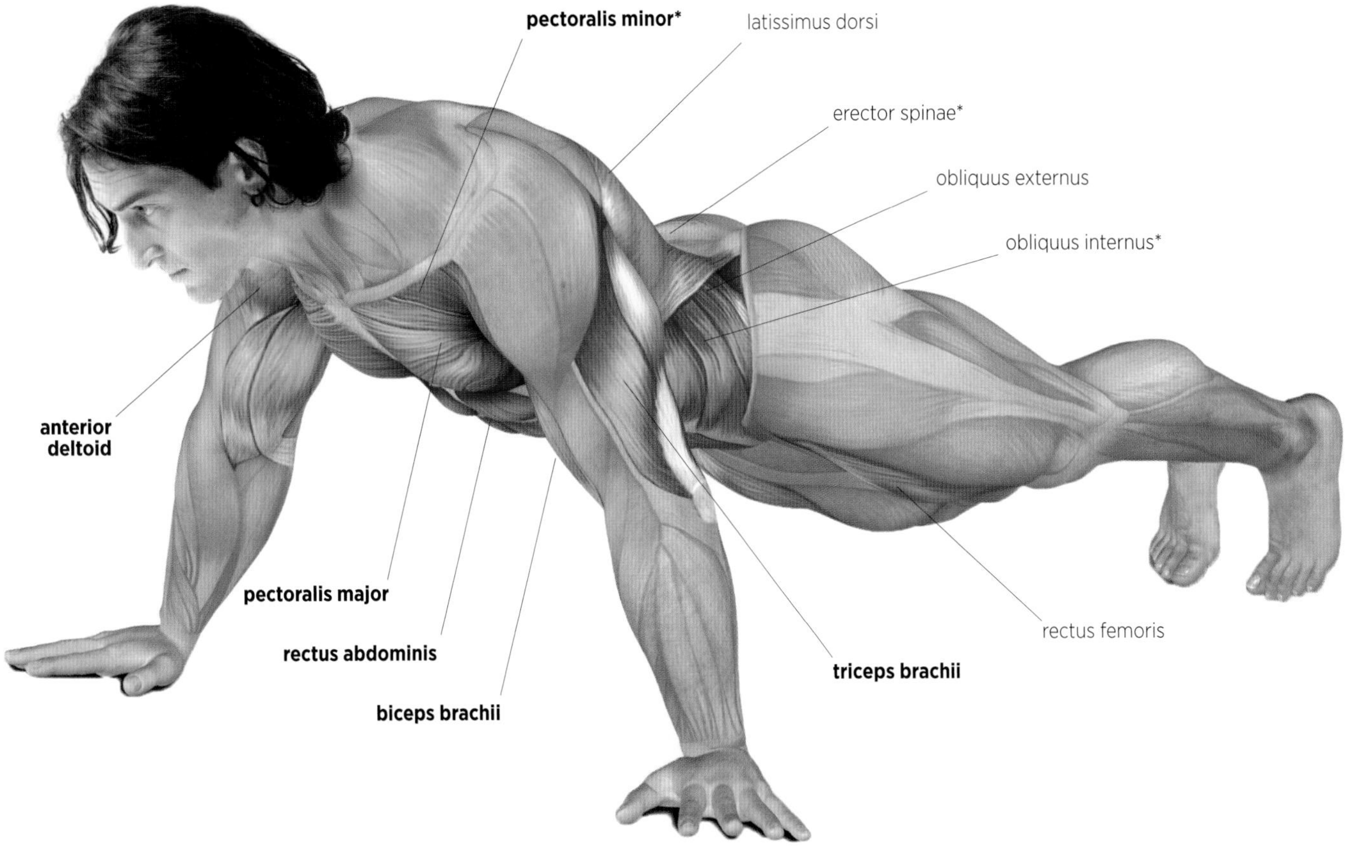

pectoralis minor*
latissimus dorsi
erector spinae*
obliquus externus
obliquus internus*
anterior deltoid
pectoralis major
rectus abdominis
biceps brachii
triceps brachii
rectus femoris

Dive-Bomber Push-Up

This upper-body and core exercise gets its name from the swooping movement you make as you move though the exercise. It will effectively strengthen your arms, shoulders, chest, back, and abdominals.

HOW TO DO IT

- Stand with your feet shoulder-width apart. Bend forward to place your hands on the floor, also shoulder-width apart. Raise your hips so that your body forms an inverted V.
- With a controlled movement, swoop your hips toward the floor while simultaneously raising your chest.
- Continue rising upward until you're looking toward the ceiling and your back is arched.
- Swoop back down, and then repeat the entire sequence for the recommended repetitions.

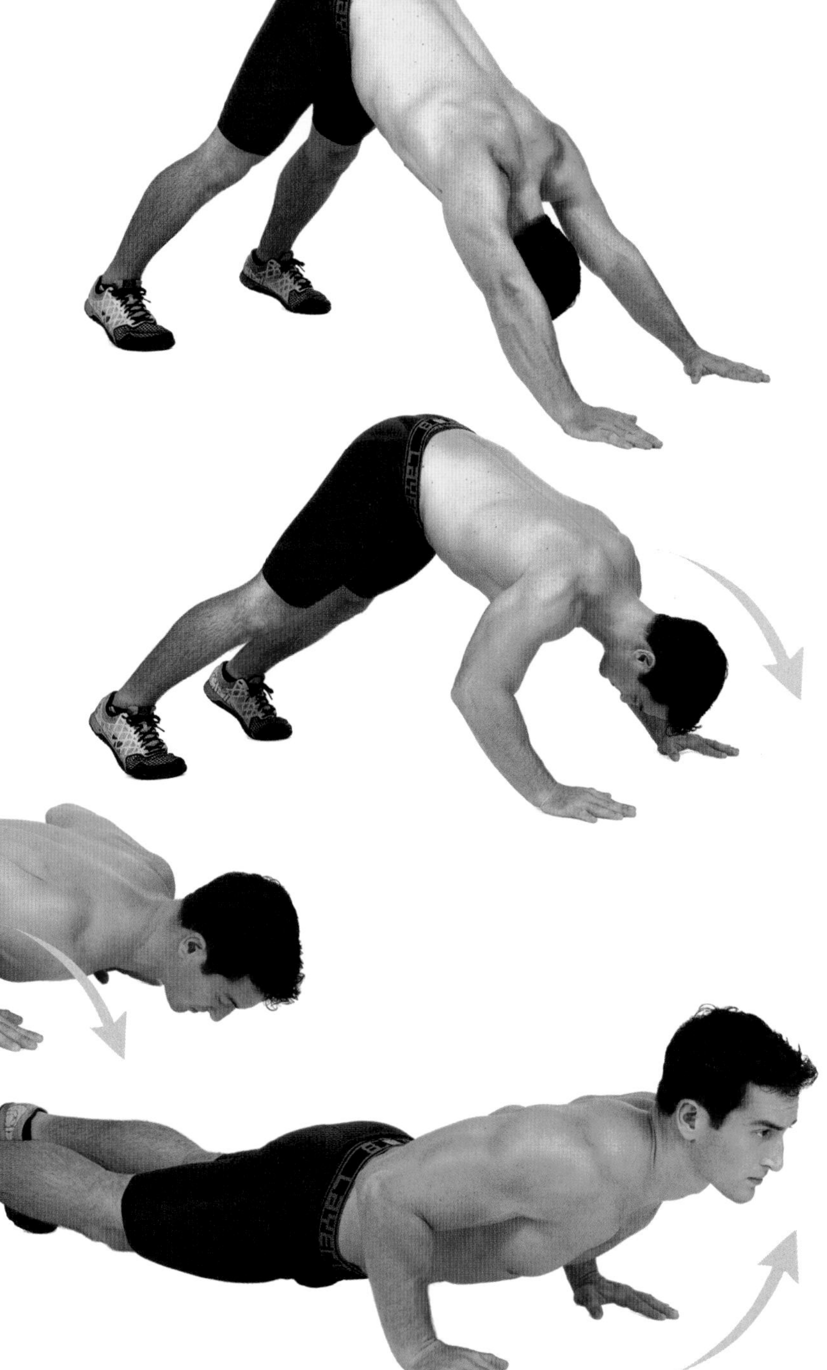

DO IT RIGHT

- Plant your hands firmly on the floor, securely grounding your fingers.
- Move with control.

FACT FILE

TARGETS
- Pectorals
- Deltoids
- Hamstrings
- Back
- Abdominals

TYPE
- Dynamic

BENEFITS
- Strengthens legs, wrists, arms, and spine
- Stretches chest, shoulders, thighs, and abdomen
- Improves posture

CAUTIONS
- Back injury
- Wrist injury or carpal tunnel syndrome

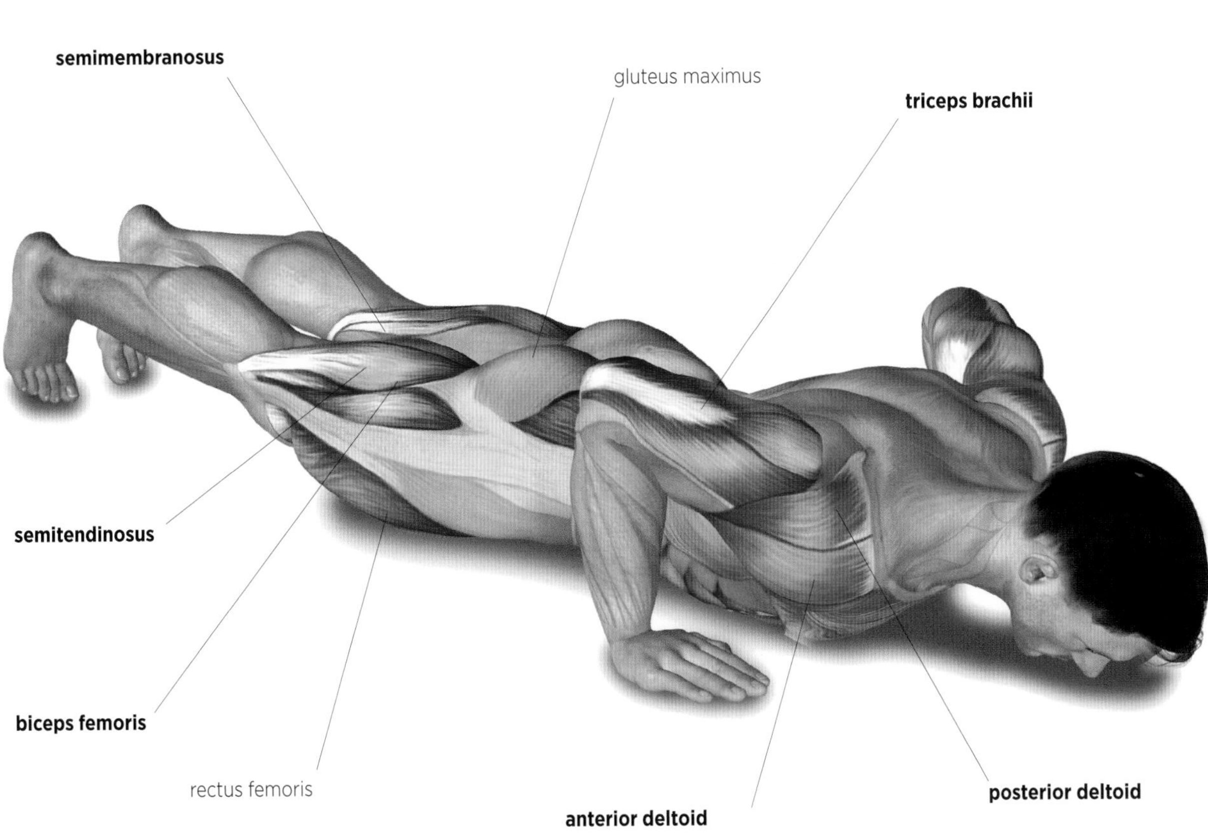

Annotation Key

Bold text indicates target muscles
Light text indicates other working muscles
* indicates deep muscles

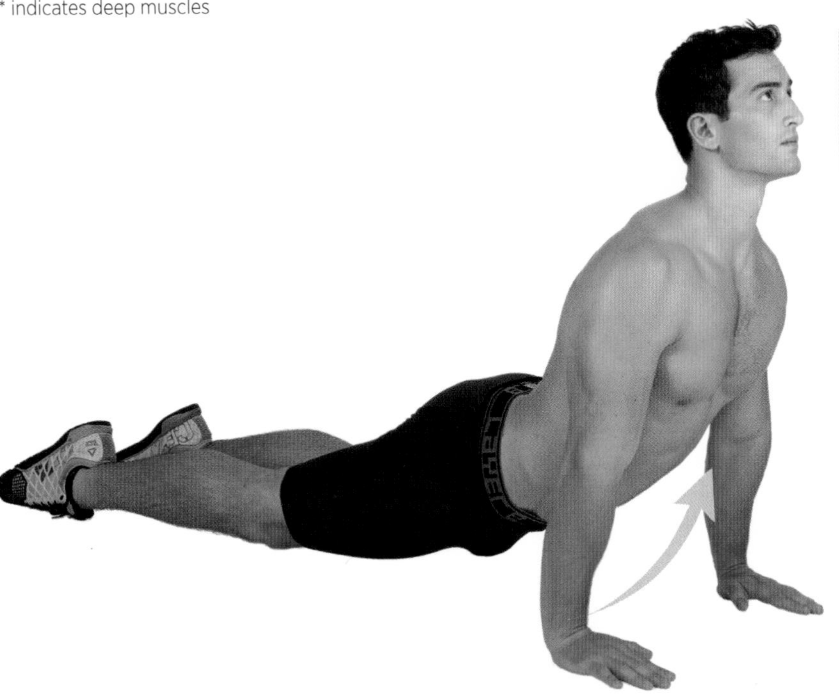

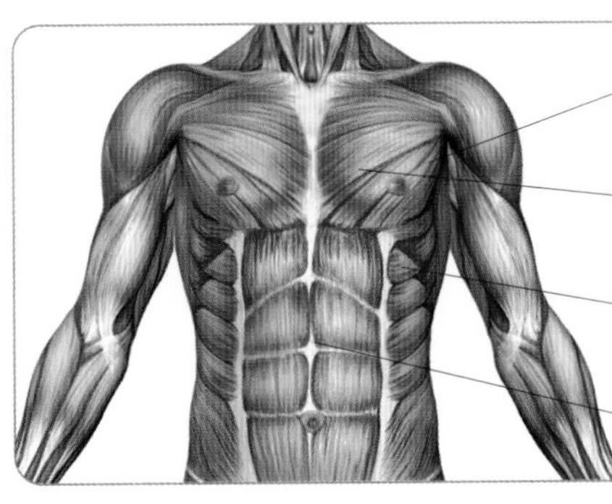

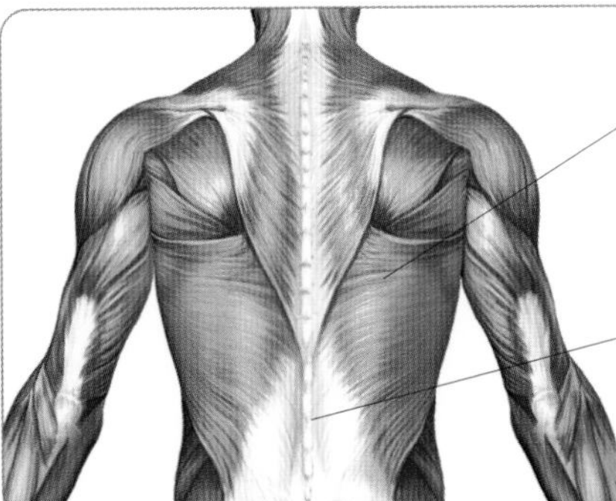

Shoulder-Tap Push-Up

The Shoulder-Tap Push-Up takes the standard push-up exercise to the next level, shifting your body weight from side to side, which further strengthens your arms. It requires good midline stability, dexterity, and chest and triceps strength.

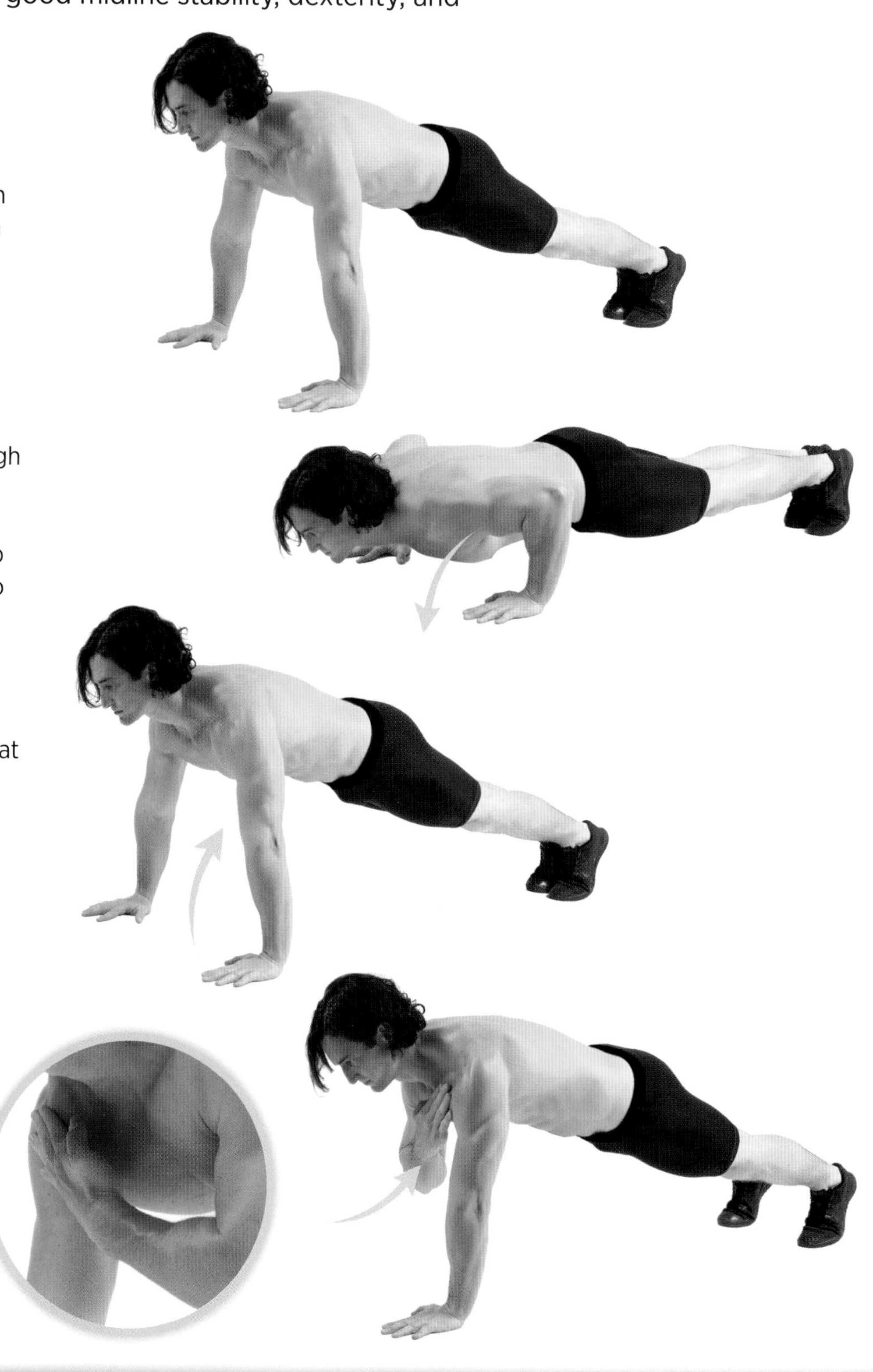

HOW TO DO IT

- Begin in a high plank position with your feet spread wider than hips-width apart and your hands planted beneath your shoulders.
- Perform a push-up, lowering yourself until your chest reaches the floor.
- While engaging your core, press your palms into the floor to return to the high plank position.
- Shift your weight onto your left arm so that you are able lift your right hand to tap your opposite (left) shoulder.
- Return your hand back to the floor.
- Repeat the entire exercise again. Repeat for the recommended repetitions, alternating arms with every rep.

DO IT RIGHT

- Keep your core engaged and your back straight.
- Completely shift your body weight before removing a hand from the ground.
- Keep your hips square to the floor, avoiding too much movement in your pelvis, even during the weight shift.

anterior deltoid
pectoralis minor*
pectoralis major
rectus abdominis

trapezius
medial deltoid
posterior deltoid
latissimus dorsi
gluteus maximus
biceps femoris

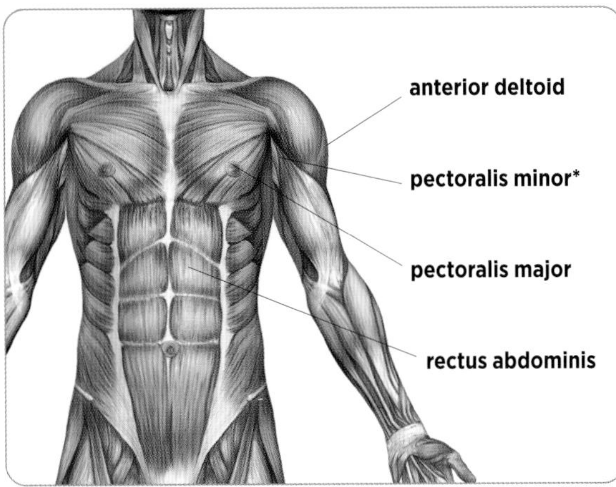

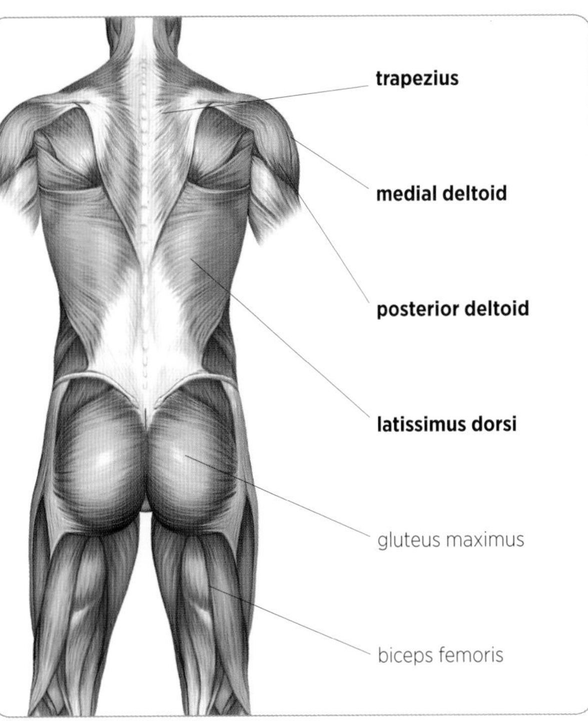

Annotation Key

Bold text indicates target muscles
Light text indicates other working muscles
* indicates deep muscles

FACT FILE

TARGETS
- Pectorals
- Triceps
- Deltoids
- Abdominals

TYPE
- Dynamic

BENEFITS
- Improves balance
- Improves coordination
- Strengthens and tones abdominals, chest, arms, and legs
- Increases midline stability

CAUTIONS
- Wrist issues
- Back issues

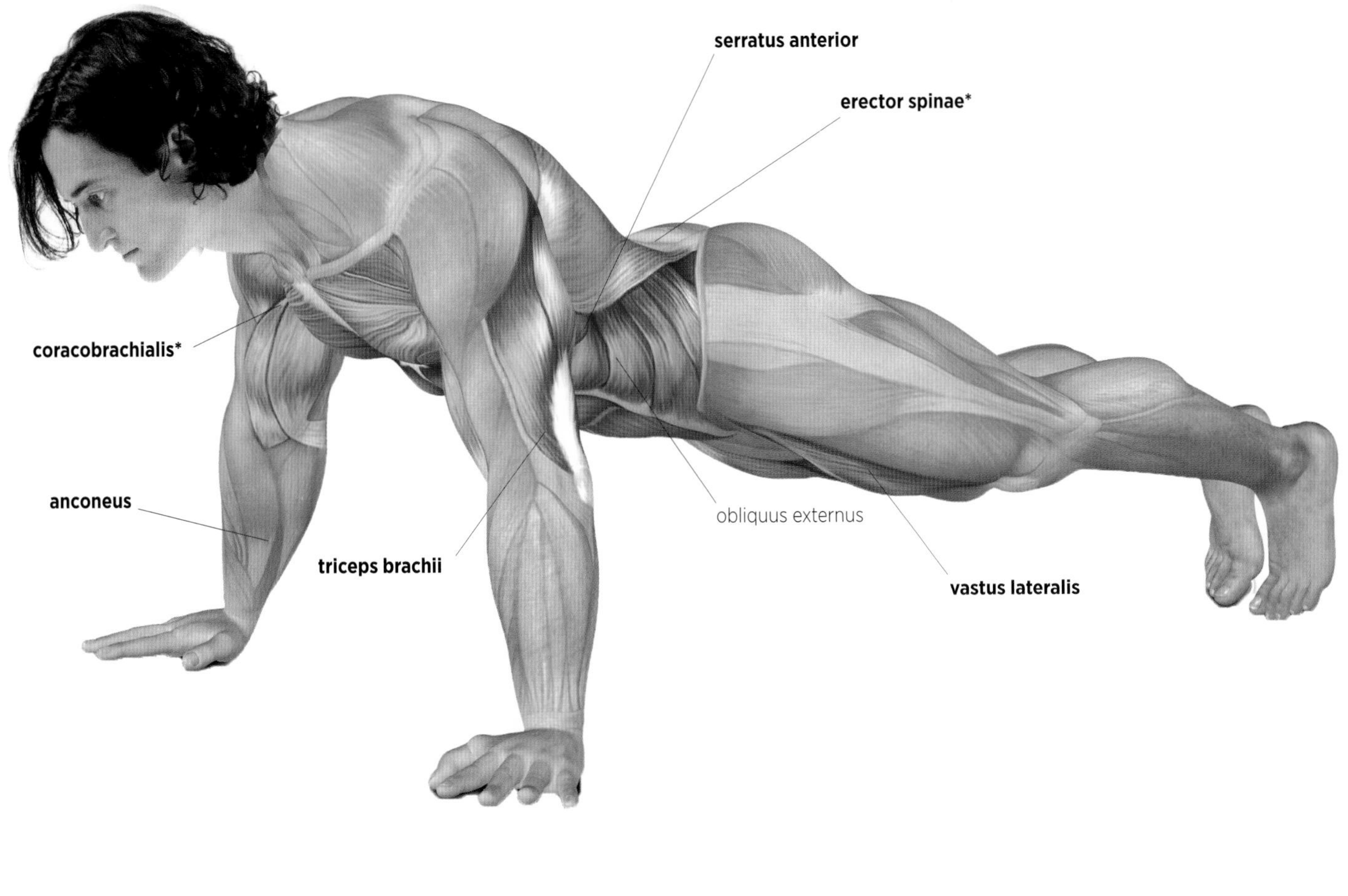

serratus anterior
erector spinae*
coracobrachialis*
anconeus
triceps brachii
obliquus externus
vastus lateralis

Push-Up Hand Walk-Over

The Push-Up Hand Walk-Over adds a dynamic element to the basic push-up. As with any push-up, this variation targets your pectorals and triceps. The added lateral movement also challenges your shoulder and core stabilizers.

DO IT RIGHT

- Keep your hands aligned under your shoulders.
- Avoid dipping your shoulders to one side.
- Avoid shifting your hips as your hands walk.
- Avoid craning your neck.

HOW TO DO IT

- Begin in a high plank position, balancing on your toes with your feet together and with your right hand on the floor and your left on an elevated box or step.
- Keeping your torso rigid and your legs straight, bend your elbows to lower your chest toward the floor to perform a push-up.
- Push back up, straightening your elbows to return to the starting position.
- Lift your right hand off the floor, and place it beside your left on the top of the box.
- Lift your left hand off the box, placing it on the floor about one shoulder-width to the left, again assuming a high plank position.
- Bend your elbows to perform another push-up, this time on the other side of the box.
- Return to the top of the box. Continue alternating sides for the recommended repetitions.

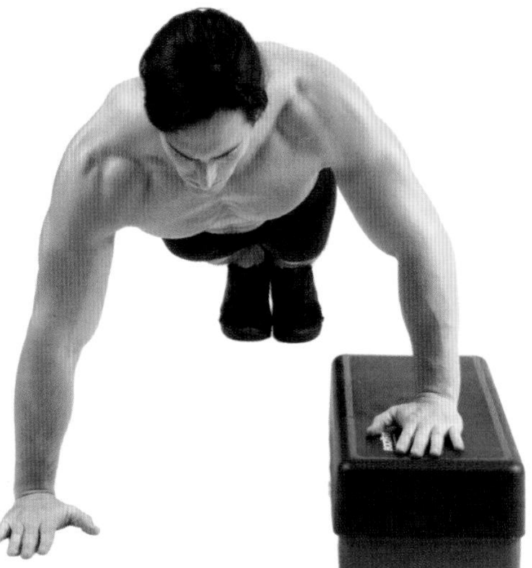

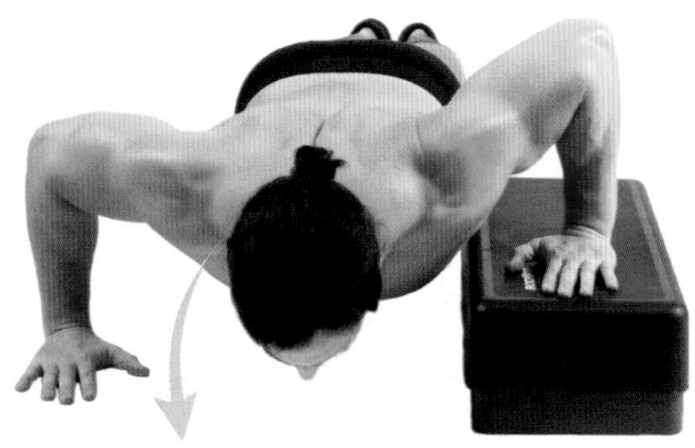

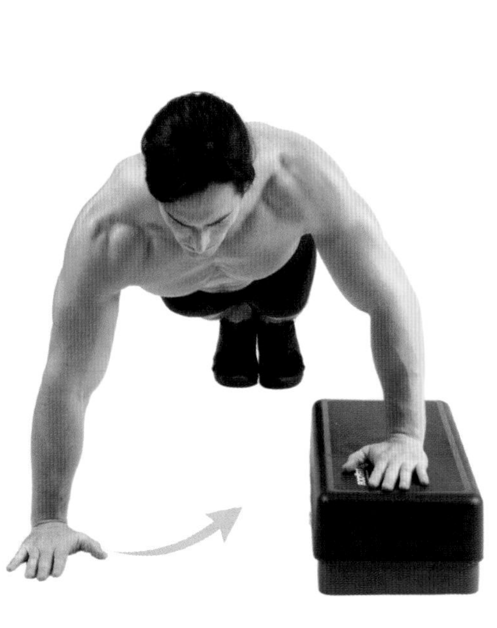

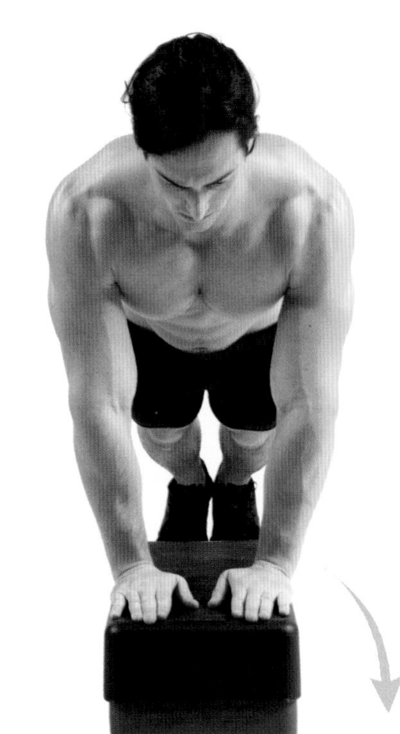

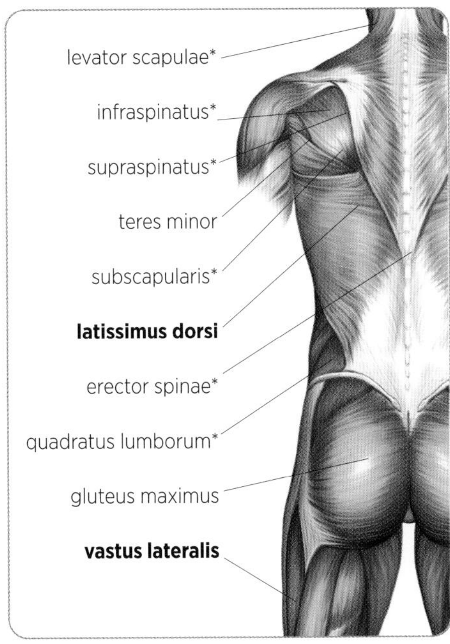

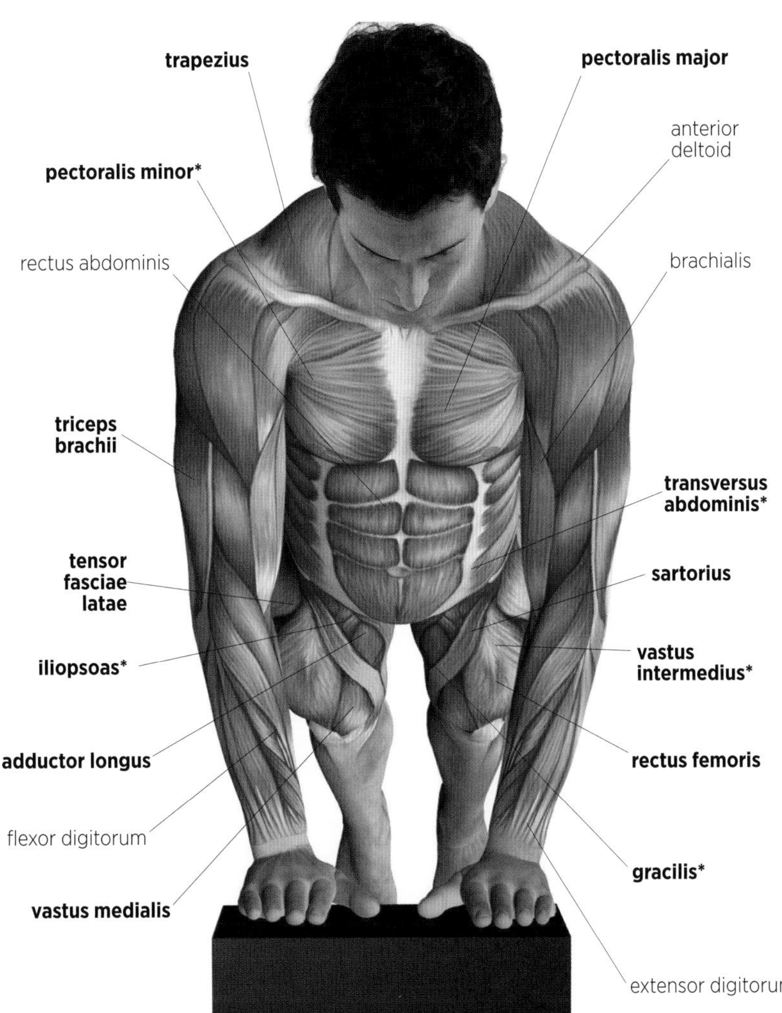

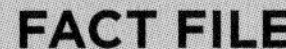

FACT FILE

TARGETS
- Chest
- Shoulders
- Back
- Arms
- Legs

TYPE
- Dynamic

BENEFITS
- Strengthens pelvic, trunk, and shoulder stabilizers
- Stabilizes entire body

CAUTIONS
- Shoulder issues
- Back issues
- Neck pain

EQUIPMENT
- Step or box

Annotation Key

Bold text indicates target muscles
Light text indicates other working muscles
* indicates deep muscles

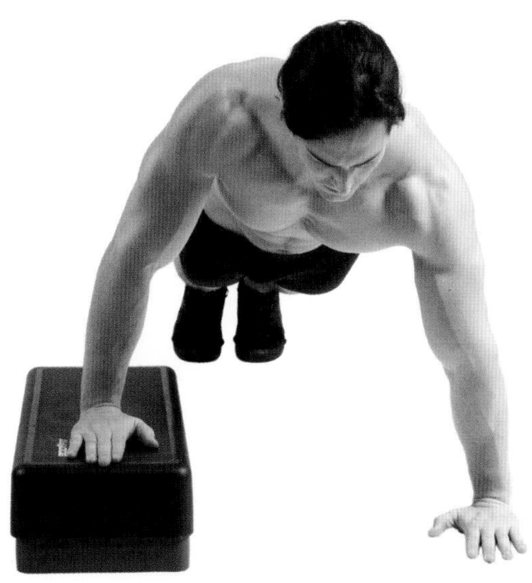

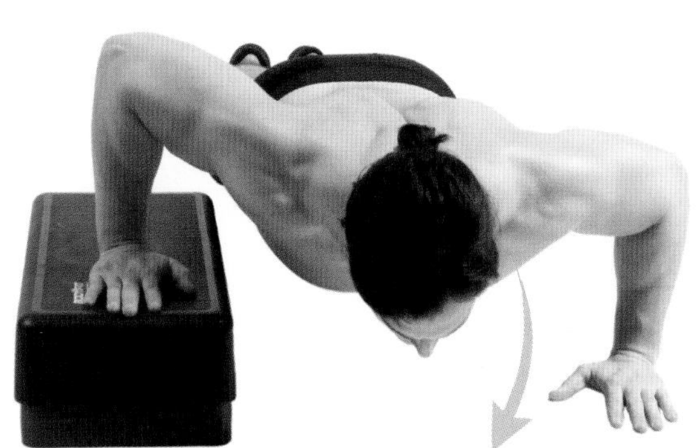

CHAPTER SEVEN

CORE EXERCISES

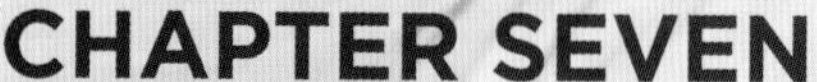

The strength of your core impacts many parts of your daily life, whether you're sitting at your desk or doing chores around the house. Core exercises train the muscles in your abdomen, lower back, pelvis, and hips to work in harmony, improving balance and stability. Some of the key benefits of core strength include reducing back stress, something that 80% of adults will experience at some point in their life; injury prevention, as your core muscles protect your internal organs and provide the support your spine needs during load-bearing exercises; and improved breathing, as a strong core will help you to breathe properly, especially during exertion. Additionally, the ability to take deep breaths provides more oxygen to tired muscles, aiding cardiovascular health.

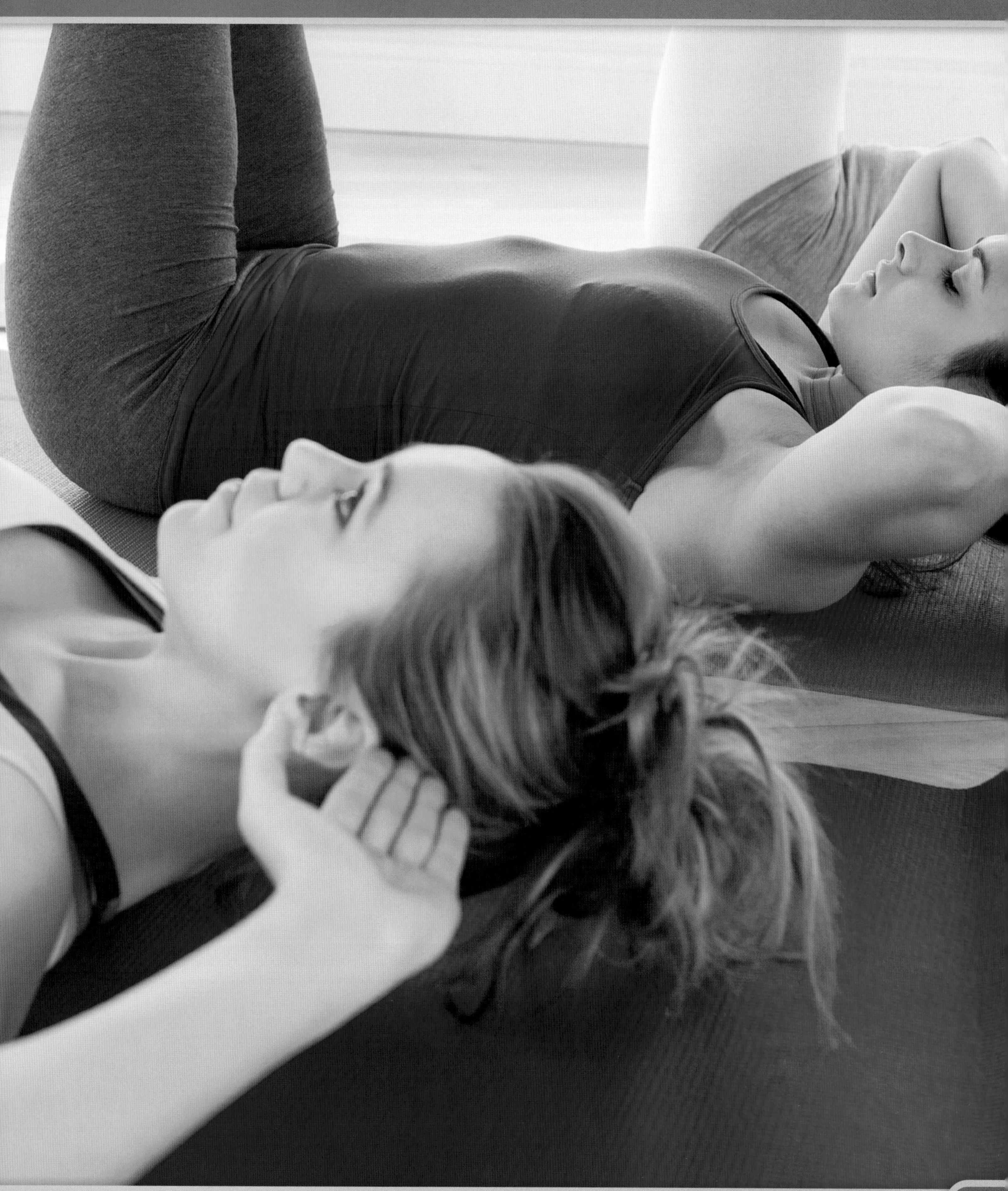

Bent-Knee Sit-Up

Similar to Crunches (pages 228–29), Bent-Knee Sit-Ups are classic exercises for abdominal-endurance training, hitting both your abs and obliques.

HOW TO DO IT

- Lie faceup with your legs bent so that your feet are tucked as close to your buttocks as possible. Either put your hands on your head or cross your arms over your chest.
- Flex your torso toward your thighs until your back is off the floor.
- Lower back down to the starting position, and then repeat for the recommended repetitions.

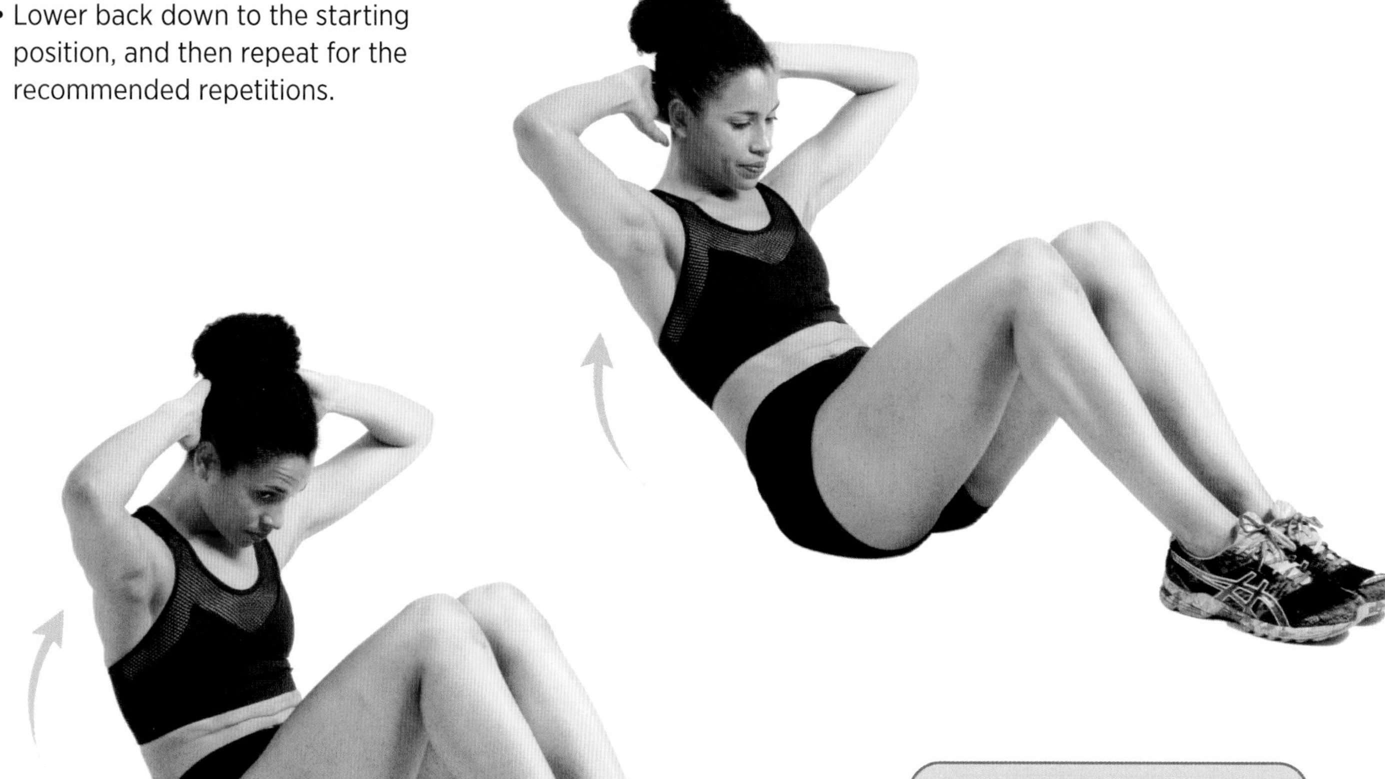

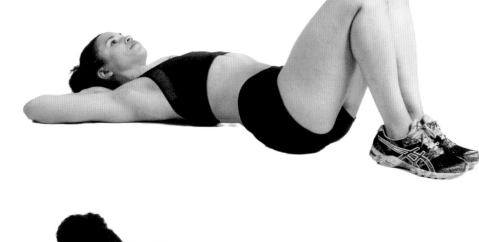

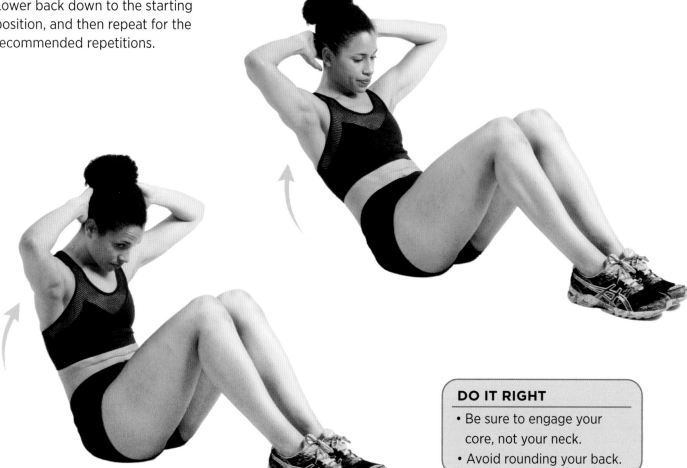

DO IT RIGHT

- Be sure to engage your core, not your neck.
- Avoid rounding your back.

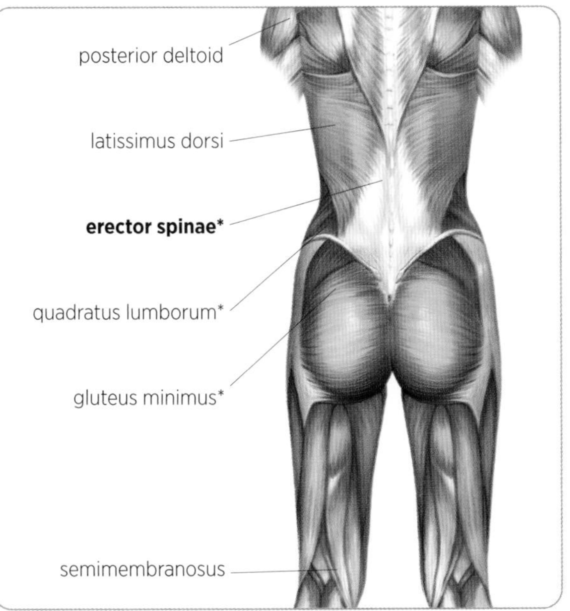

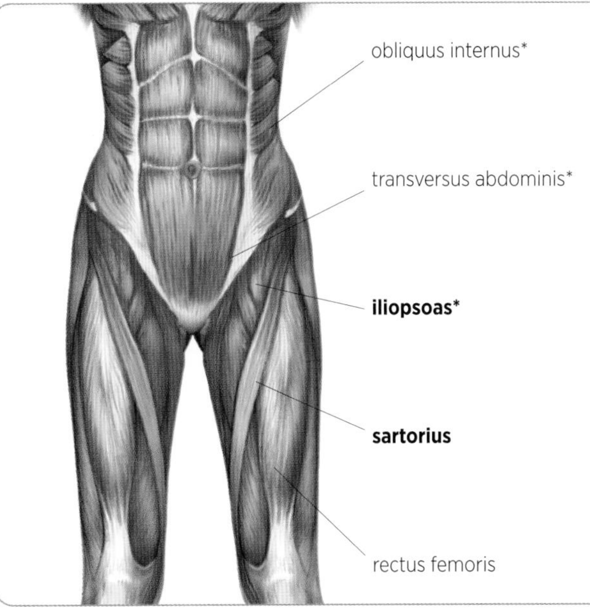

FACT FILE

TARGETS
- Abdominals
- Obliques
- Hip flexors
- Spine

TYPE
- Dynamic

BENEFITS
- Strengthens abdominals, obliques, hip flexors, and spinal erectors

CAUTIONS
- Lower-back issues
- Neck issues

posterior deltoid
latissimus dorsi
erector spinae*
quadratus lumborum*
gluteus minimus*
semimembranosus

obliquus internus*
transversus abdominis*
iliopsoas*
sartorius
rectus femoris

Annotation Key

Bold text indicates target muscles
Light text indicates other working muscles
* indicates deep muscles

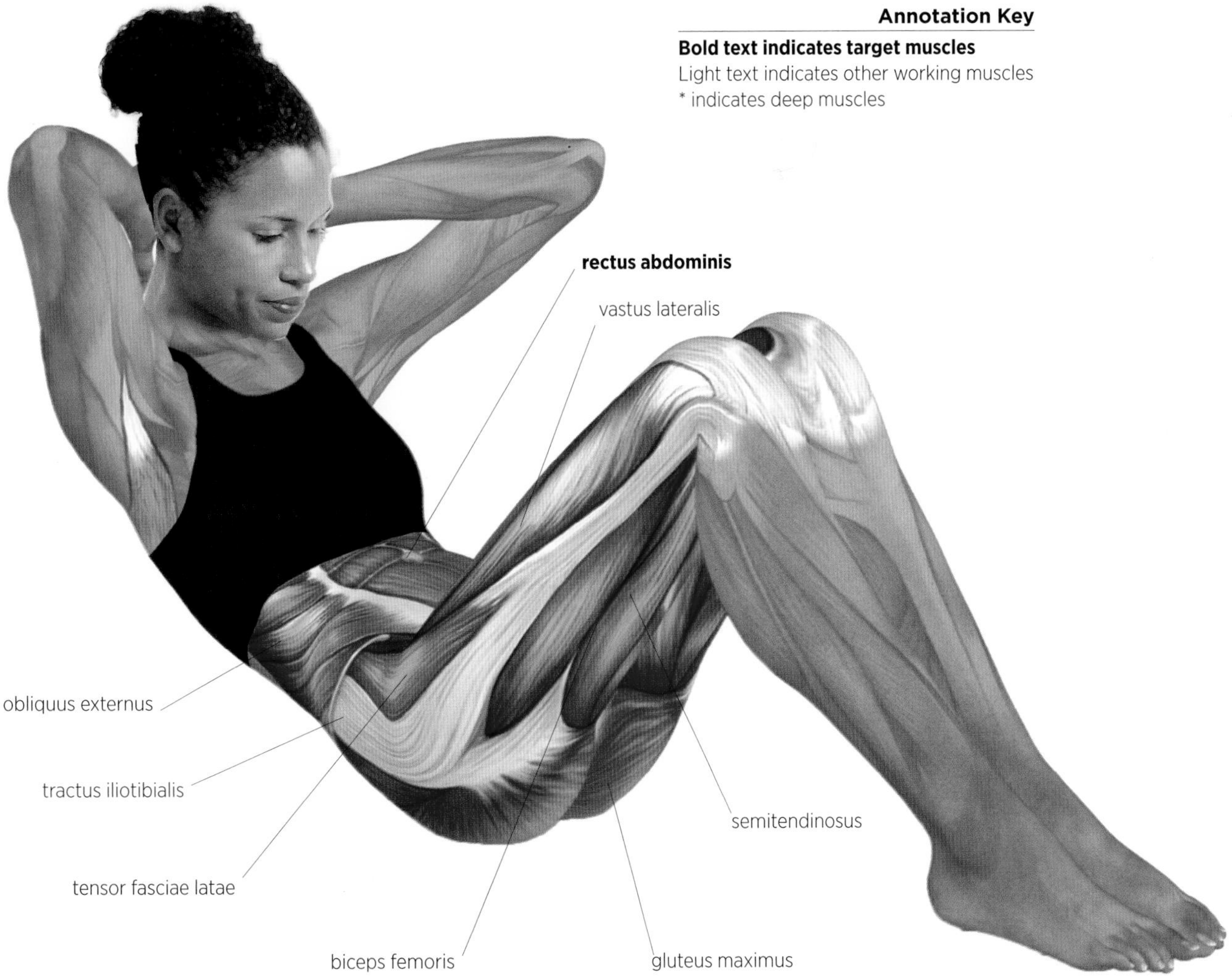

rectus abdominis
vastus lateralis
obliquus externus
tractus iliotibialis
tensor fasciae latae
biceps femoris
gluteus maximus
semitendinosus

Bicycle Crunch

The Bicycle Crunch targets your upper abdominals and your obliques, strengthening and toning these muscles. Resist the urge to "cycle" too quickly; a smooth, controlled pace is most effective.

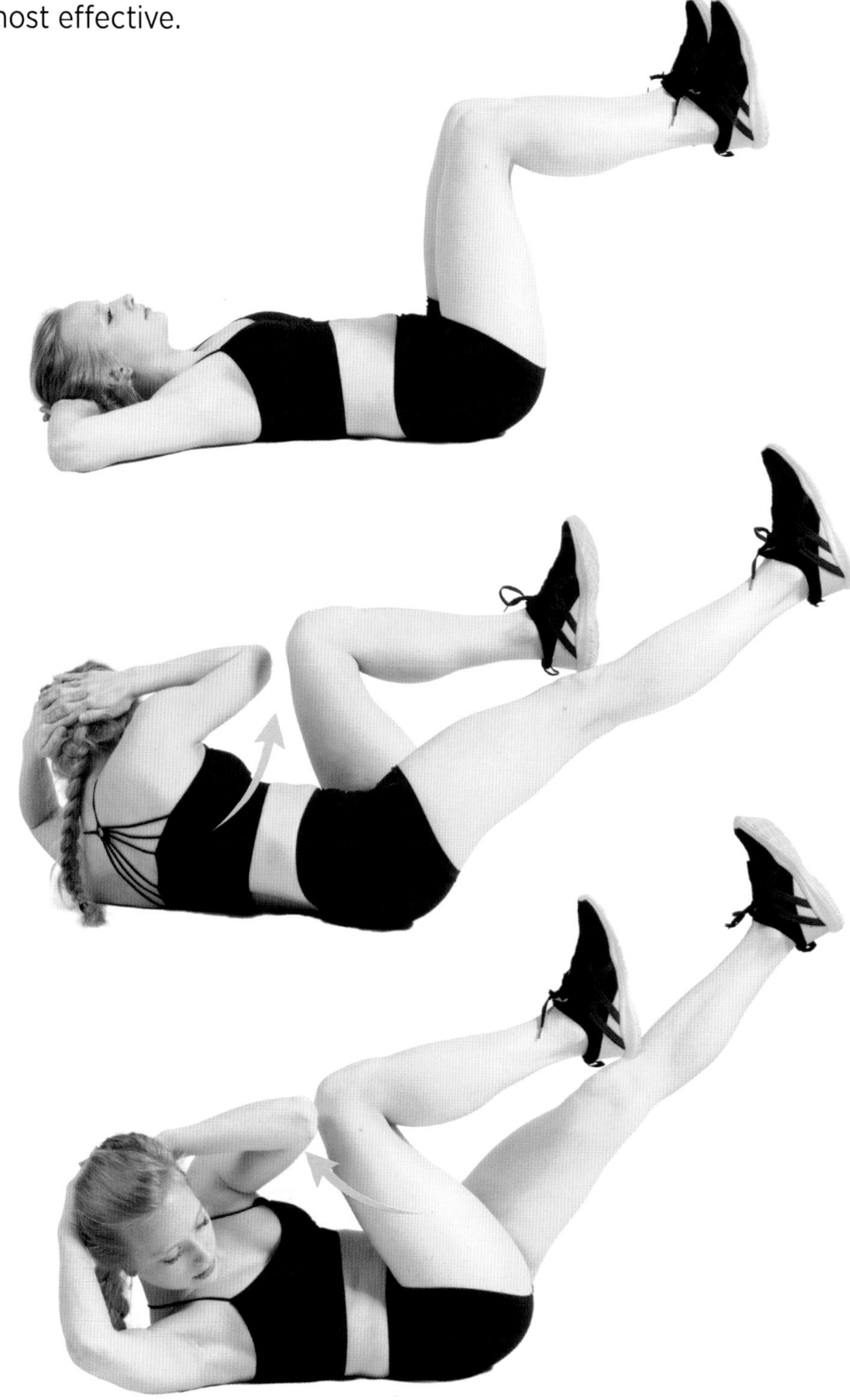

HOW TO DO IT

- Lie faceup with fingers at your ears, your elbows flared outward, and your legs bent to form a 90-degree angle.
- Begin to lift your shoulders and upper torso off the floor as you raise your right elbow diagonally. At the same time, bring your left knee toward your elbow and extend your right leg diagonally forward until your right elbow and left knee meet.
- Lower, and then repeat on the other side. Continue alternating sides for the recommended repetitions.

DO IT RIGHT

- Raise your elbow and opposite knee equally so that they meet in the middle.
- Avoid raising your lower back off the floor.
- Avoid rushing through the movement.

obliquus internus*
iliopsoas*
pectineus*
vastus intermedius*
rectus femoris
gracilis*
vastus medialis

biceps femoris
semitendinosus
semimembranosus

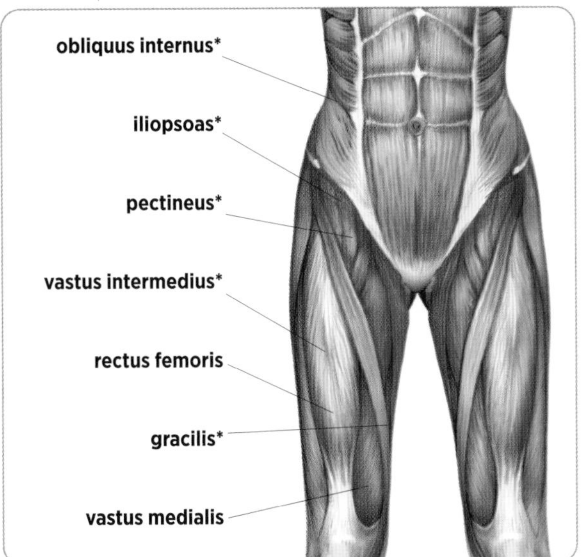

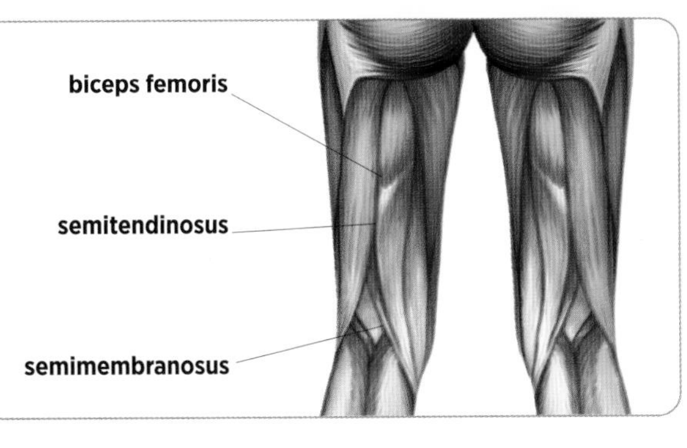

MODIFICATION

EASIER: Bend both knees and place both feet on the floor, keeping them anchored there throughout the exercise. Leading with your abdominals, raise your entire torso off the floor as you bring your left elbow to your right knee. Lower and repeat, alternating sides.

FACT FILE

TARGETS
- Abdominals
- Obliques
- Hip flexors
- Spine

TYPE
- Dynamic

BENEFITS
- Strengthens abdominals
- Stabilizes core
- Tones obliques and midsection

CAUTIONS
- Lower-back issues
- Neck issues

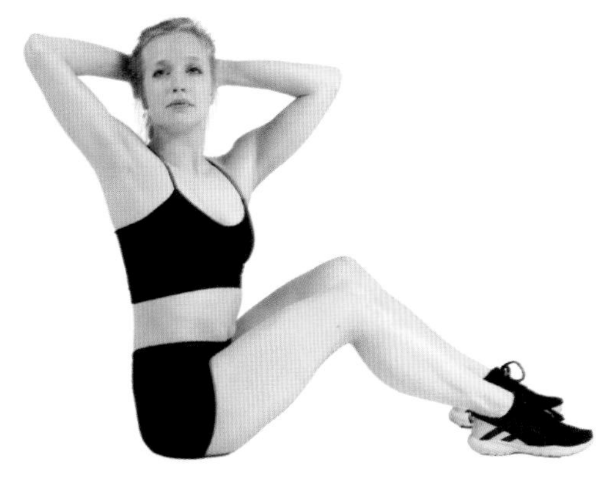

Annotation Key
Bold text indicates target muscles
Light text indicates other working muscles
* indicates deep muscles

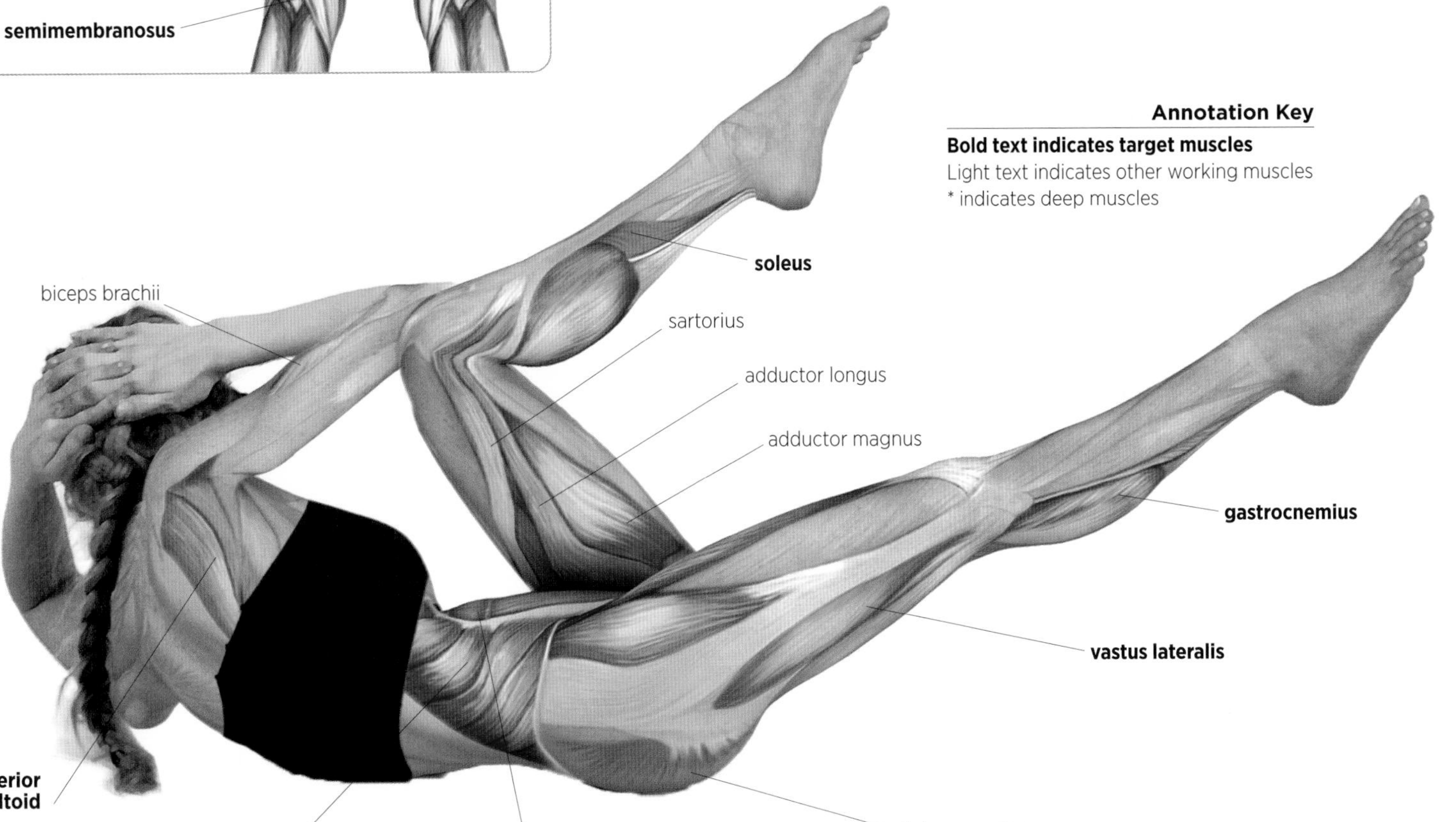

soleus
biceps brachii
sartorius
adductor longus
adductor magnus
gastrocnemius
vastus lateralis
posterior deltoid
obliquus externus
rectus abdominis
gluteus maximus

V-Up

The challenging V-Up has multiple benefits. Its full range of motion targets both your upper and lower rectus abdominis, and it also works to strengthen your lower-back muscles and tighten your quads.

HOW TO DO IT

- Lie faceup with your legs straight and your arms extended behind your head.
- Simultaneously raise your arms and legs so that your fingertips are nearly touching your feet, while maintaining a flat back.
- Lower back down to the starting position, and then repeat for the recommended repetitions.

DO IT RIGHT

- Keep your arms and legs straight.
- Avoid using a jerking motion as you raise or lower your arms and legs.

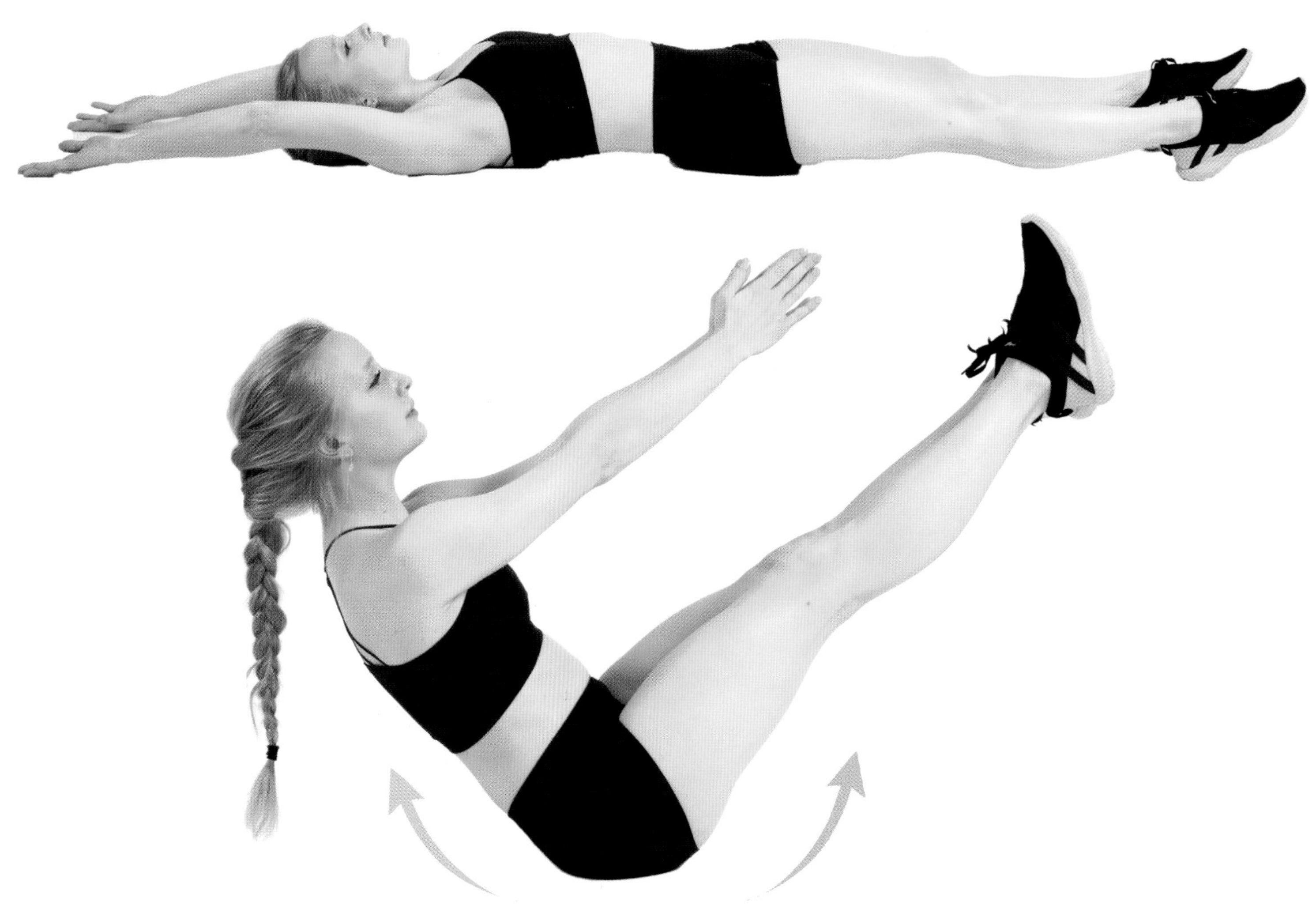

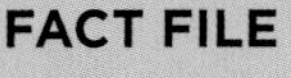

FACT FILE

TARGETS
- Abdominals
- Lower back

TYPE
- Dynamic

BENEFITS
- Strengthens core
- Increases spinal mobility

CAUTIONS
- Lower-back issues
- Neck issues

MODIFICATION

HARDER: Grasp a medicine ball in your hands, keeping it in place throughout the exercise.

transversus abdominis*
iliopsoas*
pectineus*
adductor longus
vastus intermedius*
rectus femoris
vastus medialis

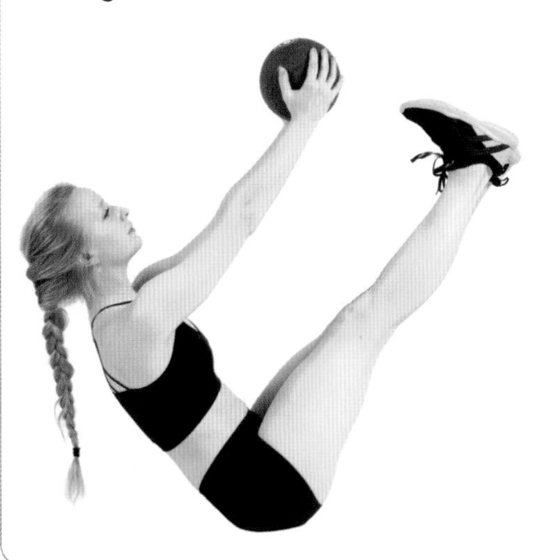

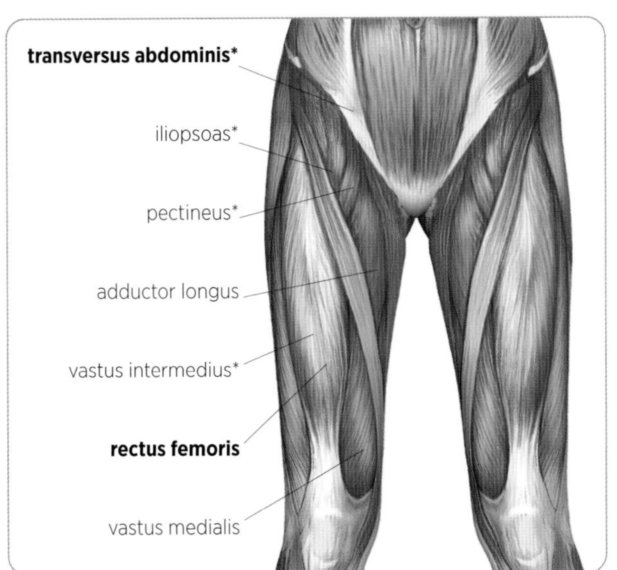

Annotation Key
Bold text indicates target muscles
Light text indicates other working muscles
* indicates deep muscles

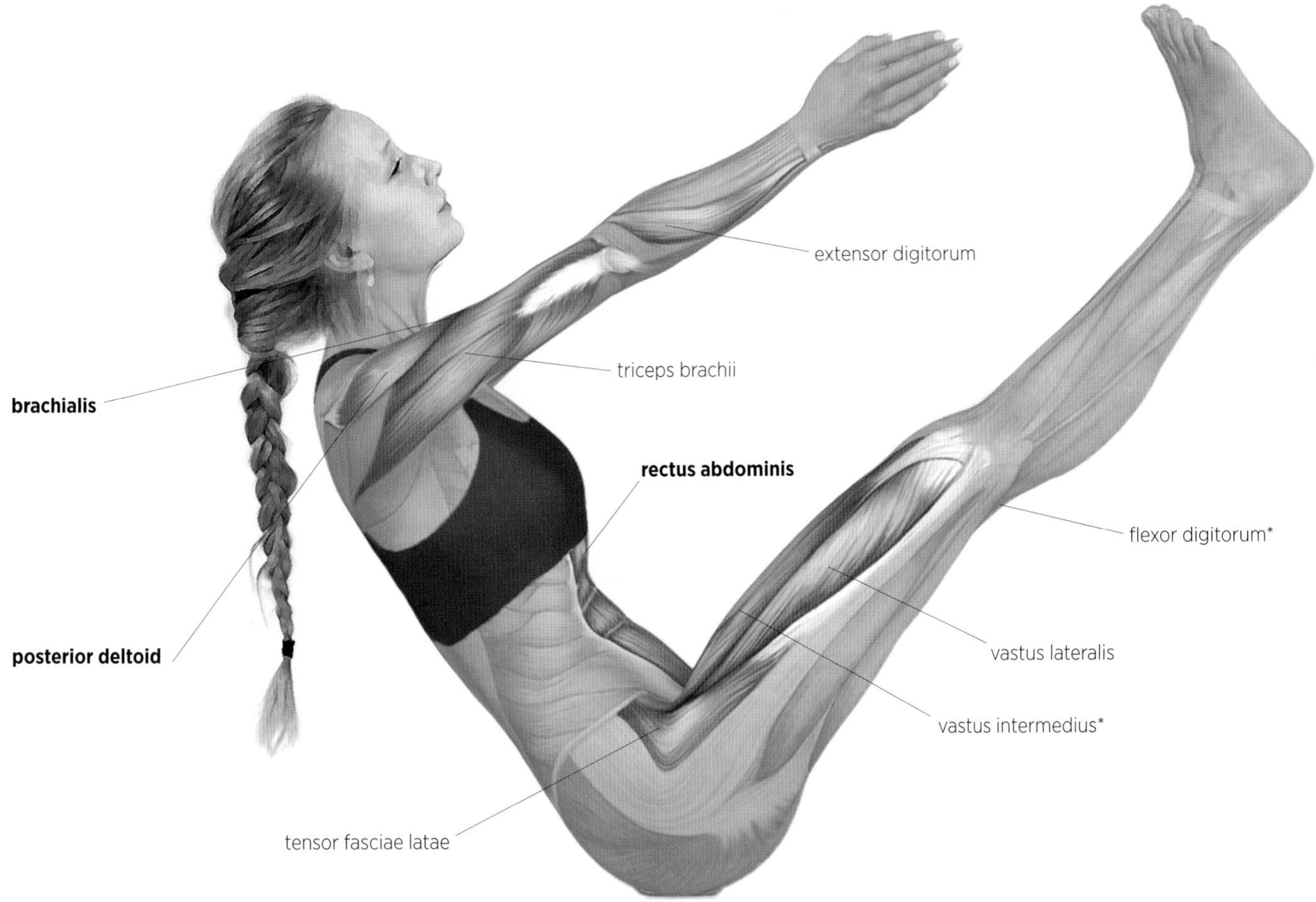

extensor digitorum
triceps brachii
brachialis
rectus abdominis
flexor digitorum*
posterior deltoid
vastus lateralis
vastus intermedius*
tensor fasciae latae

Knees to Chest

Inspired by boot-camp training, Knees to Chest targets your lower abdominals and hip flexors. As with many military-style exercises, it is a multiphase exercise featuring four movements performed to a counting beat.

HOW TO DO IT

- Lie faceup with your legs straight and your head raised off the floor. Place both hands under your buttocks to straighten your lumbar spine, and then lift both legs so that your feet are about 6 inches off the floor. Your knees should be bent slightly.

- Keeping your feet together, bring both knees to your chest for count 1, and then straighten your legs for count 2.

- Repeat this movement for counts 3 and 4 to complete one rep. Repeat for the recommended repetitions.

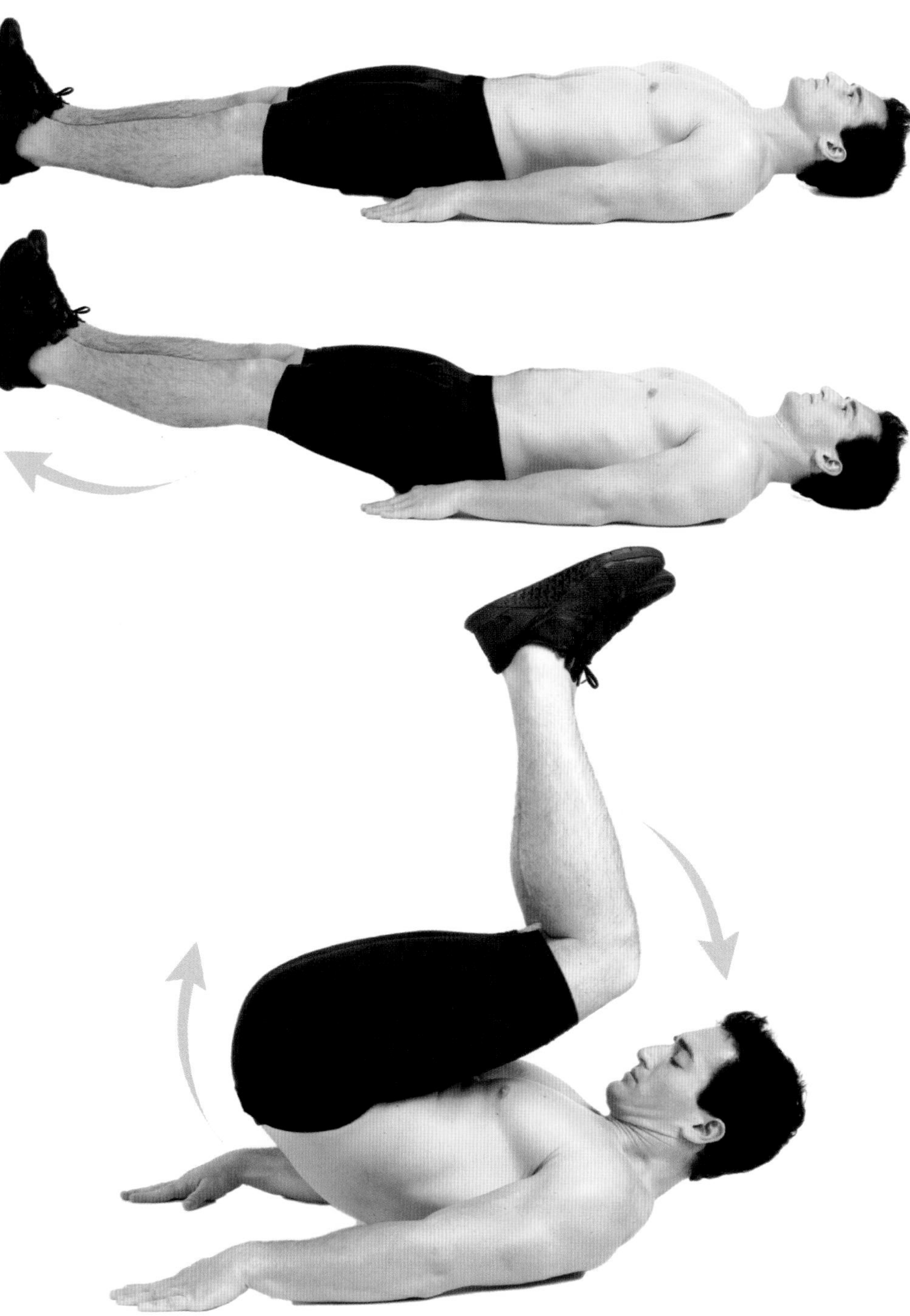

DO IT RIGHT

- Keep your hands under your butt to protect your lower back from excess extension.
- Avoid resting your head on the floor.

FACT FILE

TARGETS
- Abdominals
- Hip flexors

TYPE
- Dynamic

BENEFITS
- Strengthens abdominals and hip flexors
- Increases endurance

CAUTIONS
- Lower-back pain

Annotation Key

Bold text indicates target muscles

Light text indicates other working muscles

* indicates deep muscles

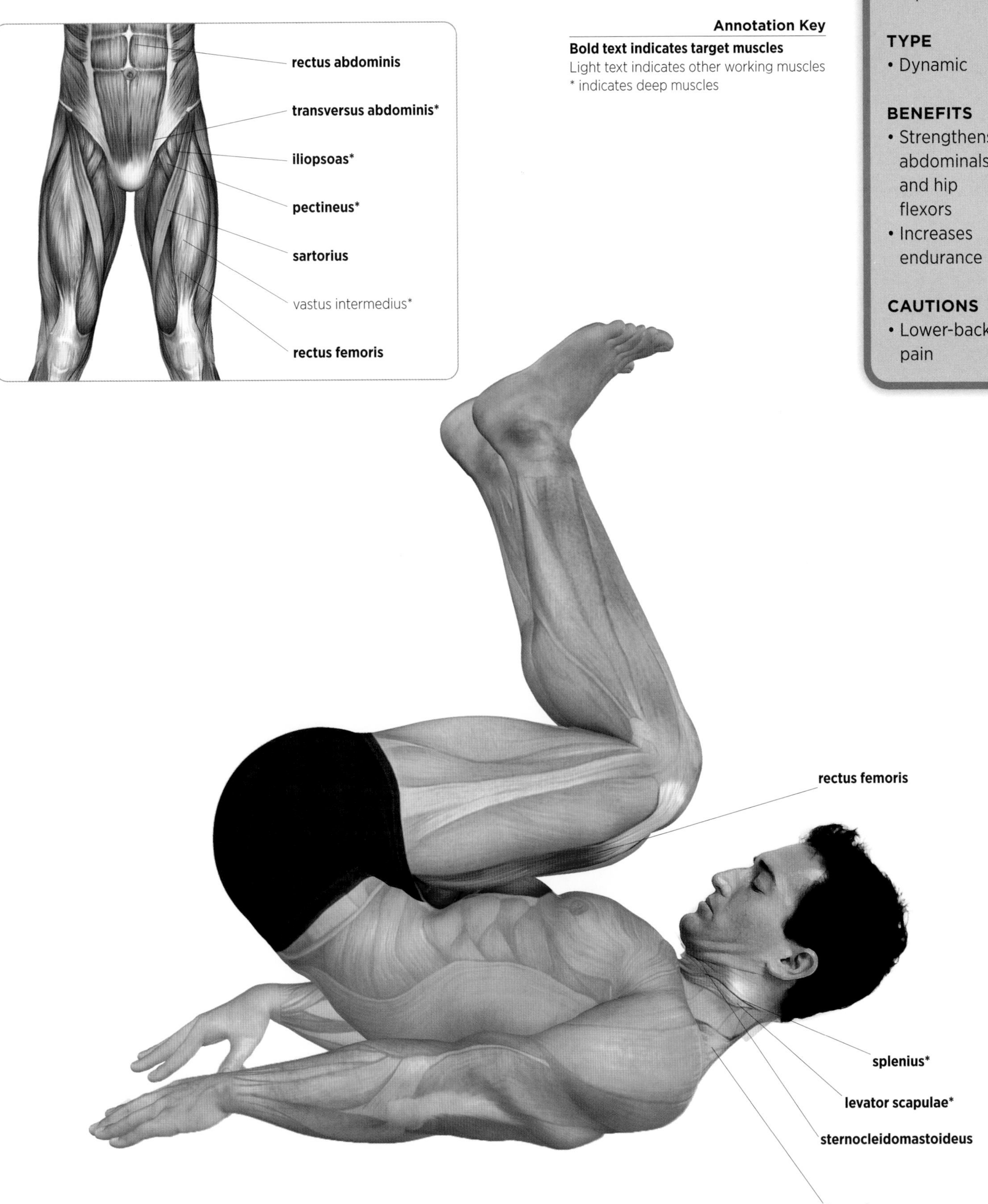

Double Leg Lift

It may look simple, but the Double Leg Lift challenges your hard-to-reach, inner-core muscles. Both strengthening and stabilizing, this Pilates exercise targets both your internal and external abdominals.

HOW TO DO IT

- Lie faceup with your legs together and your arms down at your sides. Lift your legs so that they form a 30-degree angle with the floor, and point your toes.
- Pull in your abdominals, and lower your legs to the floor.
- Keeping your back flat, pull your abdominals in again, and lift your legs back up. Continue lifting and lowering your legs for the recommended repetitions.

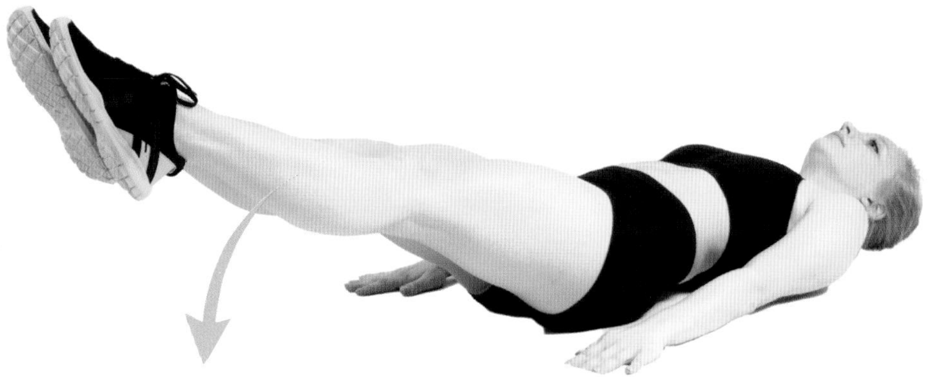

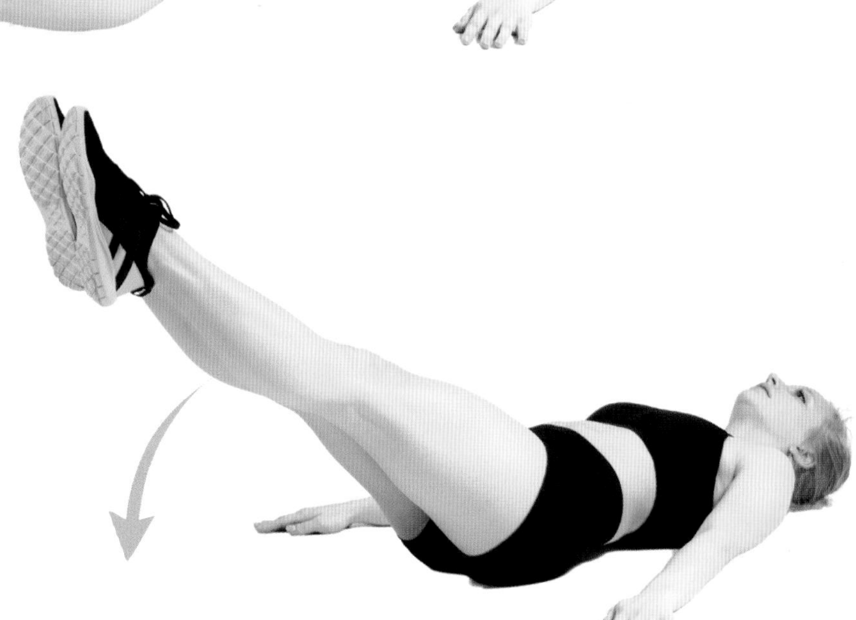

DO IT RIGHT

- Keep your back flat on the floor.
- Avoid dropping your legs; move slowly and with control.
- Use your abdominals to drive the movement.

FACT FILE

TARGETS
- Abdominals
- Hip flexors

TYPE
- Dynamic

BENEFITS
- Strengthens internal and external abdominals
- Stabilizes core

CAUTIONS
- Lower-back pain

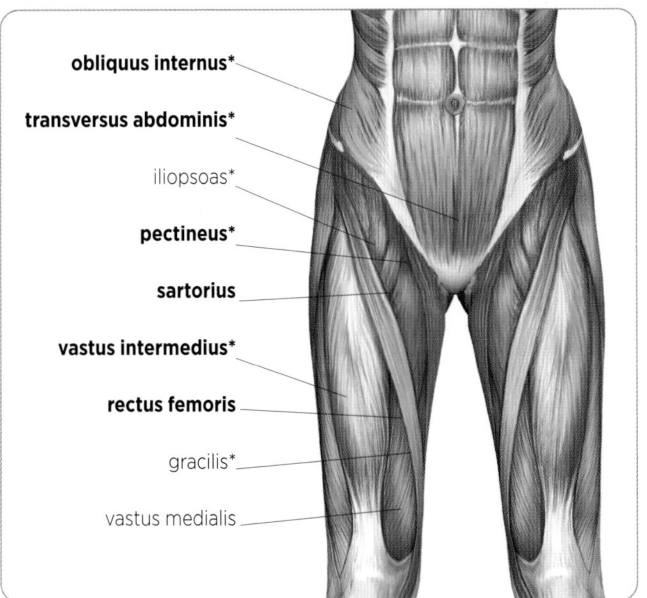

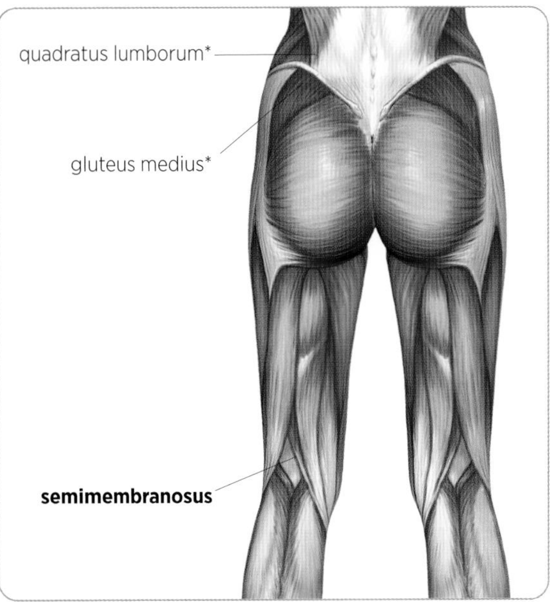

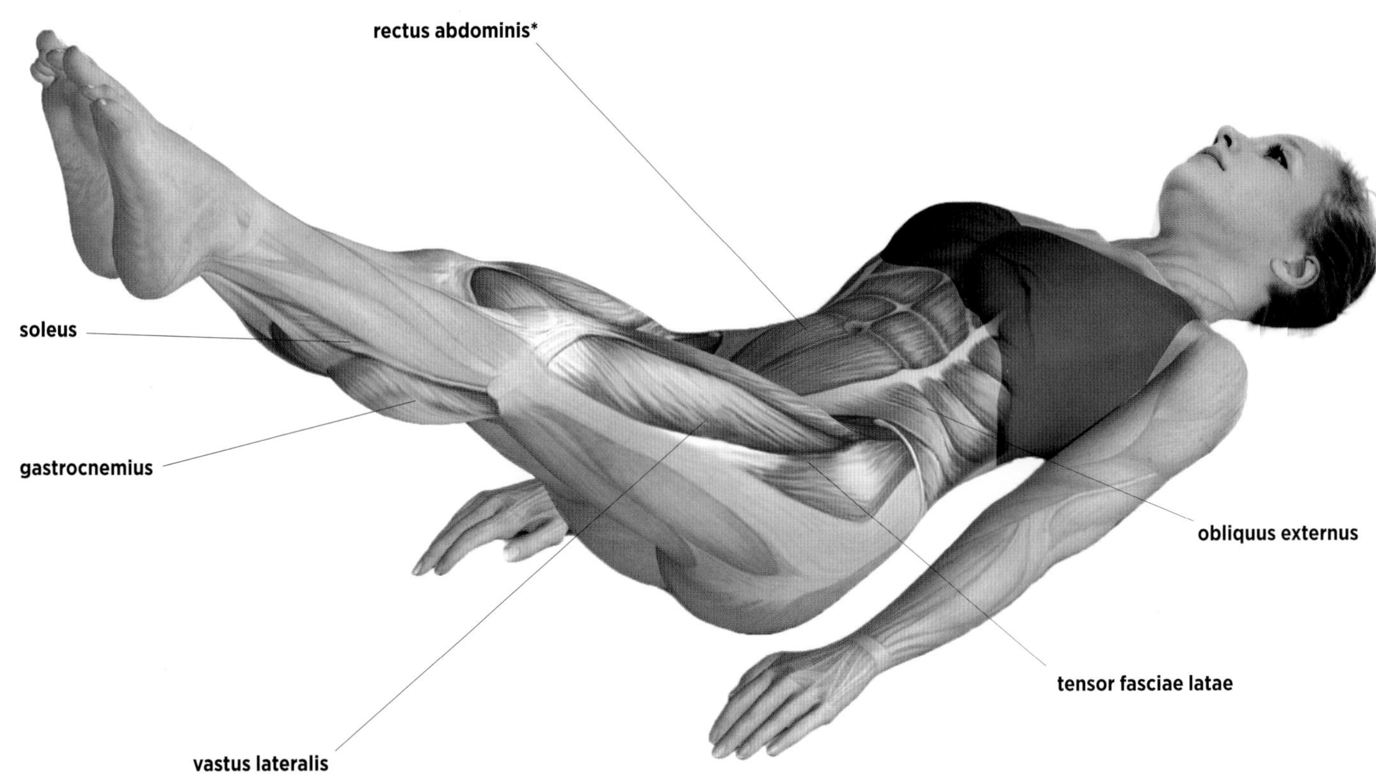

Metronome

Metronomes are wonderful for engaging your core musculature in a twisting motion. With its focus on your obliques, as well as your transverse abdominis, you will get a fantastic core workout.

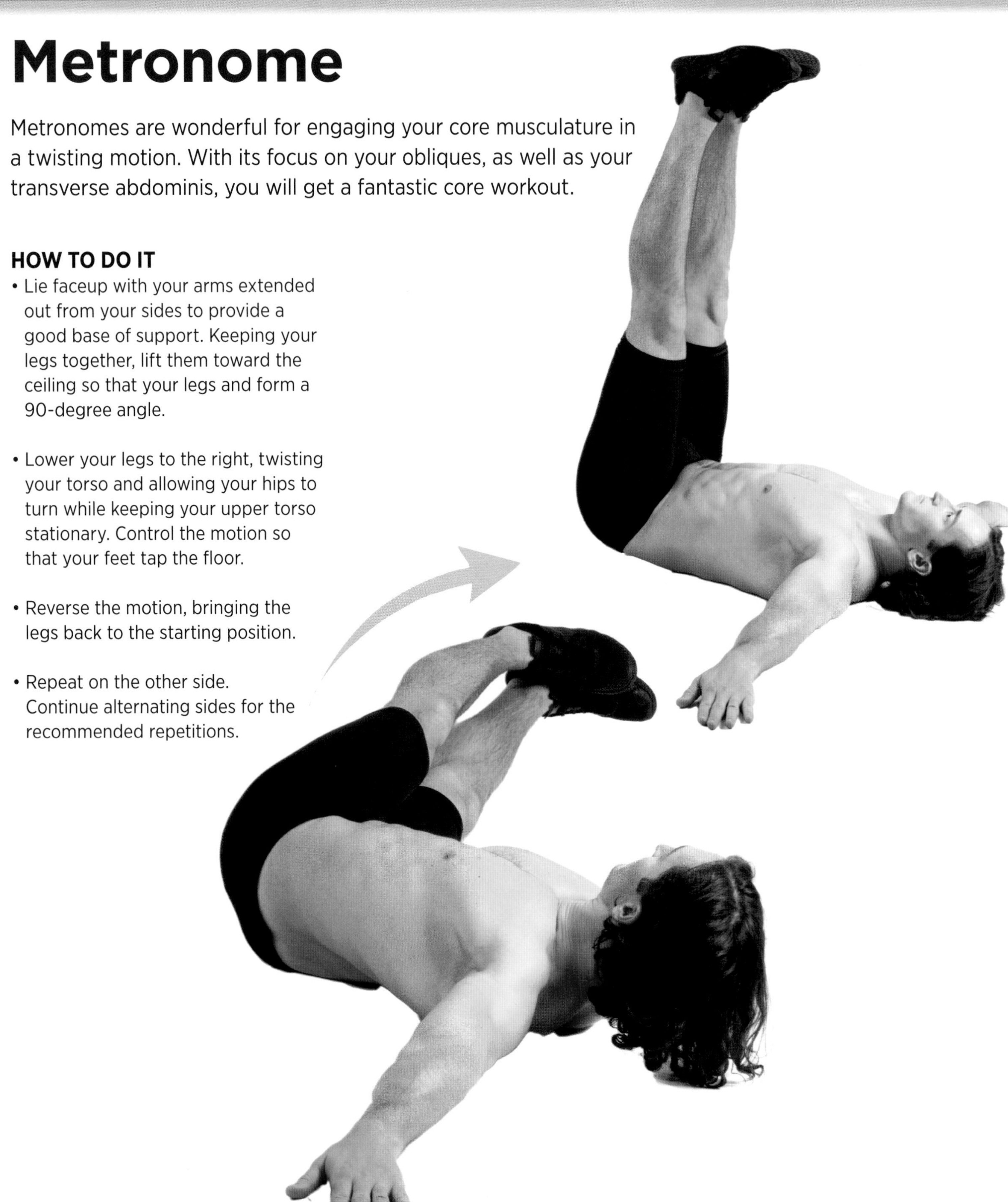

HOW TO DO IT

- Lie faceup with your arms extended out from your sides to provide a good base of support. Keeping your legs together, lift them toward the ceiling so that your legs and form a 90-degree angle.
- Lower your legs to the right, twisting your torso and allowing your hips to turn while keeping your upper torso stationary. Control the motion so that your feet tap the floor.
- Reverse the motion, bringing the legs back to the starting position.
- Repeat on the other side. Continue alternating sides for the recommended repetitions.

FACT FILE

TARGETS
- Abdominals
- Hip flexors

TYPE
- Dynamic

BENEFITS
- Strengthens and tones abdominal muscles
- Engages several different abdominal fibers
- Improves flexibility

CAUTIONS
- Lower-back issues

DO IT RIGHT
- Keep your legs straight.
- Lower your legs only as far down as you can while still keeping both shoulders on the floor.
- Keeps your hips flexed to 90 degrees throughout hip rotation; don't allow your legs to drop.

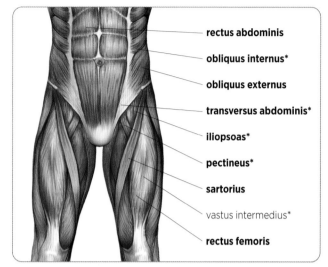

rectus abdominis
obliquus internus*
obliquus externus
transversus abdominis*
iliopsoas*
pectineus*
sartorius
vastus intermedius*
rectus femoris

Annotation Key
Bold text indicates target muscles
Light text indicates other working muscles
* indicates deep muscles

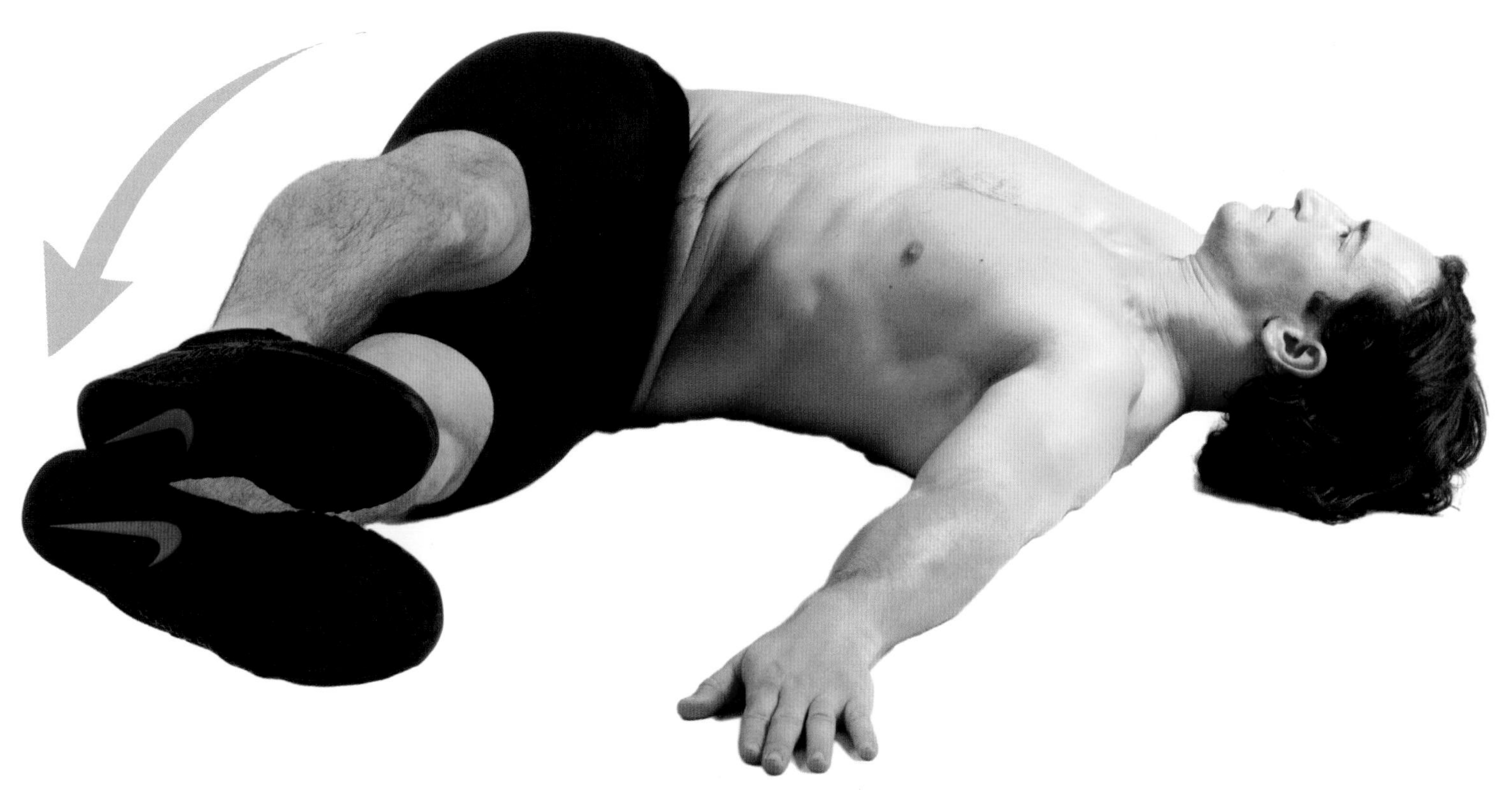

Hollow Hold to Superman

This advanced exercise hits every core muscle group, making this the one-stop shop for a stronger core and well-defined abdominals. Combining the benefits of the Hollow Hold gymnastic exercise and the Superman back extension, it will engage all your abdominal muscles, including your obliques, as well as the deep muscles in your back.

HOW TO DO IT

- Lie faceup with your legs and arms extended.
- To perform the Hollow Hold, engage your core, pulling your navel toward your spine. Lift your legs off the floor, and elevate your shoulder blades. Keep your arms outstretched overhead.
- Using only your obliques, roll over so that you end up facing down, keeping your arms and legs elevated off the floor by engaging your lower-back extensor muscles. This is the Superman position.
- Using only your core, rotate back to the starting position. Repeat on the other side. Continue alternating sides for the recommended repetitions.

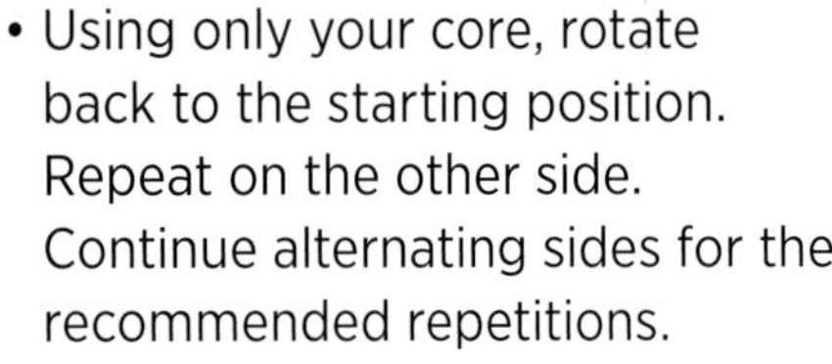

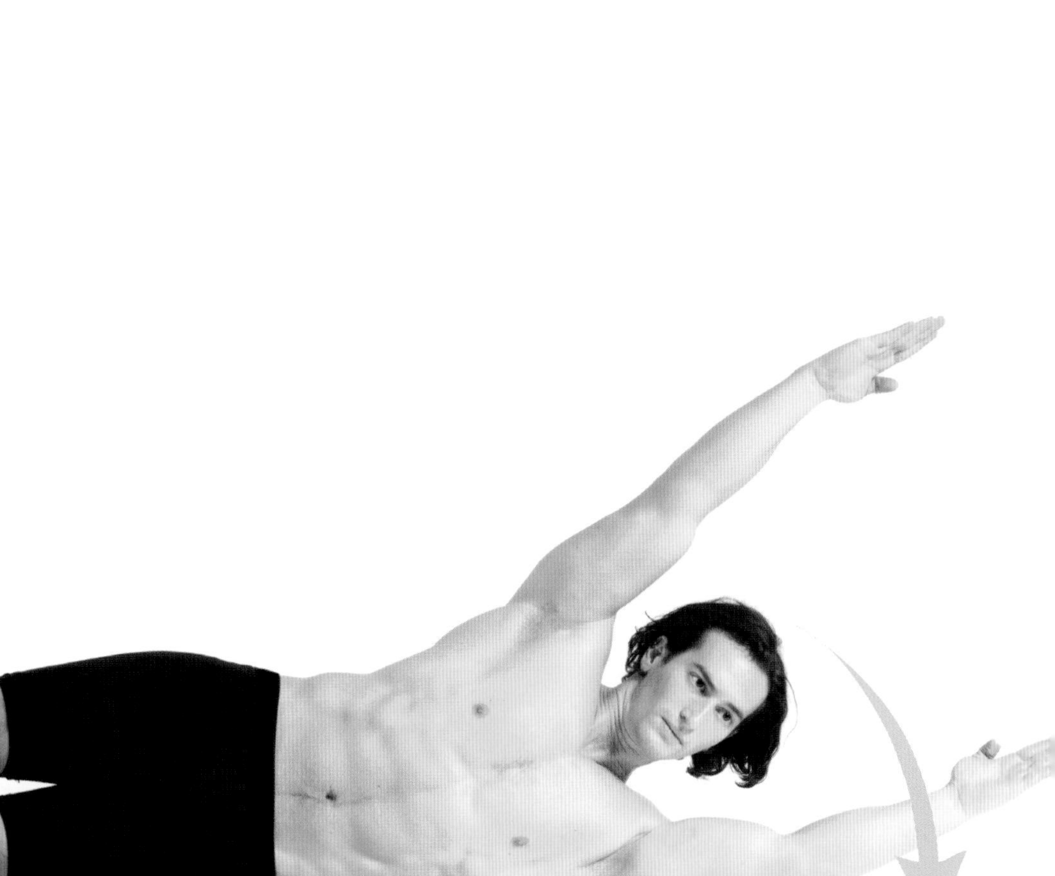

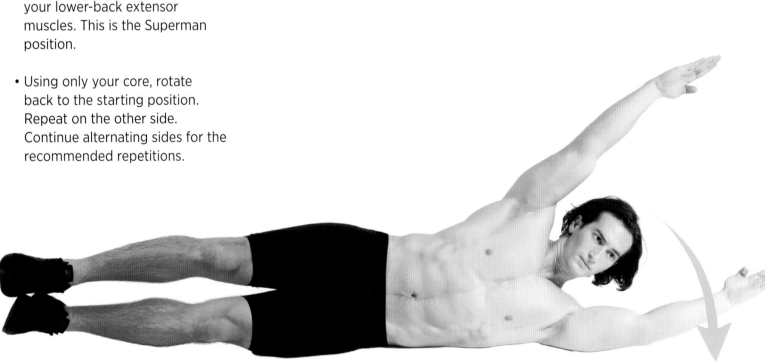

FACT FILE

TARGETS
- Abdominals
- Back
- Hip flexors
- Glutes

TYPE
- Dynamic

BENEFITS
- Strengthens and tones abdominals and back extensors
- Improves coordination

CAUTIONS
- Lower-back issues

DO IT RIGHT
- Keep your core engaged.
- Press your lower back into the floor while in the Hollow Hold, avoiding excessive spinal arching.
- Perform in both directions to engage both sides symmetrically.

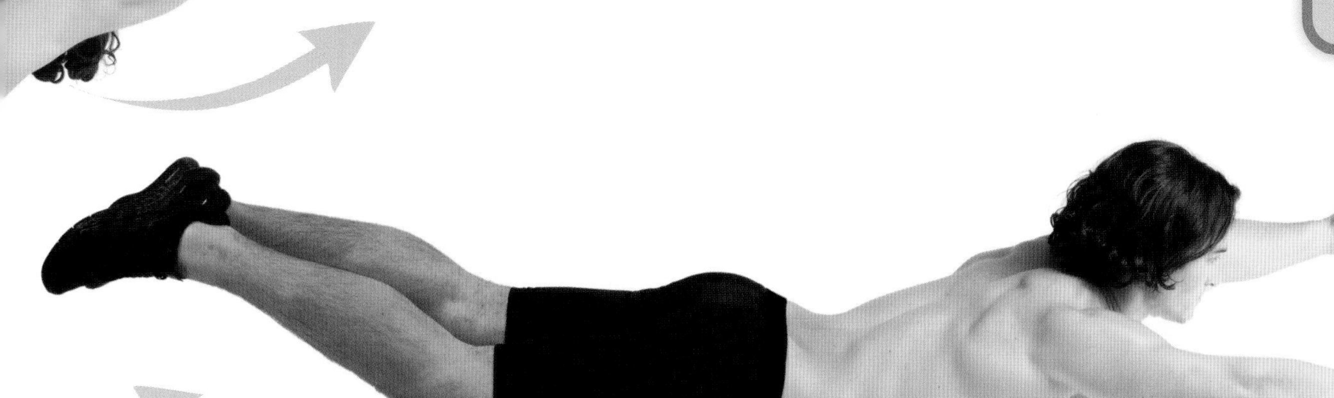

Annotation Key

Bold text indicates target muscles
Light text indicates other working muscles
* indicates deep muscles

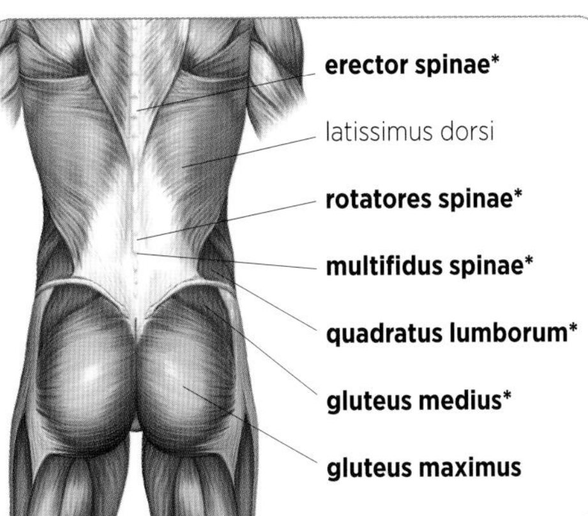

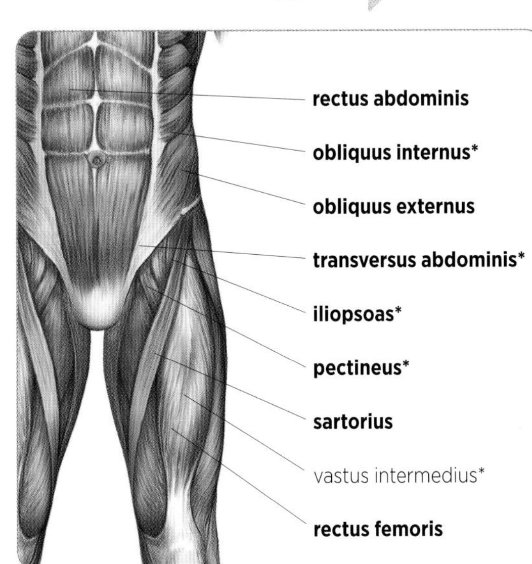

Crunch

A straightforward lift-up Crunch is one of the best ways to tone and fire up your abdominal muscles. Doing this gives the added bonus of stabilizing your spine and so relieving backache.

HOW TO DO IT

- Lie on your back with your legs bent and your hands behind your head, elbows flared outward.
- Contracting your abdominals, raise your head and shoulders off the floor.
- Lower, and repeat for the recommended repetitions.

DO IT RIGHT

- Lead with your abs, as if a string were hoisting you up by your belly button.
- Try to keep your feet planted on the floor.
- Keep your elbows flared outward.
- Avoid using your neck to drive the movement.

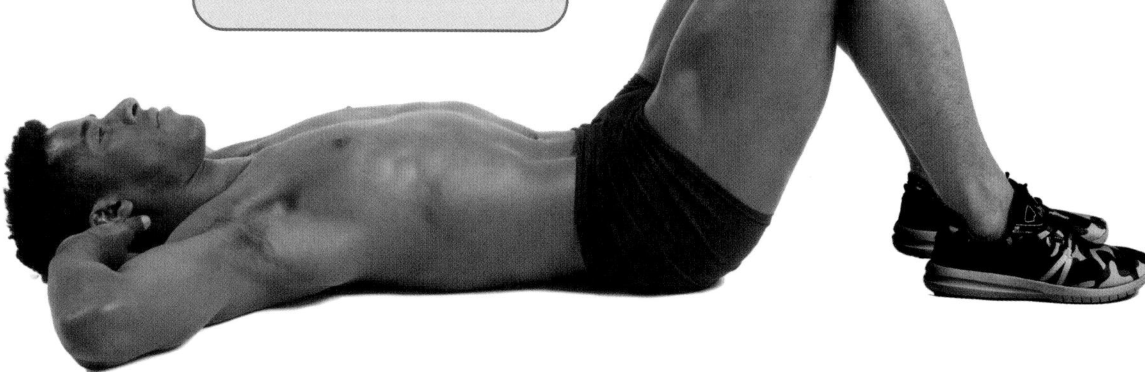

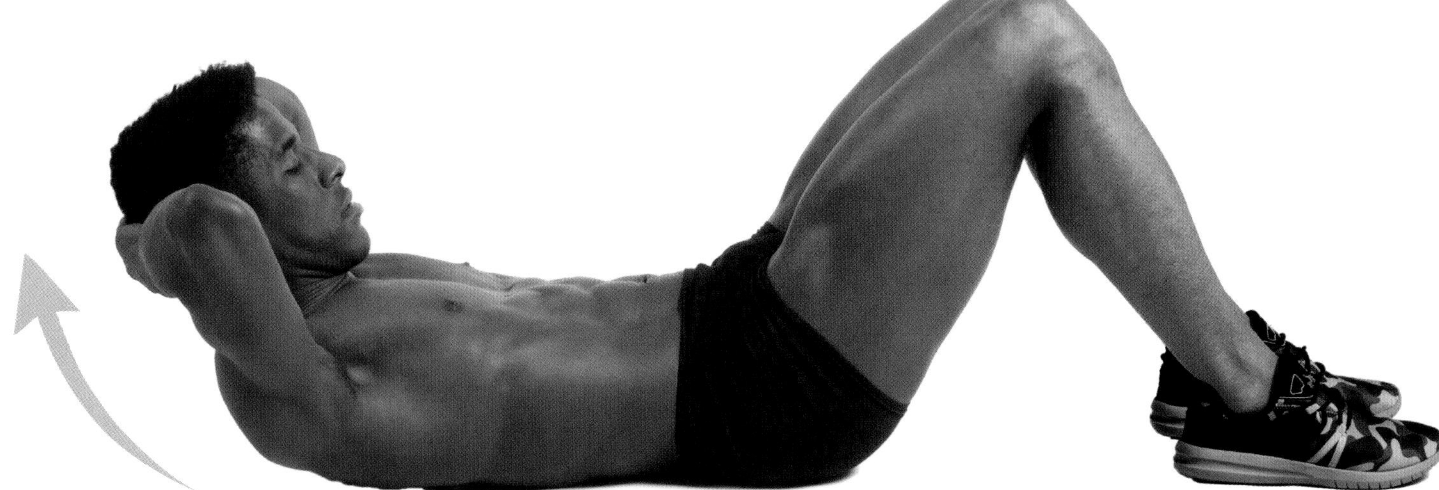

FACT FILE

TARGETS
- Front and side abdominals

TYPE
- Static

BENEFITS
- Strengthens and helps to define abdominals

CAUTIONS
- Lower-back issues
- Neck pain

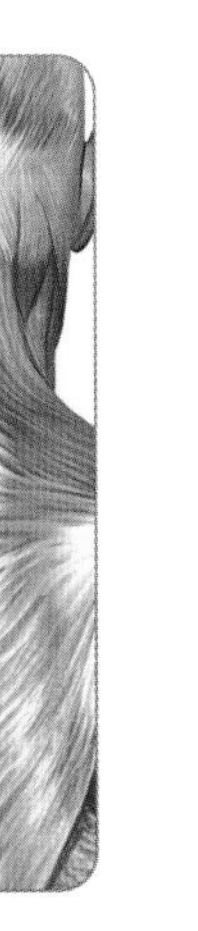

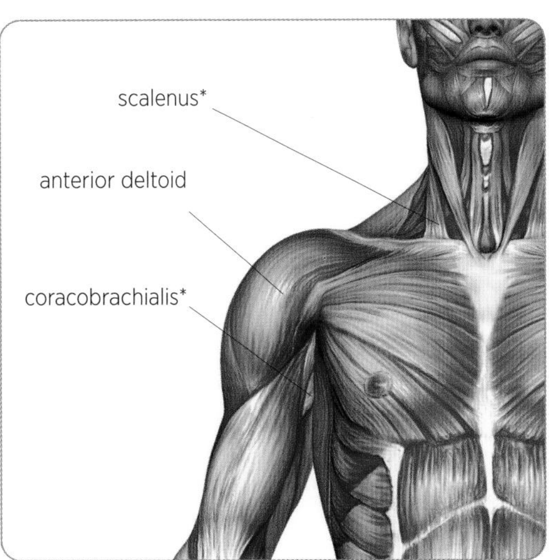

Annotation Key

Bold text indicates target muscles
Light text indicates other working muscles
* indicates deep muscles

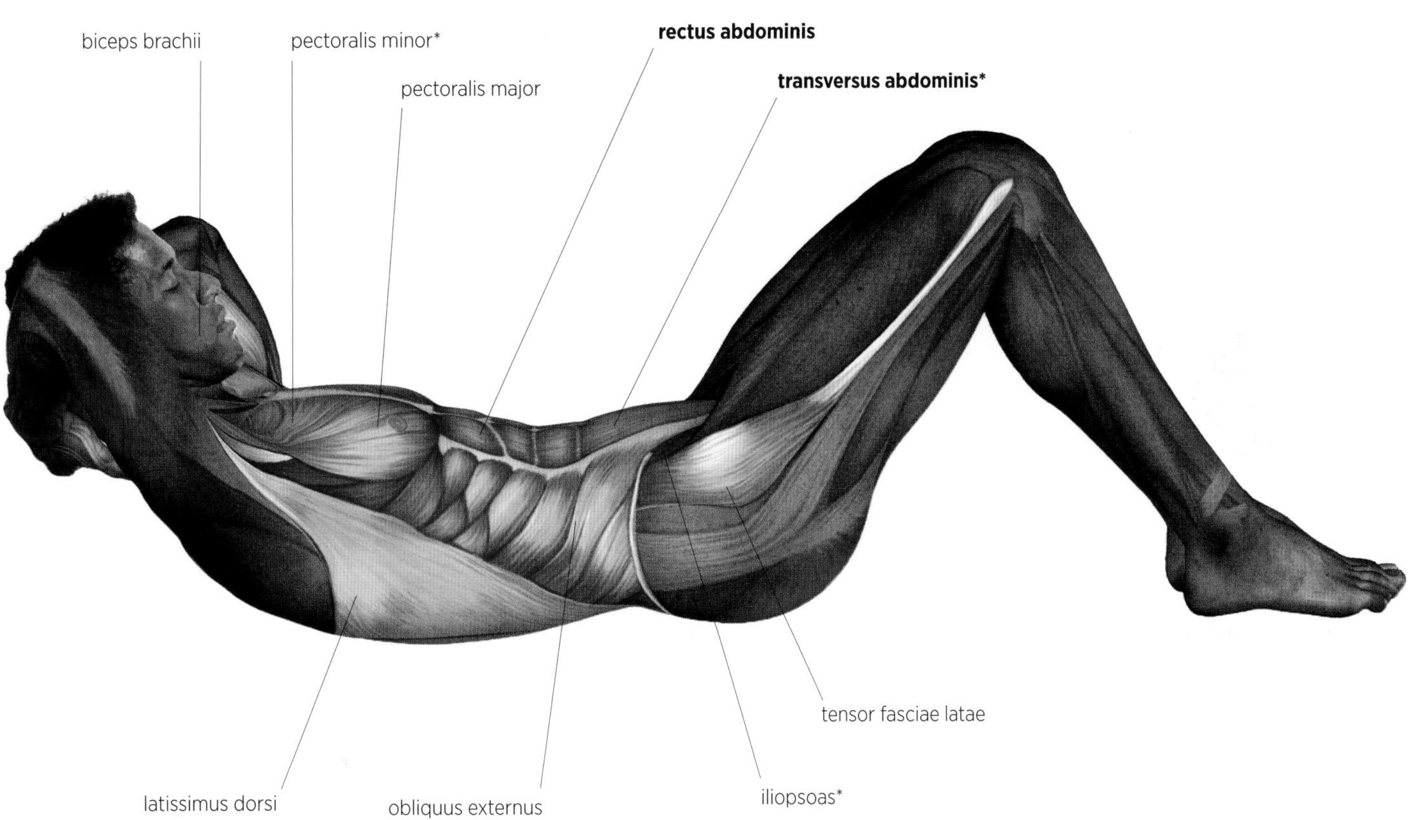

Penguin Crunch

The Penguin Crunch really works your obliques and upper abdominals. Because it incorporates lateral movement of the abdominals, it is a great way to prepare for sports that require rotational movement, such as swimming.

HOW TO DO IT

- Lie on your back with your head elevated and your arms straight at your sides and raised off the floor. Bend your knees.
- Holding your torso in a flexed position, lean to the right, and reach your right hand forward. Hold for the recommended time, and then pull it back.
- Repeat on the opposite side. Alternate sides for the recommended repetitions.

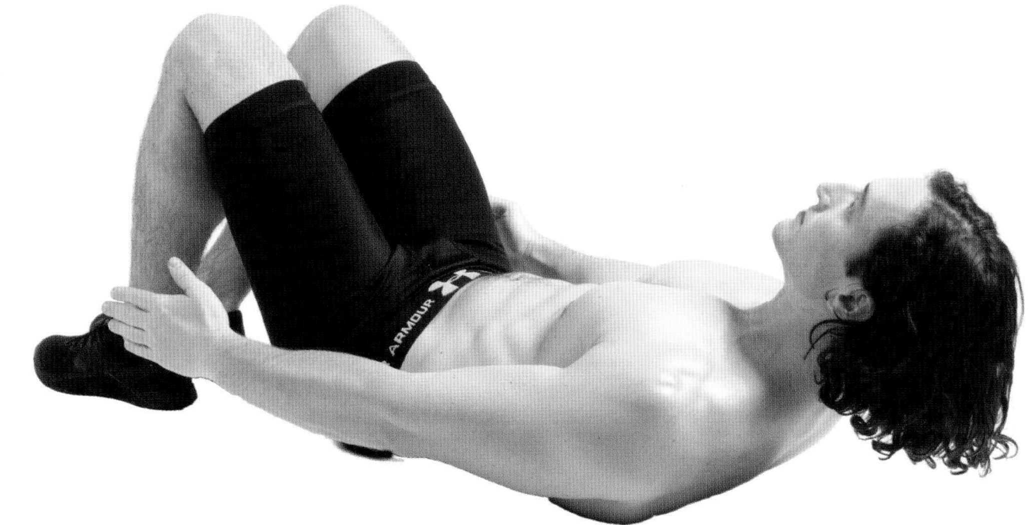

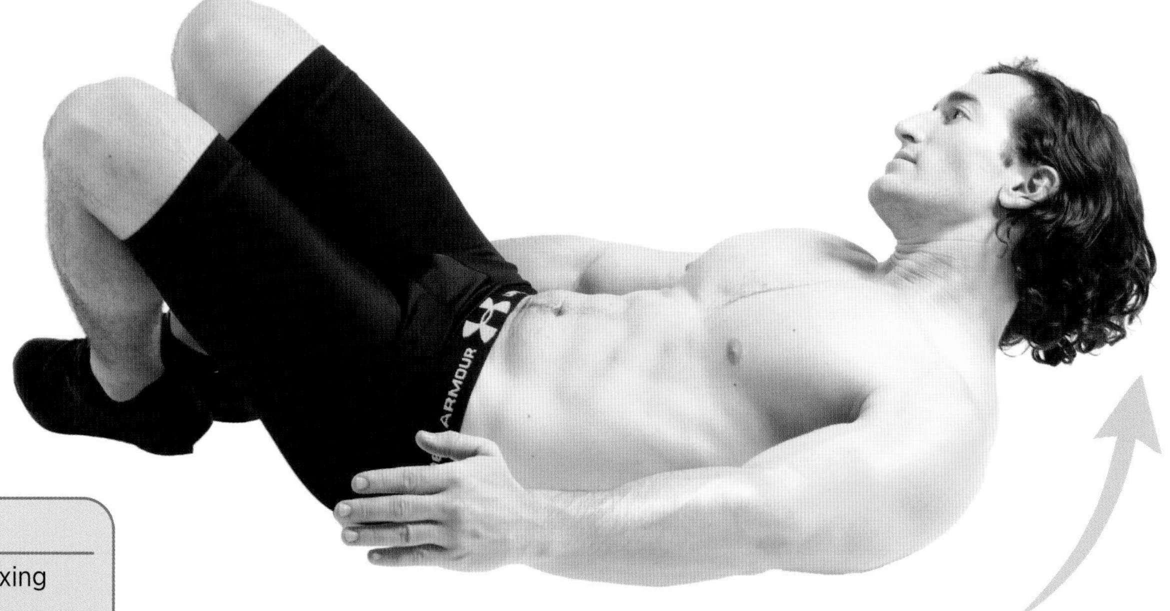

DO IT RIGHT

- Concentrate on flexing your obliques.
- As you reach, pull in using your midsection.
- Avoid overusing your neck and/or back muscles.

FACT FILE

TARGETS
- Upper and deep abdominals
- Obliques

TYPE
- Dynamic

BENEFITS
- Strengthens core
- Streamlines the abdominals, especially the obliques

CAUTIONS
- Lower-back issues

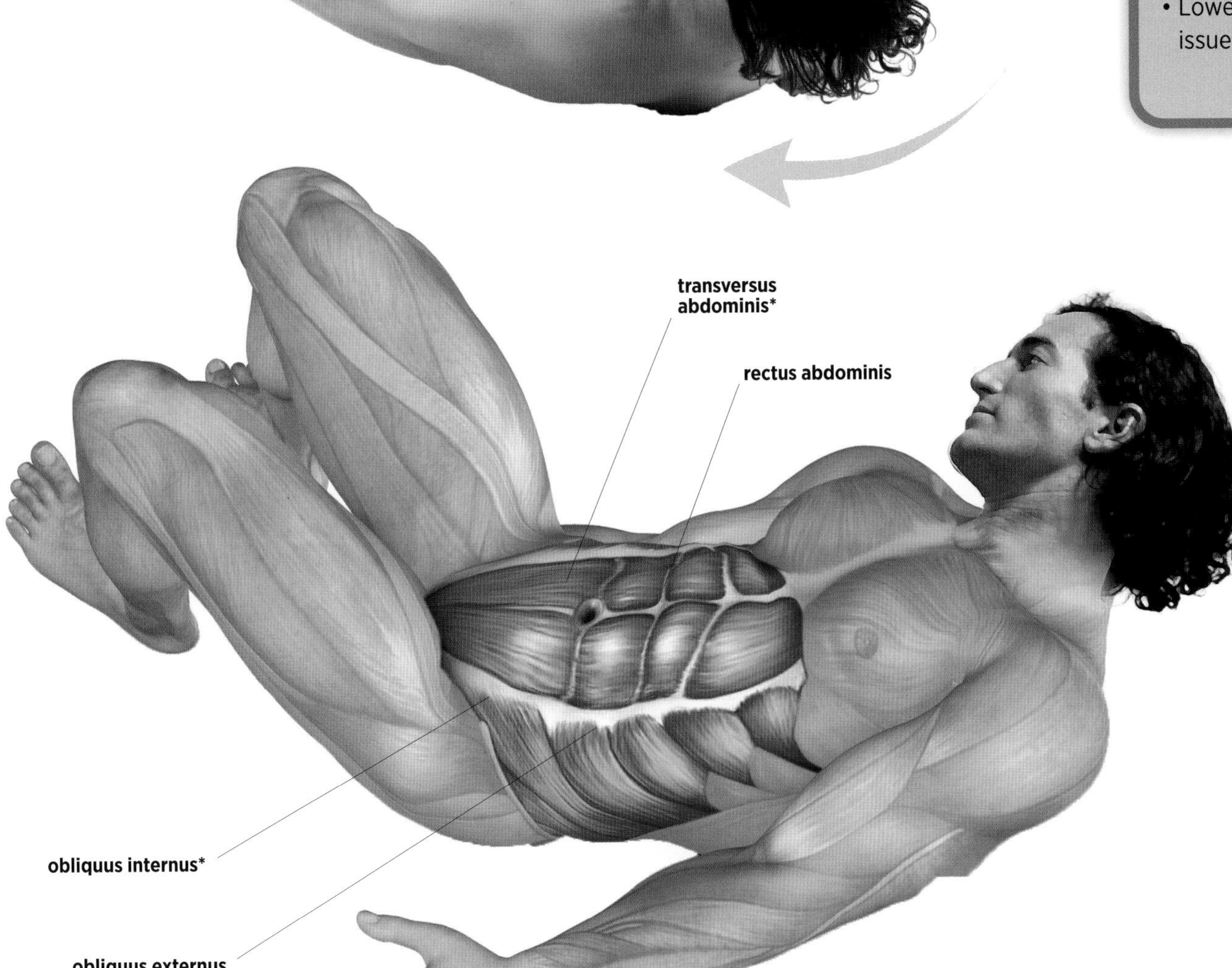

Annotation Key

Bold text indicates target muscles

Light text indicates other working muscles

* indicates deep muscles

Scissors

In Scissors, your legs are like scissor blades and your core like the handles. Keeping your handles stable frees your blades to cut through the air precisely. This is a great way to build up your core.

HOW TO DO IT

- Lie on your back, with your pelvis lengthened along the floor but not jammed right into it. Place your arms along your sides, and fold your knees in toward your chest.
- Curl your head and neck off the floor, extending your legs to the ceiling one at a time. Both buttocks should remain anchored to the floor throughout the exercise.
- Extend both arms toward your left leg so you can grasp it with both hands while the leg remains straight. At the same time, lower your right leg halfway to the floor.
- Start to switch legs by reaching both of them up to the ceiling so that they cross each other in midair.
- Take hold of your extended right leg, and lower your left leg halfway to the floor.
- Alternate legs for the recommended repetitions.

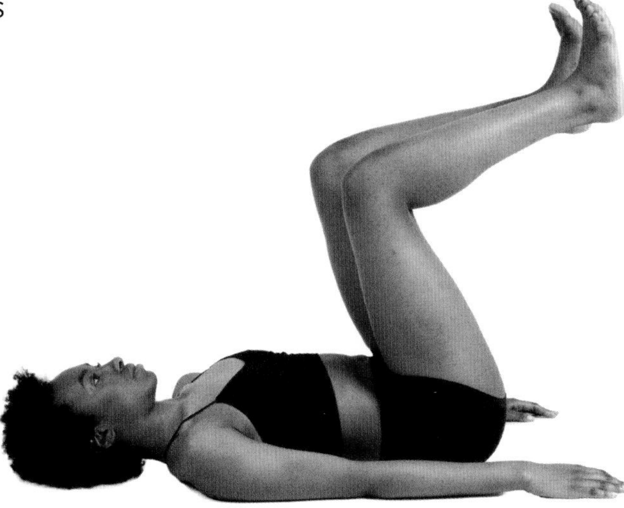

DO IT RIGHT

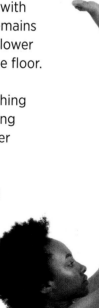

- Keep your core muscles engaged and active.
- Stabilize your shoulders by pressing your shoulder blades down your back.
- Keep your buttocks firmly planted into the floor.
- Keep your legs lengthened.
- Avoid pulling your shoulders forward while grasping your leg.
- Avoid bending your knees.
- Avoid using your arms to pull your leg toward you, rather than using your abdominal muscles to lift your upper body toward your leg.

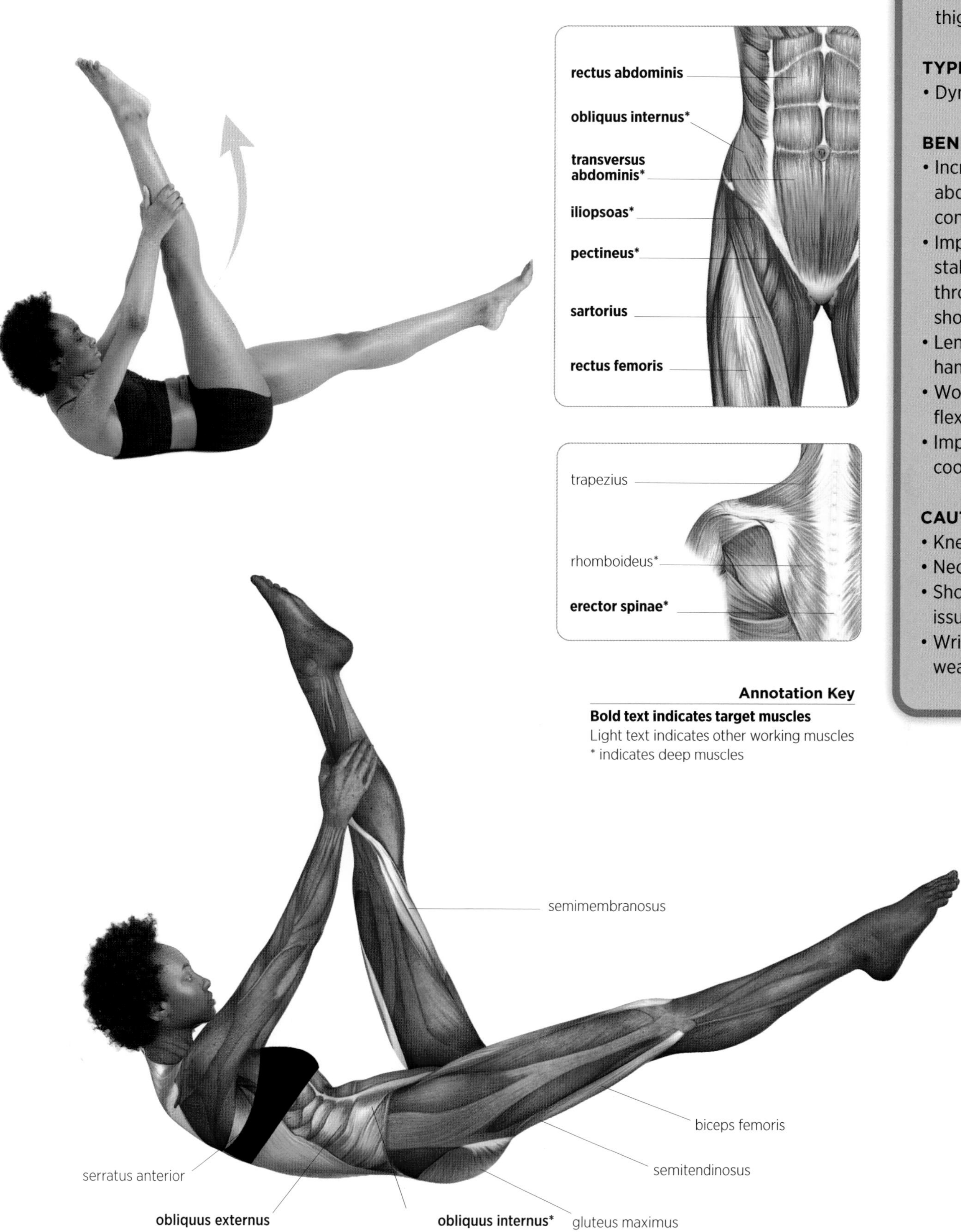

Annotation Key

Bold text indicates target muscles

Light text indicates other working muscles

* indicates deep muscles

FACT FILE

TARGETS
- Abdominals
- Back
- Front of thighs

TYPE
- Dynamic

BENEFITS
- Increases abdominal control
- Improves stabilization through shoulder area
- Lengthens hamstrings
- Works hip flexors
- Improves coordination

CAUTIONS
- Knee pain
- Neck issues
- Shoulder issues
- Wrist weakness

Thigh Rock-Back

The Thigh Rock-Back drives through the thighs and core. It builds particular strength in the quads center-front of your thighs and the central abdominals. Keeping your body straight teaches stability and focus.

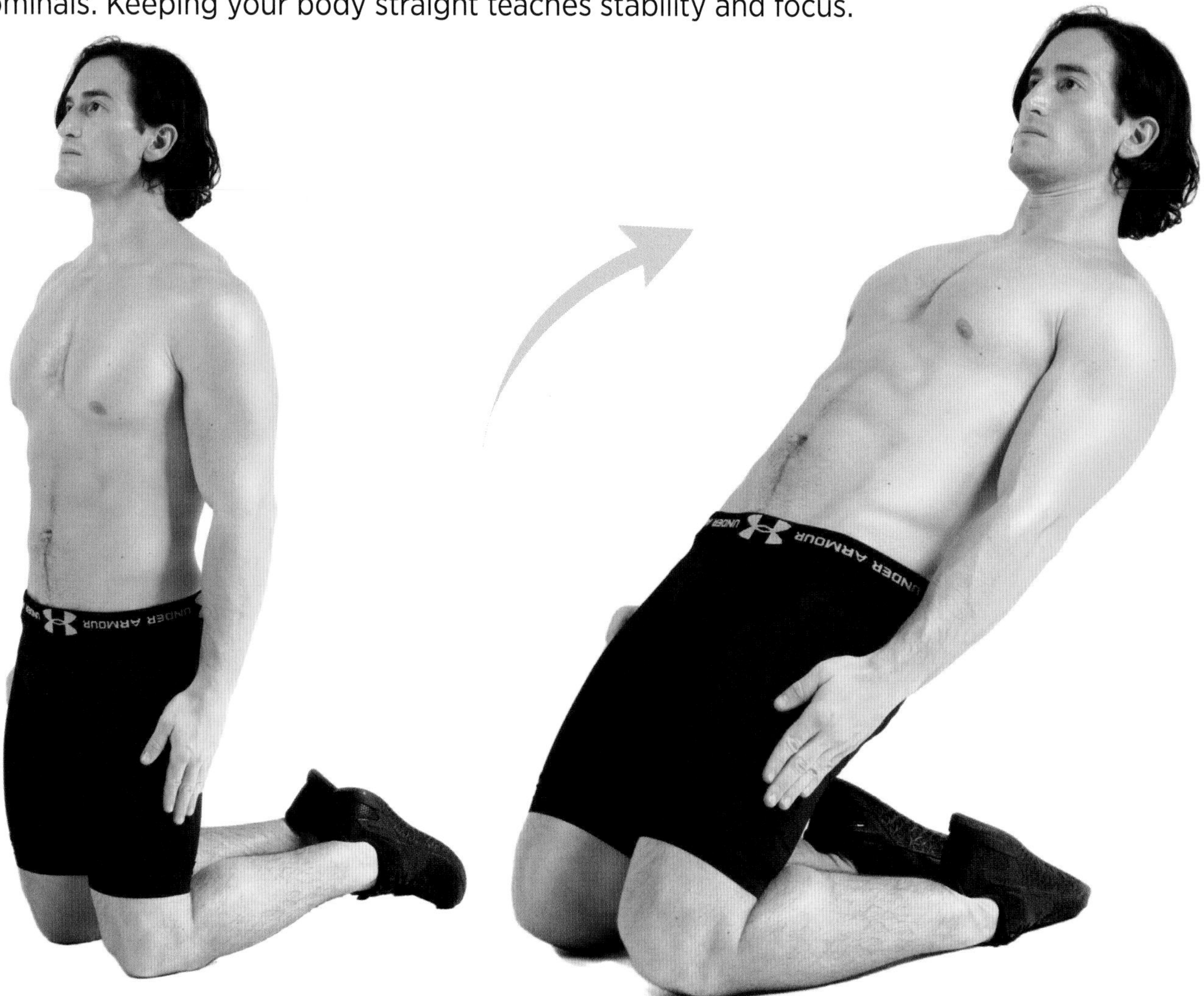

HOW TO DO IT

- Kneel on the floor with your back straight and your knees slightly apart, your arms by your sides. Pull in your abdominals, drawing your navel toward your spine.
- Lean back, keeping your hips open and aligned with your shoulders, stretching the front of your thighs.
- Once you have leaned back as far as you can, squeeze your glutes and slowly bring your body back to the upright position. Repeat for the recommended repetitions.

DO IT RIGHT

- Keep a straight line between your torso and your knees.
- Ensure your abdominals are controlling the movement.
- Keep your glutes tight.
- Avoid rocking so far back that you cannot return to the starting position.
- Avoid bending in your hips.

FACT FILE

TARGETS
- Thighs
- Abdominals

TYPE
- Dynamic

BENEFITS
- Stretches thighs
- Strengthens abdominals
- Increases ankle's range of motion

CAUTIONS
- Lower-back issues

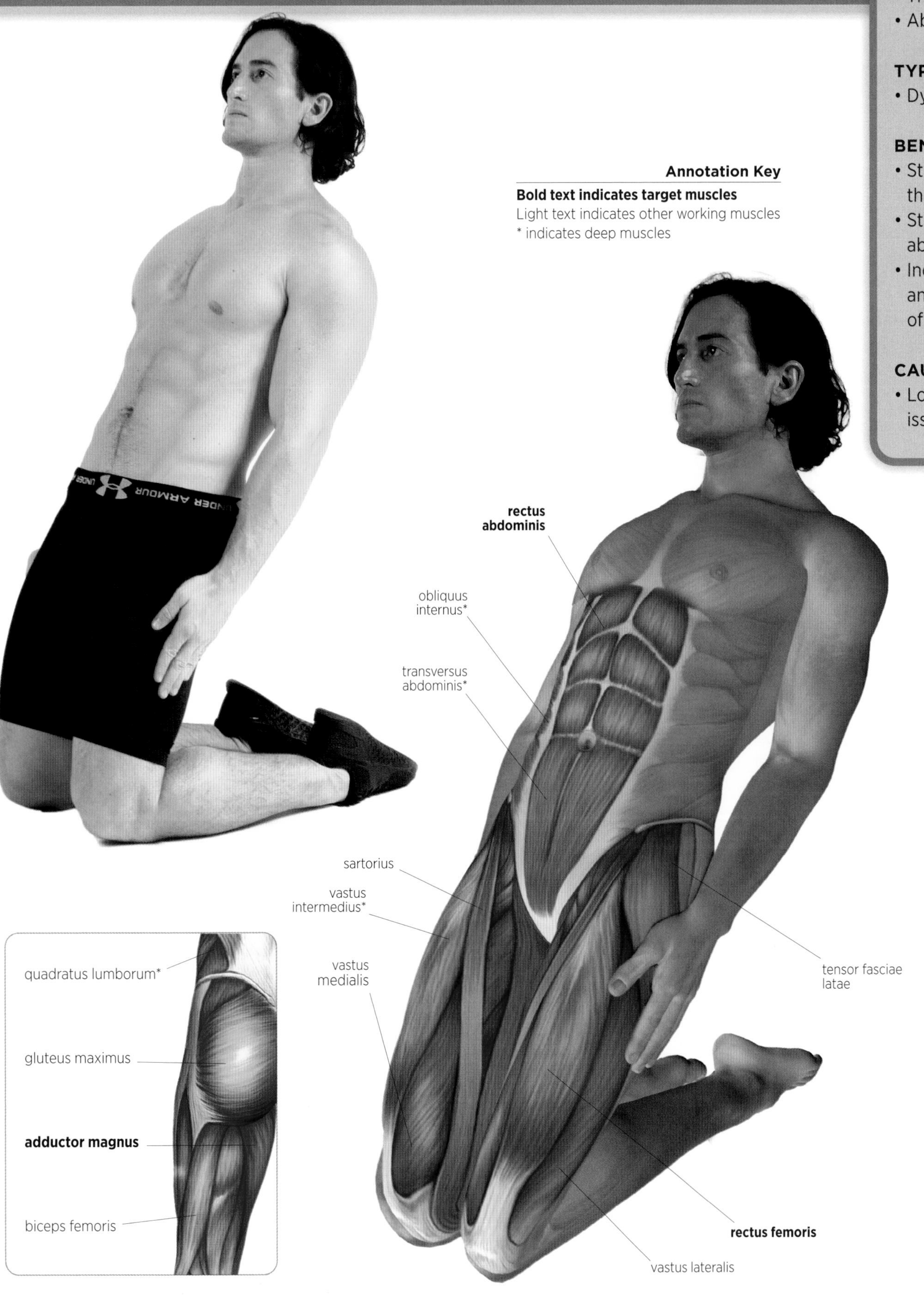

Reverse Crunch

The Reverse Crunch challenges your abdominals that little bit more compared to the simpler Crunch that uses an upper-body lift (pages 228–29). It works by using your lower-body weight for resistance.

HOW TO DO IT

- Lie on your back with your arms extended along your sides and your feet off the floor. Your legs should be slightly bent. This is your starting position.

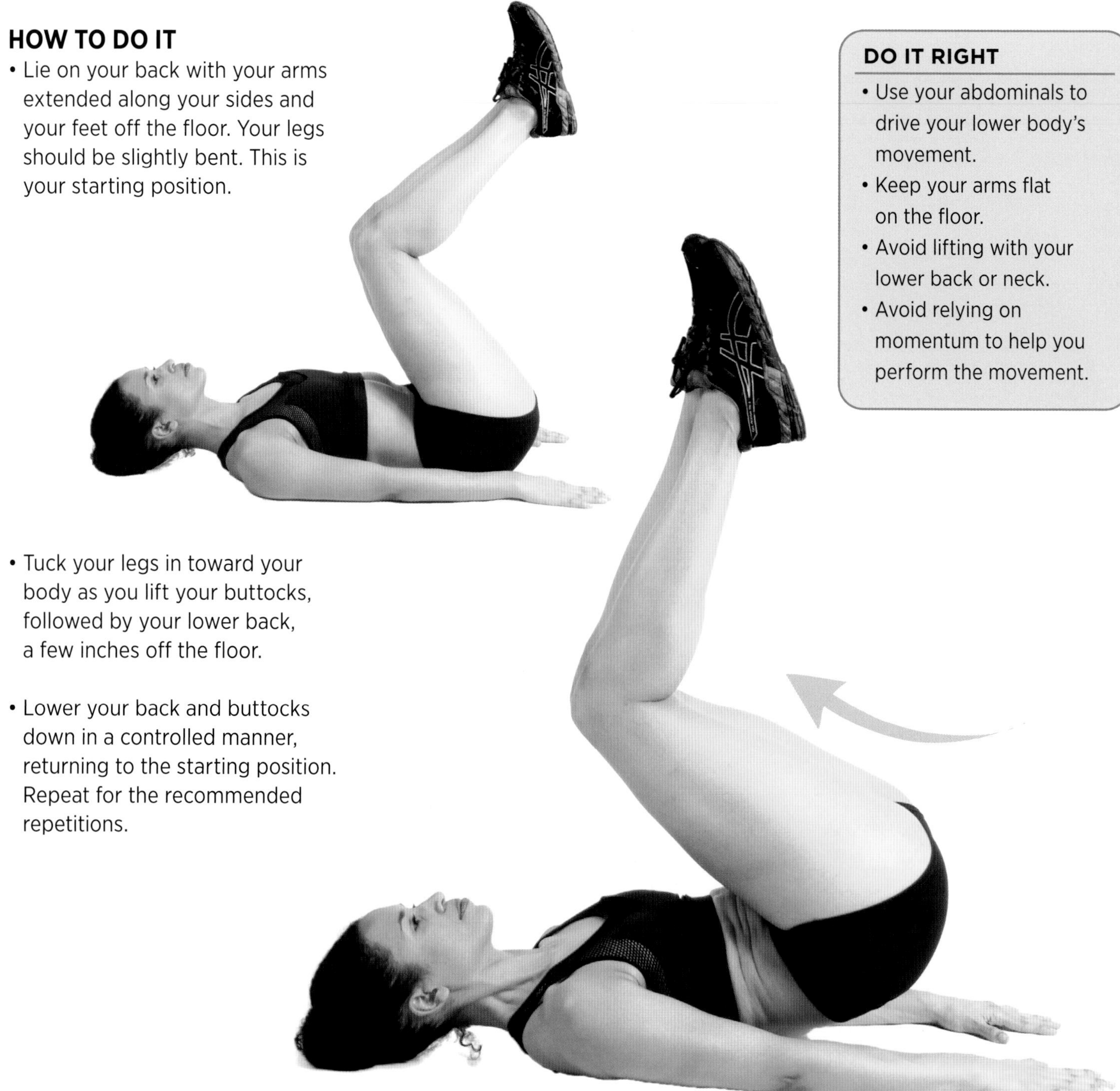

- Tuck your legs in toward your body as you lift your buttocks, followed by your lower back, a few inches off the floor.

- Lower your back and buttocks down in a controlled manner, returning to the starting position. Repeat for the recommended repetitions.

DO IT RIGHT

- Use your abdominals to drive your lower body's movement.
- Keep your arms flat on the floor.
- Avoid lifting with your lower back or neck.
- Avoid relying on momentum to help you perform the movement.

FACT FILE

TARGETS
- Abdominals: upper front and sides

TYPE
- Static

BENEFITS
- Strengthens and tones abdominals

CAUTIONS
- Hip issues
- Lower-back issues

MODIFICATION

HARDER: Once you can do a controlled basic Reverse Crunch without difficulty, try lifting a little farther. Take great care with going too high, though, as the spine and neck could become very vulnerable.

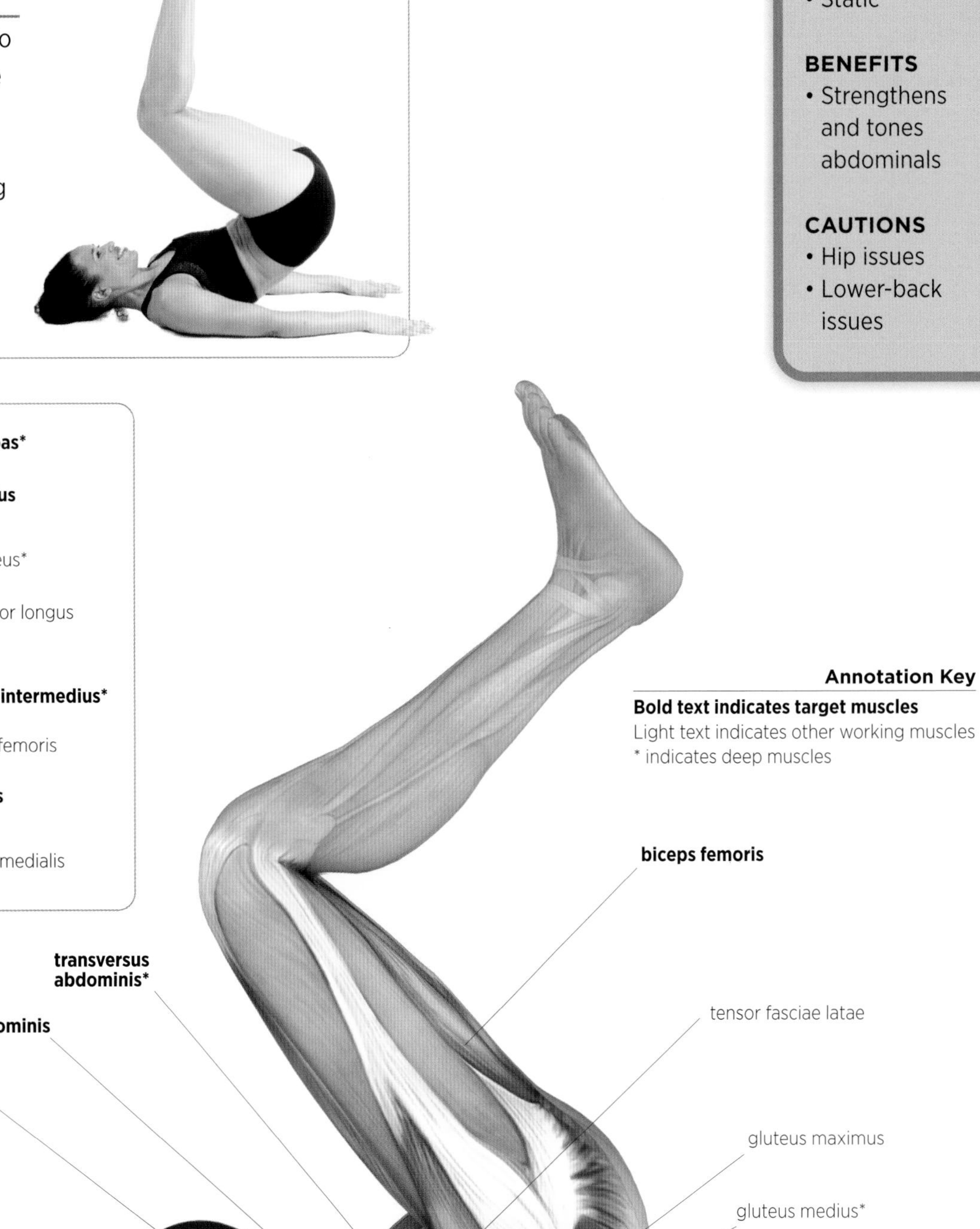

Annotation Key

Bold text indicates target muscles
Light text indicates other working muscles
* indicates deep muscles

Leg Levelers

Leg Levelers is a straightforward way to bring a wide range of muscles into play, from your shoulders to your thighs. This is an excellent routine for your core.

DO IT RIGHT

- Keep your hands under your buttocks to protect your lower back from excess extension.
- Avoid resting your head on the ground.

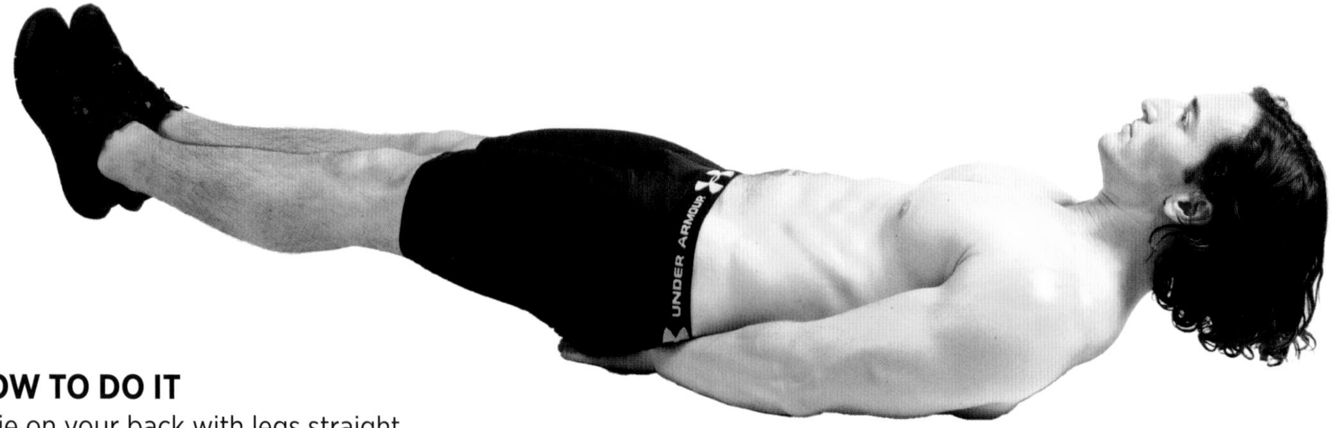

HOW TO DO IT

- Lie on your back with legs straight and your head raised off the floor. Place both hands under your buttocks to straighten the lumbar spine, and then lift both legs so that your feet are about 6 inches off the ground. Your knees should be bent slightly.
- Keeping your legs together, raise them until they form a 45-degree angle with the ground. Hold for the recommended time.
- Lower your legs back to 6 inches and hold for the recommended time. Repeat this up-and-hold and then down-and-hold sequence for the recommended repetitions.

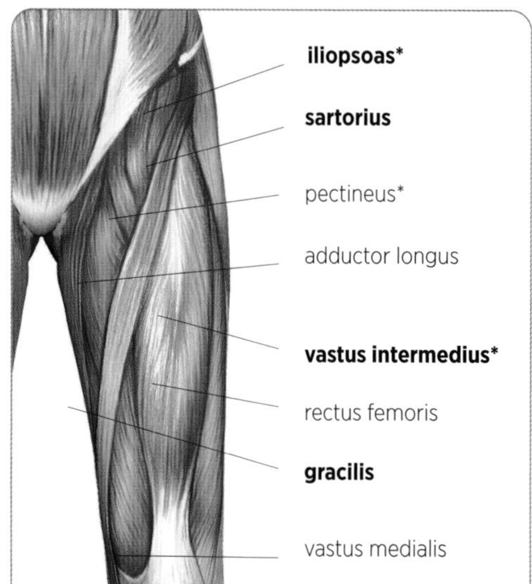

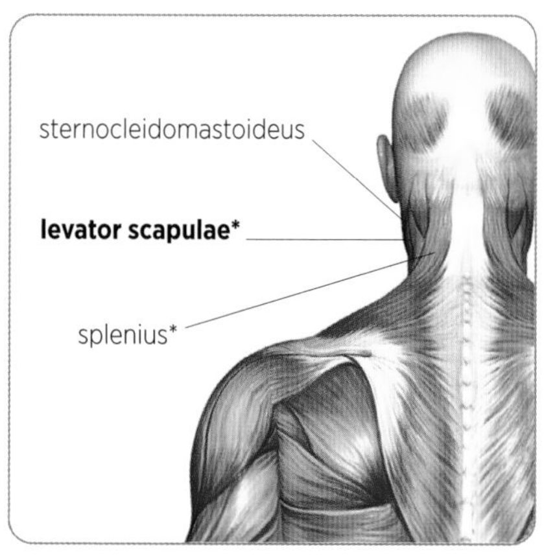

Annotation Key

Bold text indicates target muscles
Light text indicates other working muscles
* indicates deep muscles

FACT FILE

TARGETS
- Core
- Hip flexors
- Thighs

TYPE
- Static

BENEFITS
- Strengthens abdominals and hip flexors
- Increases running and swimming endurance

CAUTIONS
- Lower-back issues/pain

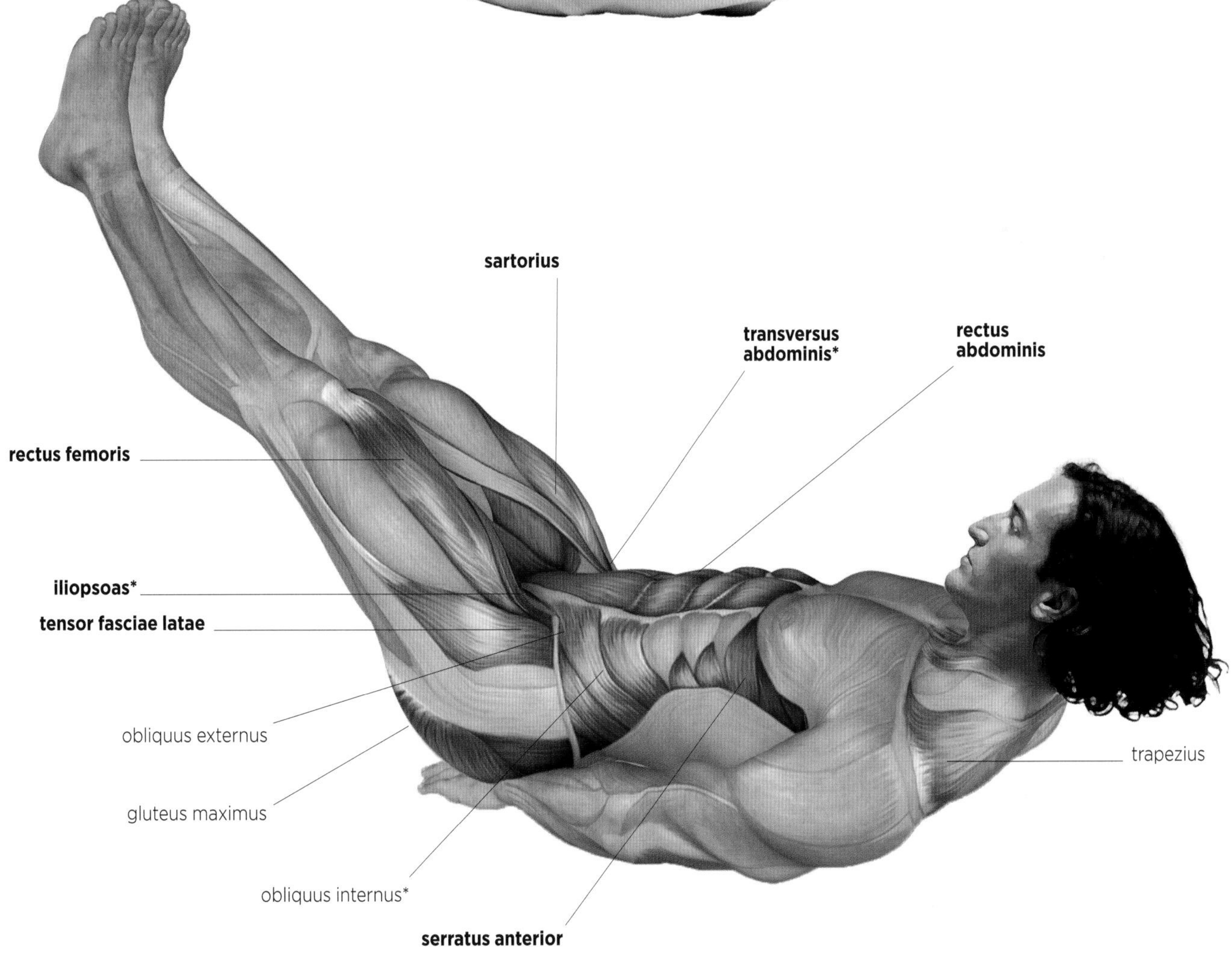

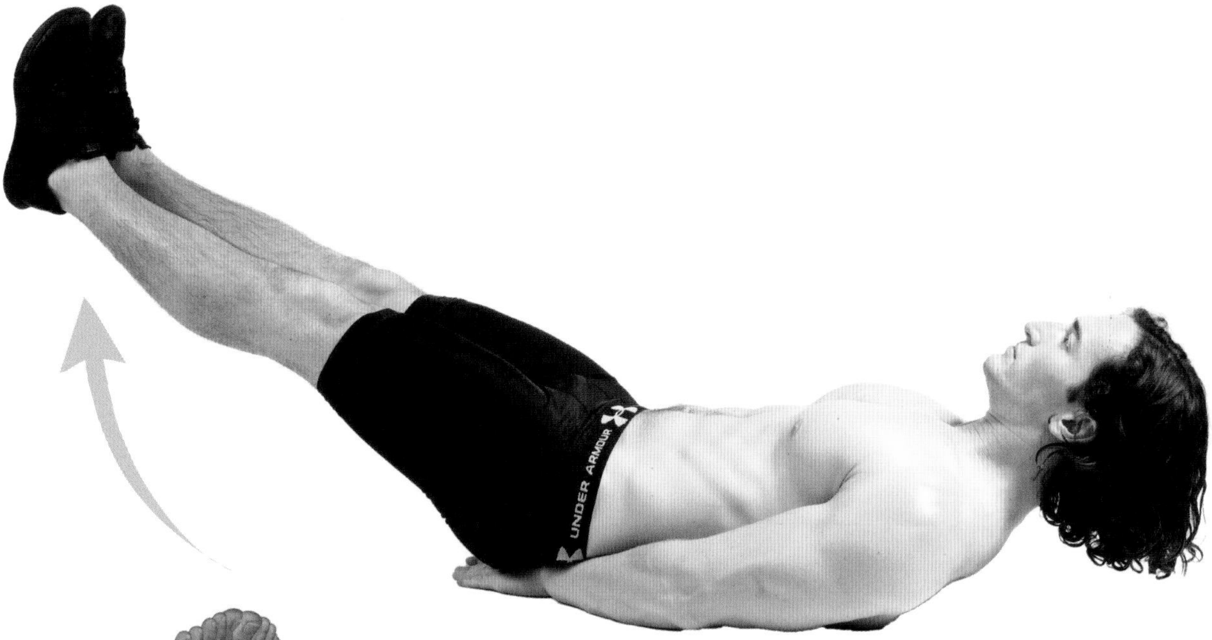

Body Saw

As the name suggests, this exercise is all about moving your body back and forth like a saw. The more your body stays in a straight line, the more power you build in your abdominals and lower back.

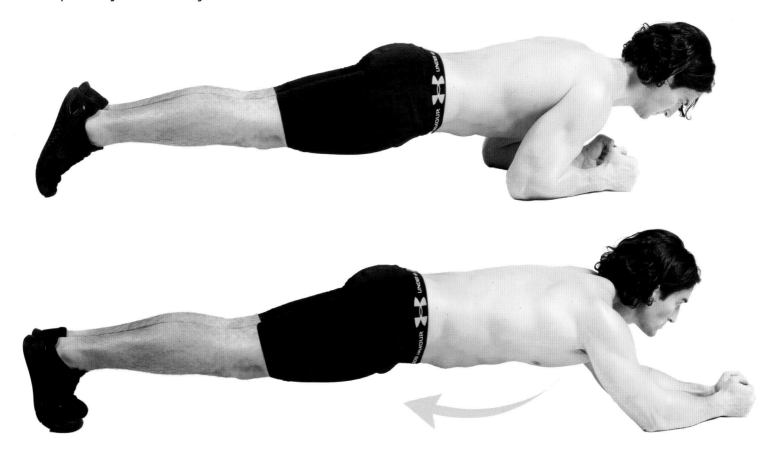

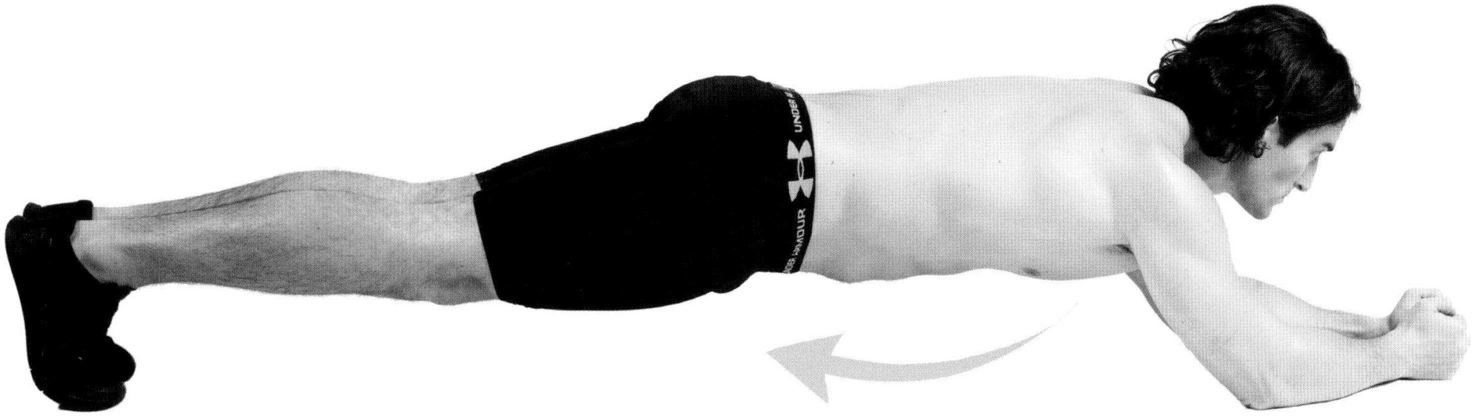

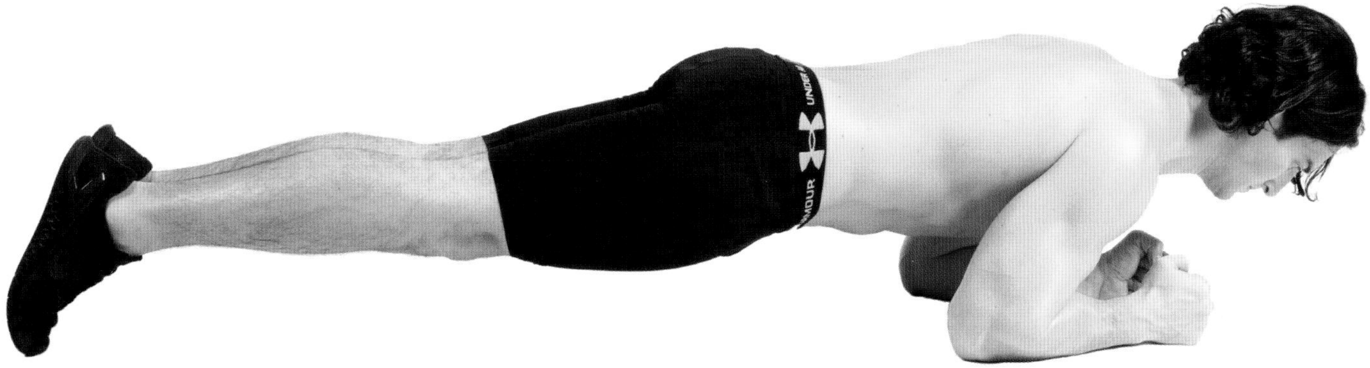

HOW TO DO IT

- Begin facedown, balancing on your toes and your forearms.
- Shift your body backward, pressing into the floor with your forearms as your feet change position.
- Shift your body forward to return to your starting position. Repeat the back-and forth sequence for the recommended repetitions.

DO IT RIGHT

- Keep your body in one straight line.
- Gaze toward the floor.
- Avoid arching your back, or curving it forward.

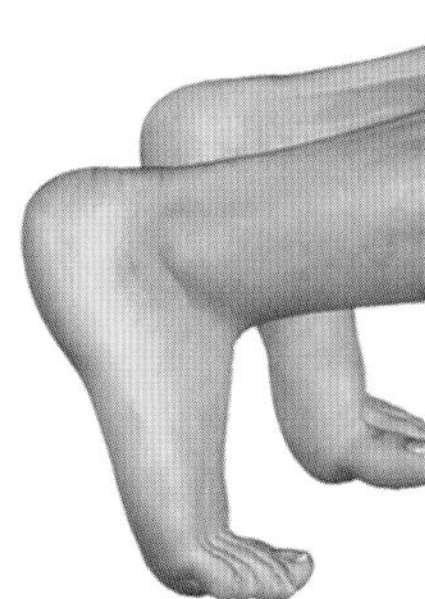

FACT FILE

TARGETS
- Abdominals
- Back
- ITB (Iliotibial Band)

TYPE
- Static

BENEFITS
- Stabilizes core
- Strengthens abdominals

CAUTIONS
- Shoulder issues
- Lower-back issues

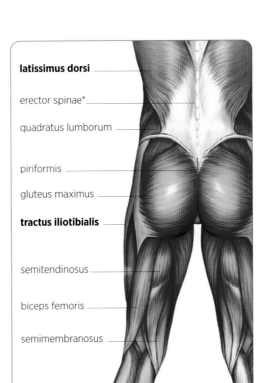

latissimus dorsi
erector spinae*
quadratus lumborum
piriformis
gluteus maximus
tractus iliotibialis
semitendinosus
biceps femoris
semimembranosus

Annotation Key

Bold text indicates target muscles
Light text indicates other working muscles
* indicates deep muscles

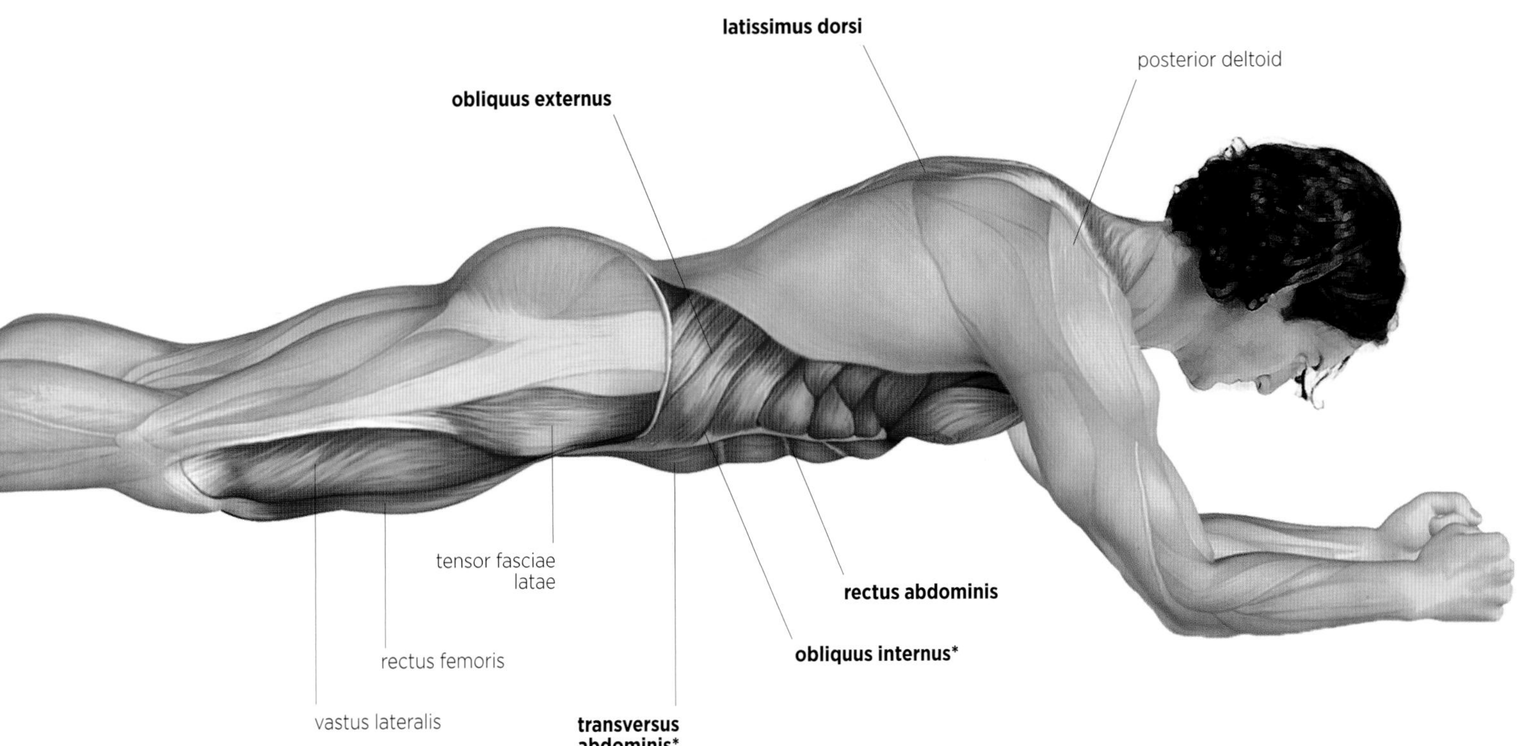

Fire-Hydrant In-Out

Fire Hydrant In-Out is a hardworking core-stabilizing exercise, as well as a great abdominal strengthener. It targets your glutes, with assistance from your abdominal muscles. It also powers up your inner thighs and hamstrings.

HOW TO DO IT

- Begin on your hands and knees, with your palms on the floor and spaced shoulder-width apart. Your spine should be in a neutral position: straight but relaxed.
- Keeping your right leg bent at a 90-degree angle, raise it laterally (to the side).
- Now straighten your right leg until it is fully extended behind you.
- Bend your right knee and bring your leg back into its 90-degree position, and then lower it to meet your left leg. Repeat for the recommended repetitions. Repeat on the opposite side.

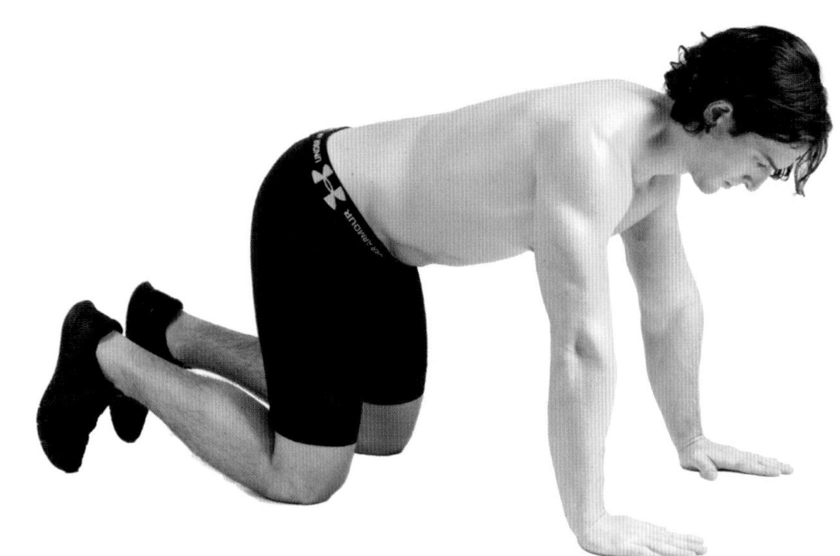

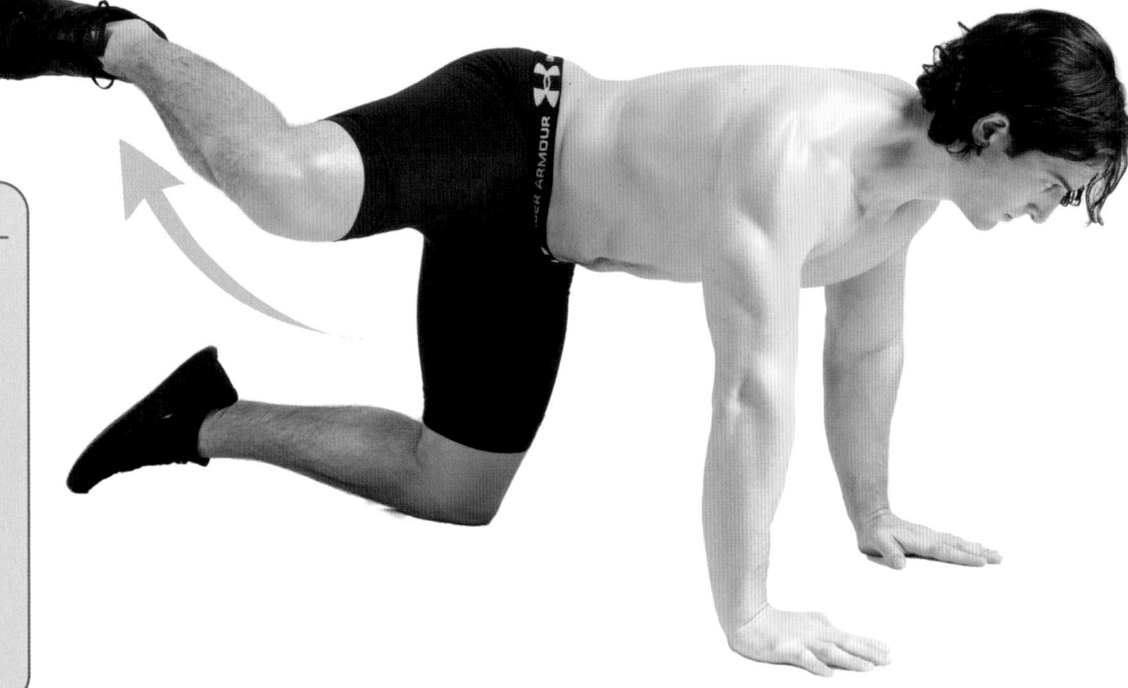

DO IT RIGHT

- Press your hands into the floor to keep your shoulders from sinking.
- Squeeze your glutes with your leg fully extended.
- Avoid lifting your hip as you lift your bent leg to the side.
- Avoid rushing; make sure you feel each part of the repetition.

FACT FILE

TARGETS
- Core
- Abdominals
- Glutes

TYPE
- Static

BENEFITS
- Stabilizes pelvis
- Strengthens glutes

CAUTIONS
- Wrist pain
- Knee issues

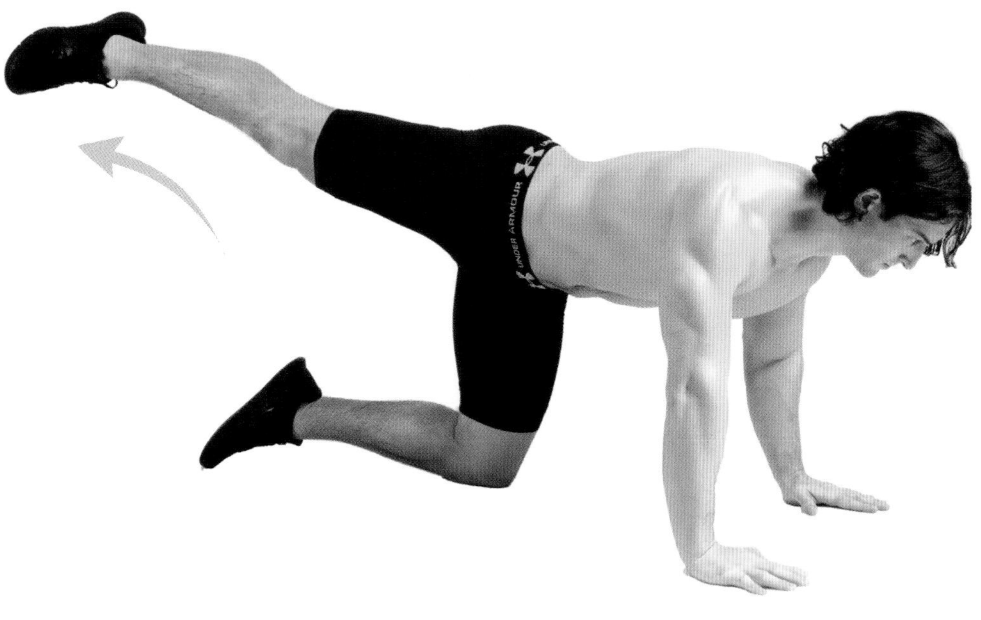

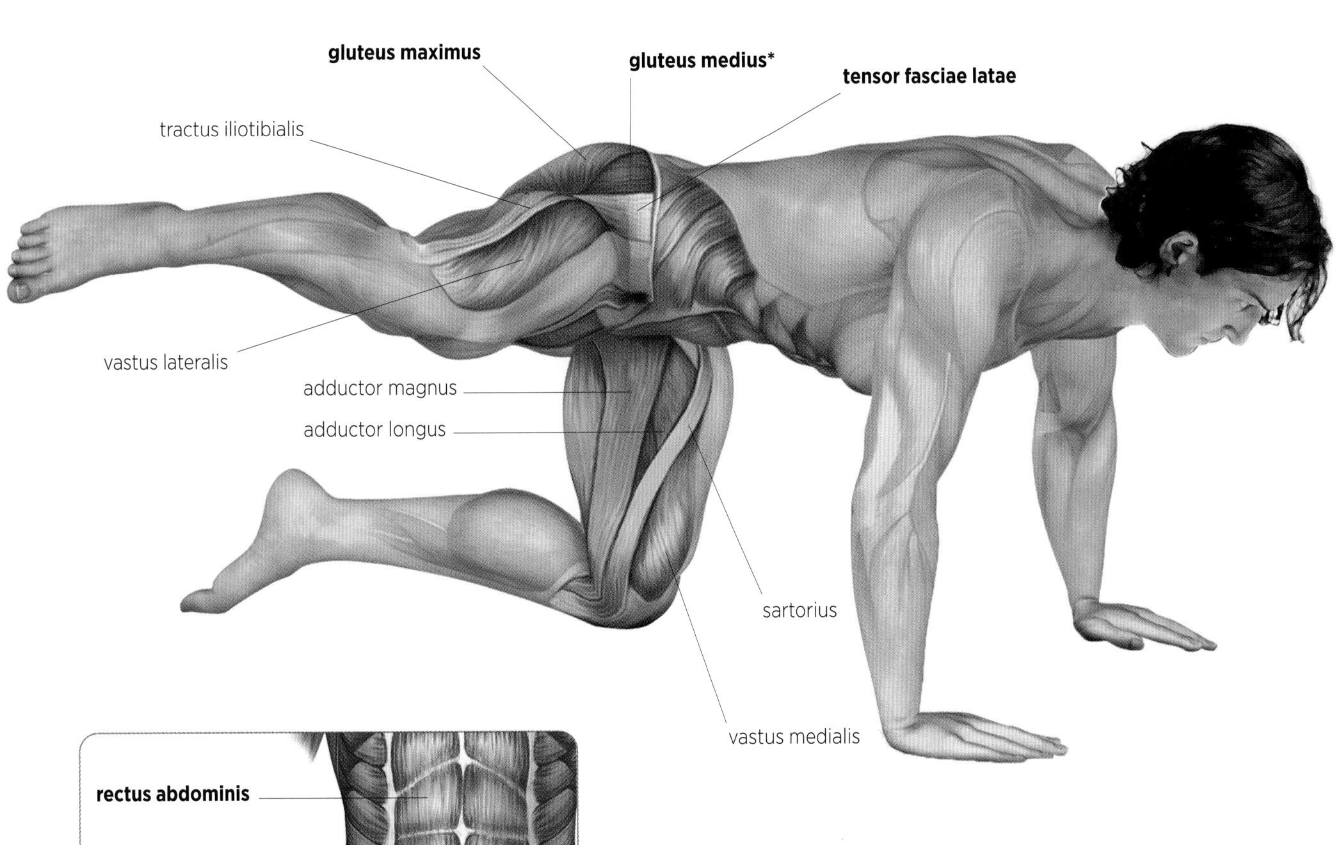

Annotation Key

Bold text indicates target muscles
Light text indicates other working muscles
* indicates deep muscles

Single-Leg V-Up

Regular practice of Single-Leg V-Up will make your abdominal muscles stronger, which it turn makes the exercise's upward motion smoother and easier. This is a great way to prepare your core muscles for all kinds of workouts.

HOW TO DO IT

- Lie on your back, with your arms extended over your head, hovering just above the floor behind you, palms up. Bend your knees and press them together. Anchor your feet into the floor.
- Slowly and with control, extend your right leg, straightening it from your hip and out through your foot.

DO IT RIGHT

- Keep your neck stretched out.
- Maintain a tight core and a level pelvis.
- When balancing, your arms should be parallel to your extended leg.
- Avoid arching your back or rolling your shoulders forward.
- Avoid relying on momentum to propel you up or down.
- Avoid allowing your stomach to bulge outward.

- Initiating the movement from your lower abdomen, raise your torso to form a 45-degree angle with the floor as you bring your arms up and over your head to reach forward.
- With control, curl your spine down to the floor as you bring your arms up overhead and behind you again, keeping your knees pressed together.
- Repeat for the recommended repetitions. Repeat on the opposite side.

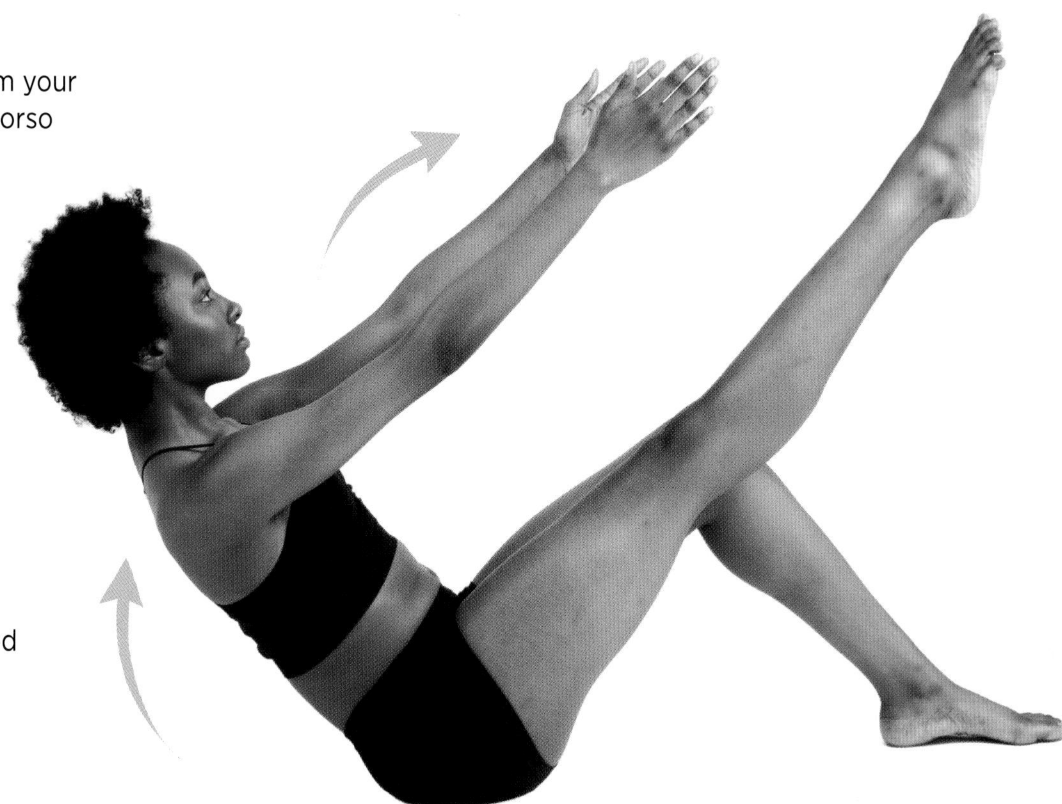

FACT FILE

TARGETS
- Abdominals
- Thighs
- Hip flexors

TYPE
- Dynamic

BENEFITS
- Strengthens and tones abdominals
- Mobilizes spine

CAUTIONS
- Herniated disc
- Lower-back issues
- Osteoporosis

MODIFICATION

HARDER: For a really tough workout for your core, try raising both legs at the same time. Proceed carefully so that this doesn't cause any back issues.

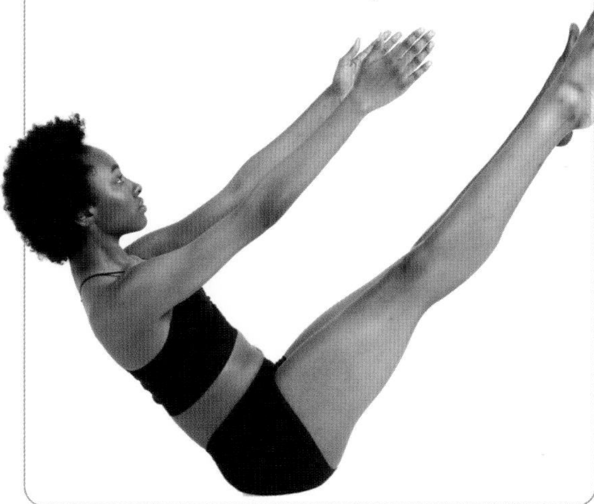

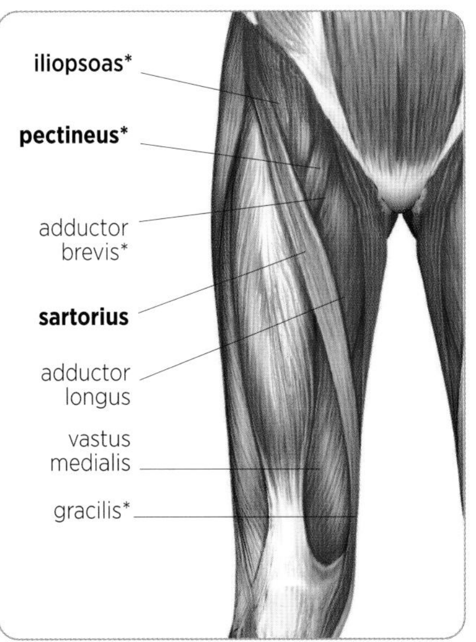

Annotation Key
Bold text indicates target muscles
Light text indicates other working muscles
* indicates deep muscles

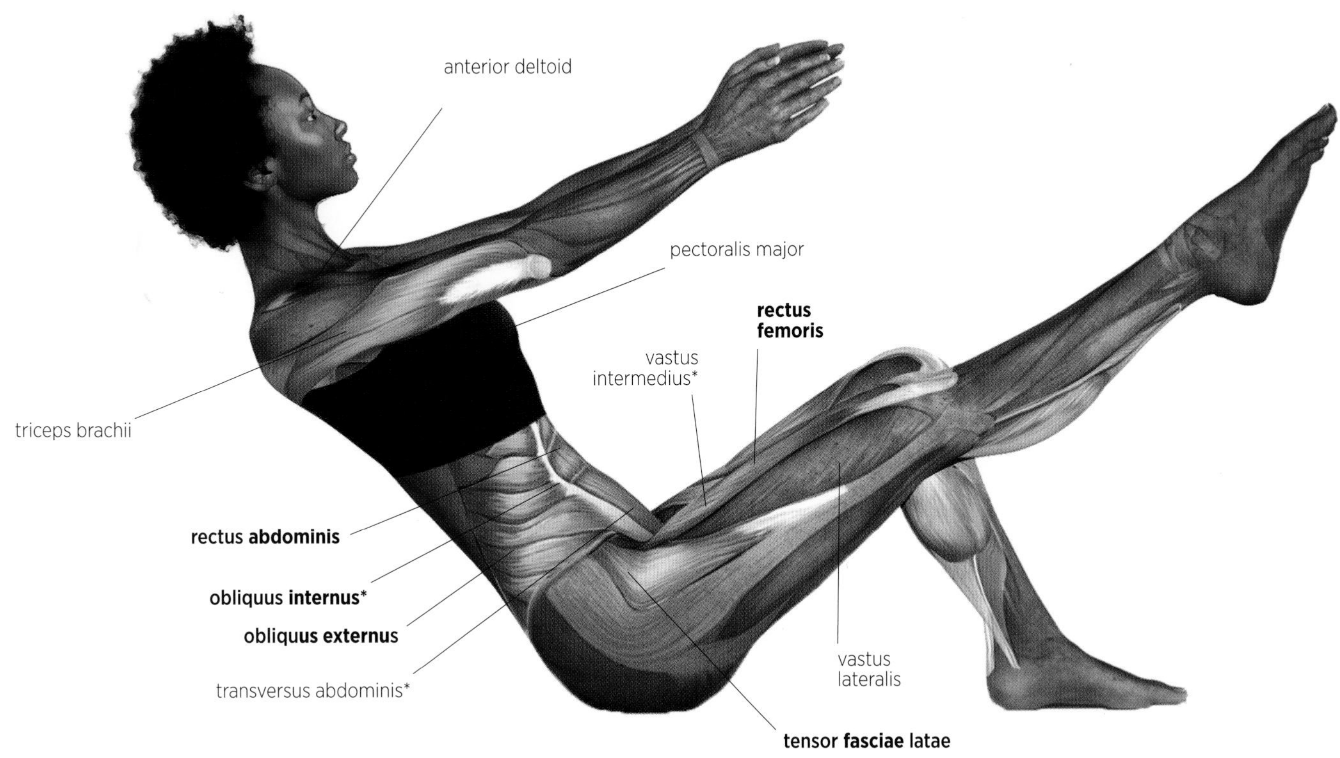

Reverse Bridge Ball Roll

This variation on a Reverse Bridge Stretch, which is practiced on a Swiss Ball, is a great chest opener, core strengthener, and oblique stretch. For an easier variation and greater stability, plant your feet wide apart in front of the ball.

HOW TO DO IT

- Lie supine with your lower back on a Swiss ball and your feet together. Keep your knees bent at 90 degrees and your feet planted on the floor in front of the ball. Stretch your arms out to your sides, palms facing upward.

- Move your upper body across the ball to your left, rolling across the ball so it is beneath your left shoulder.

- Hold for the recommended time, and then slowly roll back to the starting position, with the Swiss ball centered between your shoulder blades. Repeat on the opposite side, and perform the recommended repetitions.

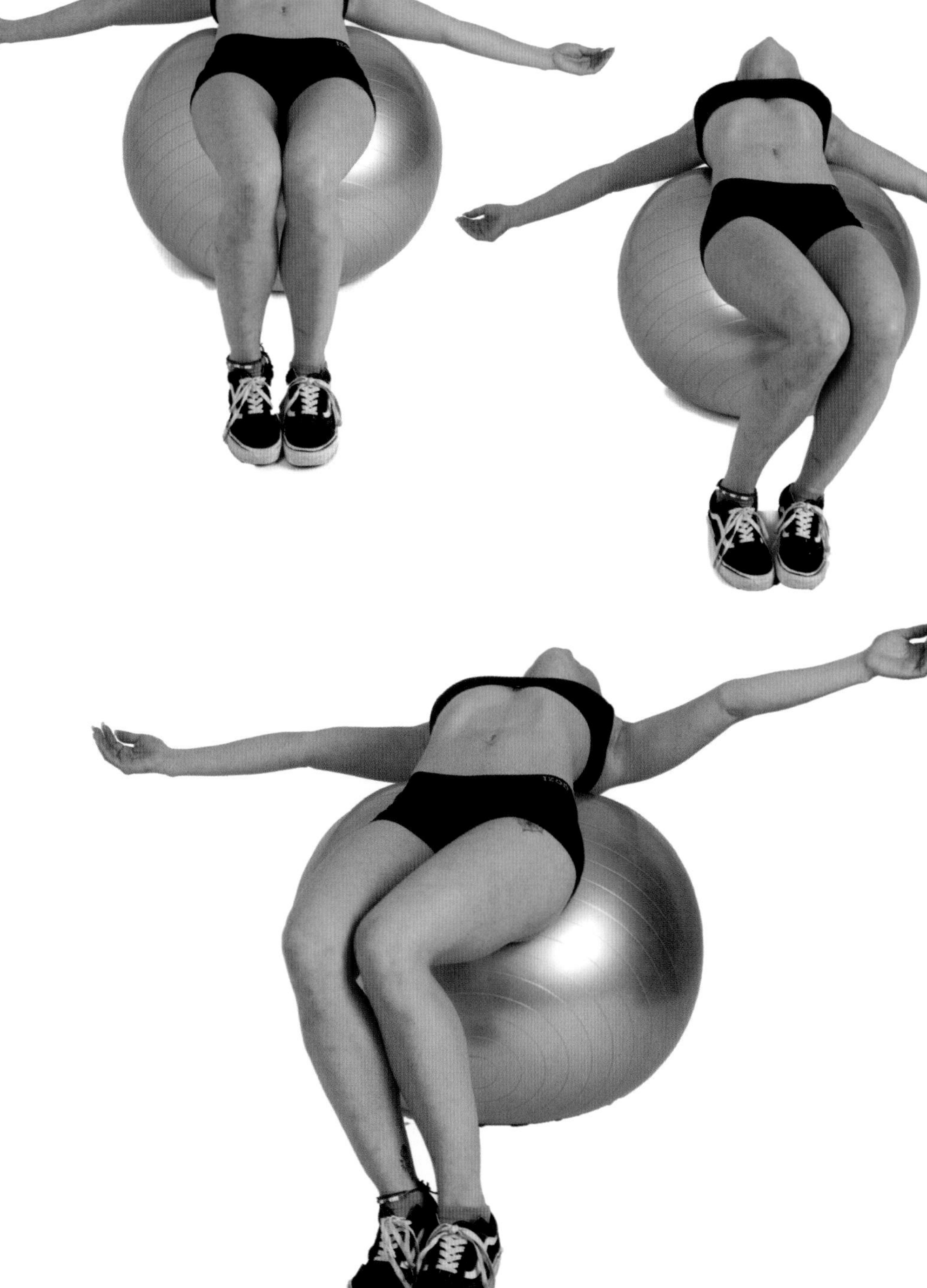

DO IT RIGHT

- Exhale as you roll to the side, and inhale as you return to the starting position.
- Hold your body stable as you roll across the ball, keeping your core engaged.
- If necessary, increase the space between your feet to maintain your balance.
- Avoid allowing your pelvis to drop—your body should form a straight line from your shoulders to your knees.

FACT FILE

TARGETS
- Obliques
- Abdominals

TYPE
- Isometric

BENEFITS
- Stabilizes core
- Strengthens obliques and abdominals

CAUTIONS
- Neck pain
- Lower-back pain
- Spinal problems

EQUIPMENT
- Swiss ball

MODIFICATION

EASIER: Rather than keeping your feet together, position them about shoulder-width apart.

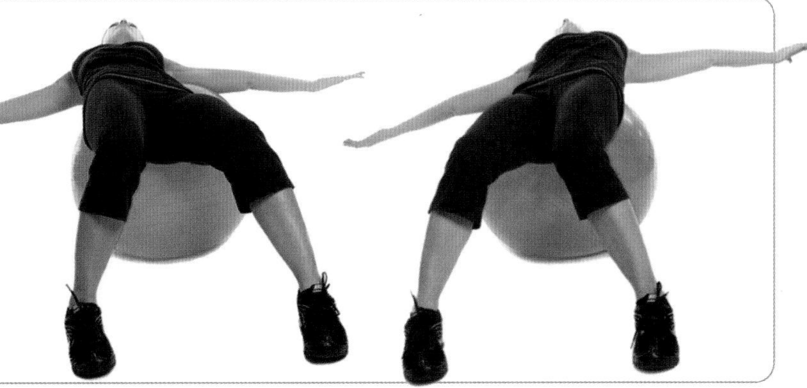

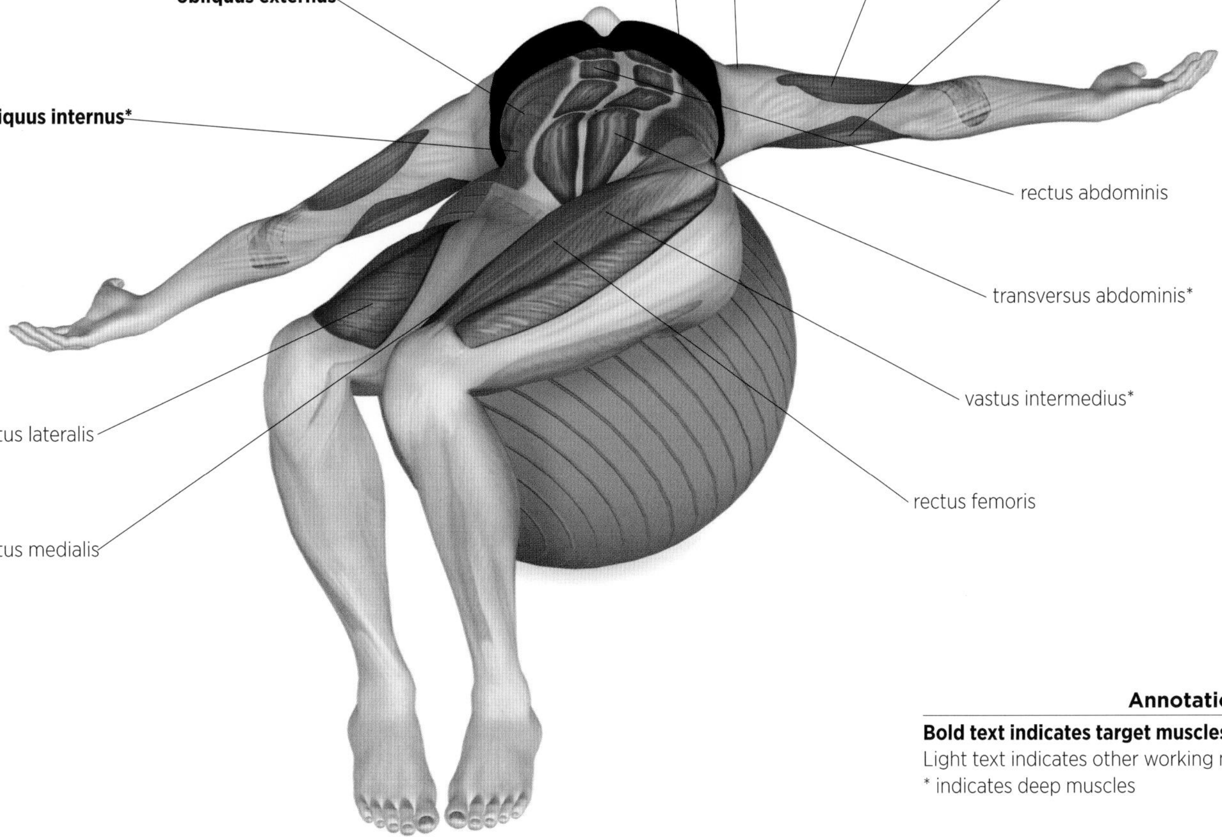

serratus anterior
anterior deltoid
biceps brachii
triceps brachii
obliquus externus
obliquus internus*
rectus abdominis
transversus abdominis*
vastus intermedius*
vastus lateralis
rectus femoris
vastus medialis

Annotation Key

Bold text indicates target muscles
Light text indicates other working muscles
* indicates deep muscles

Jackknife Pull

The Jackknife is a real test for the abdominal muscles. Your legs and hips will also benefit from this Pilates exercise, and you should find yourself becoming more flexible as you perfect this pose.

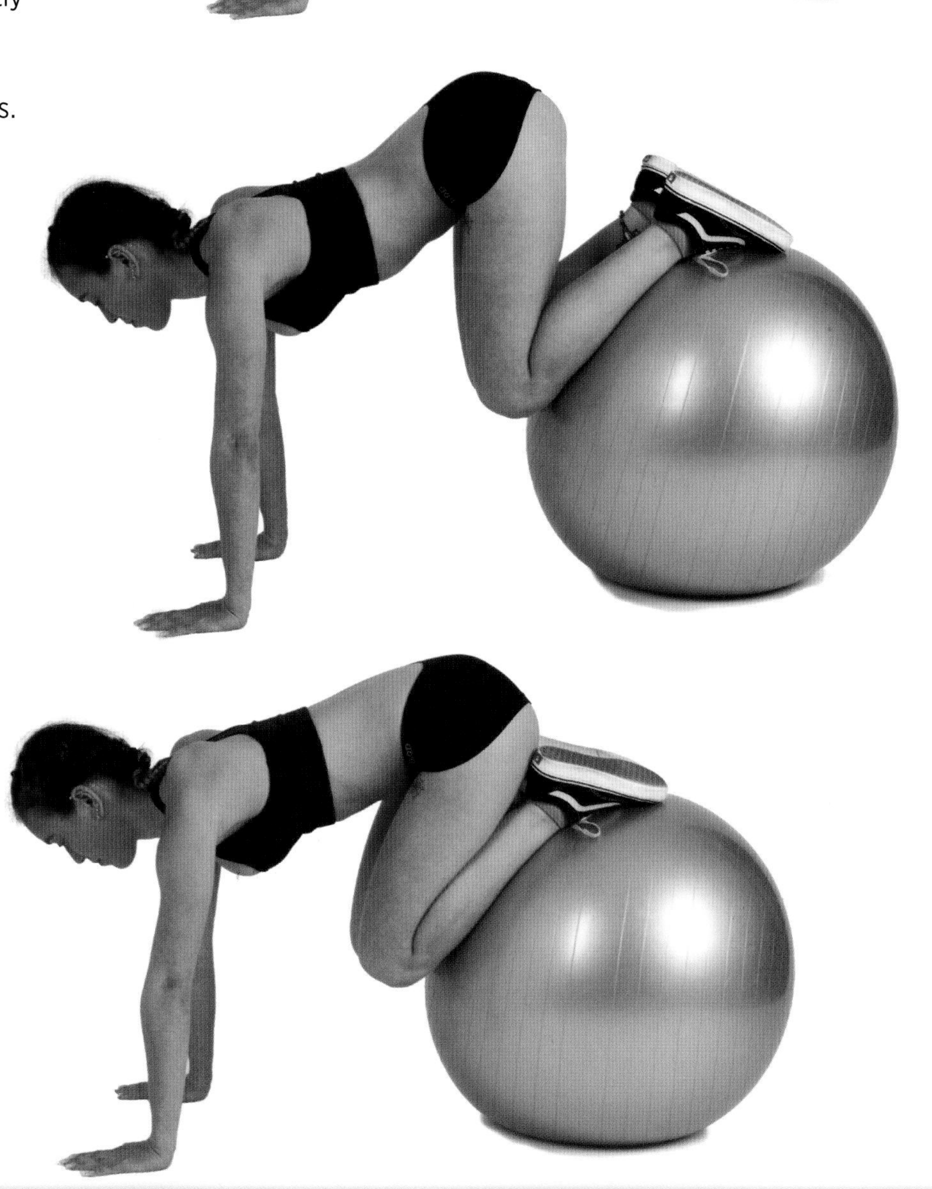

HOW TO DO IT

- Start by rolling forward on the Swiss ball, walking your hands forward until your body is straight.
- Hold the position.
- Using your knees, shins and feet, gently roll the ball forward and hold.
- Perform the recommended repetitions.

DO IT RIGHT

- Aim to keep your limbs as straight as possible throughout this stretch.
- Inhale while lowering your body and legs, and exhale as you lift.
- Avoid letting your hands leave the floor.

FACT FILE

TARGETS
- Abdominals
- Obliques
- Hip flexors

TYPE
- Dynamic

BENEFITS
- Abdominal strengthener
- Core stabilizer

CAUTIONS
- Neck problems
- Shoulder pain

EQUIPMENT
- Swiss ball

subscapularis*
rhomboideus*

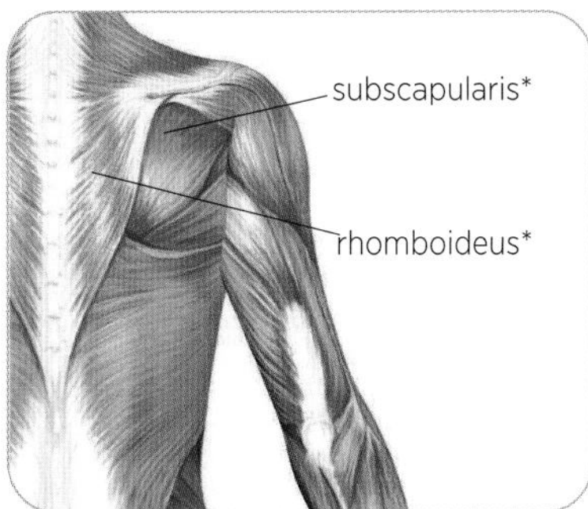

rectus abdominis
transversus abdominis*
sartorius

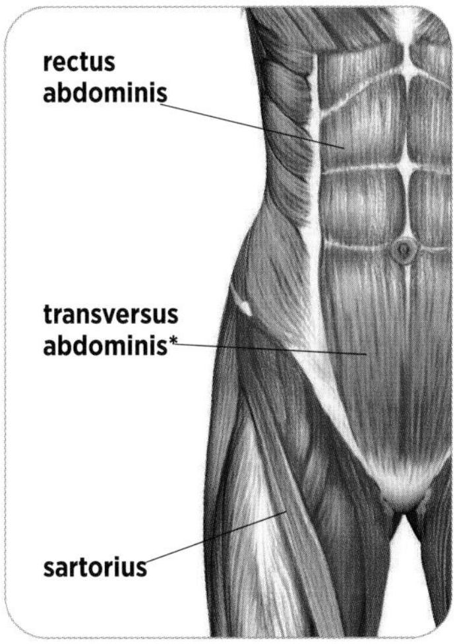

Annotation Key

Bold text indicates target muscles

Light text indicates other working muscles

* indicates deep muscles

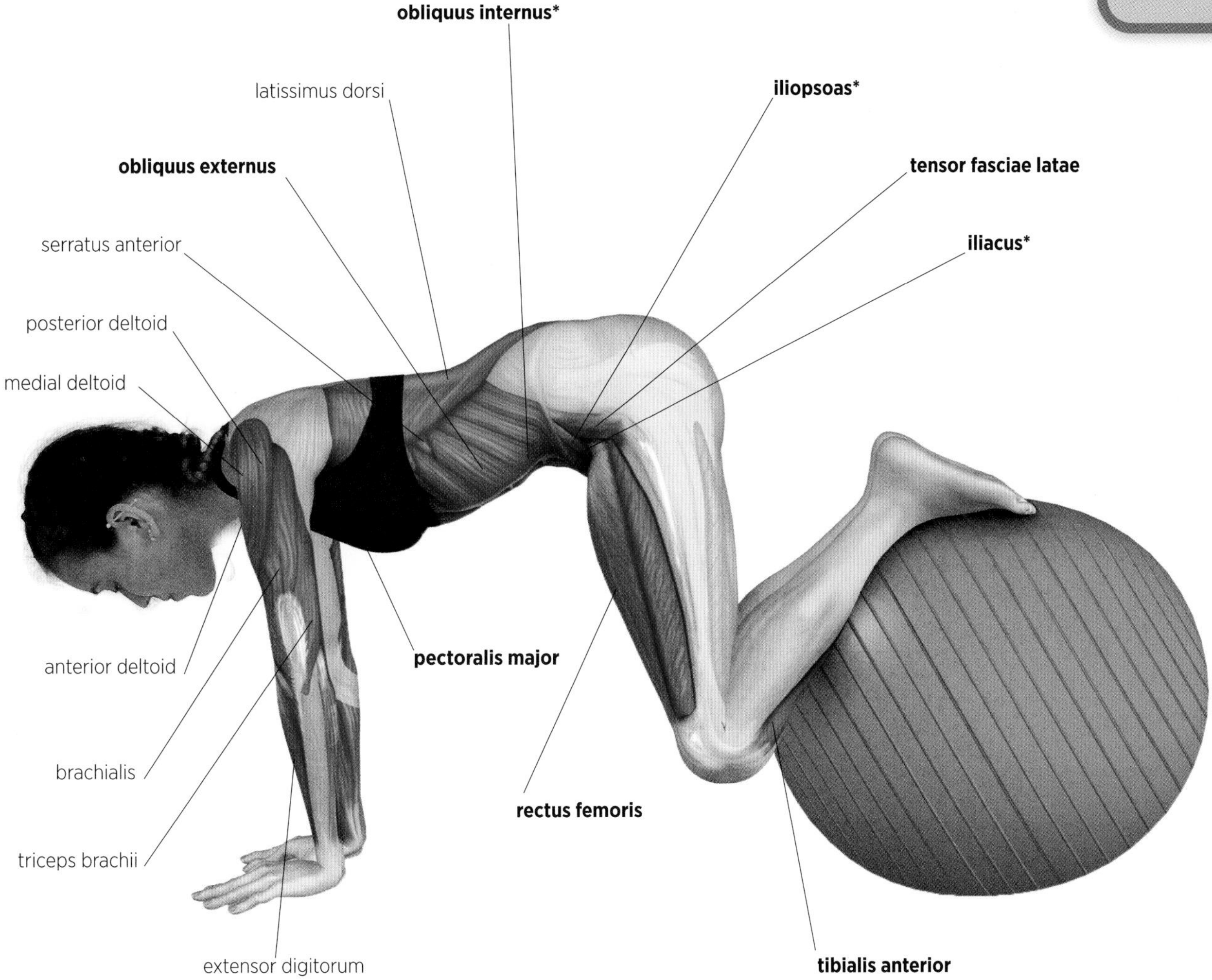

obliquus internus*
latissimus dorsi
iliopsoas*
obliquus externus
tensor fasciae latae
serratus anterior
iliacus*
posterior deltoid
medial deltoid
anterior deltoid
pectoralis major
brachialis
rectus femoris
triceps brachii
extensor digitorum
tibialis anterior

Hip Circles

Performing hip circles on a Swiss Ball can help loosen your pelvic muscles, releasing any built-up tension in your hip joints. In addition, hip circles work the upper body and challenge your core, while relieving pain in your lower-back.

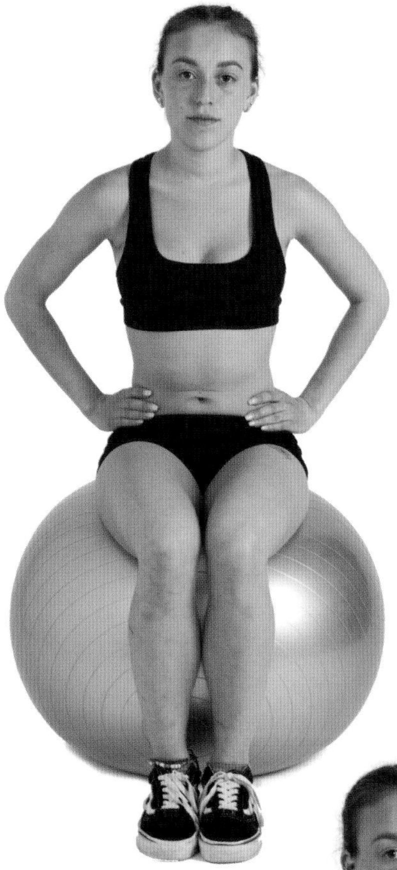

HOW TO DO IT

- Sit on a Swiss ball with your feet together and your hands on your hips.
- Tighten your abdominal muscles.
- Use your pelvis to rotate the ball slowly to the right in small counterclockwise circles.
- Return to the starting position, and then repeat in the opposite direction.

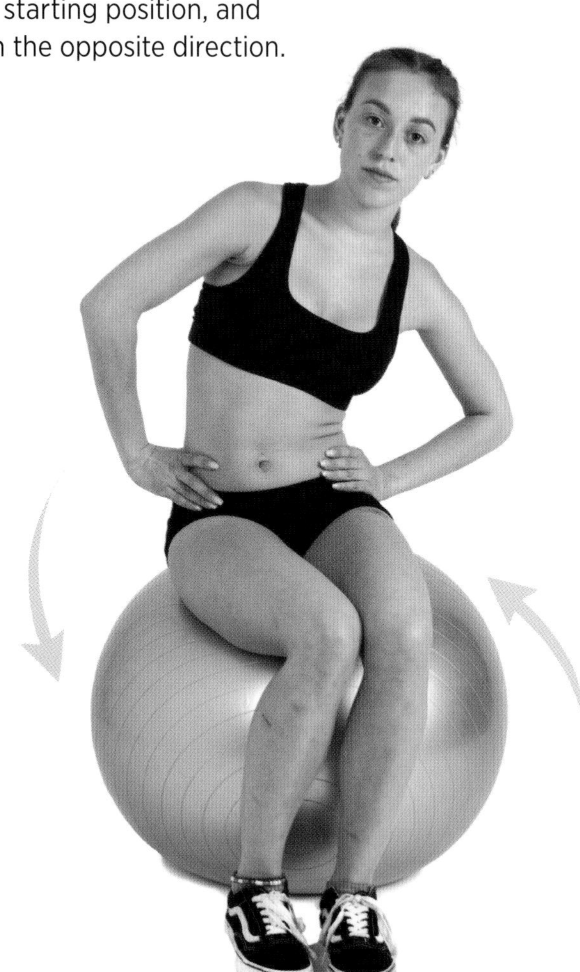

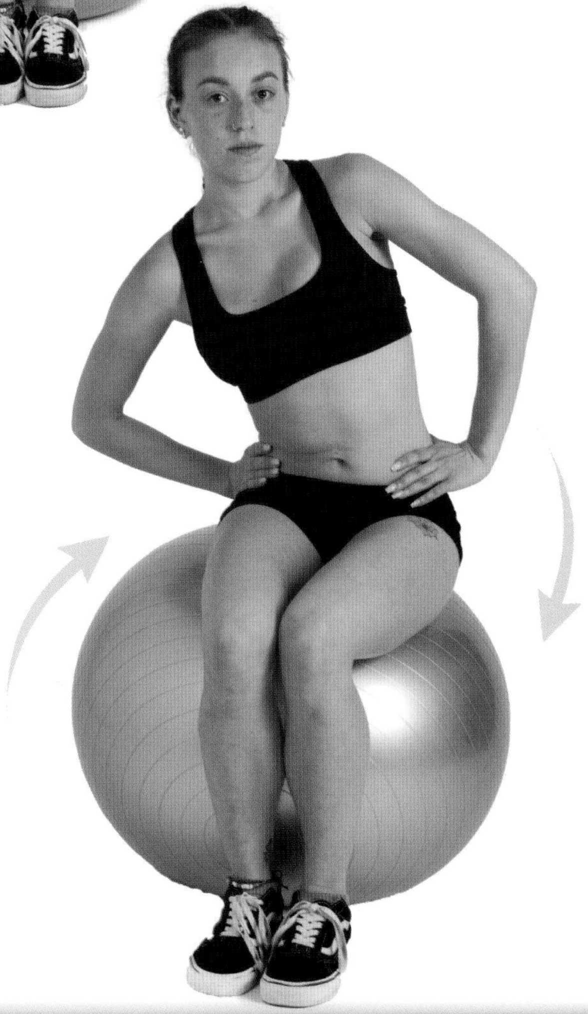

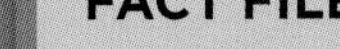

FACT FILE

TARGETS
- Lower-back
- Hips
- Abdominals

TYPE
- Static

BENEFITS
- Stabilizes core
- Stretches lower-back
- Strengthens abdominals

CAUTIONS
- Severe lower-back pain
- Hip problems

EQUIPMENT
- Swiss ball

Annotation Key

Bold text indicates target muscles
Light text indicates other working muscles
* indicates deep muscles

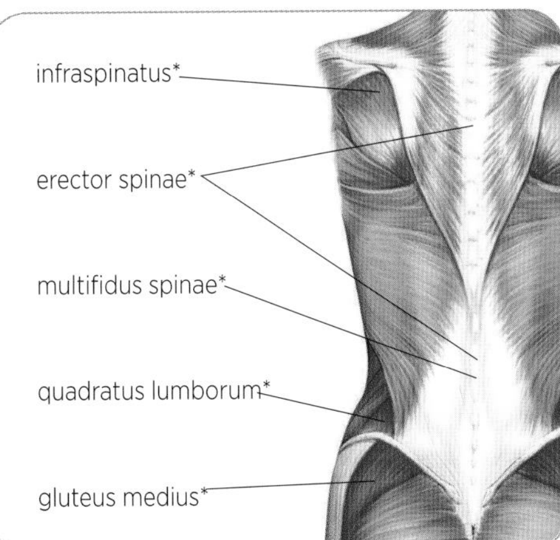

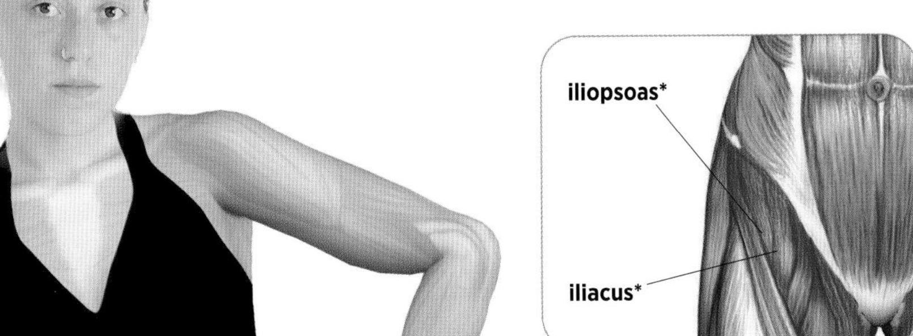

rectus abdominis

obliquus externus

transversus abdominis*

vastus intermedius*

DO IT RIGHT
- Keep your circles small.
- If you feel a crunching in your neck, you are moving too widely.
- Avoid using your legs to initiate the movement.

Swiss Ball Rollout

The Swiss Ball Rollout stabilizes your cores muscles, which prepares them for many everyday movements. When performing this exercise, you more effectively activate the rectus abdominis and obliques than when performing sit-ups and crunches.

HOW TO DO IT

- Kneel in front of a Swiss ball, and place your hands on it at about hip height.
- Slowly roll the ball forward, extending your body as you go.
- While keeping a flat back and remaining anchored on your knees, continue to roll forward until you are completely stretched out.
- To return to the starting position, engage your abdominal and lower-back muscles and roll back to the starting position. Repeat for the recommended repetitions.

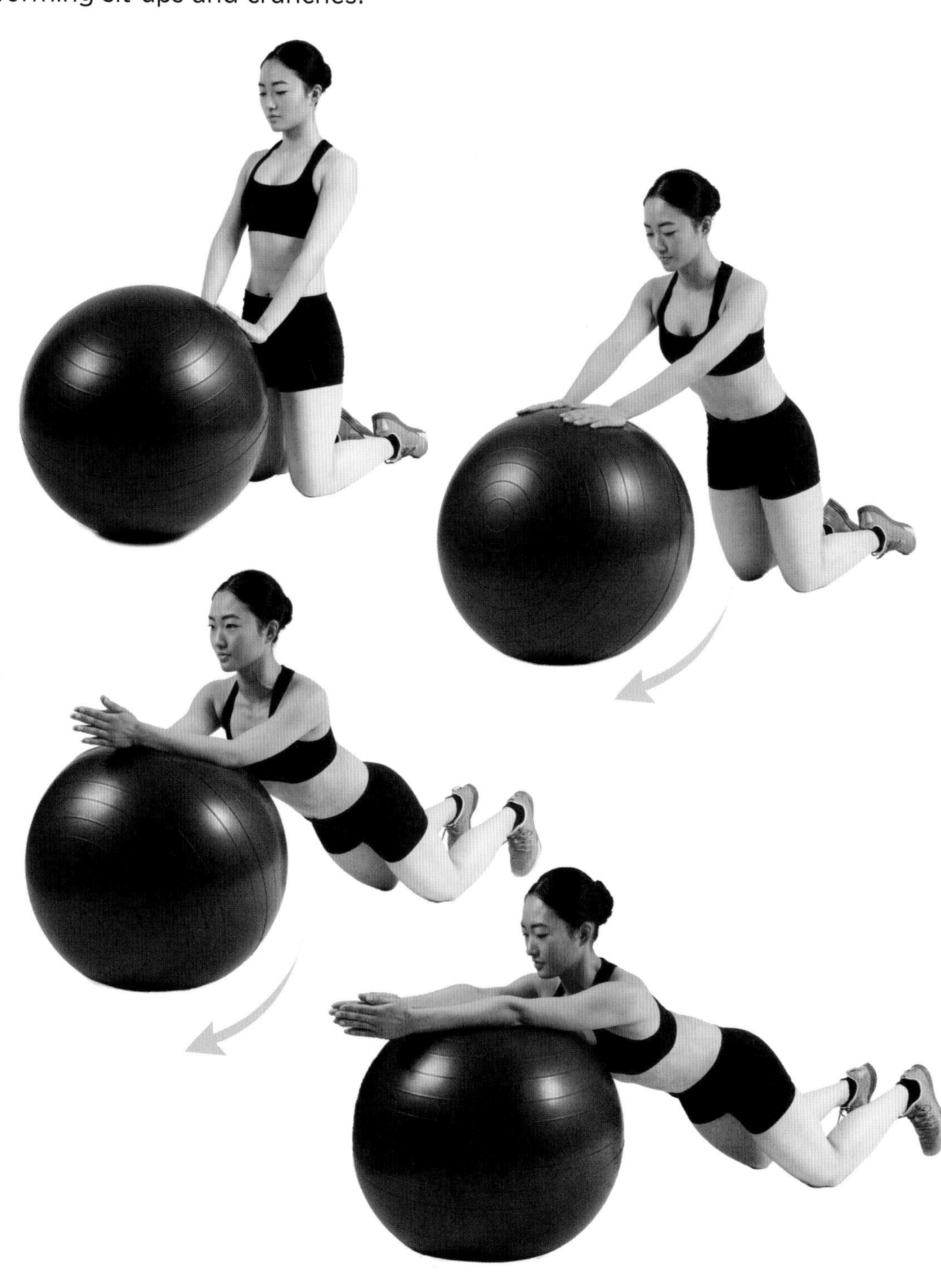

DO IT RIGHT

- Keep your abdominals contracted and tight.
- Keep your body elongated throughout the movement.
- Avoid bridging your back.
- Avoid allowing your hips or lower back to sag.

serratus anterior
iliopsoas*
pectineus*

teres major
multifidus spinae*
quadratus lumborum*

FACT FILE

TARGETS
- Abdominals
- Obliques
- Lower back

TYPE
- Static

BENEFITS
- Stabilizes core
- Strengthens abdominals, obliques, and back

CAUTIONS
- Shoulder issues
- Knee issues

EQUIPMENT
- Swiss ball

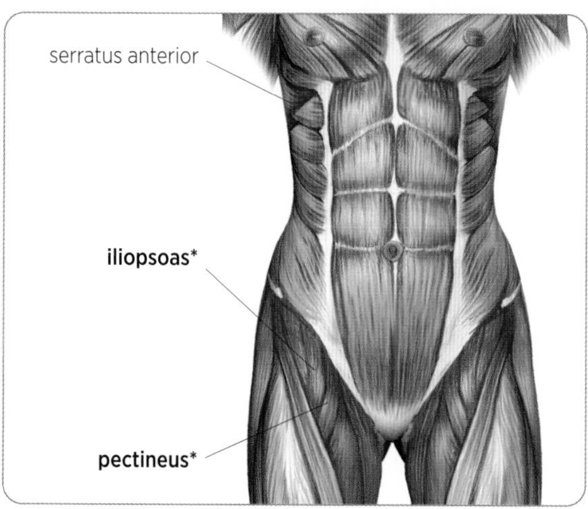

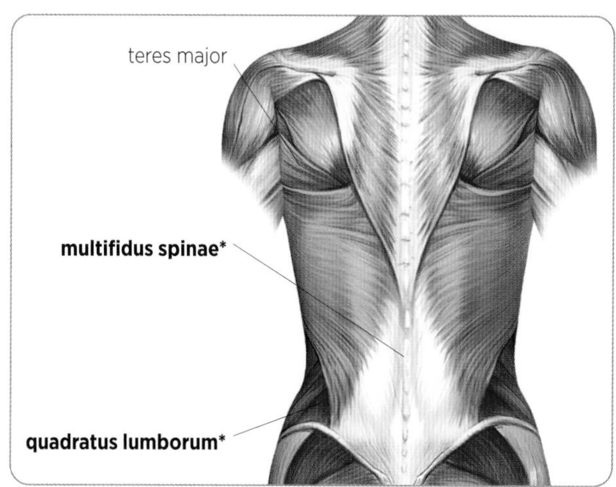

Annotation Key

Bold text indicates target muscles
Light text indicates other working muscles
* indicates deep muscles

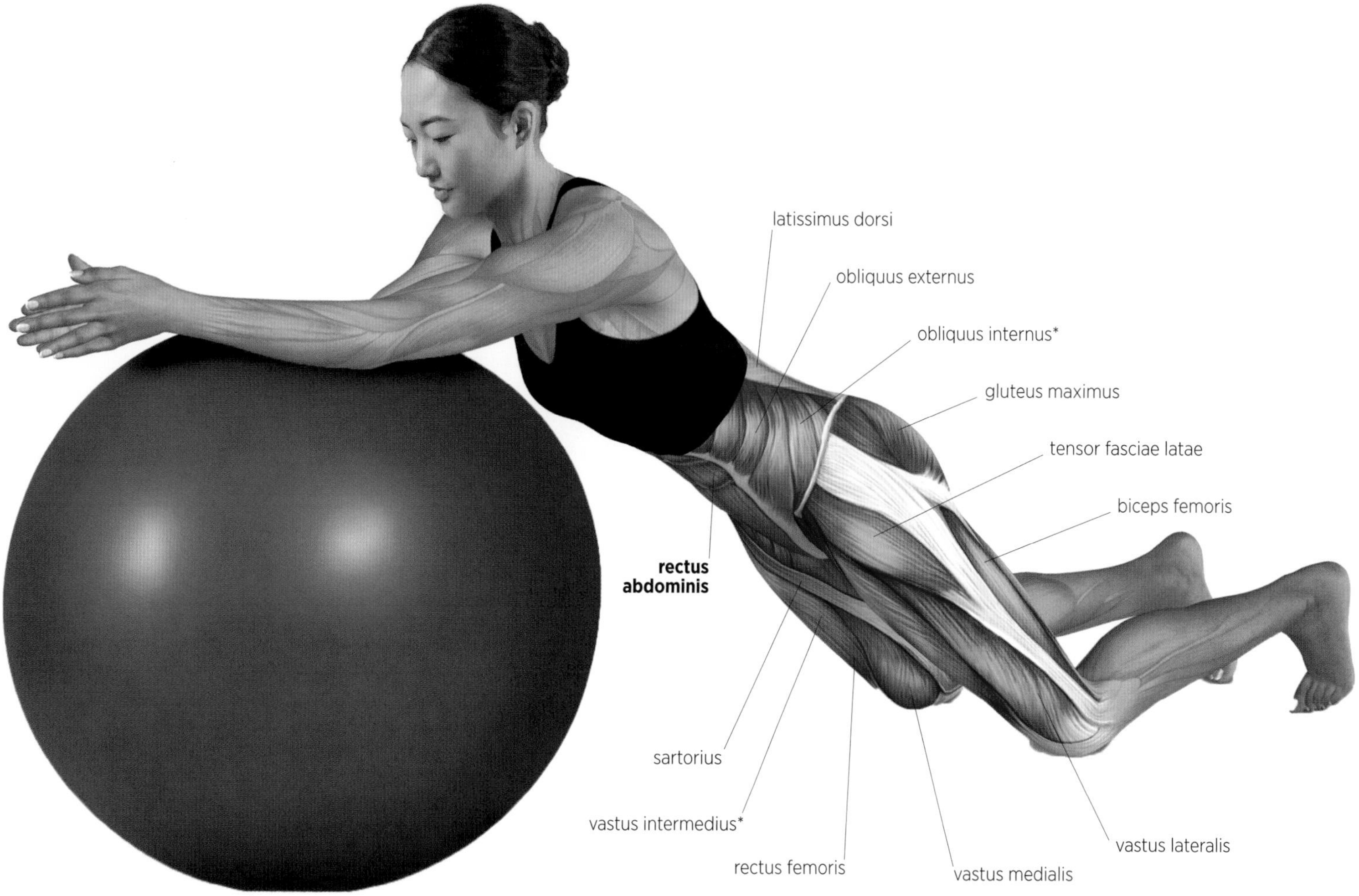

latissimus dorsi
obliquus externus
obliquus internus*
gluteus maximus
tensor fasciae latae
biceps femoris
rectus abdominis
sartorius
vastus intermedius*
rectus femoris
vastus medialis
vastus lateralis

CHAPTER EIGHT

LEG EXERCISES

Leg workouts can improve both cardiovascular health and strength, as stronger legs translate into improved endurance and core strength. Leg workouts can also help with weight loss—aerobic workouts such as running and cycling both improve general health and strengthen your legs, and the resulting muscle growth impacts your metabolism, as muscle has higher energy needs than fat. Weight loss, in turn, results in reduced stress on the leg bones and joints. Leg workouts also help to increase and maintain bone density, decreasing the risk of developing osteoporosis.

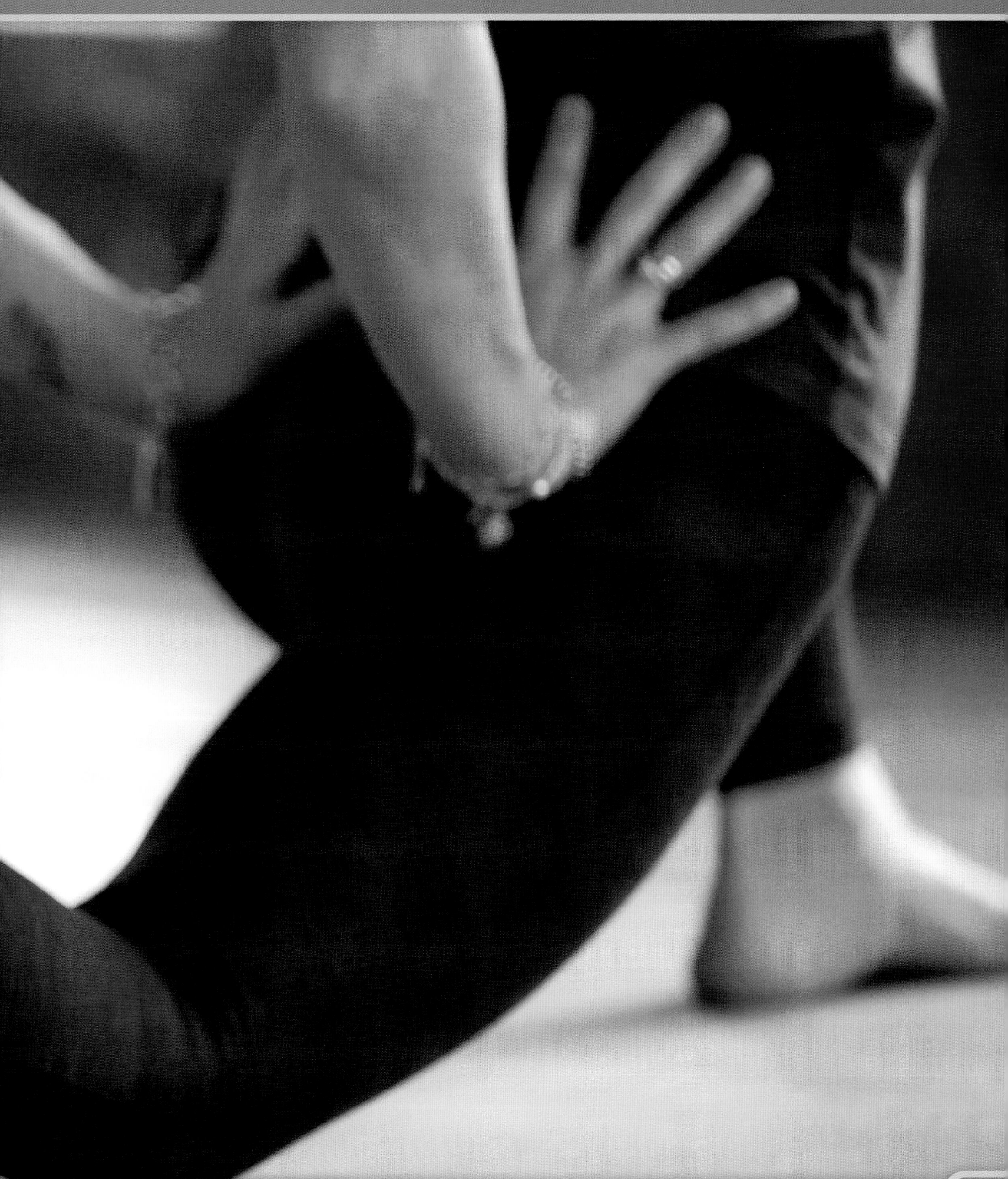

Bridge

Bridge pose is a favorite of all kinds of exercise programs because it opens up and strengthens so effectively. This is a great exercise for the upper body, while also putting your legs through their paces.

HOW TO DO IT

- Lie on your back, with your pelvis and spine aligned but feeling natural and not pressed flat to the floor. Your legs should be bent with feet on the floor, and your knees aligned with your hips and feet. Your feet shouldn't be too far away from your buttocks, and firmly planted on the floor. Extend your arms along your sides, palms downward, and press your shoulders down your back to stabilize your shoulder blades.

- Curl your hips upward from the floor, creating a stable bridge position from your shoulders to your parallel knees. Hold this position for the recommended time.

- Curl your spine back toward the floor, starting with your cervical vertebrae and rolling down your thoracic vertebrae and farther down to your lumbar vertebrae.

- Repeat for the recommended repetitions.

DO IT RIGHT

- Maintain strongly engaged lower abdominals.
- Keep your inner thighs active to maintain parallel legs.
- Keep your hips level.
- Avoid jamming your chin into your chest.
- Avoid letting your rib cage "pop" forward and upward.
- Avoid arching, and pushing into, your lower back while in the bridge.

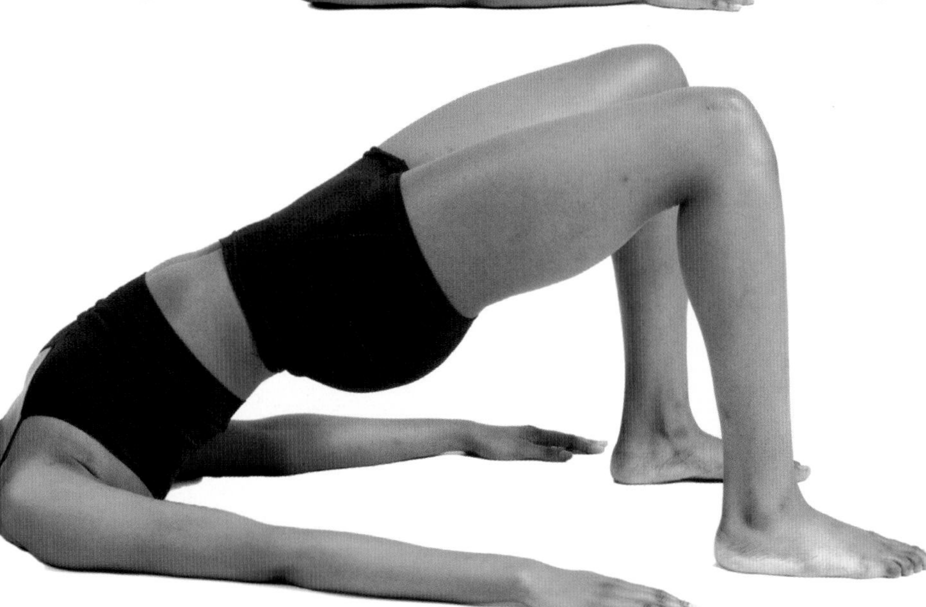

MODIFICATION

HARDER: Place a small medicine ball between your knees, squeezing it as you perform the Bridge. This increases lower-body resistance and enhances your awareness of the physical interconnections involved in the movement.

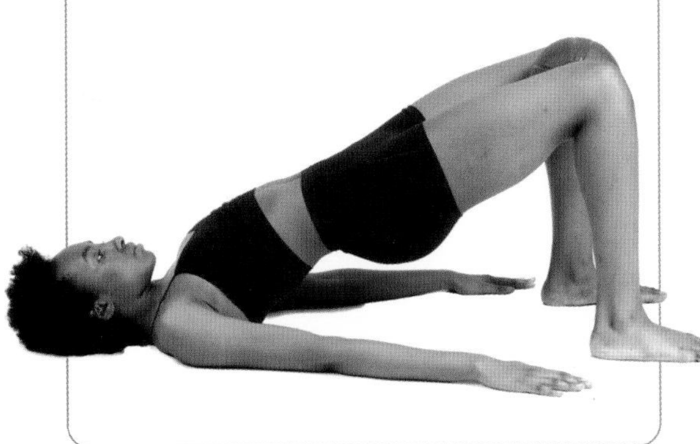

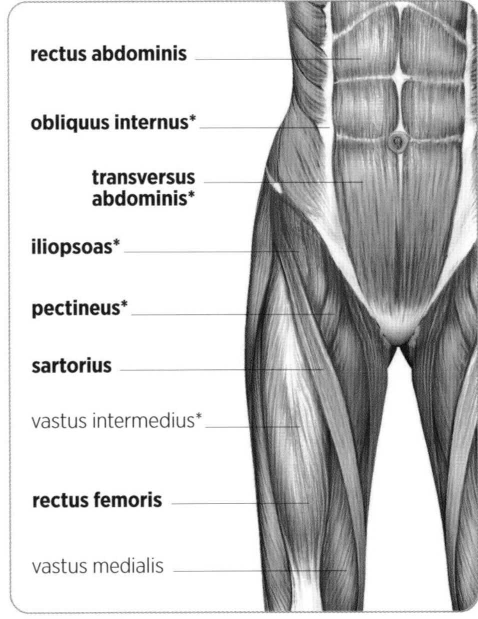

Annotation Key

Bold text indicates target muscles
Light text indicates other working muscles
* indicates deep muscles

FACT FILE

TARGETS
- Abdominals
- Hip flexors
- Chest
- Thighs
- Glutes
- Back
- Neck

TYPE
- Static

BENEFITS
- Increases shoulder stability
- Strengthens powerhouse muscles
- Opens chest and pelvic area
- Works legs

CAUTIONS
- Back injury
- Neck issues
- Shoulder issues

EQUIPMENT
- Optional: Small medicine ball for modification

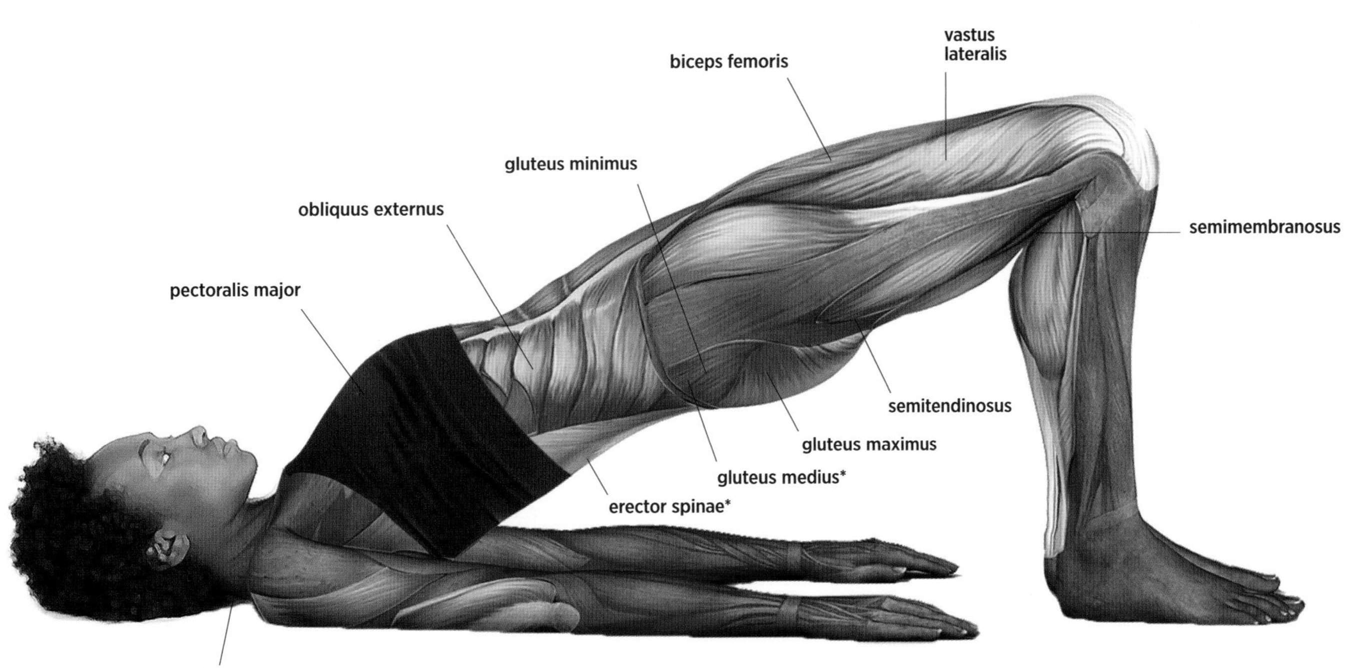

Extension Heel Beats

This exercise is especially effective for your glutes and inner-thigh adductors, but it also works much of your core and upper legs. As with all exercises performed in a prone position, keep your abdominals fully engaged.

HOW TO DO IT

- Lie on your stomach, resting your forehead on the back of your stacked hands. Slightly rotate your legs from the hip joints outward and press the inner sides of your legs and your heels together.
- Fully engage your glutes. Slightly lift your extended legs up from the floor.

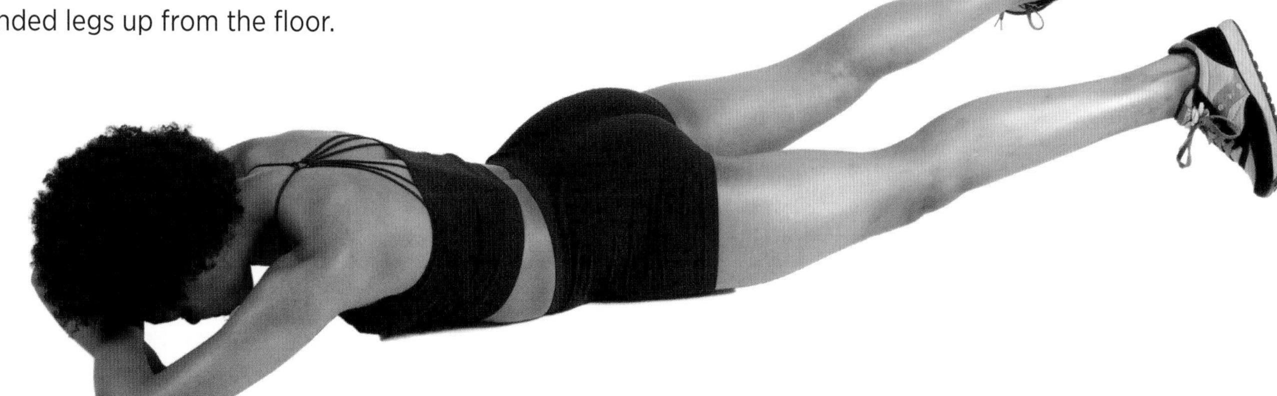

- With your feet fairly pointed, lightly beat your heels together for the recommended number of times.
- Flex your feet (that is, not pointed), and move your legs to hip-distance apart. Hold for the recommended time.
- Now stretch out your feet again and press your legs and heels together to begin another set of heel beats. Repeat for the recommended repetitions.

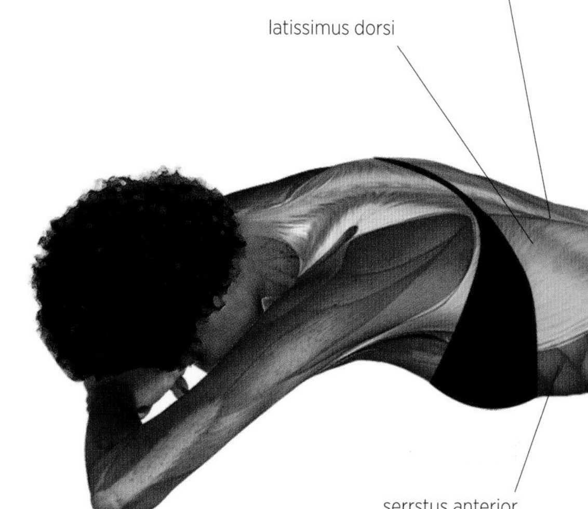

FACT FILE

TARGETS
- Adductors
- Glutes

TYPE
- Static

BENEFITS
- Strengthens and stretches leg muscles
- Increases hip-joint mobility
- Facilitates proper alignment

CAUTIONS
- Lower-back issues

DO IT RIGHT
- Stabilize your shoulder girdle.
- Keep your neck extended.
- Keep your hips firmly pressed into the floor as you press your navel toward your spine.
- Stretch your legs fully without locking your knees.
- Avoid lifting your legs so high that you feel tension in your lower back.
- Avoid altering the slightly turned-out position of your legs.

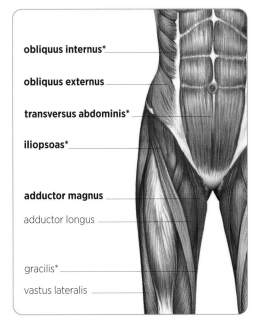

obliquus internus*
obliquus externus
transversus abdominis*
iliopsoas*
adductor magnus
adductor longus
gracilis*
vastus lateralis

Annotation Key
Bold text indicates target muscles
Light text indicates other working muscles
* indicates deep muscles

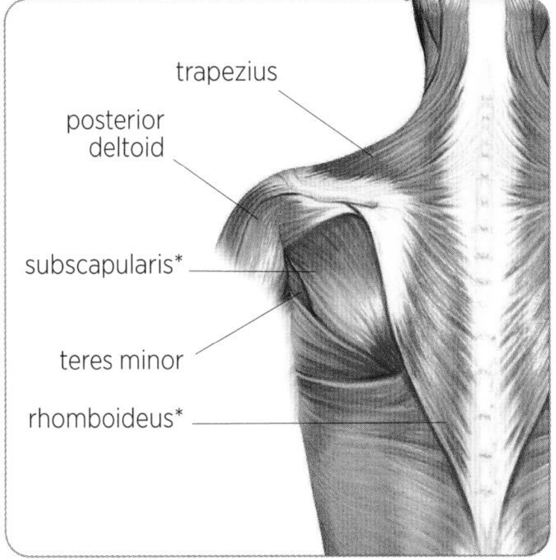

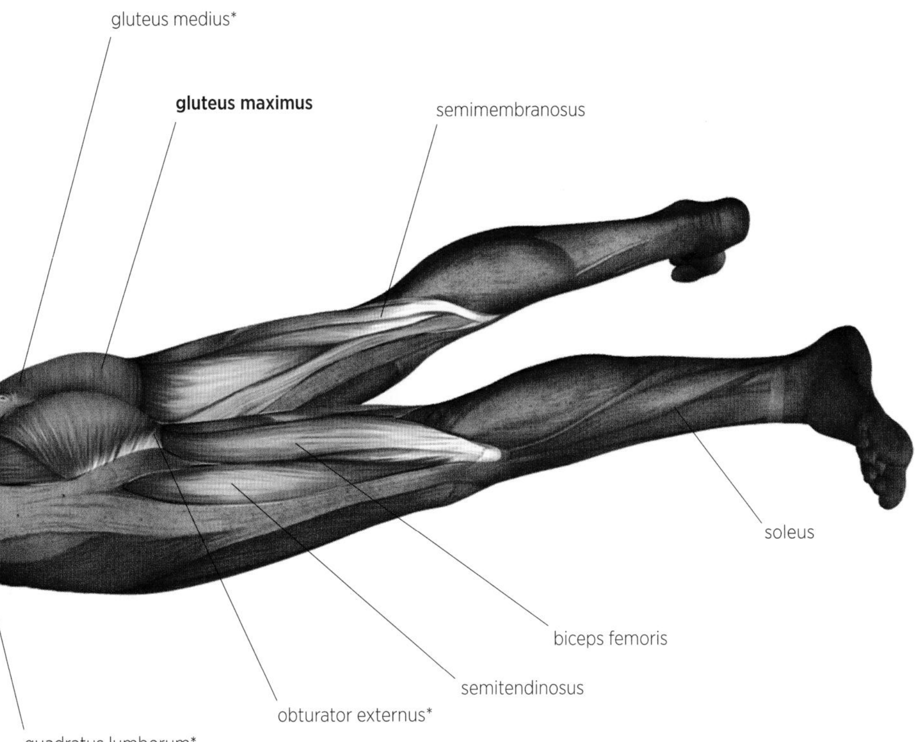

Squat

Another very simple exercise that really delivers for your buttocks and legs. The Squat works your abdominals, too, which means that it helps to stabilize your core. Plus the pose promotes better balance.

HOW TO DO IT

- Stand with your feet shoulder-width apart, your toes pointed slightly outwards and your arms extended in front of you.
- Bend your knees, while keeping your back flat. Lower yourself toward the floor until your thighs are parallel to it.
- Push through your heels to stand erect. Repeat for the recommended repetitions.

DO IT RIGHT

- Squat deep, and be sure to keep your thighs parallel to the floor.
- Avoid hyperextending your knees past your toes while squatting.

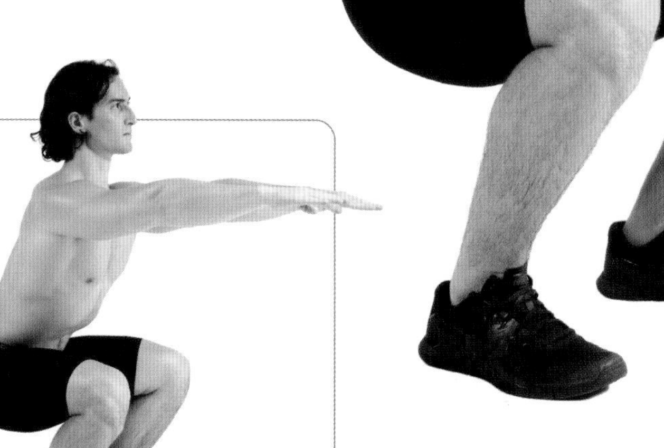

MODIFICATION

HARDER: Bringing your feet closer together increases the effort required.

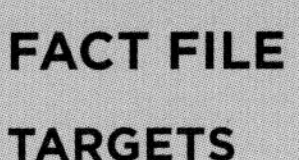

FACT FILE

TARGETS
- Quads
- Hamstrings
- Glutes

TYPE
- Static

BENEFITS
- Increases power and mass in the thighs

CAUTIONS
- Knee issues
- Lower-back pain

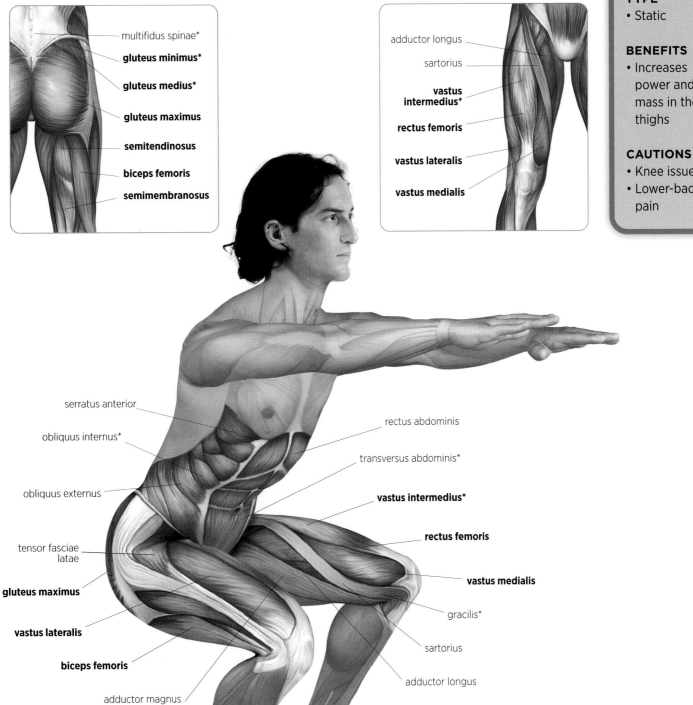

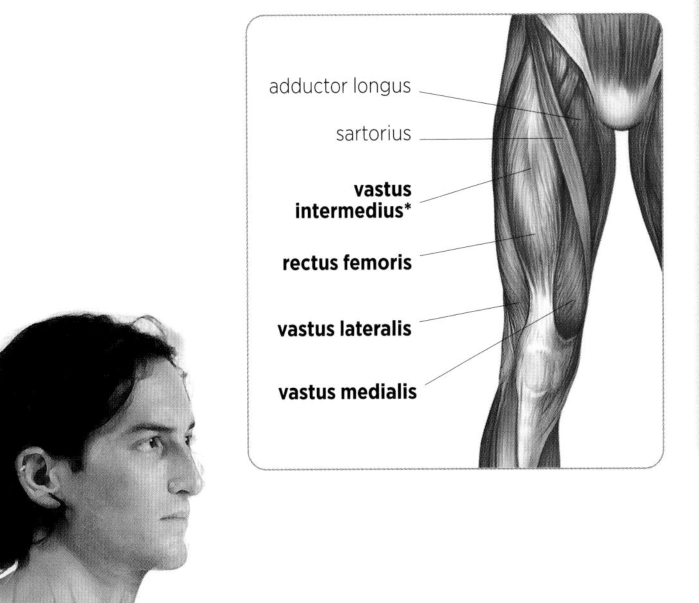

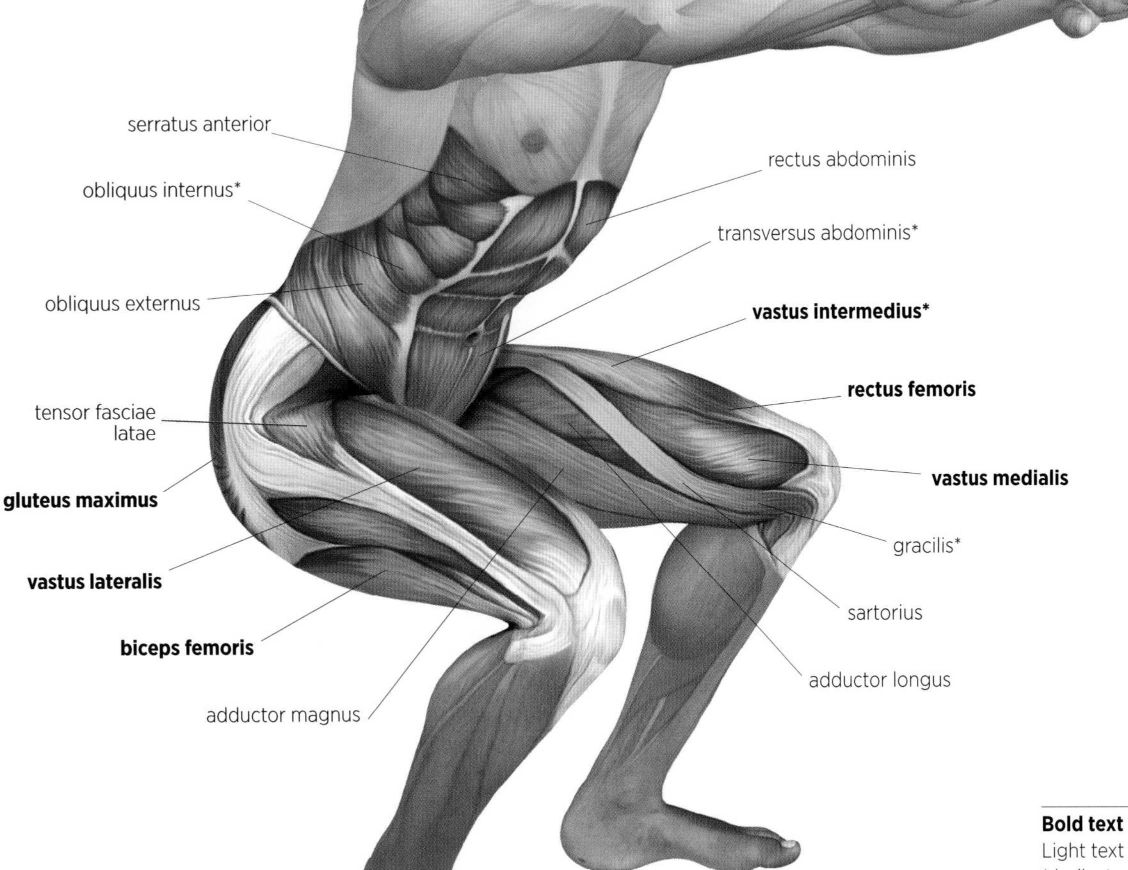

Annotation Key

Bold text indicates target muscles

Light text indicates other working muscles

* indicates deep muscles

Single-Leg Gluteal Lift

The Single-Leg Gluteal Lift develops tight, strong glutes while working many other major muscles. A key to safe success here is to use your abdominals to lift your body.

HOW TO DO IT

- Lie on your back with your arms along your sides and legs bent with your feet directly under your knees. Extend your left leg upward, pointing through your foot.
- Engage your abdominals to pop up to a one-legged, stable Bridge pose (pages 256–57). Raise your body only as high as you can go while maintaining correct alignment.
- Maintain this position, focusing on keeping your hips level, navel pressing to spine, and your raised leg extending from the hip joint.
- Lower your body back down to the floor, keeping your left leg extended.
- Repeat the bridge, with the same leg raised, for the recommended repetitions. Switch legs and repeat on the opposite side for the recommended repetitions.

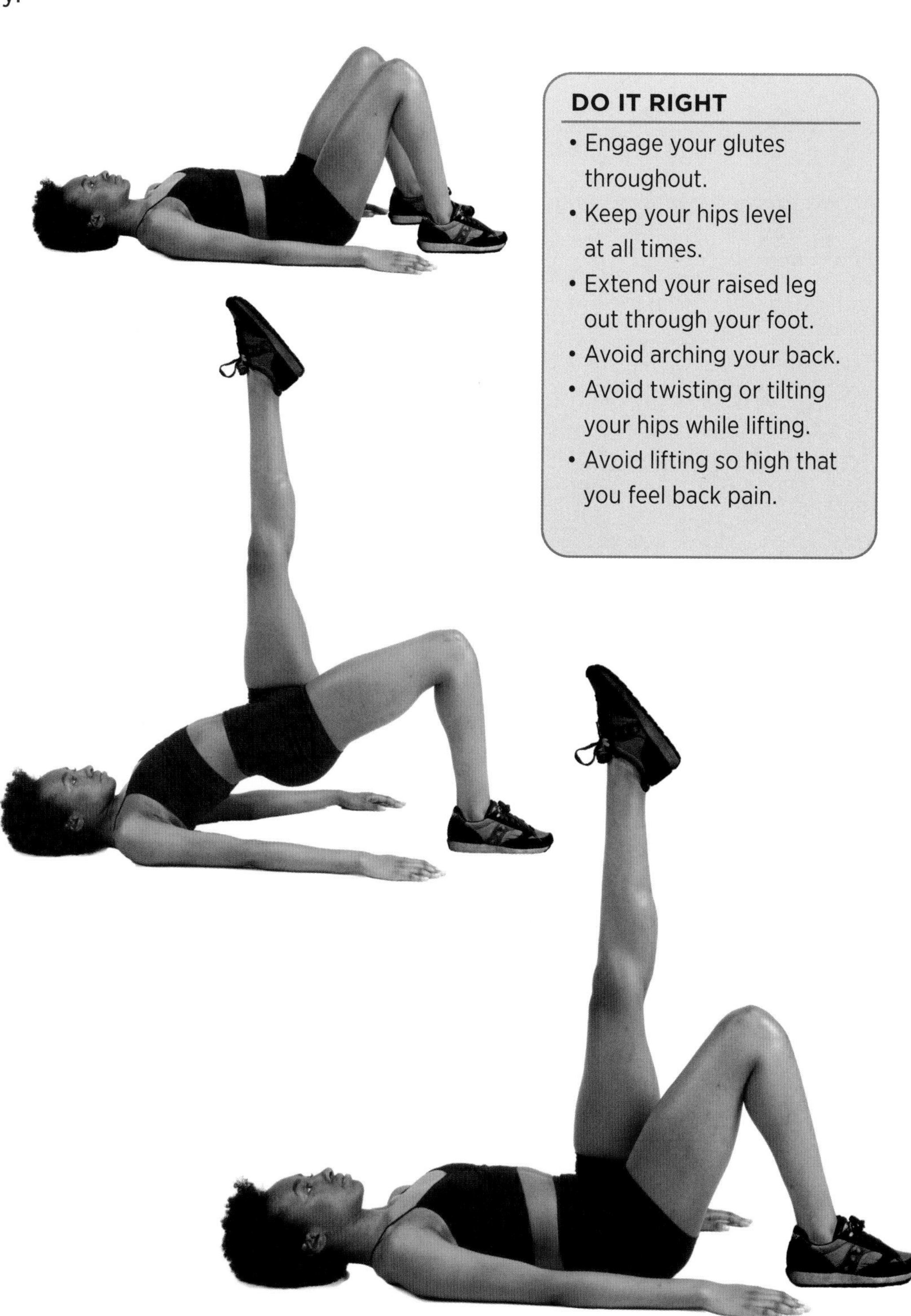

DO IT RIGHT

- Engage your glutes throughout.
- Keep your hips level at all times.
- Extend your raised leg out through your foot.
- Avoid arching your back.
- Avoid twisting or tilting your hips while lifting.
- Avoid lifting so high that you feel back pain.

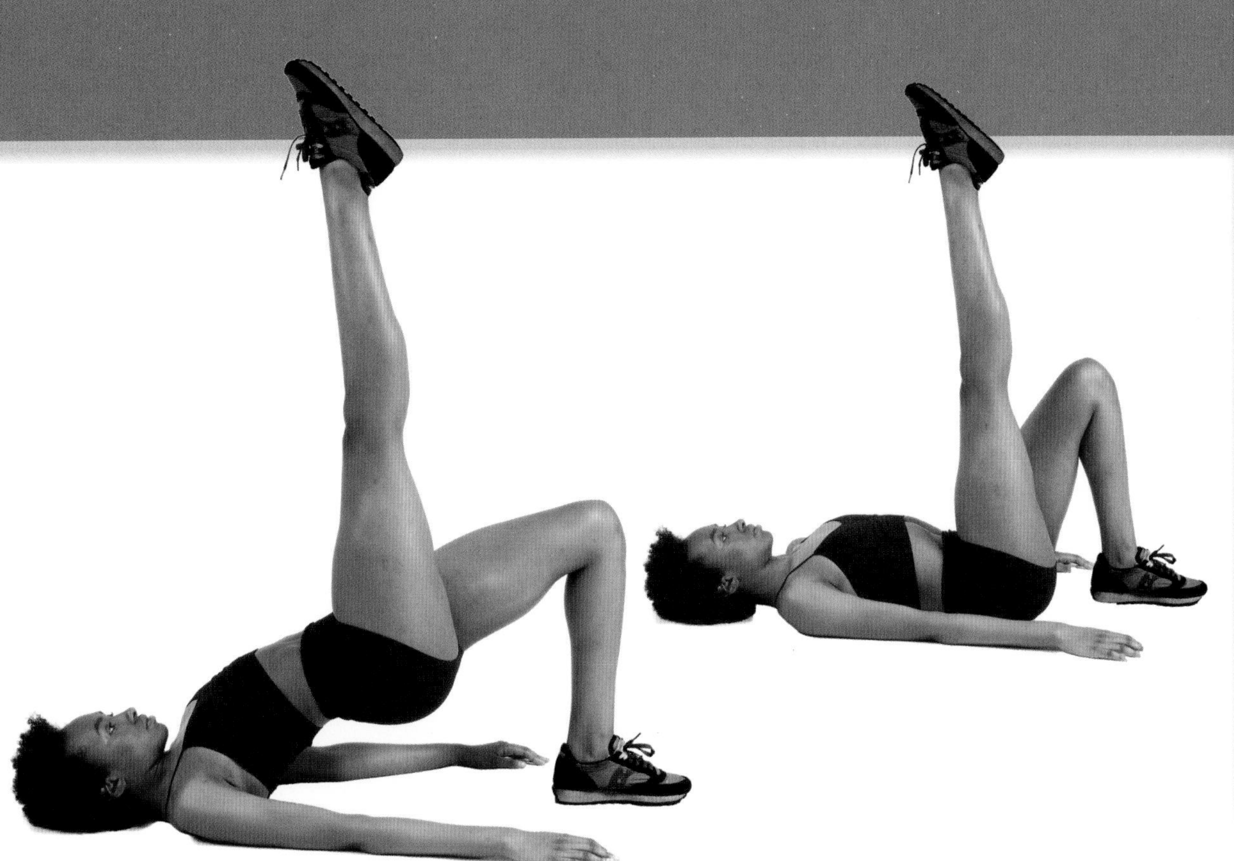

FACT FILE

TARGETS
- Glutes
- Hip flexors
- Legs
- Abdominals
- Neck, shoulders, and back

TYPE
- Static

BENEFITS
- Strengthens and tones glutes and abdominals

CAUTIONS
- Back pain/issues

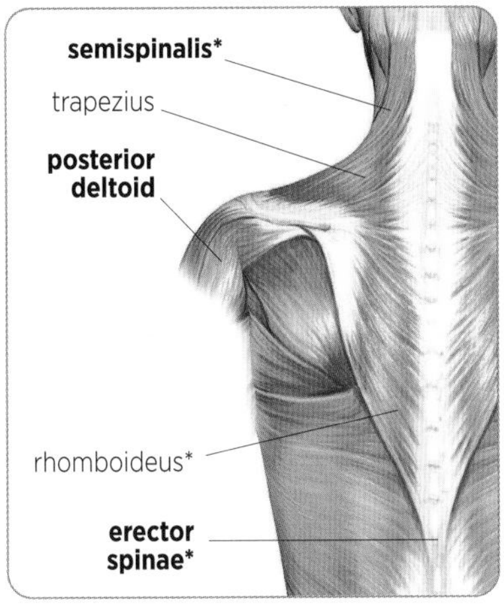

semispinalis*
trapezius
posterior deltoid
rhomboideus*
erector spinae*

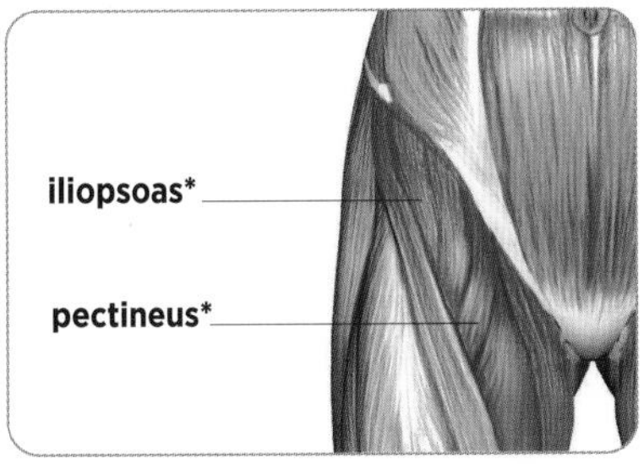

iliopsoas*
pectineus*

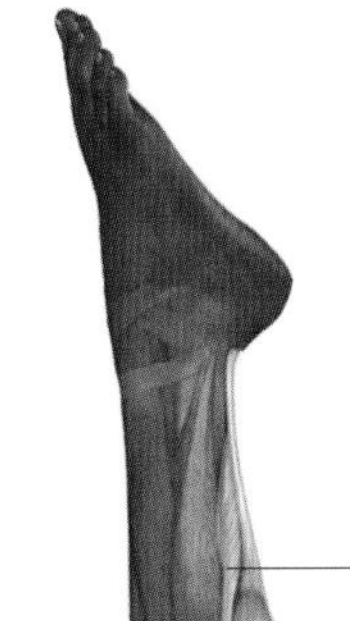

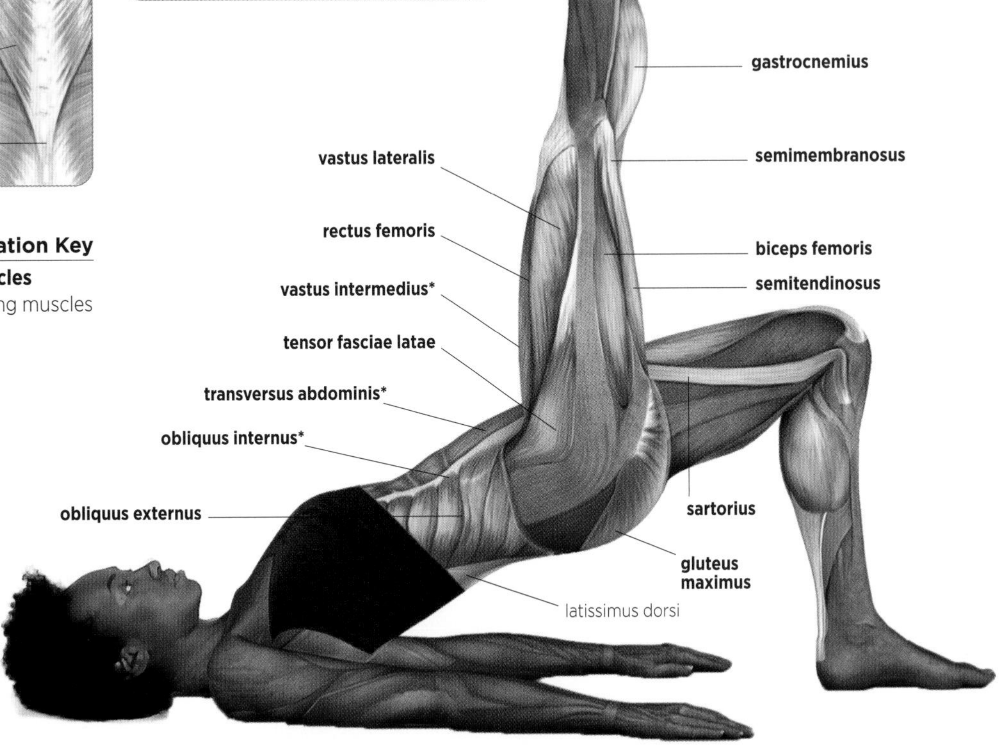

soleus
gastrocnemius
semimembranosus
vastus lateralis
rectus femoris
biceps femoris
semitendinosus
vastus intermedius*
tensor fasciae latae
transversus abdominis*
obliquus internus*
obliquus externus
sartorius
gluteus maximus
latissimus dorsi

Annotation Key

Bold text indicates target muscles
Light text indicates other working muscles
* indicates deep muscles

Lunge

The Lunge strengthens your hamstrings, thighs, and glutes, but also does so much more. This exercise is a dynamic stretch for your hip flexors and also stabilizes your hips, knees, and ankles.

HOW TO DO IT

- Stand with your feet a little way apart, up to hip-width, and your arms at the sides of your body or with your hands on your hips.
- Step your left leg forward. Keep a slight bend in your left knee.
- Bend both knees as you move into a lunge position. Lower your body, flexing your left knee and hip until your right leg is in light contact with the floor.
- Return to the starting position by straightening out your right leg and bringing your left leg back to meet your right.
- Switch legs and repeat on the opposite side. Alternate sides for the recommended repetitions.

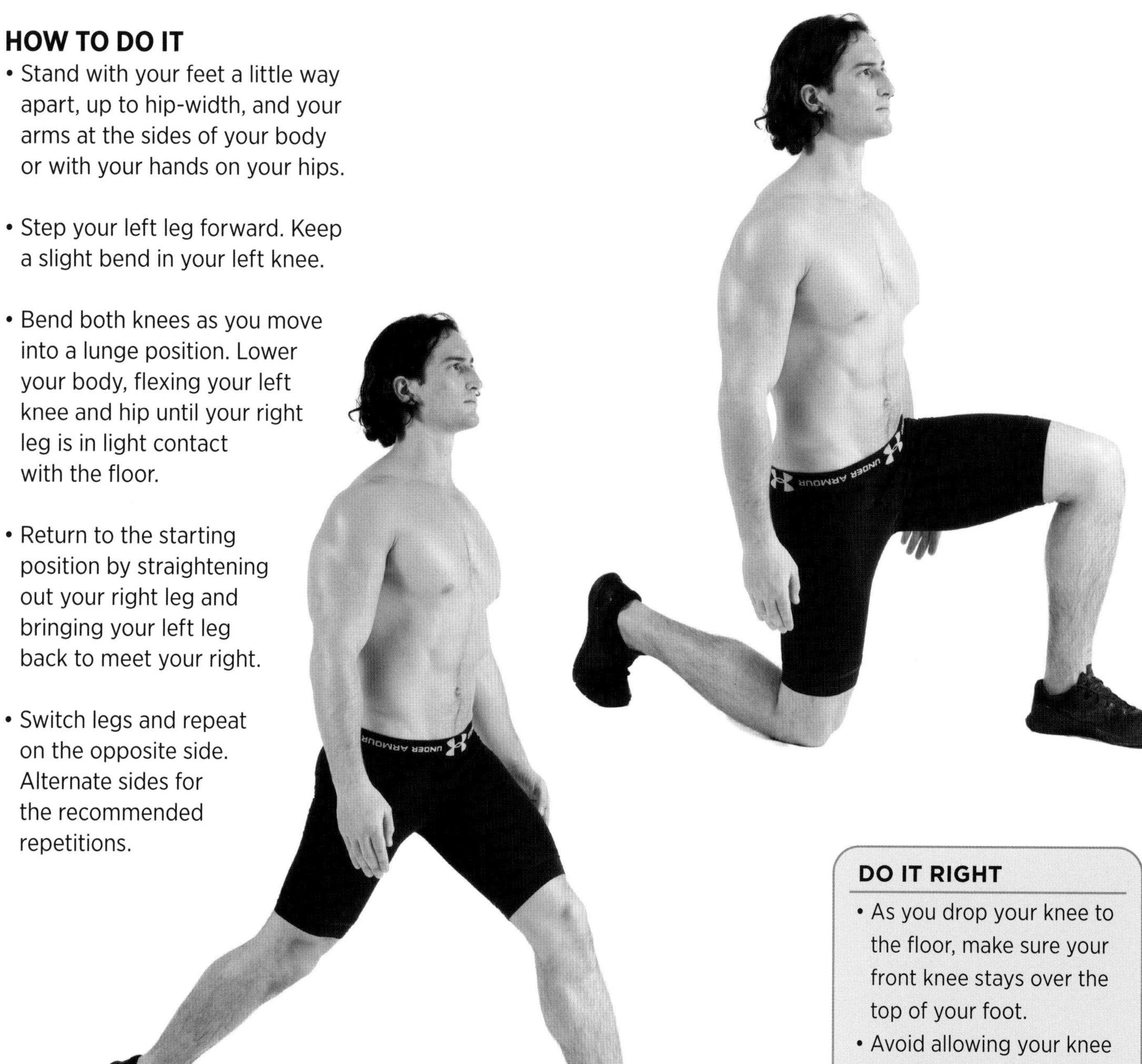

DO IT RIGHT

- As you drop your knee to the floor, make sure your front knee stays over the top of your foot.
- Avoid allowing your knee to bend forward beyond your toes; this will place stress on your knee.

FACT FILE

TARGETS
- Glutes
- Thighs and calves
- Hip flexors

TYPE
- Dynamic

BENEFITS
- Strengthens quads
- Stabilizes hip

CAUTIONS
- Knee issues

Annotation Key

Bold text indicates target muscles
Light text indicates other working muscles
* indicates deep muscles

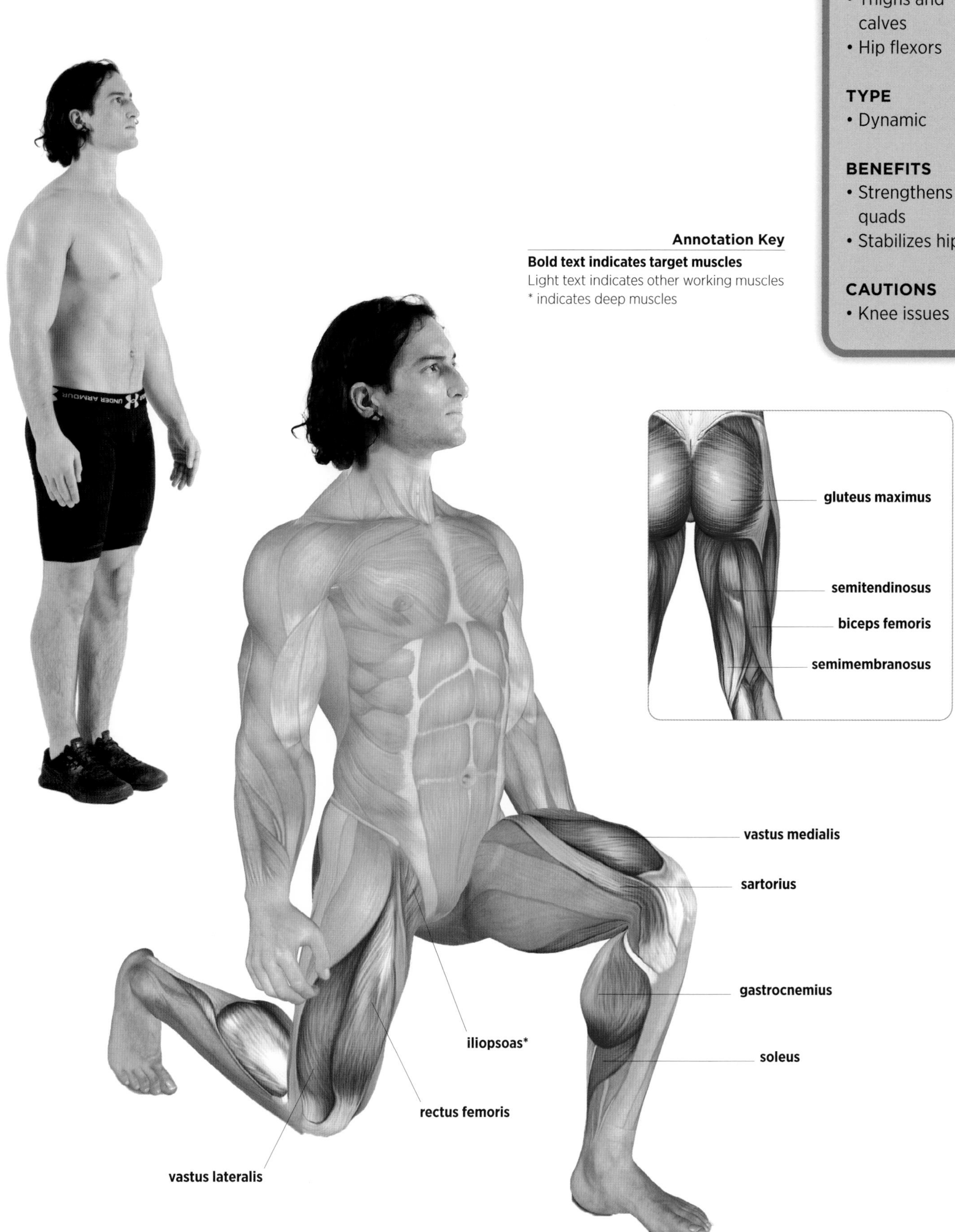

Lateral Lunge with Squat

The Lateral Lunge with Squat combines the benefits of two exercise mainstays: a sideways lunge and a squat. This isolation exercise targets the inner and outer thighs, which can help build strength and stability in the hip and lateral knee.

HOW TO DO IT

- Stand with your feet together and your hands on your hips.
- Contract your abdominals and glutes, and step out your right foot. Keeping your weight on your heels, bend your left knee and lower your hips as far as you can.
- Push off the ground with your right foot, and return to the starting position.
- Repeat on the opposite side, alternating sides for the recommended repetitions.

DO IT RIGHT

- Keep your spine in neutral position as you bend your hips.
- Relax your shoulders and neck.
- Align your knee with the toe of your bent leg.
- Lower as far as you are able, but not beyond your thighs parallel to the floor.
- Avoid lifting your heels—squat only as deeply as you can while keeping your feet flat on the floor.
- Avoid arching your back.

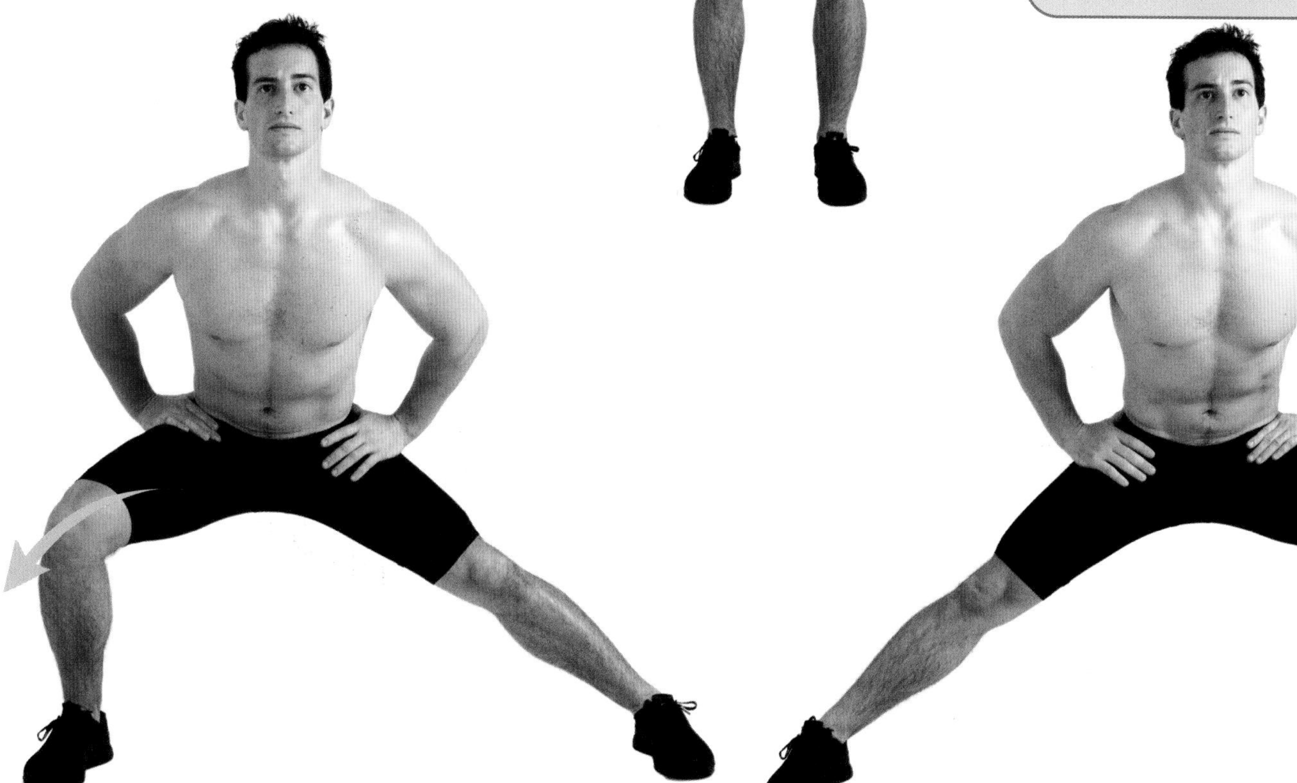

FACT FILE

TARGETS
- Thighs
- Hips
- Glutes
- Calves

TYPE
- Dynamic

BENEFITS
- Strengthens glutes, thighs, and calves
- Strengthens and stabilizes hip abductors and adductors
- Strengthens and stabilizes lateral knee muscles

CAUTIONS
- Knee pain
- Hip pain

Annotation Key
Bold text indicates target muscles
Light text indicates other working muscles
* indicates deep muscles

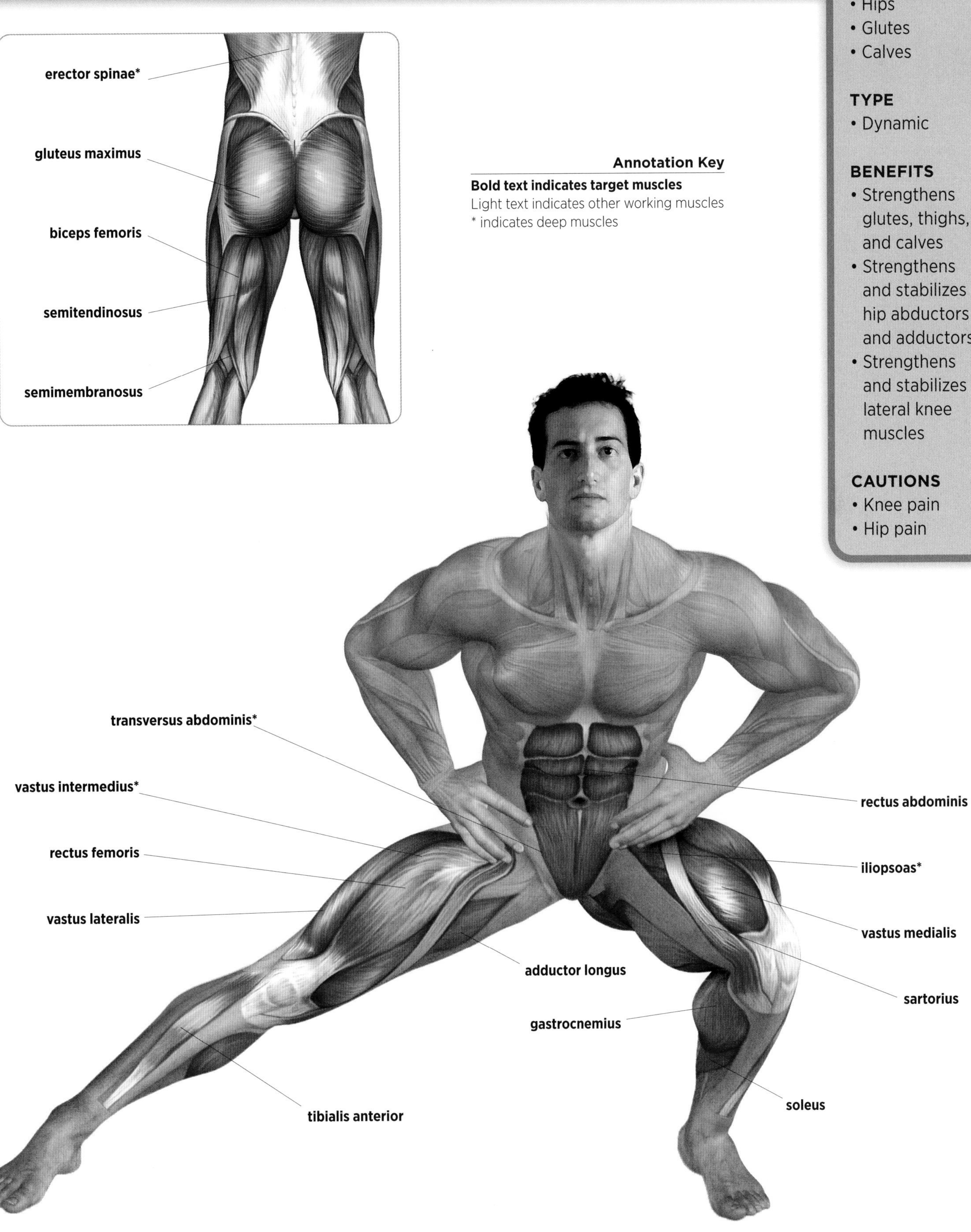

High Lunge with Twist

Like the basic High Lunge, this version is an effective strengthening exercise for your thighs, hips, and glutes. The added twist gives it a boost, stretching your obliques, chest, and shoulders.

HOW TO DO IT

- Begin in a High Lunge with your right leg forward.
- Balance your weight on your left hand, and carefully and slowly guide your right arm up toward the ceiling, twisting your torso to the right.
- Return to the center, and then repeat on the opposite side. Continue alternating sides for the recommended repetitions.

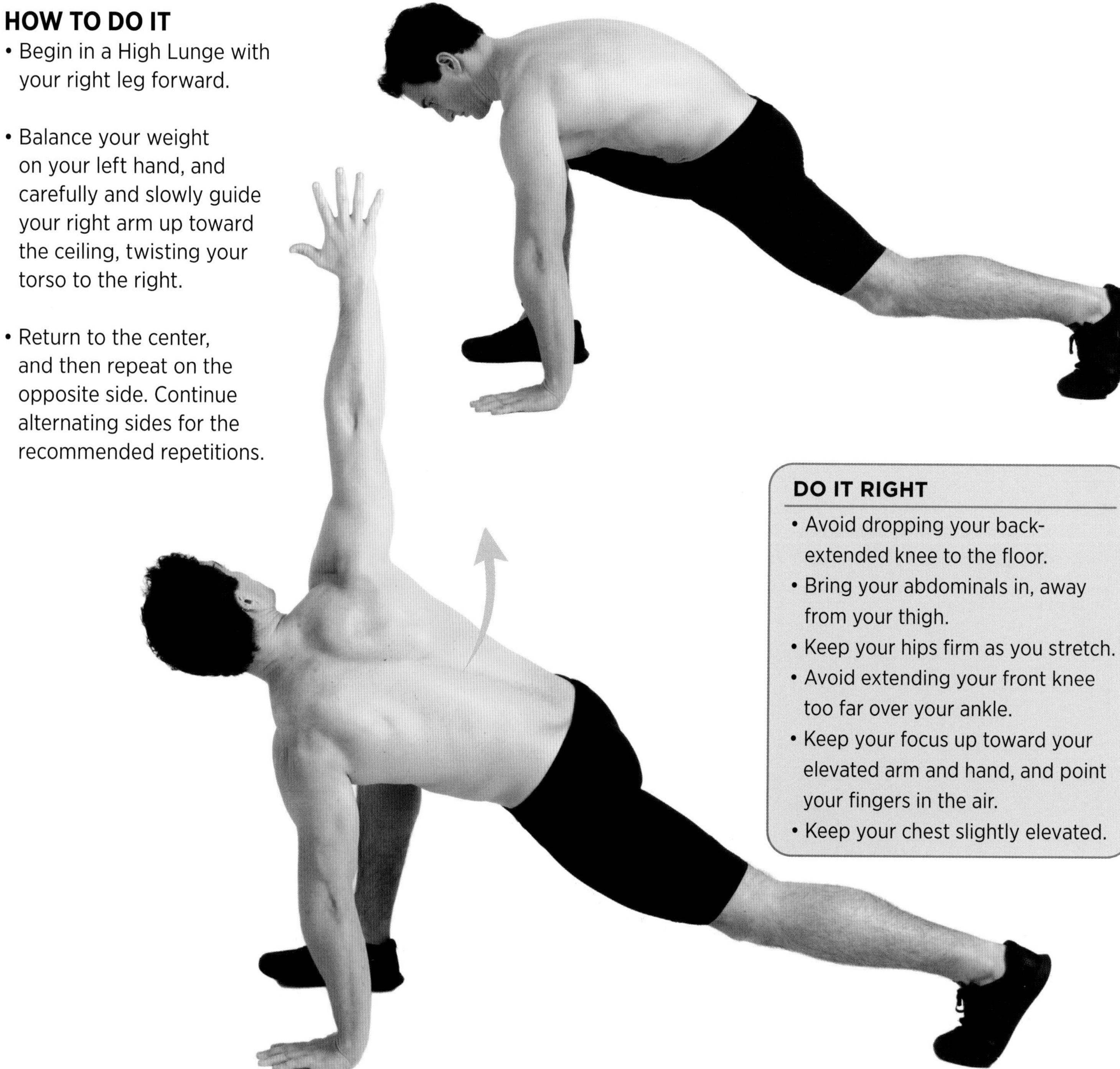

DO IT RIGHT

- Avoid dropping your back-extended knee to the floor.
- Bring your abdominals in, away from your thigh.
- Keep your hips firm as you stretch.
- Avoid extending your front knee too far over your ankle.
- Keep your focus up toward your elevated arm and hand, and point your fingers in the air.
- Keep your chest slightly elevated.

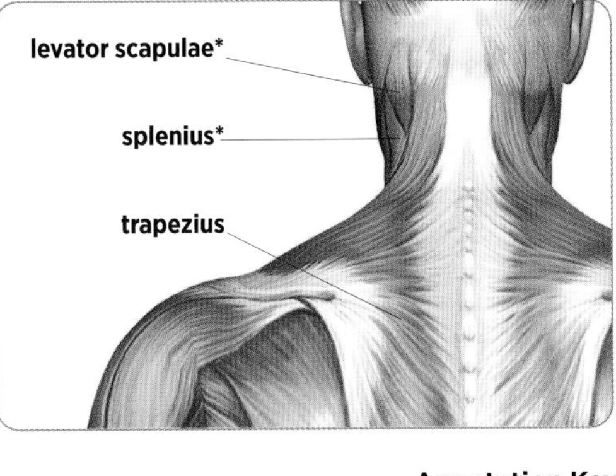

Annotation Key

Bold text indicates target muscles

Light text indicates other working muscles

* indicates deep muscles

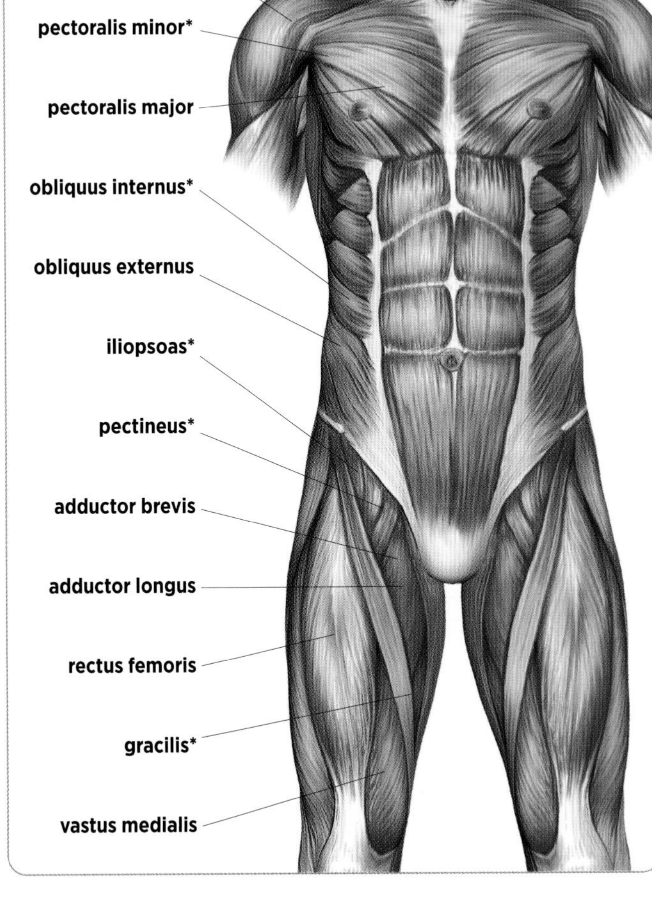

FACT FILE

TARGETS

- Quadriceps
- Gluteal area
- Hip flexors
- Hip adductors
- Hamstrings
- Obliques
- Rib cage
- Chest
- Shoulders

TYPE

- Dynamic

BENEFITS

- Stretches groins and obliques
- Strengthens abdominals, legs, and arms
- Stretches hip flexors, shoulders, and chest

CAUTIONS

- Hip issues
- Knee issues

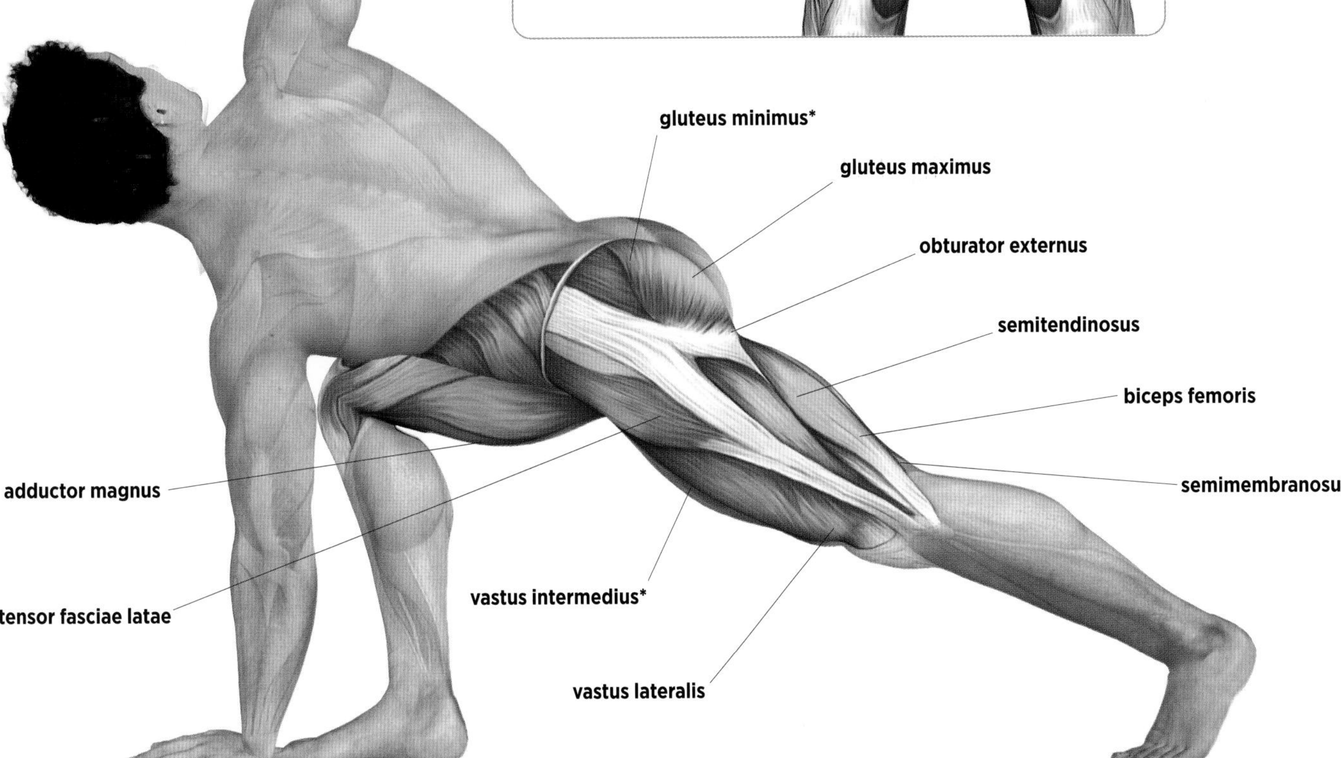

Box Jump

Jumping exercises have a lot to offer, providing strength and power benefits, as well as giving you a cardio boost. The Box Jump targets your lower body and promotes explosive power so that you can perform at top levels.

HOW TO DO IT

- Stand in front of a plyo box, aerobics step, or other low platform.
- Drop into a quarter-squat.
- Push through your heels, swing your arms, and spring up onto the box.
- Step back down, and then repeat for the recommended repetitions.

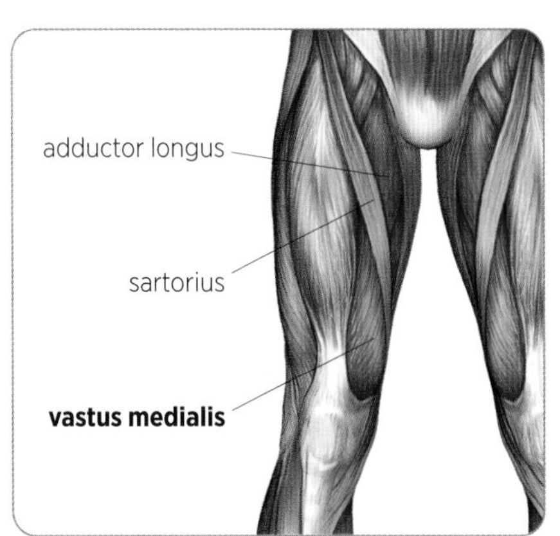

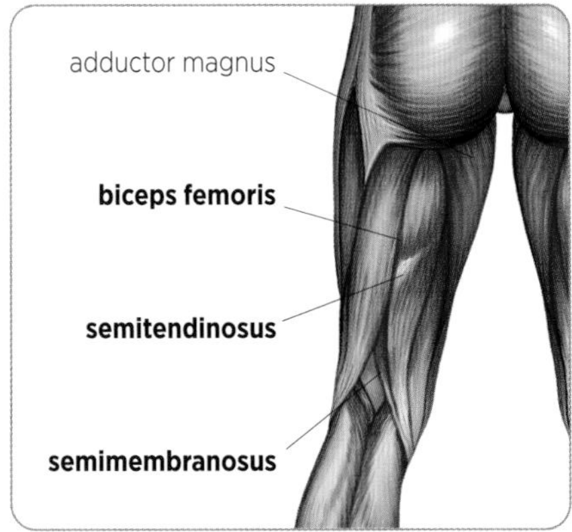

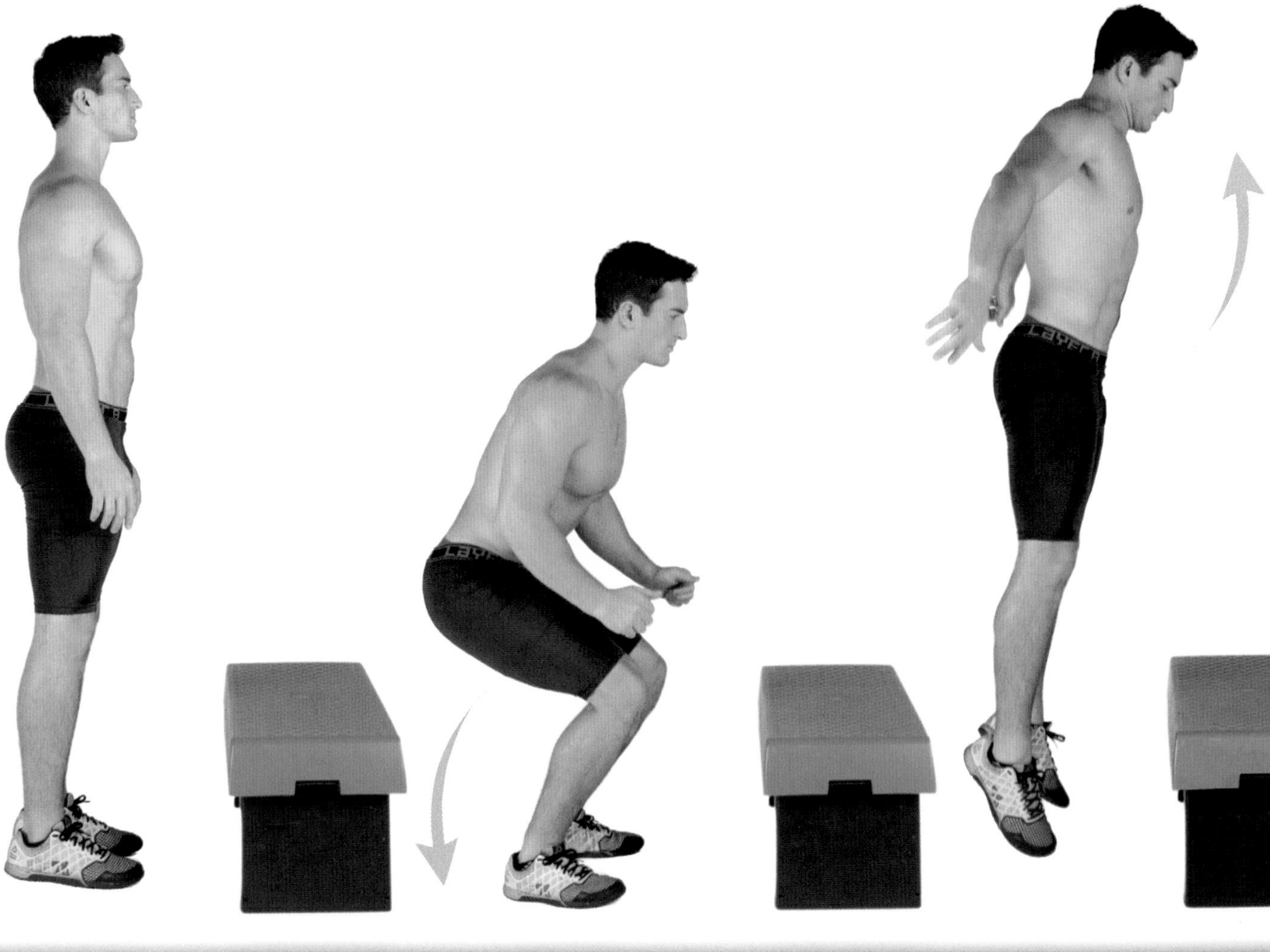

FACT FILE

TARGETS
- Quadriceps
- Hamstrings
- Glutes
- Calves

TYPE
- Dynamic

BENEFITS
- Strengthens thighs, glutes, and calves
- Produces explosive lower-body power

CAUTIONS
- Hip issues
- Knee issues
- Ankle issues

EQUIPMENT
- Plyo box, aerobics step, or other low platform

MODIFICATION

EASIER: Use a lower step.

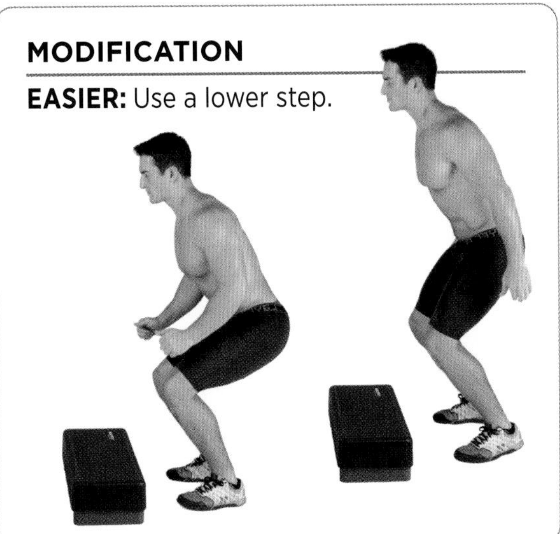

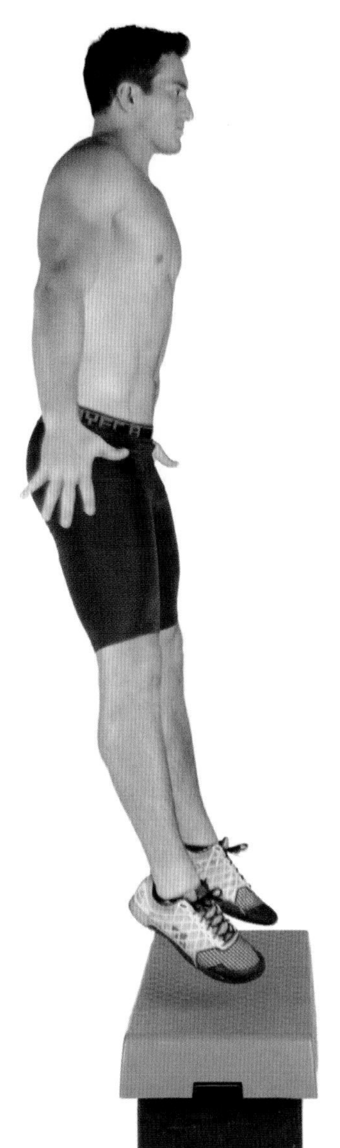

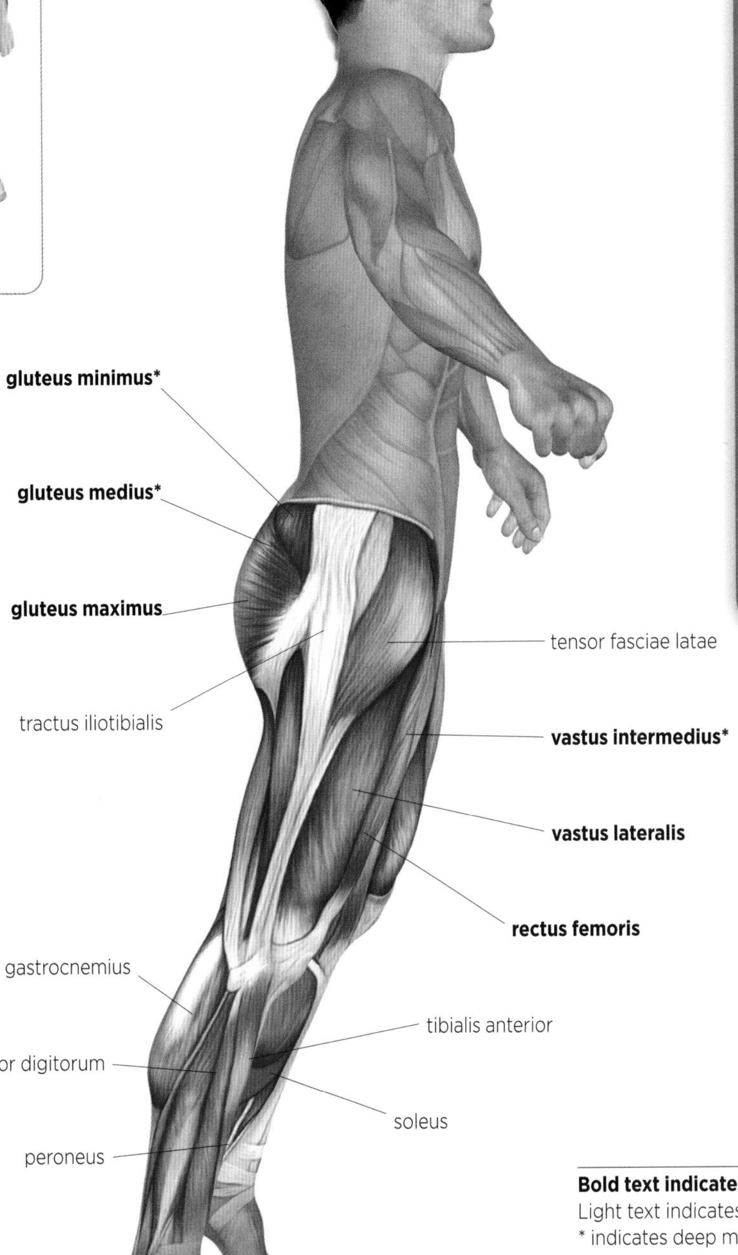

Annotation Key
Bold text indicates target muscles
Light text indicates other working muscles
* indicates deep muscles

DO IT RIGHT

- Keep a tight core throughout the movement.
- Avoid landing excessively hard.

Side Kick

Add a little cardio to your stretching routine with the Side Kick, which is also known as the Lateral Kick. It stretches your outer thigh muscles and your obliques, while also strengthening your lower body.

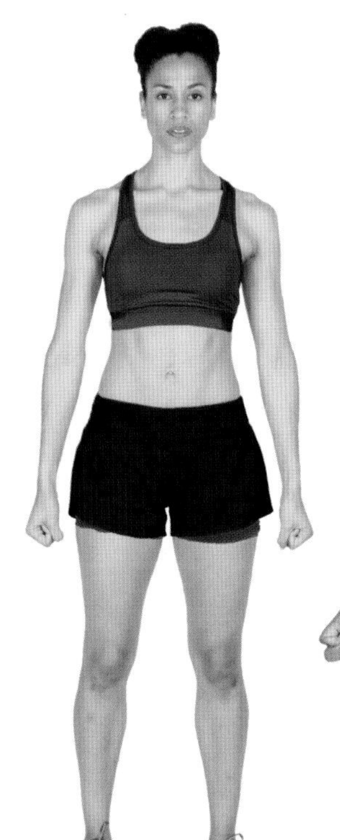

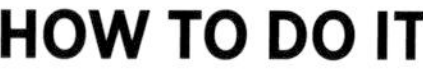

HOW TO DO IT

- Stand with feet hip-width apart and your arms at your sides.
- Kick your left leg out to the side, keeping it in line with your torso and shifting your weight to your right foot as your left foot leaves the floor. At the same time, extend both arms out to the side until they are at shoulder height, parallel to the floor.
- Return to the starting position, and then repeat on the opposite side. Alternate sides for the recommended repetitions.

DO IT RIGHT

- Kick straight out to the side, making sure your foot is in line with your shoulders.
- Avoid leaning forward or backward.
- Avoid kicking too fast; move only as quickly as you can while maintaining your form

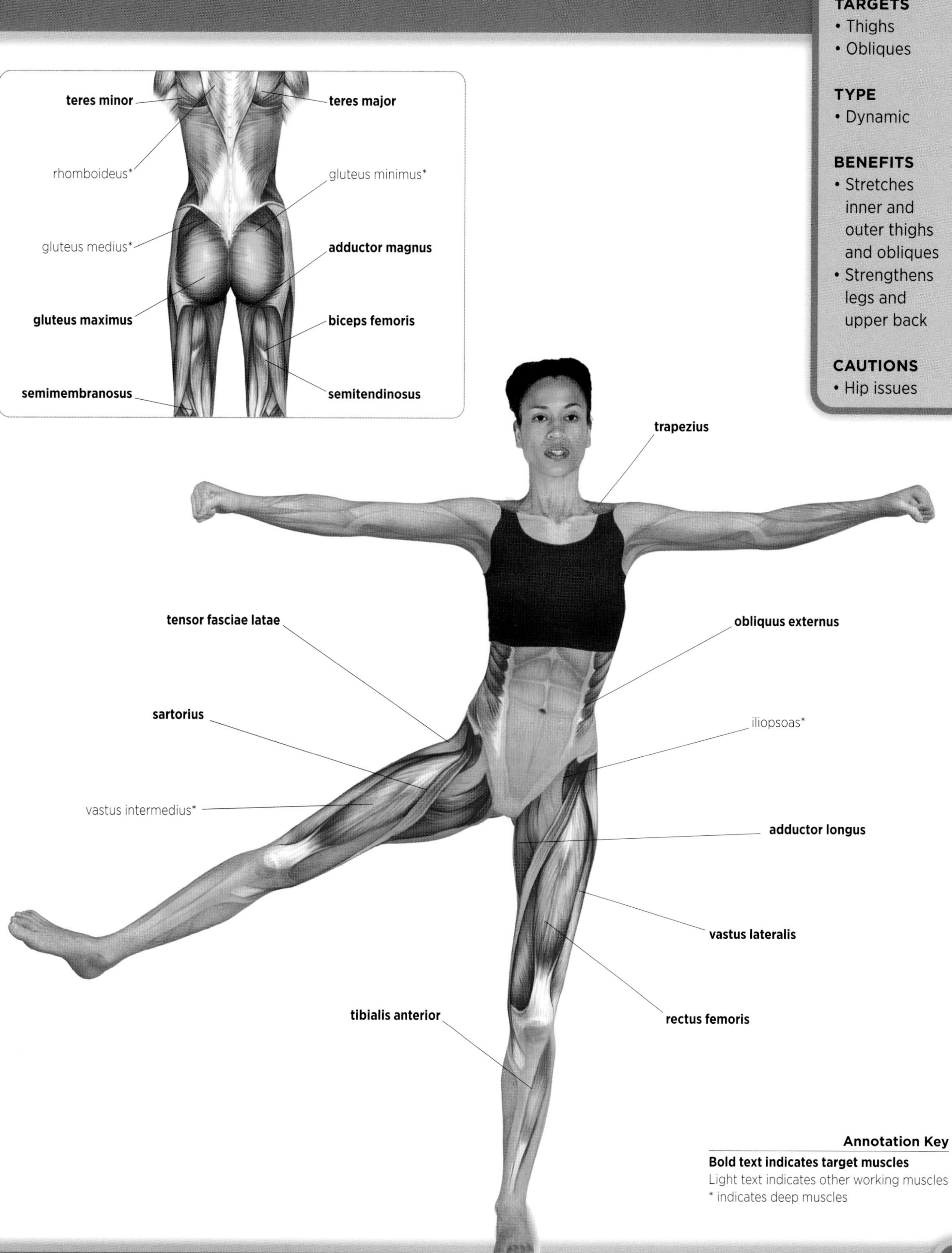

FACT FILE

TARGETS
- Thighs
- Obliques

TYPE
- Dynamic

BENEFITS
- Stretches inner and outer thighs and obliques
- Strengthens legs and upper back

CAUTIONS
- Hip issues

Annotation Key

Bold text indicates target muscles

Light text indicates other working muscles

* indicates deep muscles

Towel Hamstrings Pull

The Towel Hamstring Pull uses the physical force of friction to your advantage. This exercise works your posterior chain from a bottom-up approach, including your calves, hamstrings, glutes, and, finally, your core.

HOW TO DO IT

- Lie faceup with your legs extended, heels placed on top of towel, and your arms extended down along your sides.
- Engage your hamstrings and glutes by digging your heels into the towel and bridging upward so that your glutes are elevated off the floor, placing your hips in the air.
- Engage your hamstrings to pull your heels toward your trunk while keeping your hips in the air.
- Allow your heels to slide away from you until they return to the floor in the full extended position. Repeat for the recommended repetitions.

DO IT RIGHT

- Keep weight through your heels and on the towel.
- Avoid flaring your knees in or out, keeping them in track and parallel.
- Keep your core engaged to avoid excessive curvature of your spine.
- Perform on a low-friction surface, such as a wood floor.

FACT FILE

TARGETS
- Hamstrings
- Calves
- Glutes
- Abdominals

TYPE
- Static

BENEFITS
- Improves coordination
- Strengthens and tones lower calves, hamstrings, and glutes
- Develops core stability

CAUTIONS
- Back issues
- Hip issues

EQUIPMENT
- Towel

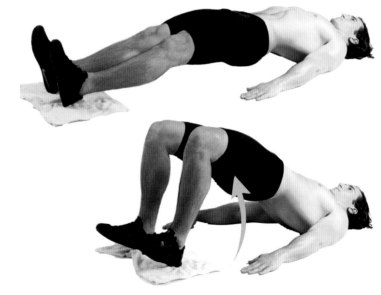

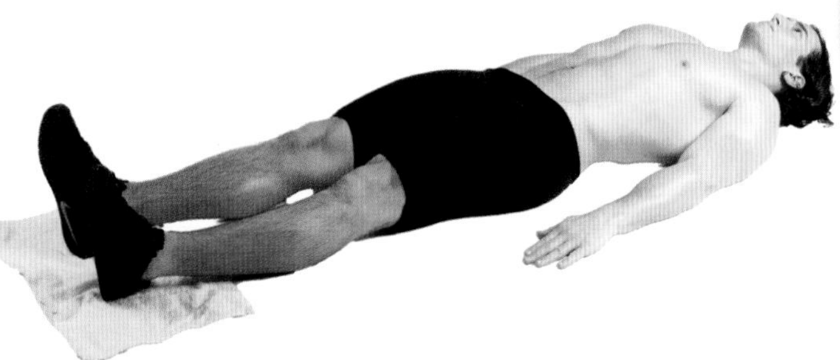

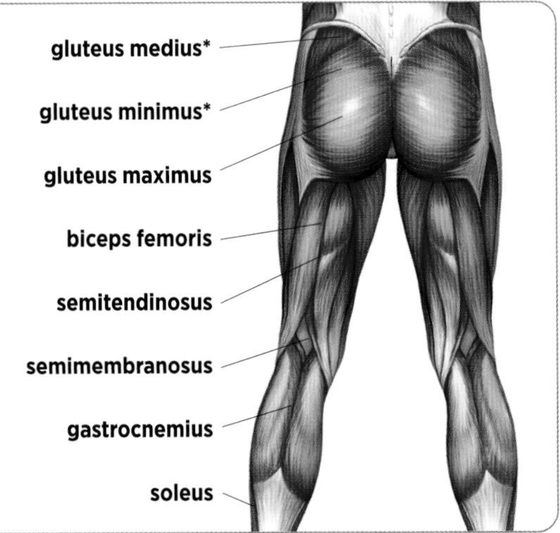

Annotation Key
Bold text indicates target muscles
Light text indicates other working muscles
* indicates deep muscles

Towel Abduction and Adduction

It may resemble cleaning the floor, but this exercise provides its own housekeeping for your inner- and outer-thigh muscles. It is essential to condition these muscles, known as your hip abductors and adductors, if your goal is to have healthier, more powerful legs.

HOW TO DO IT

- Begin by placing the towel on the floor. Standing on top of the towel, assume a wide stance, spreading your feet approximately twice your hips-width apart.
- While keeping your legs as straight as possible, draw your feet together, pulling the opposite sides of the towel together under your feet.
- Return to the starting position by pressing outward, spreading your legs apart until the towel is taught again under your feet. Repeat for the recommended repetitions.

DO IT RIGHT

- Keep your legs straight.
- Perform on a low-friction surface, such as a wood floor, or use special sliders.
- Perform smoothly and with control.

FACT FILE

TARGETS
- Hips
- Abdominals
- Glutes

TYPE
- Static

BENEFITS
- Strengthens and tones glutes, abdominals, and legs
- Improves coordination

CAUTIONS
- Hip issues

EQUIPMENT
- Towel

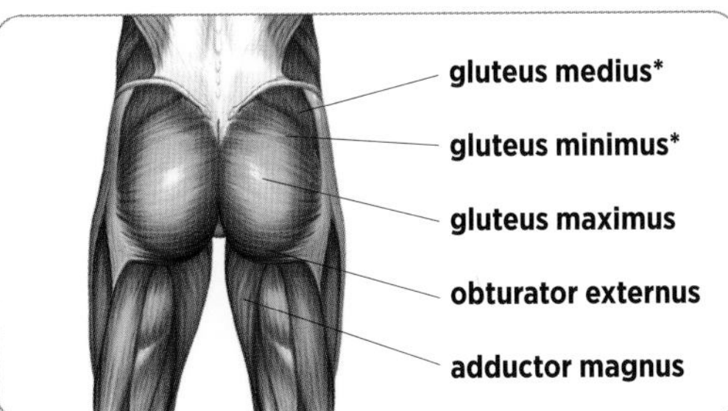

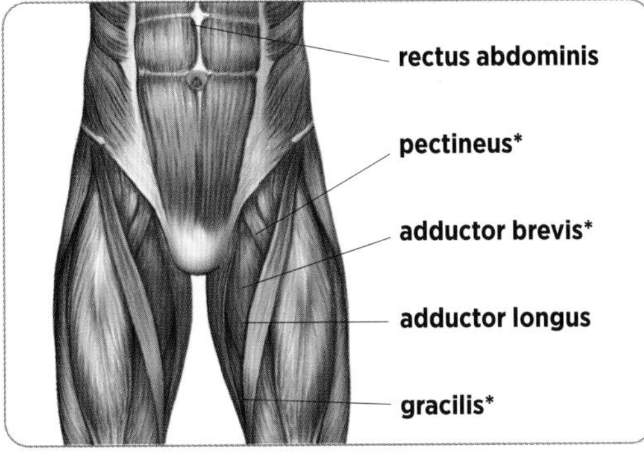

Annotation Key
Bold text indicates target muscles
Light text indicates other working muscles
* indicates deep muscles

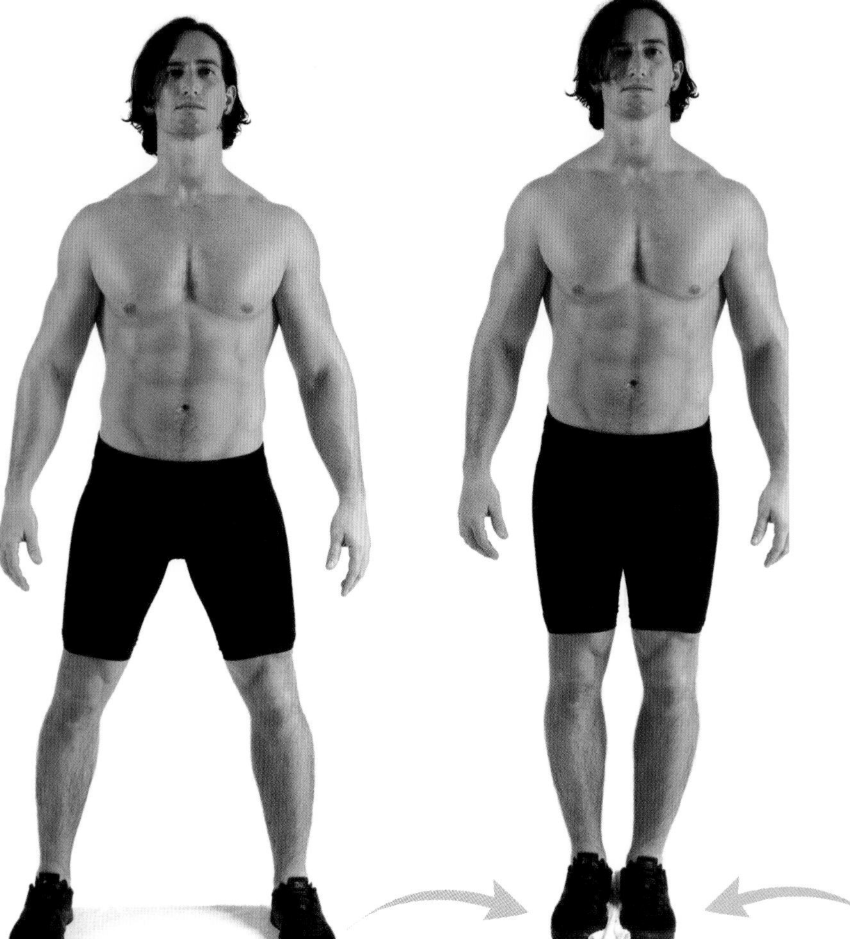

Surrender

"Never quit, never surrender!"—except maybe to this exercise. This beginner body-weight exercise will hit everything from the waist down, including your quadriceps, glutes, calves, and hips.

HOW TO DO IT

- Stand with your feet hip-width apart and your hands clasped behind your head.
- Perform a reverse lunge by flexing at your hips and knees as you step your left leg backward, dropping your knee to the floor.
- Bring your right leg down next to your left leg to come into a kneeling position with both legs.
- Step your left leg in front to again assume the lunge position, this time with your left foot forward.
- Press down into the floor with both feet, performing a lunge to return to the starting position. Continue alternating sides for the recommended repetitions.

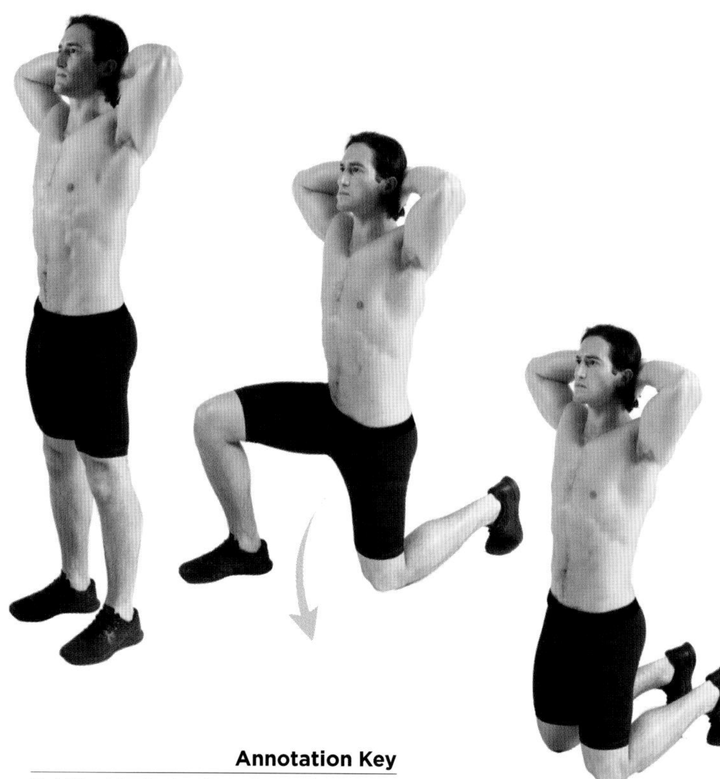

DO IT RIGHT

- Keep your back upright, focusing your gaze slightly higher than the horizon.
- Do not use your hands to assist your movements.
- Track your knees over your toes, avoiding any inward or outward deviation of the knee or ankle of your front leg.

Annotation Key

Bold text indicates target muscles

Light text indicates other working muscles

* indicates deep muscles

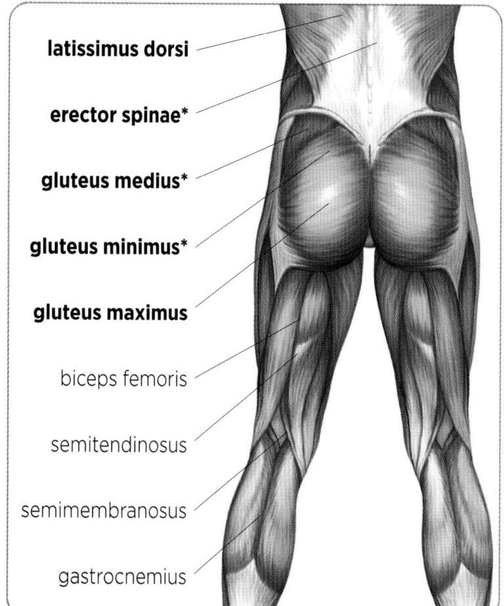

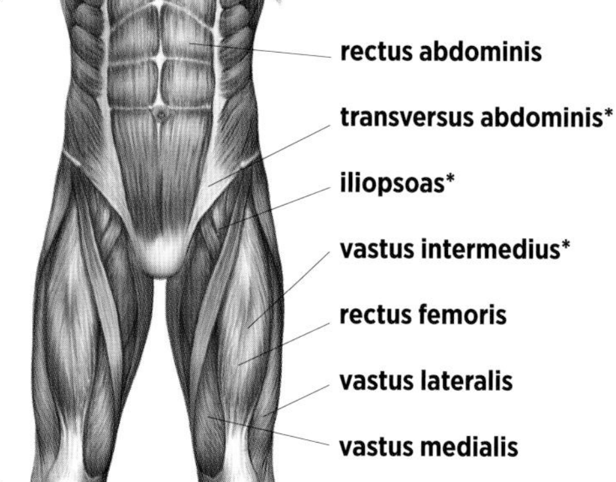

FACT FILE

TARGETS
- Hip flexors
- Quadriceps
- Glutes
- Abdominals
- Back

TYPE
- Dynamic

BENEFITS
- Strengthens and tones core and legs
- Increases lower-extremity muscular endurance
- Improves coordination

CAUTIONS
- Hip issues
- Knee issues

Unilateral Leg Raise

In this variation of the Unilateral Knee-to-Chest stretch, you straighten your leg upward as you bring your leg to your chest. This requires additional flexibility in the muscles running along the back of your leg and targets the lower-back more deeply.

HOW TO DO IT

- Lie on your back and bend your right knee in toward your chest.
- With your hands placed on your hamstrings near your knee, extend and straighten your right leg toward the ceiling.
- Point both feet.
- Switch your hand position, so your right hand is on your right calf muscle, and your left hand is on your hamstrings. Gently bring your thigh toward your chest, increasing the intensity of the stretch.
- Slowly release your leg back down to the starting position, and then repeat on the opposite side.

FACT FILE

TARGETS
- Lower-back
- Groin
- Glutes
- Hamstrings

TYPE
- Static

BENEFITS
- Lower-back stress release
- Glute and hamstring stretch
- Hip opener

CAUTIONS
- Hip injury
- Lower-back pain

semimembranosus
semitendinosus
biceps femoris
soleus
gastrocnemius
erector spinae*
gluteus medius*
gluteus minimus*
gluteus maximus

Annotation Key
Bold text indicates target muscles
Light text indicates other working muscles
* indicates deep muscles

DO IT RIGHT
- Keep your lower-back on the floor, tucking in your pelvis.
- Keep your back grounded.
- Avoid lifting your head or upper back.
- Avoid holding your breath.

Split Squat with Overhead Press

A multipurpose exercise, the Split Squat with Overhead Press combines the single-leg strengthening move of a staggered-stance squat with the upper-body toning of an upward press. This exercise will challenge your quads, glutes, hamstrings, upper back, and shoulders.

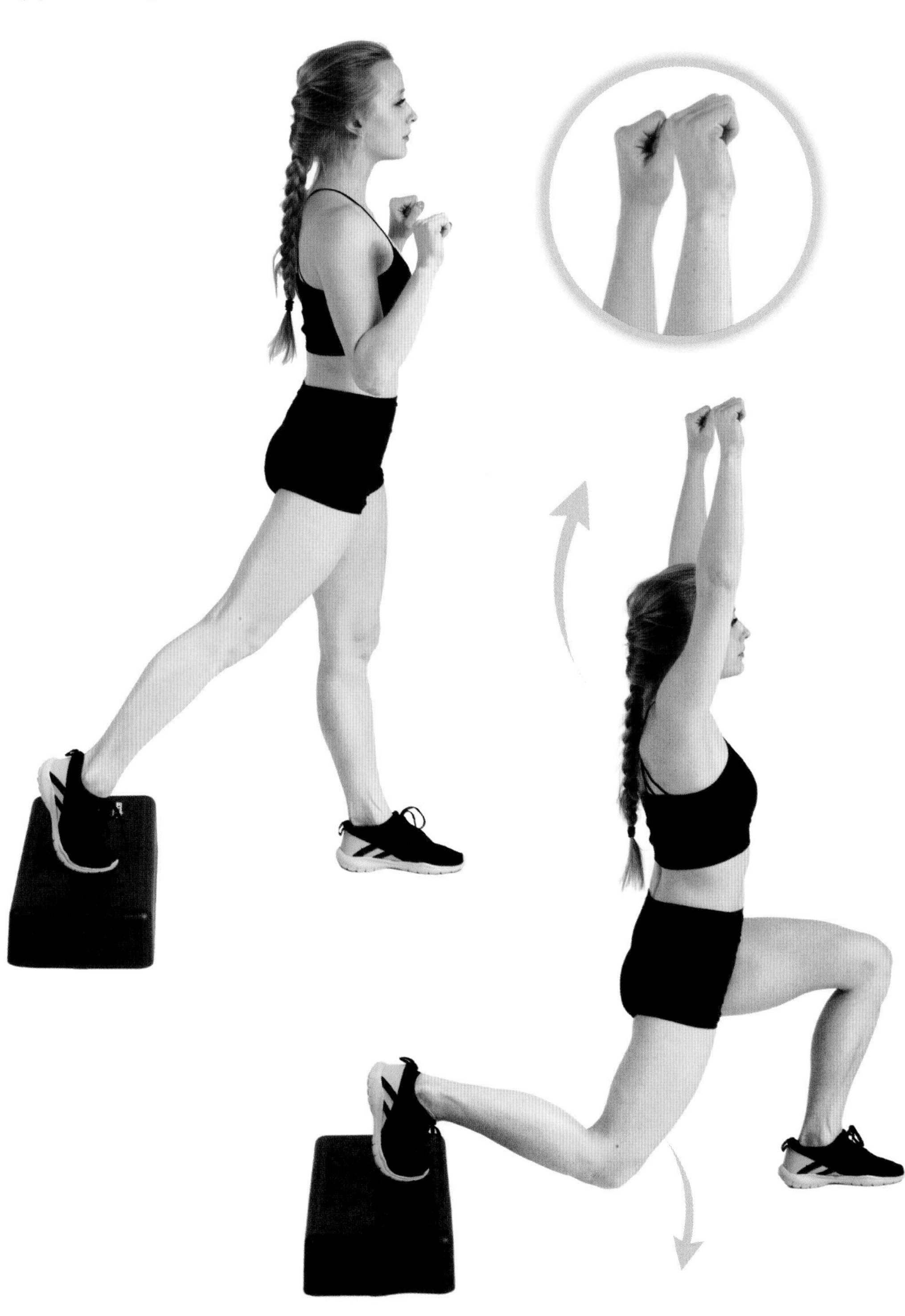

HOW TO DO IT

- Stand with your right leg behind you with the ball of your foot resting on a step.
- With your elbows bent to form right angles, raise both arms to shoulder height. Position your hands as if your were grasping a bar using an overhand grip.
- Bend both knees into a split squat position. Simultaneously, extend your arms over your head.
- Return to the starting position, and then repeat on the opposite side. Repeat for the recommended repetitions.

DO IT RIGHT

- Keep your back straight and your core upright.
- Press your shoulders back and down.
- Avoid arching your back as you raise your arms.
- Avoid letting your abdominals bulge outward.
- Avoid tensing your neck.

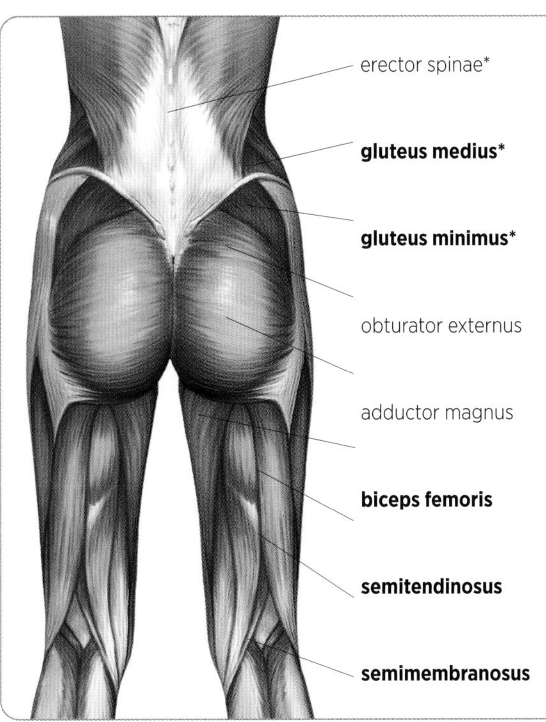

Annotation Key

Bold text indicates target muscles
Light text indicates other working muscles
* indicates deep muscles

MODIFICATION

HARDER: Hold a pair of dumbbells above your head as your execute the exercise.

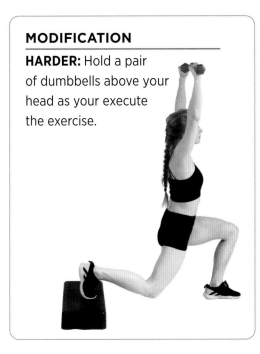

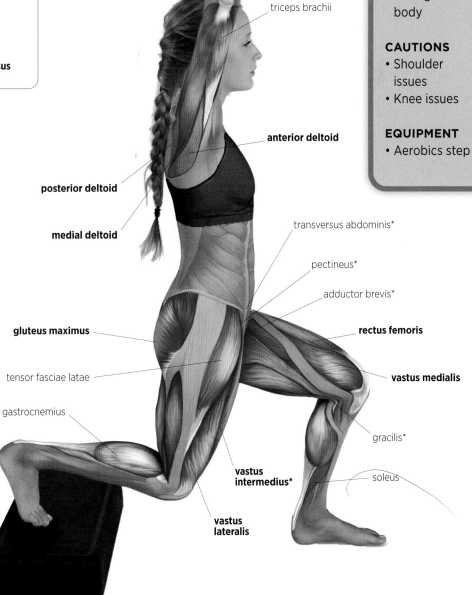

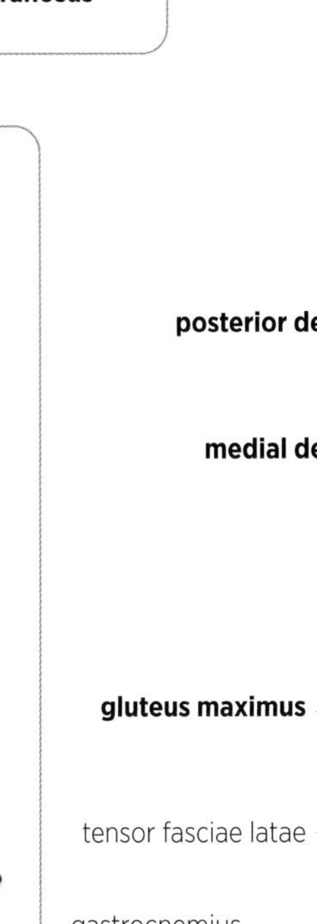

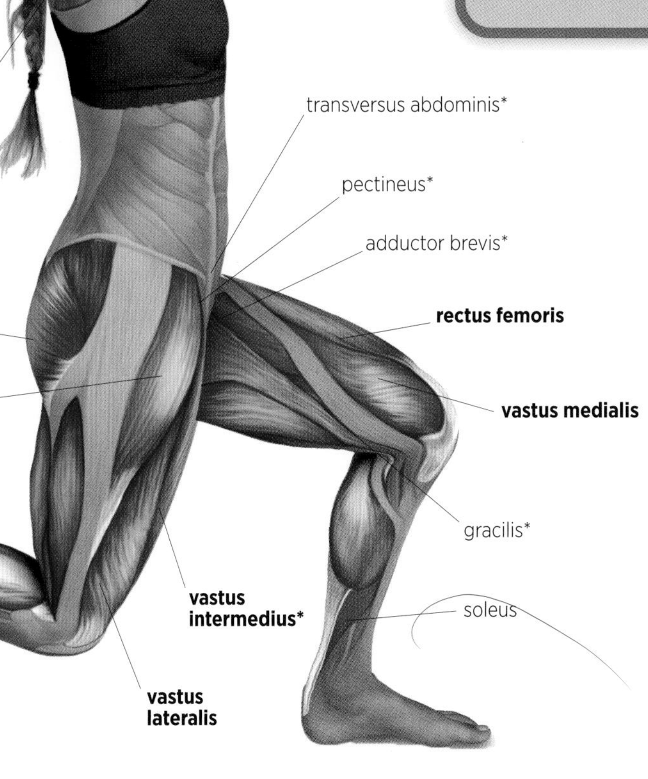

FACT FILE

TARGETS
- Glutes
- Quadriceps
- Hamstrings
- Shoulders
- Upper back

TYPE
- Dynamic

BENEFITS
- Strengthens glutes, thighs, shoulders, and upper back
- Improves range of motion throughout body

CAUTIONS
- Shoulder issues
- Knee issues

EQUIPMENT
- Aerobics step

Lateral-Extension Reverse Lunge

Backward lunges can be easier than forward ones because your knees take less strain, plus keeping your weight on your forward leg stabilizes the pose. This exercise is certainly great for the glutes, quads, and hamstrings.

HOW TO DO IT

- Stand with your feet a little way apart, up to hip-width, and your arms at the sides of your body or with your hands on your hips.
- Step your right leg backward. Keep a slight bend in your right knee and rest the ball of your foot on the floor.
- Bend both knees as you move into a lunge position. Lower your body, flexing your left knee and hip until your right leg is almost in contact with the floor. Raise your arms to the sides until they are level with your shoulders.
- Return to the starting position by straightening out your left leg and bringing your right leg forward to meet your left.
- Switch legs and repeat on the opposite side. Alternate sides for the recommended repetitions.

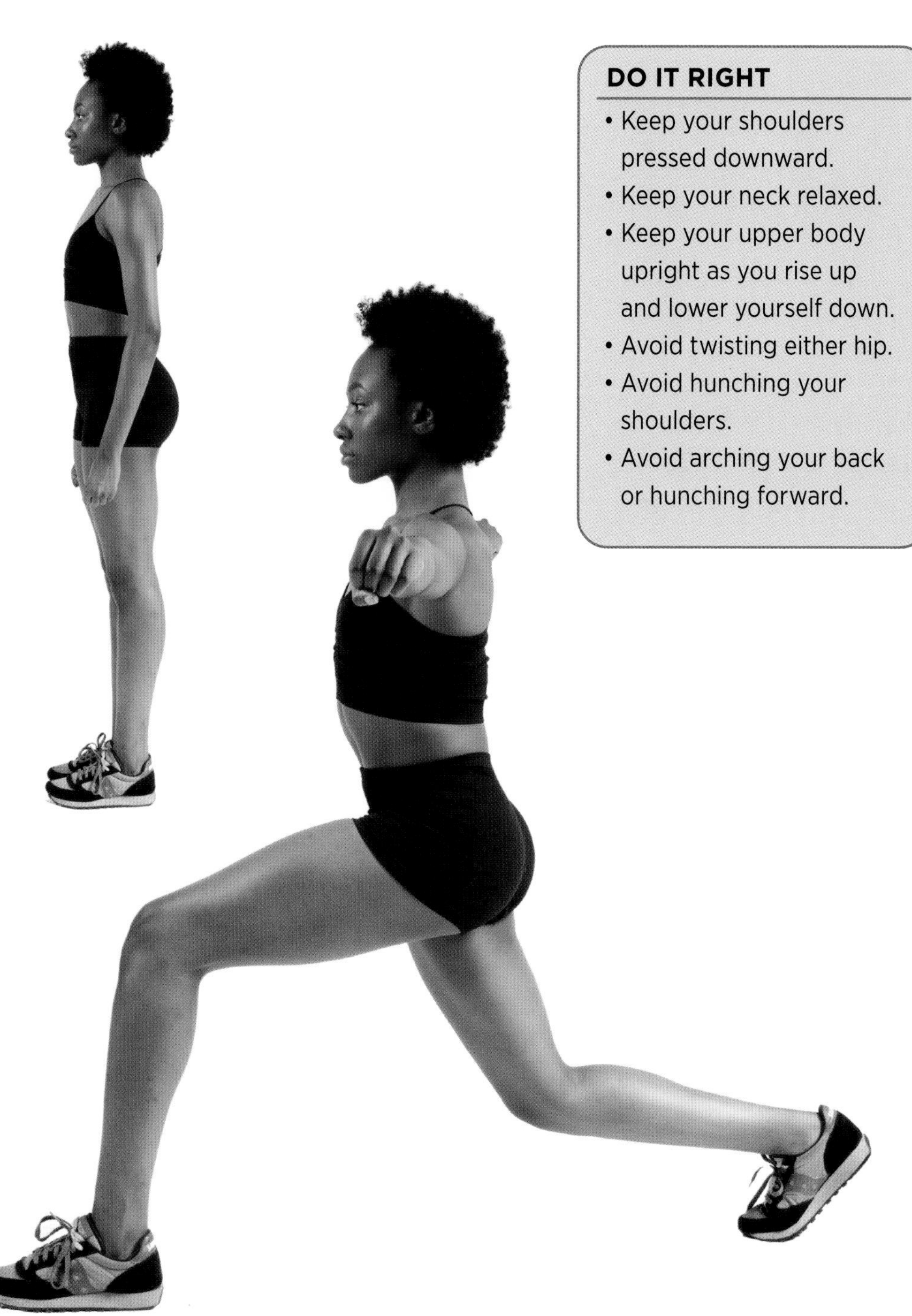

DO IT RIGHT

- Keep your shoulders pressed downward.
- Keep your neck relaxed.
- Keep your upper body upright as you rise up and lower yourself down.
- Avoid twisting either hip.
- Avoid hunching your shoulders.
- Avoid arching your back or hunching forward.

FACT FILE

TARGETS
- Glutes
- Thighs
- Back
- Shoulders

TYPE
- Dynamic

BENEFITS
- Strengthens glutes and legs
- Boosts performance in baseball, rugby, and soccer

CAUTIONS
- Ankle issues

EQUIPMENT
- Optional: Dumbbells for modification

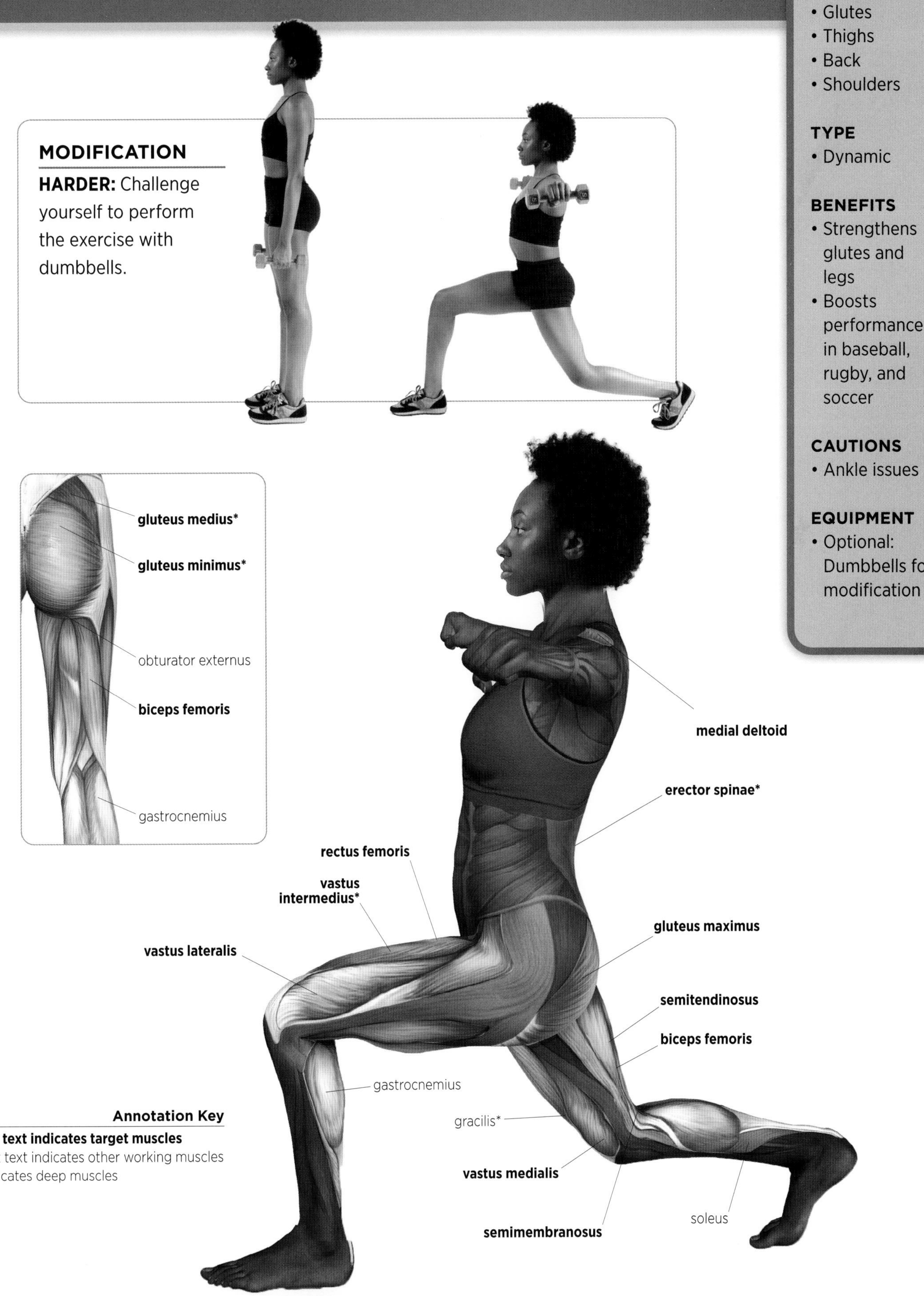

Skater's Lunge

If you want to strengthen your glutes and quads, then look no further than this simple exercise. Skater's Lunge will also give a thorough workout to your hamstrings.

HOW TO DO IT

- Stand with your legs wider than shoulder-width apart and your toes pointing forward.
- Slide to your left side into a side lunge as you bend forward slightly, with your hands placed on your left thigh, and your right leg straight.
- Repeat on the opposite side. Alternate sides for the recommended time.

DO IT RIGHT

- Push through the heel to drive the exercise.
- Move with control, keeping a steady, quick pace.
- Avoid hyperextending your knee past your toes.

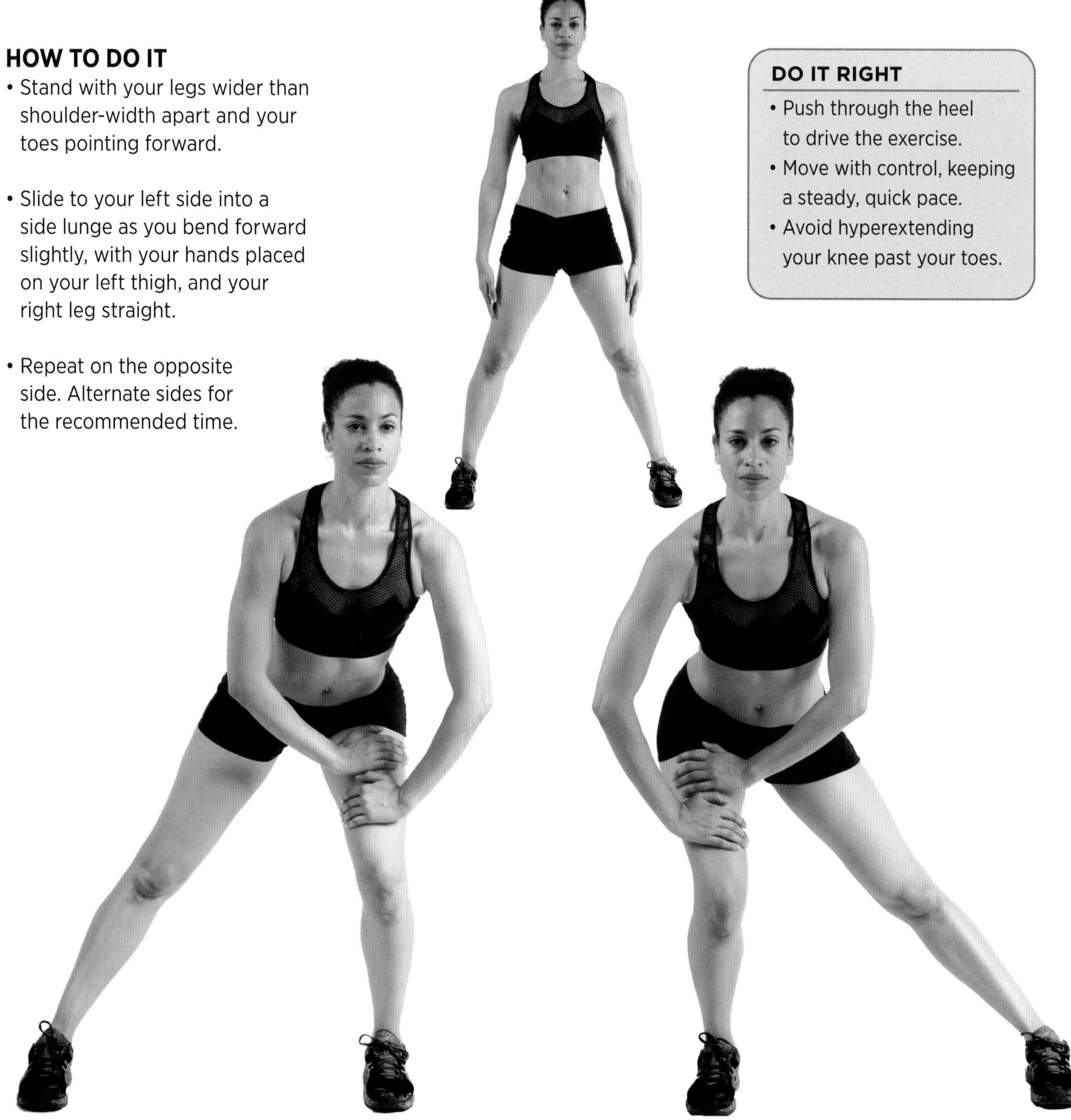

FACT FILE

TARGETS
- Glutes
- Quads
- Hamstrings

TYPE
- Dynamic

BENEFITS
- Strengthens and tones leg muscles

CAUTIONS
- Hip issues
- Knee pain

EQUIPMENT
- Optional: Dumbbells or kettlebells for modification

MODIFICATION

HARDER: Perform the exercise while grasping a dumbbell in each hand, or holding a kettlebell at each shoulder.

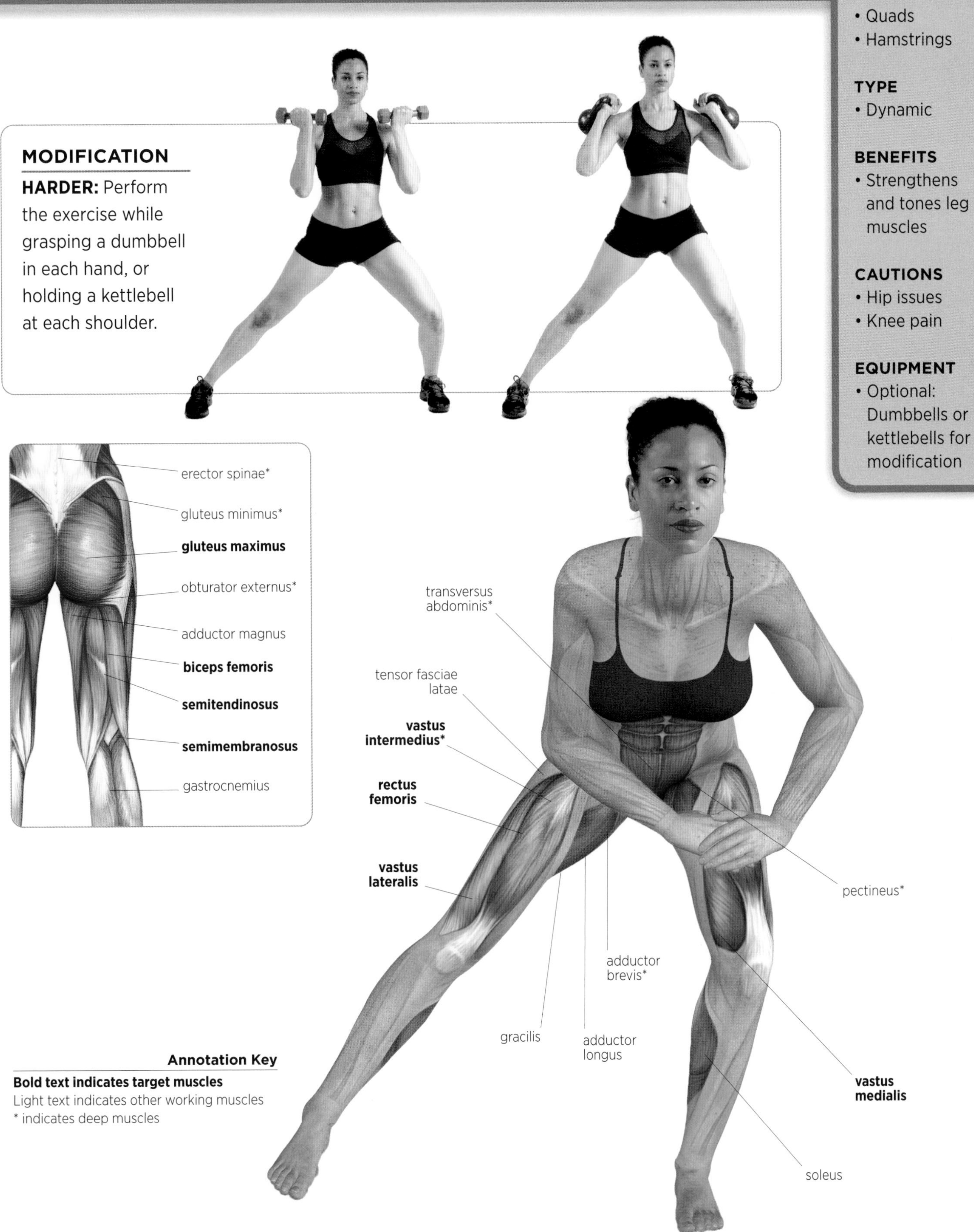

Annotation Key

Bold text indicates target muscles
Light text indicates other working muscles
* indicates deep muscles

Step-Down

For such a simple step-down movement, this exercise achieves a great amount. Strengthening your thighs and glutes, it also improves movement range in your hips and pelvis while stabilizing your core.

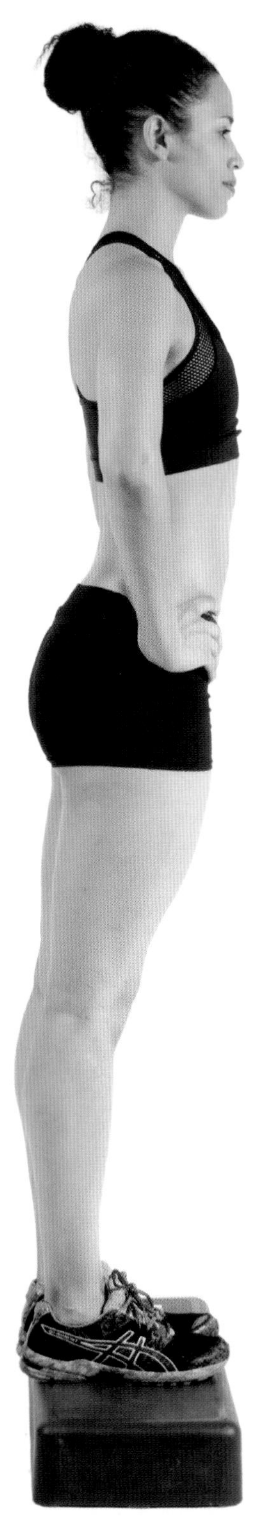

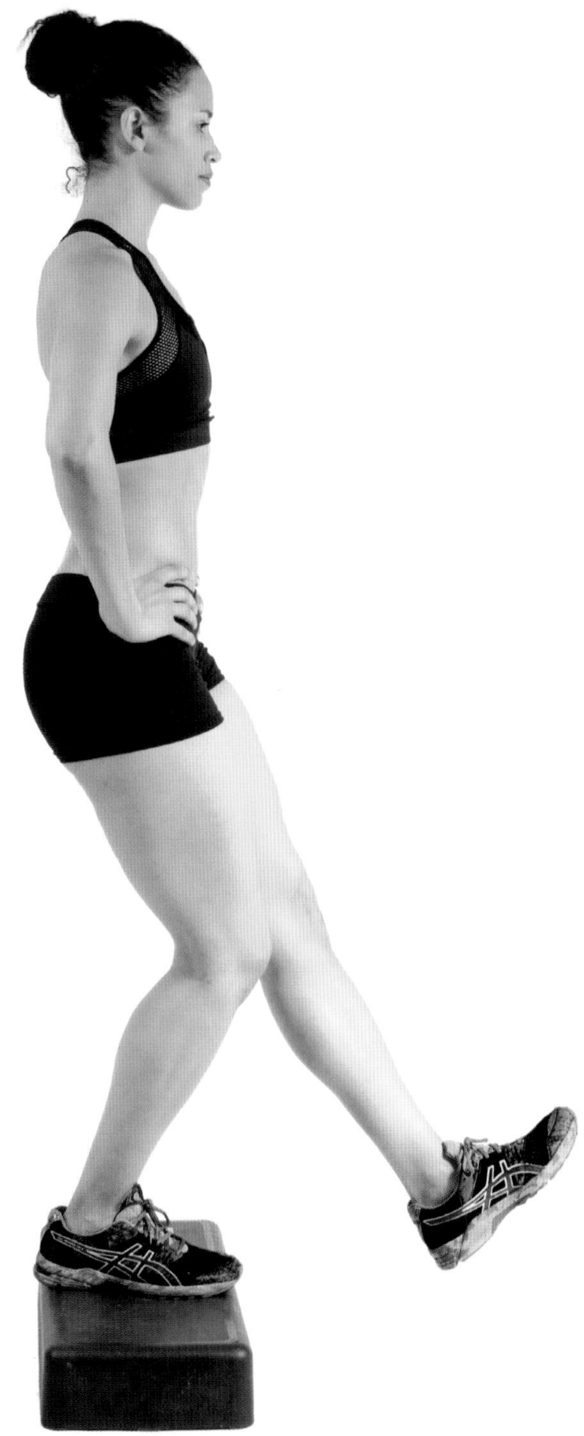

HOW TO DO IT

- Stand facing forward on a plyo box or platform.
- Bend your right leg. Simultaneously step your left leg downward, flexing the foot. Bring the heel of your left foot to rest on the floor.
- Without rotating your torso or knee, press upward through your right leg to return to your starting position. Alternate sides for the recommended repetitions.

DO IT RIGHT

- Hold the wall or a rail for support if desired.
- Move slowly and with control.
- Focus on maintaining good form.
- Avoid letting your knee twist inward; keep it in line with your middle toe.
- Avoid rushing.

FACT FILE

TARGETS
- Quads
- Hamstrings
- Leg mobilizers
- Glutes
- Lower back
- Shoulders

TYPE
- Static

BENEFITS
- Strengthens pelvic and knee stabilizers
- Boosts performance in running and rock climbing

CAUTIONS
- Ankle pain/ injury

EQUIPMENT
- Plyo box or platform

medial deltoid

anterior deltoid

rectus abdominis

obliquus externus

transversus abdominis*

gluteus medius*

gluteus maximus

tensor fasciae latae

vastus intermedius*

rectus femoris

biceps femoris

vastus lateralis

gastrocnemius

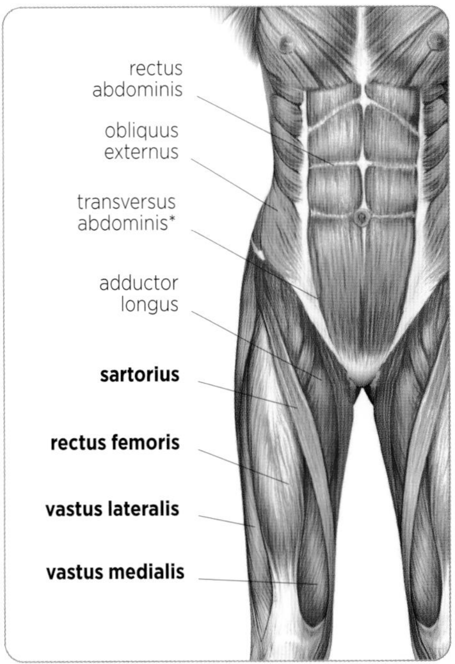

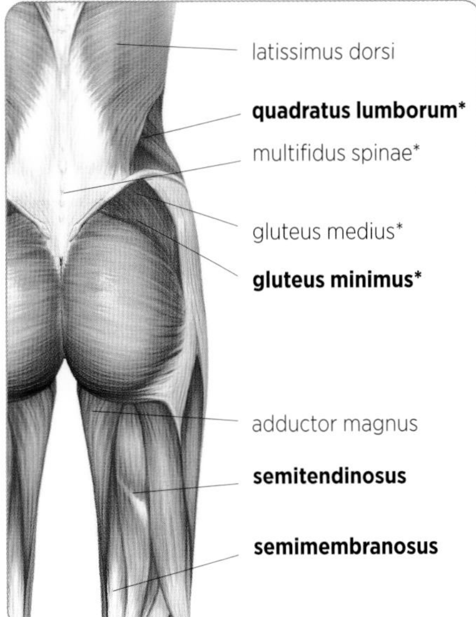

Annotation Key

Bold text indicates target muscles

Light text indicates other working muscles

* indicates deep muscles

Step-Up

The Step-Up strengthens, tones, and sculpts your quads, glutes, hip flexors, and hamstrings. At the same time, this balance movement improves pelvic and leg stability while adding a cardio benefit.

HOW TO DO IT

- Stand in front of a step, bench, or other stable platform.
- Step onto the bench with your right leg, making sure your foot is flat against the bench.
- Lean forward slightly and push yourself upward through the heel of your right foot, so that your left leg comes up onto the bench too.
- Step down with your right leg, and then repeat the same sequence with the opposite leg. Continue stepping up and down, alternating sides, for the recommended repetitions.

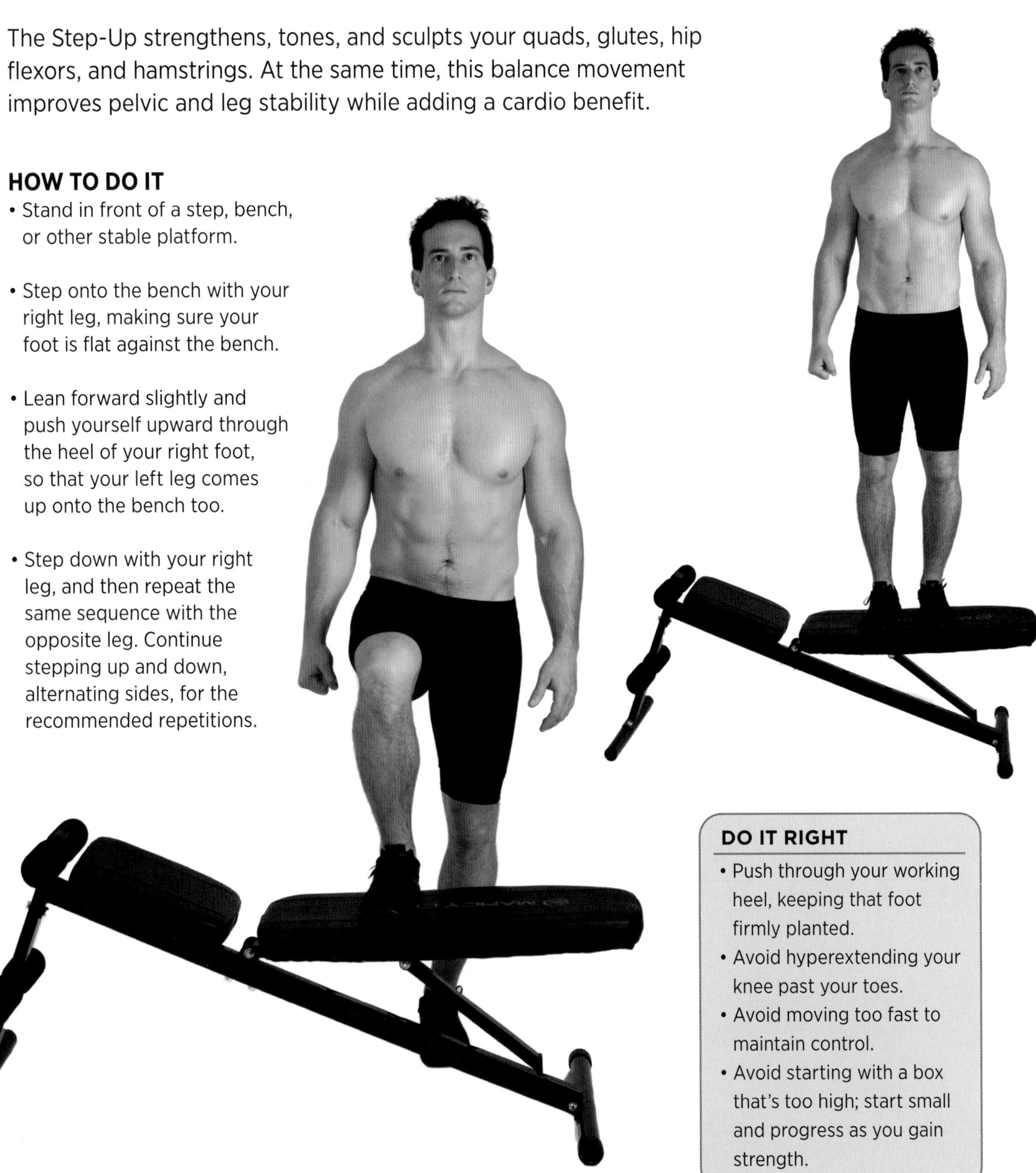

DO IT RIGHT

- Push through your working heel, keeping that foot firmly planted.
- Avoid hyperextending your knee past your toes.
- Avoid moving too fast to maintain control.
- Avoid starting with a box that's too high; start small and progress as you gain strength.

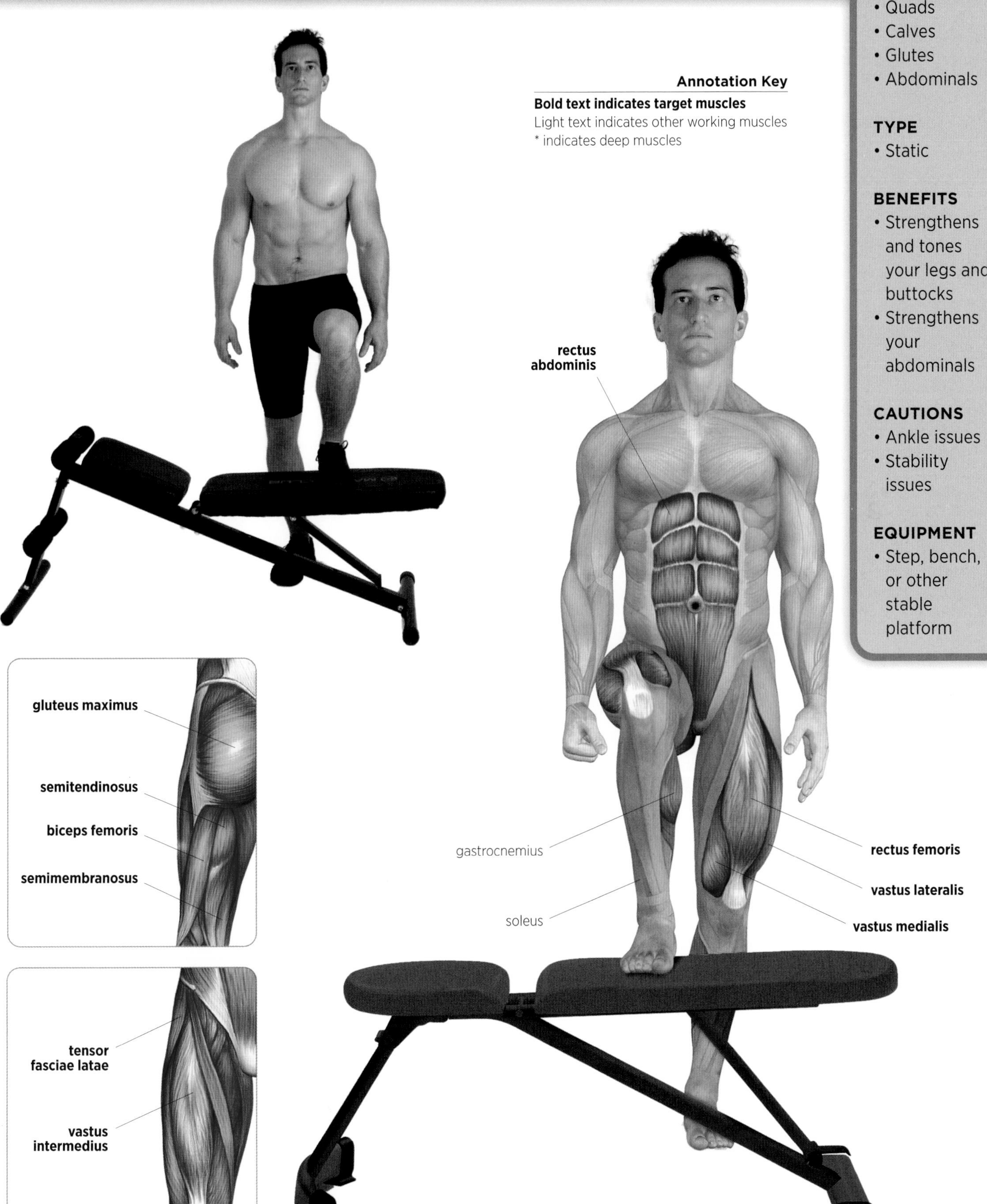

FACT FILE

TARGETS
- Hamstrings
- Quads
- Calves
- Glutes
- Abdominals

TYPE
- Static

BENEFITS
- Strengthens and tones your legs and buttocks
- Strengthens your abdominals

CAUTIONS
- Ankle issues
- Stability issues

EQUIPMENT
- Step, bench, or other stable platform

Side Adductor Stretch

The Side Adductor Stretch uses lateral movement to improve your stability, upper-leg strength, and overall flexibility. This exercise engages virtually all the muscles of your lower body.

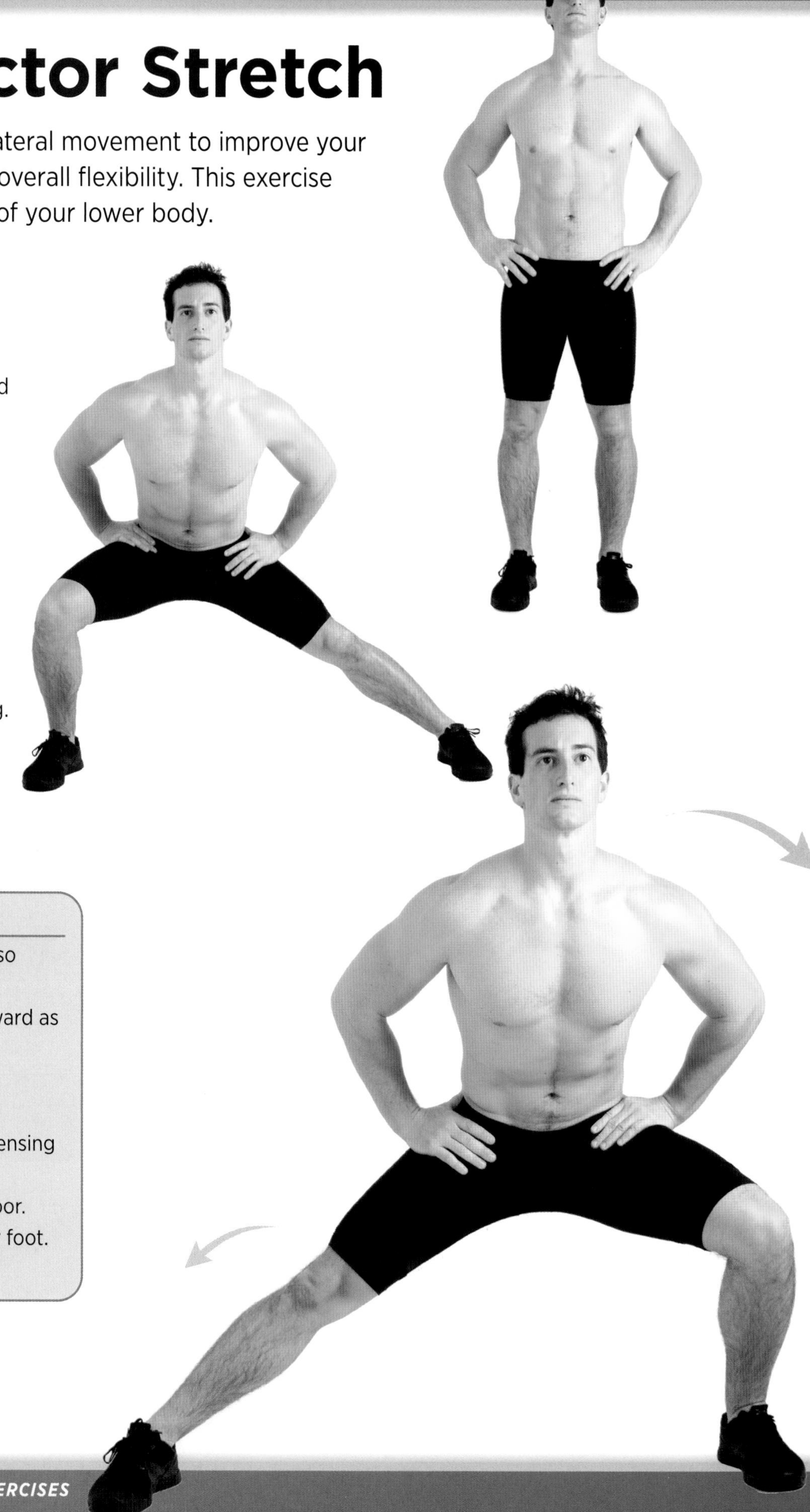

HOW TO DO IT

- Stand upright and position your feet more than hip-width apart, toes turned slightly outward.
- Rest your hands on your lower thighs for support.
- Keeping your torso steady, gradually bend your knees outward.
- Without moving your torso, shift your weight to your left side, bending your knee while straightening your right leg.
- Hold for the recommended time, release the stretch, and repeat on the opposite side.

DO IT RIGHT

- Keep your spine neutral and your torso facing forward.
- Let your shoulders come slightly forward as you stretch.
- Anchor your feet to the floor.
- Avoid rounding your spine.
- Avoid hunching your shoulders and tensing your neck.
- Avoid letting either foot lift off the floor.
- Keep your bent knee in line with your foot.

FACT FILE

TARGETS
- Hip flexors
- Adductors

TYPE
- Static

BENEFITS
- Stretches hip flexors
- Works the adductors
- Opens the hips

CAUTIONS
- Hip issues
- Lower-back pain
- Knee problems

Annotation Key

Bold text indicates target muscles

Light text indicates other working muscles

* indicates deep muscles

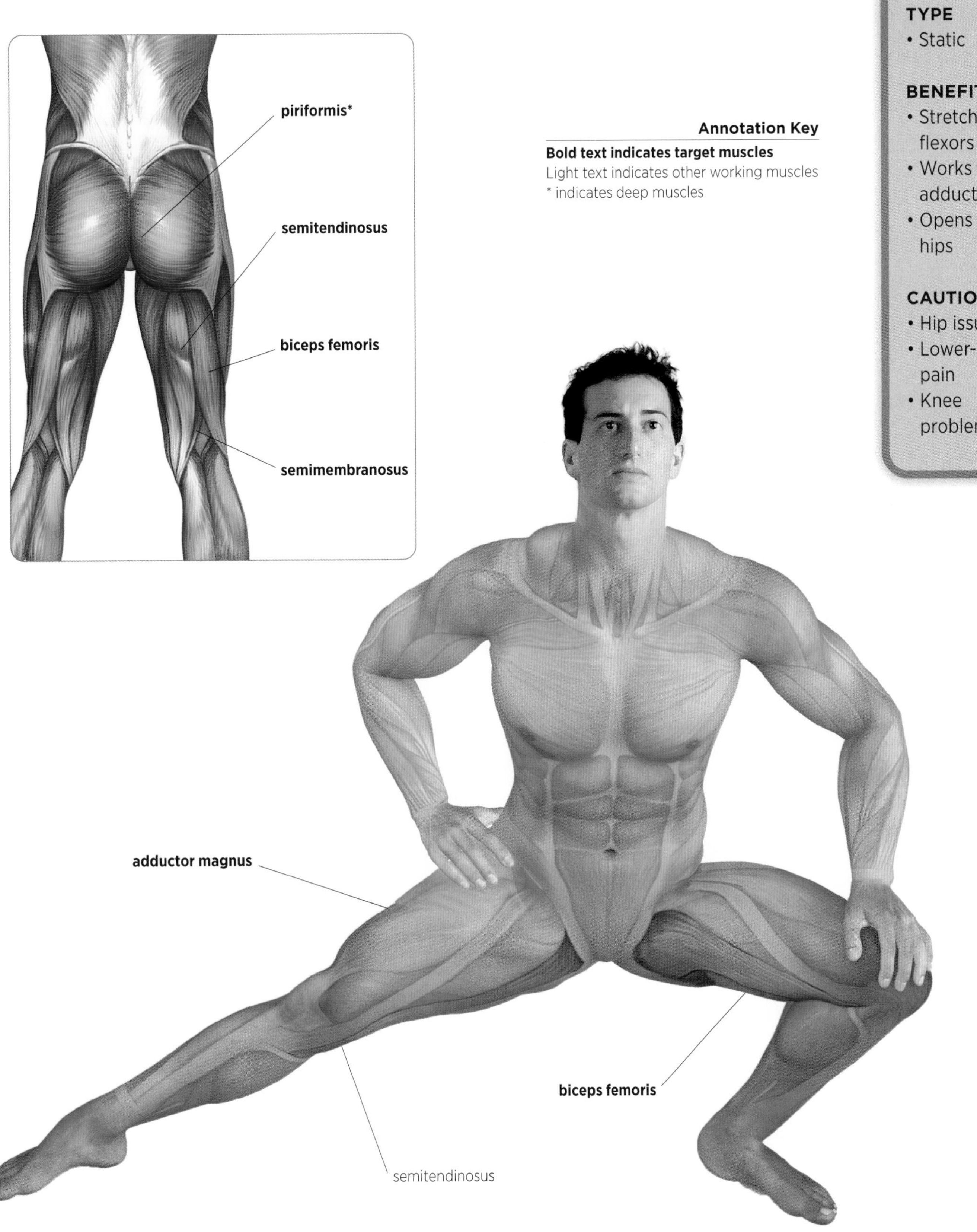

Clamshells

Clamshells strengthen your medial glutes and bring more power and stability to your hips. This exercise is commonly prescribed by physical therapists as a remedy for hip tightness and lower-back pain.

HOW TO DO IT

- Lie on your right side with your knees bent, aligning your shoulders, hips, and ankles. Bend your right arm and tuck your forearm under your head, keeping your head in line with your spine.

- Flex your feet, with your left toes pointing outward. Contract your glutes as you hinge open your hip and raise your left knee, keeping your heels together.

- Raise and extend your upper leg, with your foot flexed and toes facing forward.

- Return to the starting position. Perform the recommended repetitions, and repeat on the opposite side.

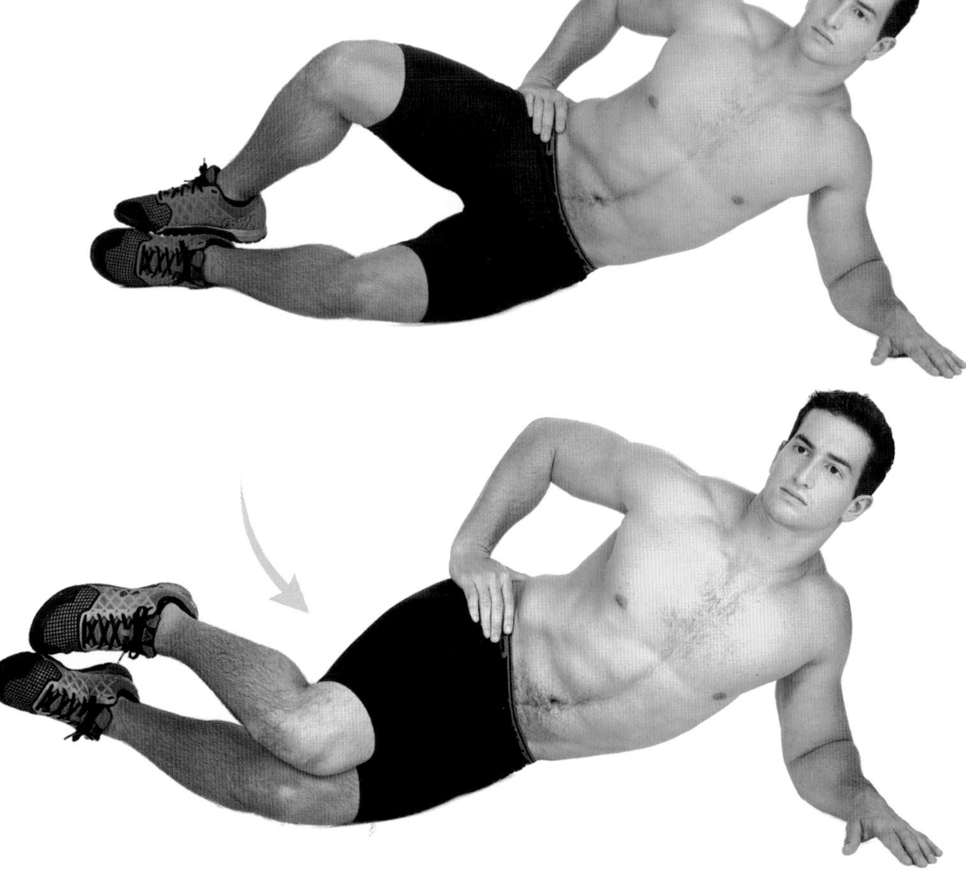

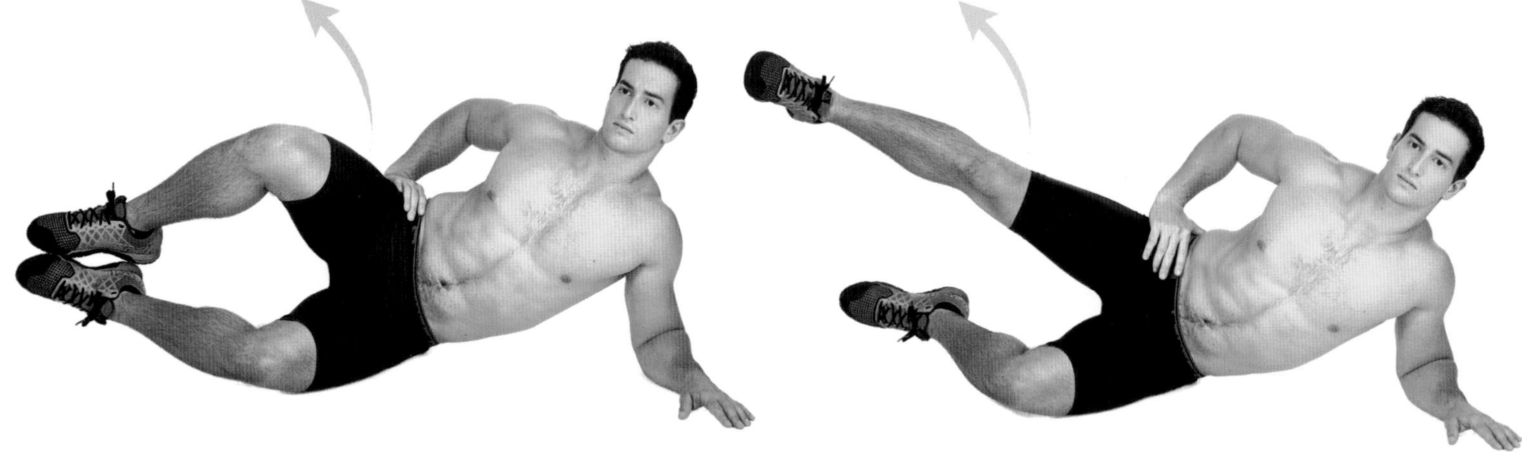

FACT FILE

TARGETS
- Glutes
- Inner thighs

TYPE
- Dynamic

BENEFITS
- Increases hip stability
- Strengthens glutes and hamstrings
- Alleviates lower-back pain

CAUTIONS
- Lower-back injury
- Intense hip pain
- Intense knee pain

Annotation Key

Bold text indicates target muscles
Light text indicates other working muscles
* indicates deep muscles

DO IT RIGHT
- Focus on moving only your upper leg.
- Your upper leg should move as if it were on a hinge.
- Keep your spine stable.
- Avoid any pelvic movement.

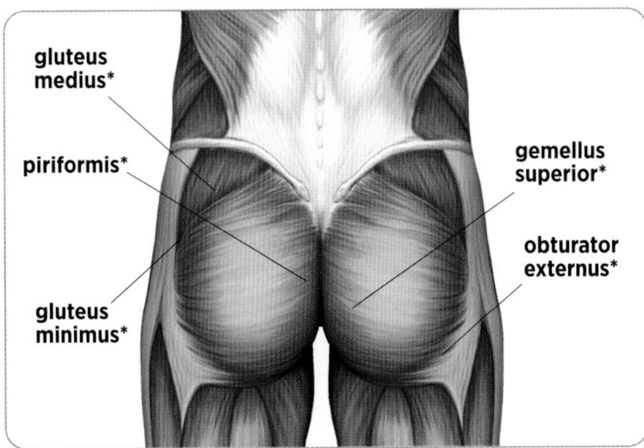

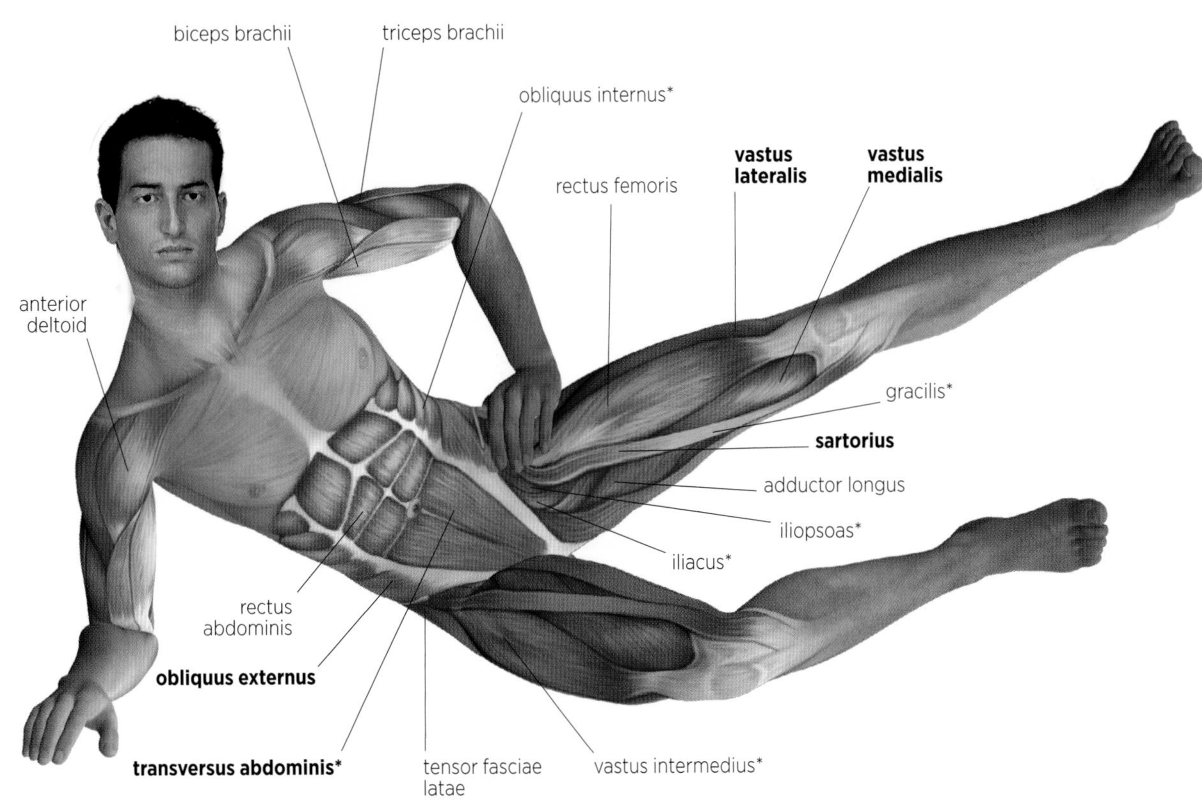

Swiss Ball Hamstrings Curl

The Swiss Ball Hamstrings Curl is a challenging exercise that targets your hamstrings and glutes. Choose a ball size that you are comfortable with, keeping in mind that the larger the ball, the greater the muscle contraction.

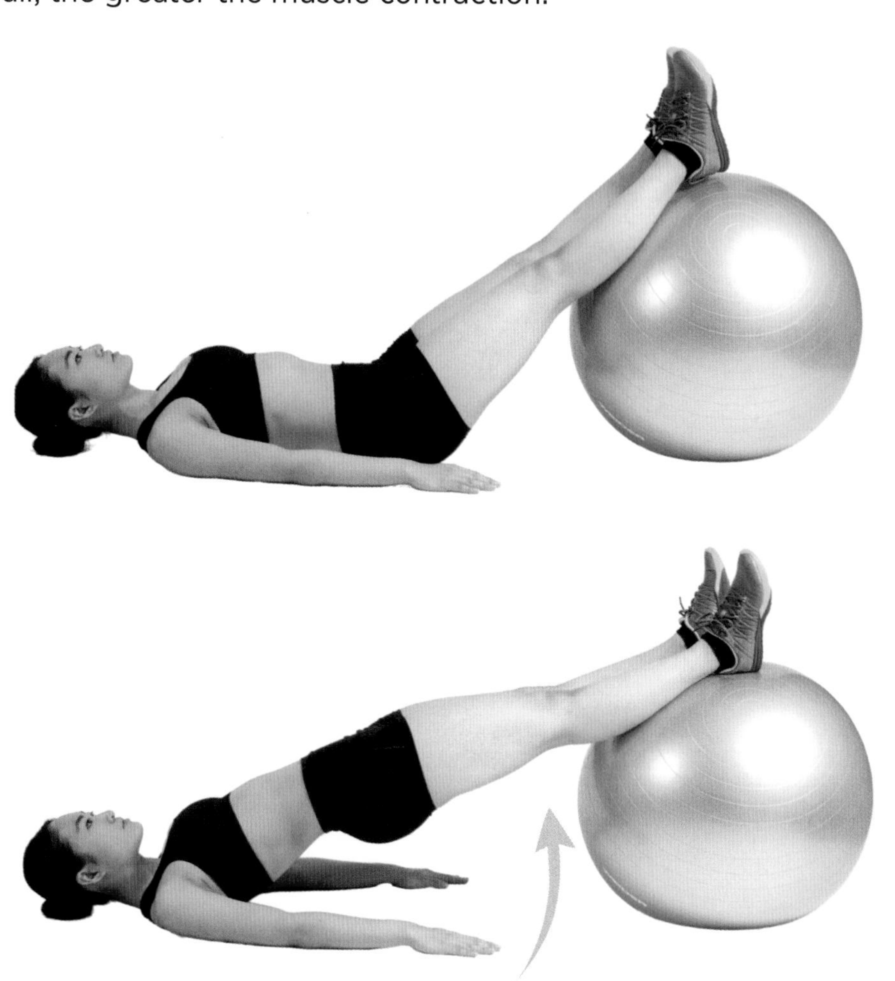

HOW TO DO IT

- Lie on your back with your arms along your sides, angled slightly away from your body. Extend your legs, and rest your lower legs and ankles on top of a Swiss ball.
- Pressing downward with your feet, bend your knees as you roll the ball toward you. Curl your pelvis, and raise your lower body off the floor. Hold for a few moments.
- With control, return to the starting position. Repeat for the recommended repetitions.

DO IT RIGHT

- Position your legs on the ball to form a 45-degree angle with the rest of your body before you curl.
- Move smoothly, maintaining control of the ball.
- Keep your arms anchored to the floor.
- Engage your abdominals, and squeeze your glutes.
- Avoid rushing through the movement.
- Avoid arching your back in the curl position.

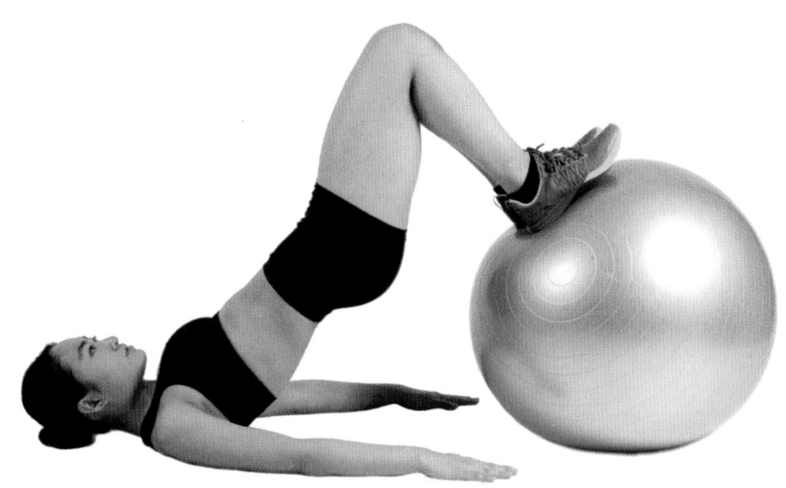

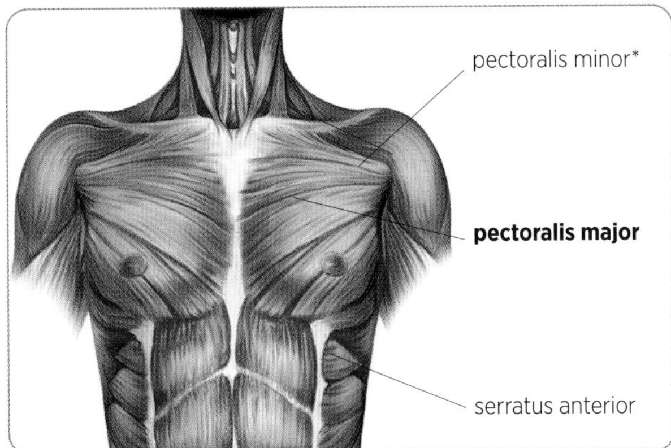

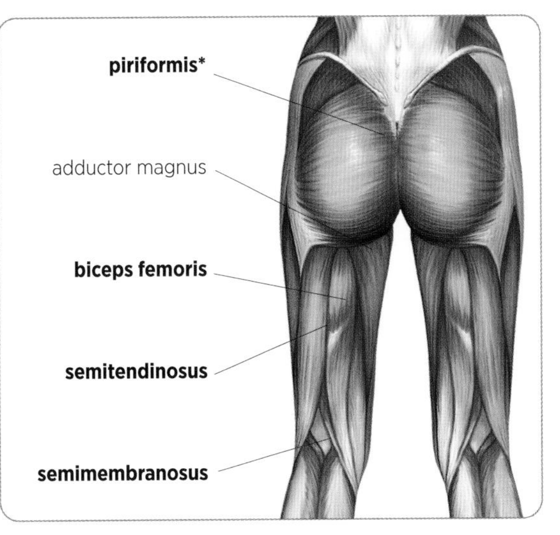

Annotation Key

Bold text indicates target muscles
Light text indicates other working muscles
* indicates deep muscles

FACT FILE

TARGETS
- Glutes
- Hamstrings

TYPE
- Dynamic

BENEFITS
- Strengthens glutes and hamstrings
- Stretches chest and spine

CAUTIONS
- Lower-back issues
- Neck issues
- Shoulder issues

EQUIPMENT
- Swiss ball

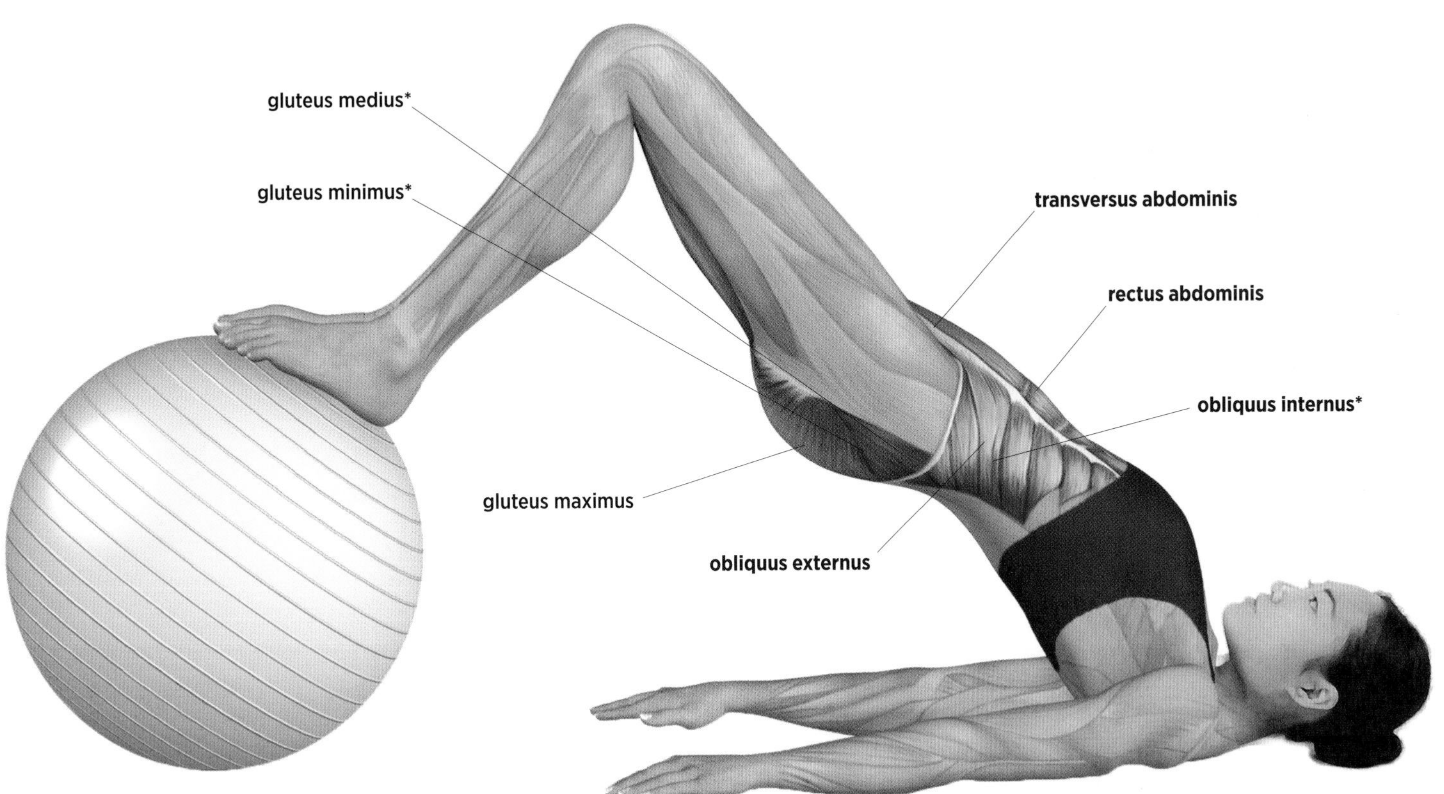

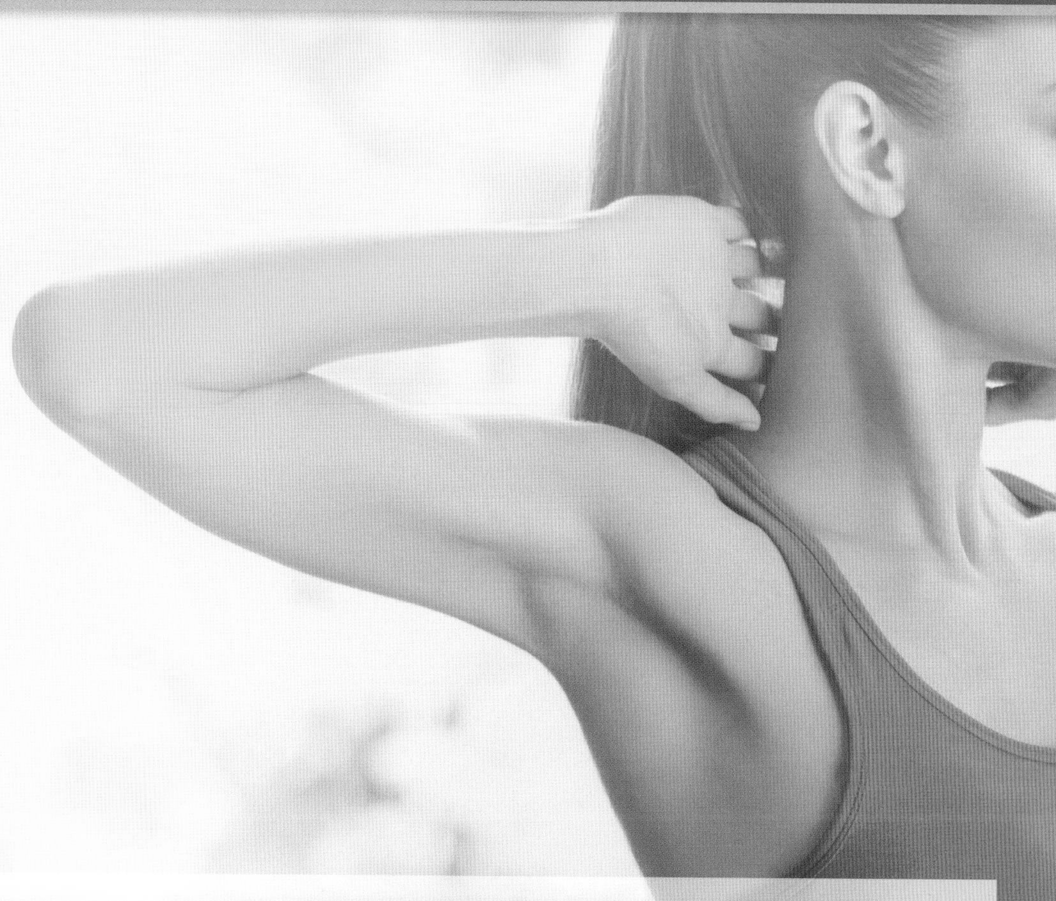

CHAPTER NINE

TOTAL-BODY EXERCISES

Complex, multi-joint exercises engage more muscle groups at once. Whether your goal is building strength, losing weight, or becoming more fit, increasing exercise complexity results in increased neuromuscular and cardiovascular challenge, and therefore greater gains. Major muscle groups working together in compound exercises burn more calories, increase strength, build more muscle, and maximize the efficiency of your workouts. By focusing on multi-joint exercises that work your entire body, you're stimulating the same muscles with one exercise that would otherwise require multiple targeted exercises.

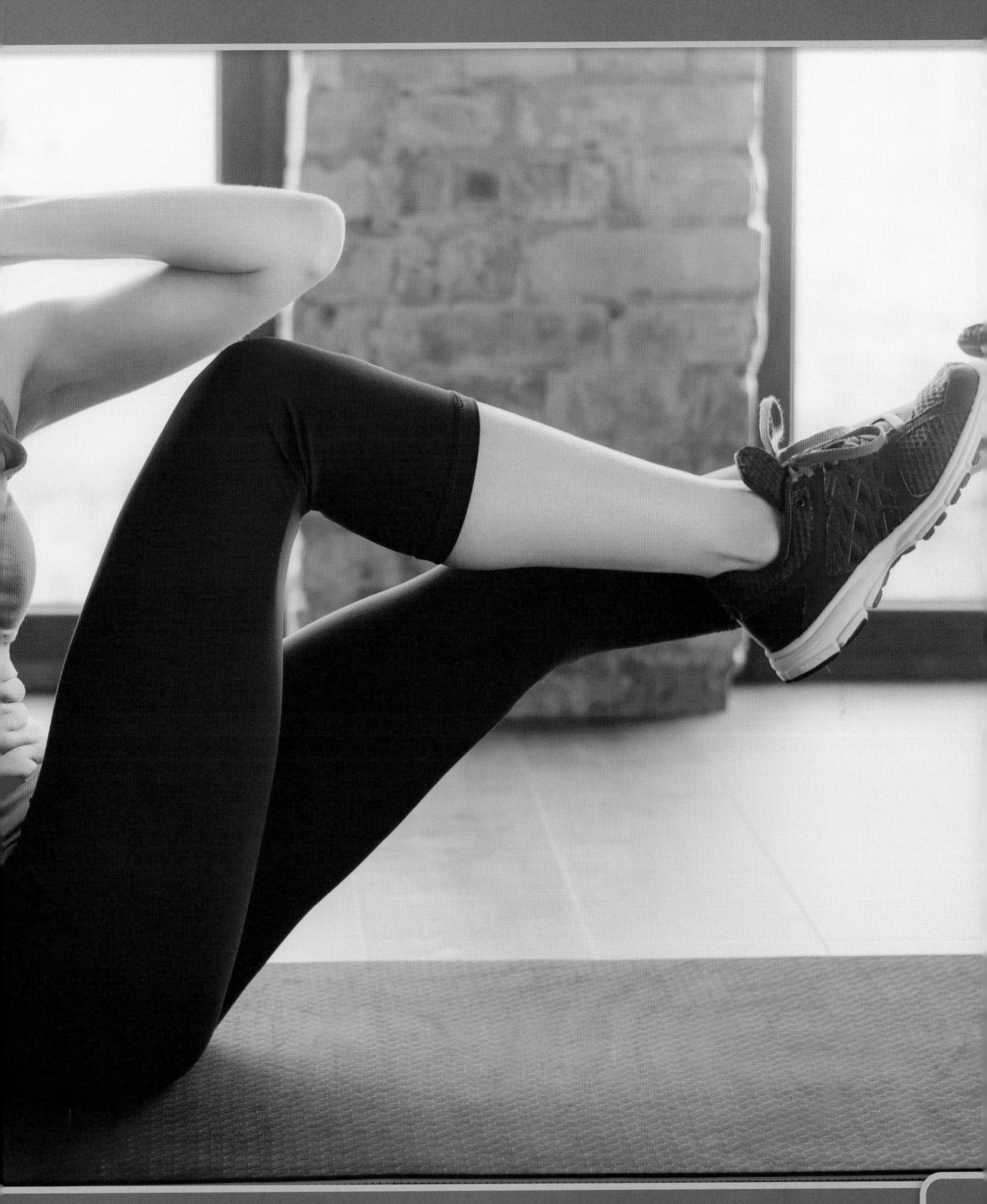

Slalom Skier

The Slalom Skier is an intense cardio exercise that gets your heart pumping and burns calories. It also strengthen the muscles of your chest, shoulders, arms, and legs.

HOW TO DO IT

- Begin in a high plank position with your feet together.
- Jump both feet to the left so that they land outside your left arm. Tuck your knees toward your chest while you jump.
- Jump your feet back to the leaning rest position, and then jump both feet back across your body to the right, landing with both feet outside your right arm and both knees bent toward your chest.
- Immediately jump back to the left. Both left and right equal one repetition. Continue alternating sides for the recommended repetitions.

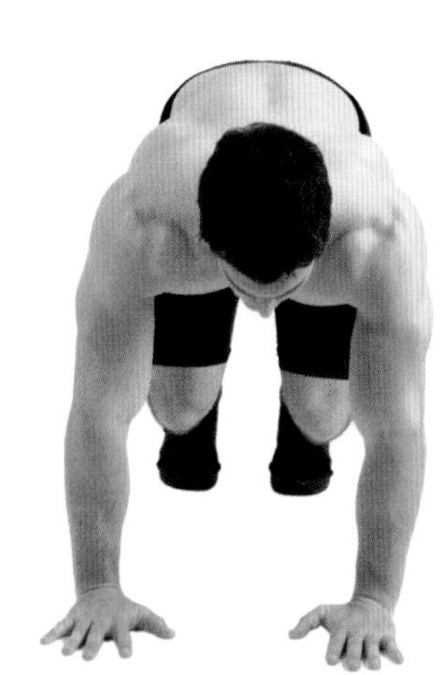

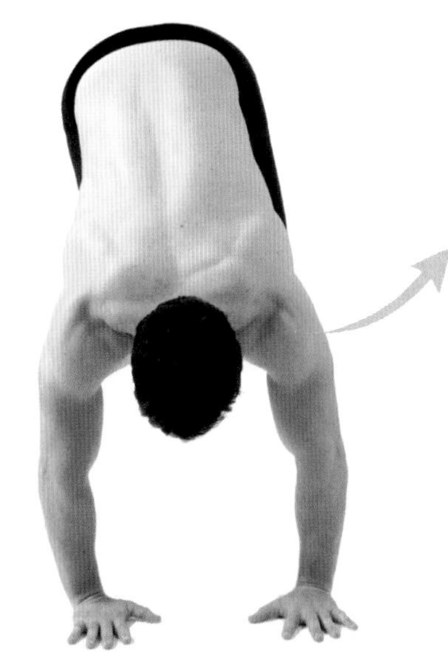

DO IT RIGHT

- When you jump your feet, bend your knees as though they were coming to your chest.
- Avoid jumping your feet too high, which places all of your body weight on your wrists.

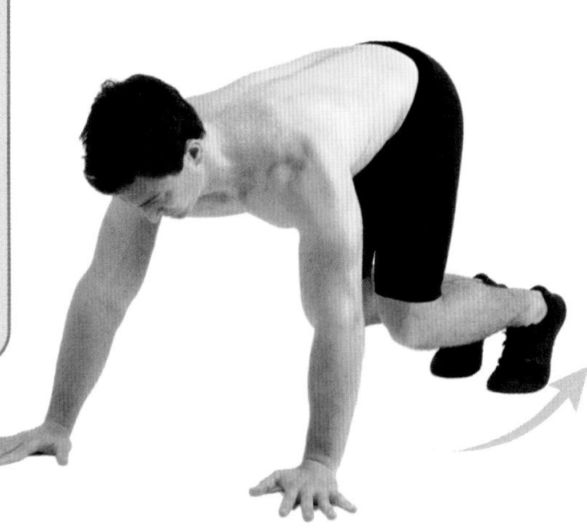

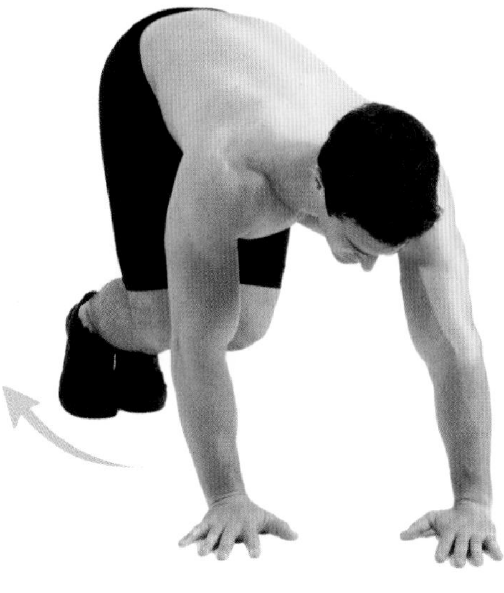

gluteus medius*
gluteus minimus*
adductor magnus
biceps femoris
semitendinosus
semimembranosus

pectoralis major
pectoralis minor*
biceps brachii

FACT FILE

TARGETS
- Chest
- Shoulders
- Arms
- Glutes
- Thighs
- Calves

TYPE
- Dynamic

BENEFITS
- Strengthens upper body and core
- Increases agility
- Improves coordination
- Increases cardiovascular endurance

CAUTIONS
- Wrist issues

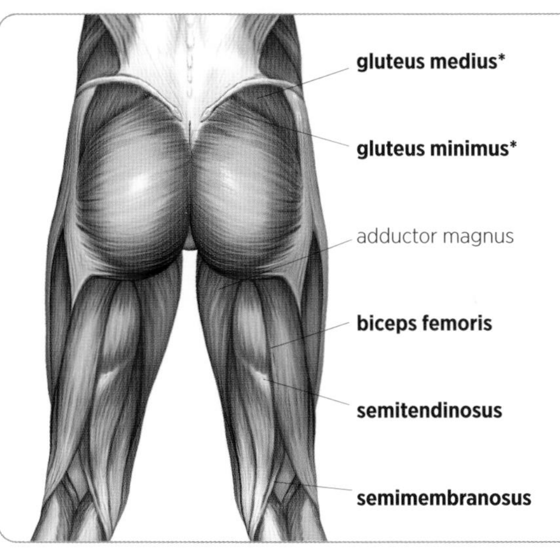

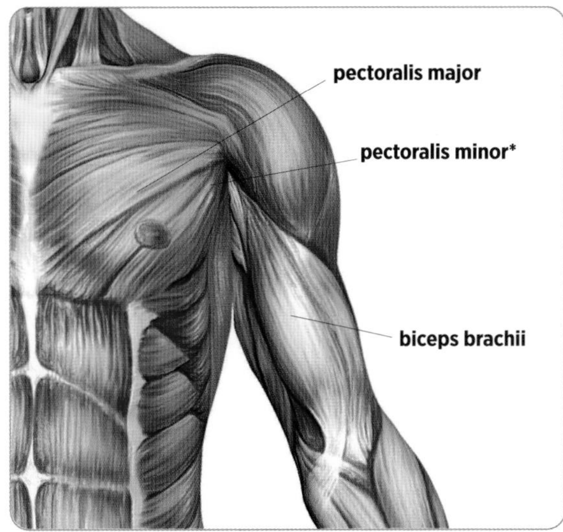

Annotation Key

Bold text indicates target muscles
Light text indicates other working muscles
* indicates deep muscles

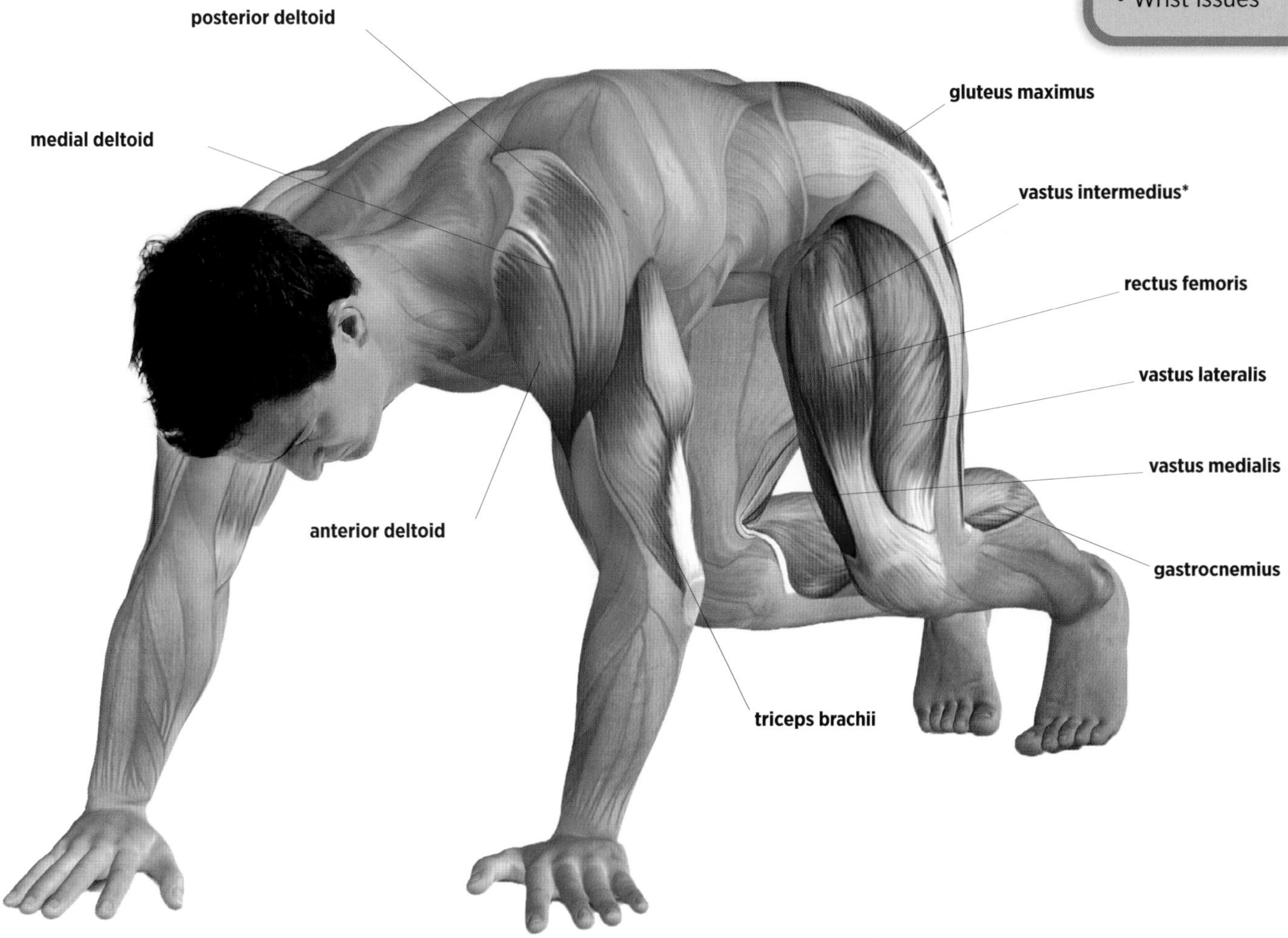

posterior deltoid
medial deltoid
anterior deltoid
triceps brachii
gluteus maximus
vastus intermedius*
rectus femoris
vastus lateralis
vastus medialis
gastrocnemius

Mountain Climber

The explosive Mountain Climber builds upper-body strength while giving your cardiovascular system an intense workout. It also helps hone your balance, coordination, and agility.

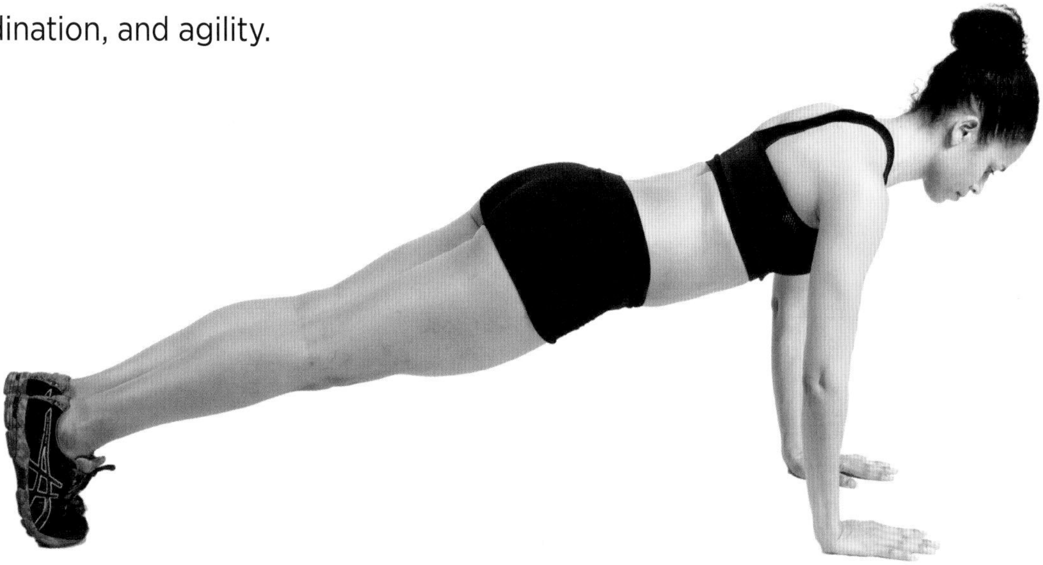

HOW TO DO IT

- Begin in a high plank position with your hands shoulder-width apart, your palms on the floor, your feet together, and your back straight.
- Bring your right knee in toward your chest. Rest the ball of your foot on the floor.
- Jump to switch your feet in the air, bringing your left foot in and your right foot back.
- Continue alternating your feet as fast as you can safely go for the recommended repetitions or time.

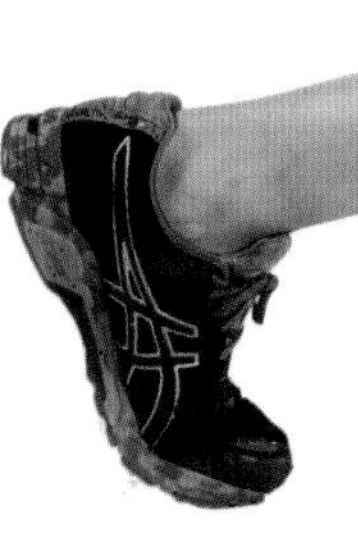

DO IT RIGHT

- Keep your back straight.
- Flare your hands out to ease shoulder stress.
- Avoid small leg movements; attempt to bring each knee to your chest.

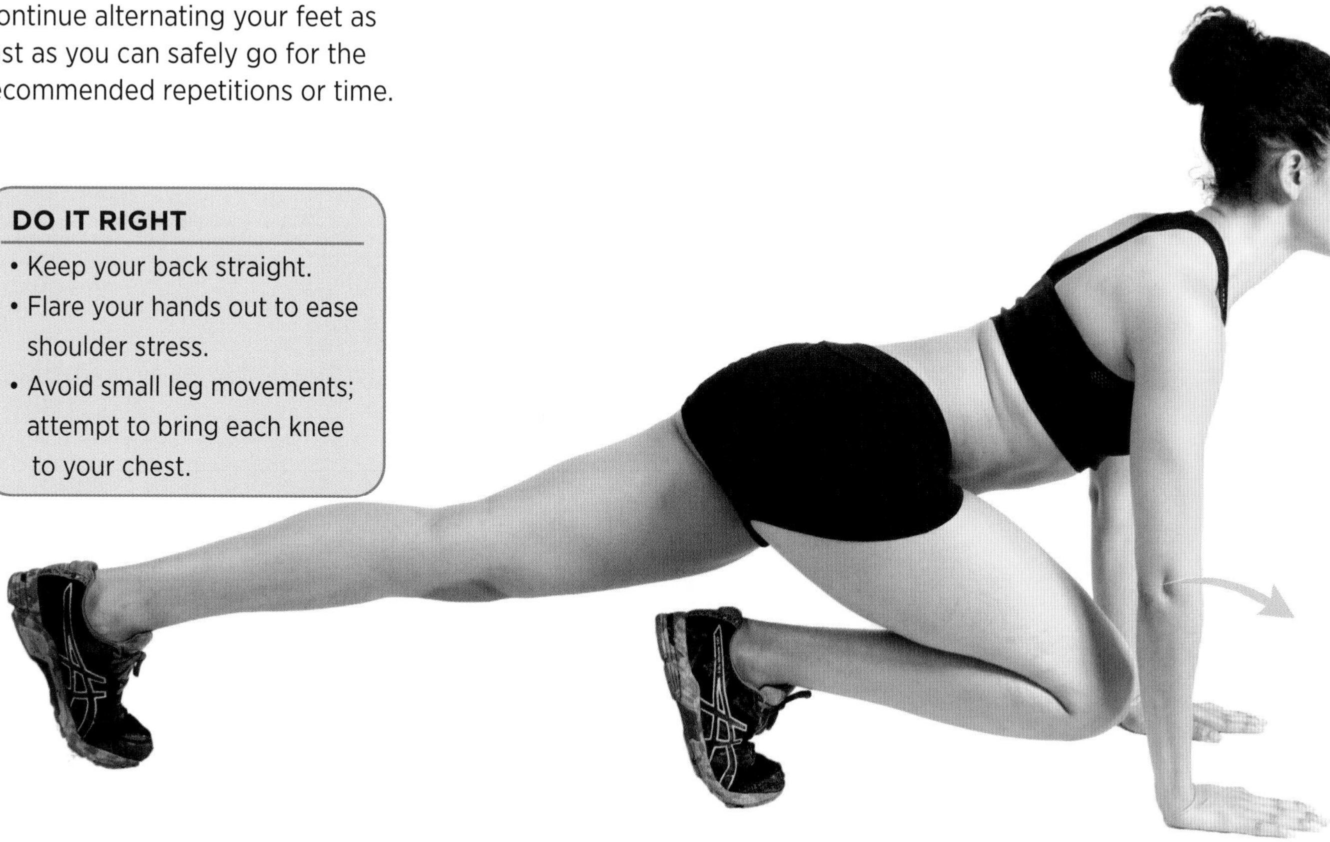

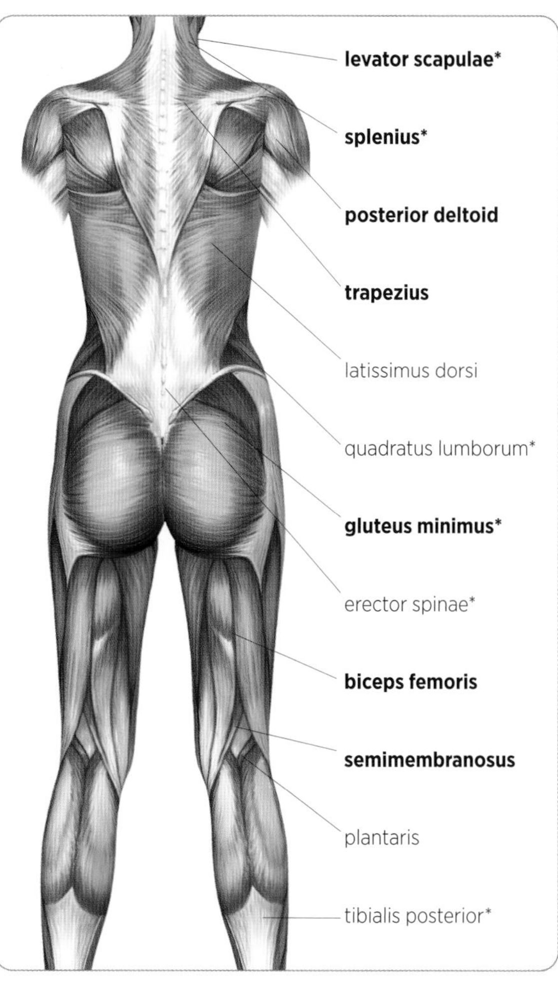

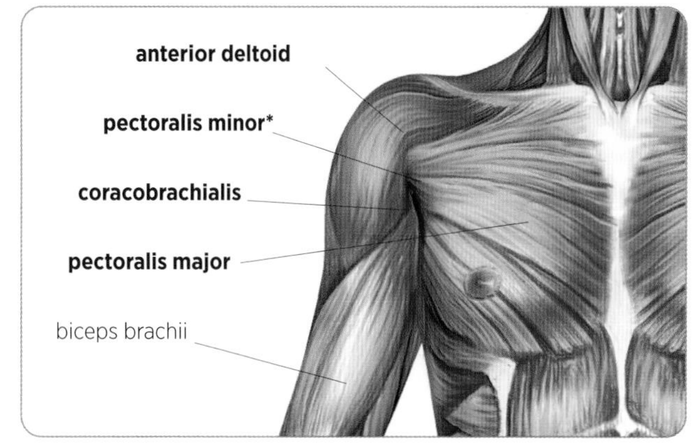

Annotation Key

Bold text indicates target muscles

Light text indicates other working muscles

* indicates deep muscles

FACT FILE

TARGETS

- Pectorals
- Triceps
- Deltoids
- Abdominals
- Back
- Hip flexors
- Quadriceps
- Hamstrings
- Glutes

TYPE

- Dynamic

BENEFITS

- Warms up muscles
- Improves coordination
- Strengthens and tones abdominals, chest, arms, and legs
- Increases cardiovascular endurance

CAUTIONS

- Shoulder issues
- Wrist issues

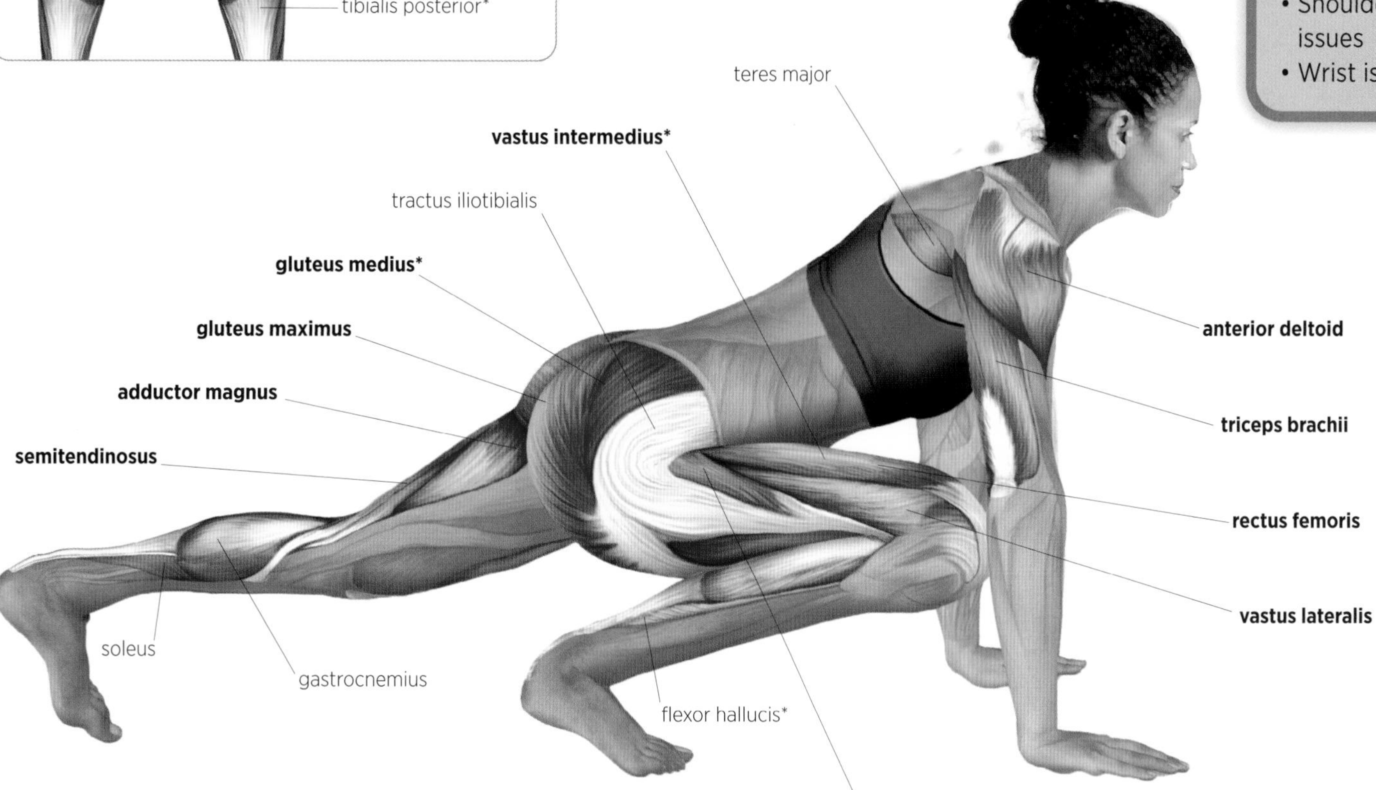

Roll-Up

A whole new way to get up in the morning, the Roll-Up is a dynamic full-body exercise that requires core control, lower-extremity power, and balance. This exercise will dynamically challenge your core.

HOW TO DO IT

- Lie faceup with your legs extended and your arms down by your sides.
- Flexing your shoulders, bring your arms above your head.
- With one explosive motion, swing your arms overhead to shoulder height and draw your knees in toward your stomach as you dynamically perform a sit-up. Place your feet on the floor as close to your buttocks as possible.
- Transfer your weight to your feet to come into a low squat. Once you establish balance, press your heels into the floor to rise into a standing position with your legs completely straight.
- Return to the starting position, and then repeat for the recommended repetitions.

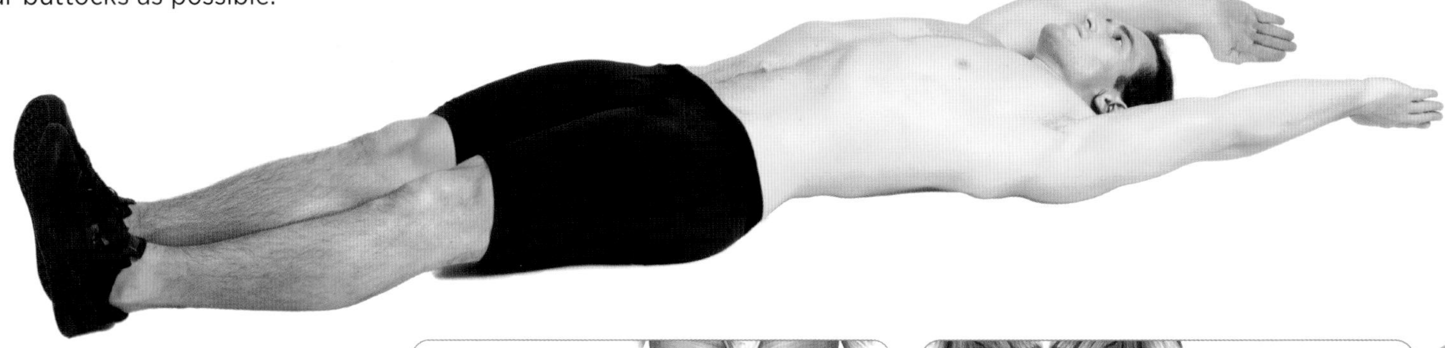

DO IT RIGHT

- Keep your body tight as you roll up.
- Throw your arms forward to transfer your body weight in front of you.
- Keep your back in a neutral position as you come up from the squat.

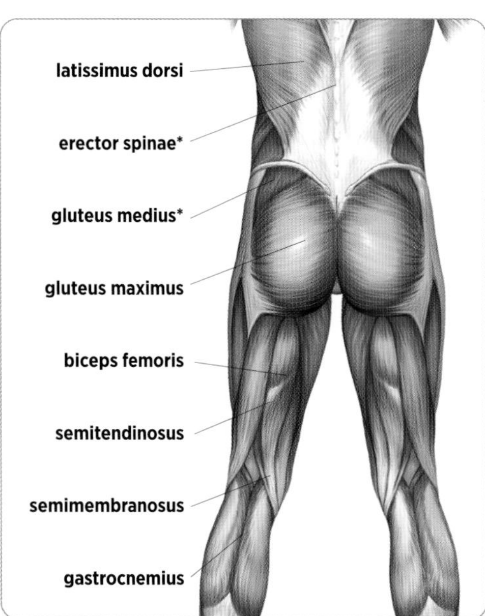

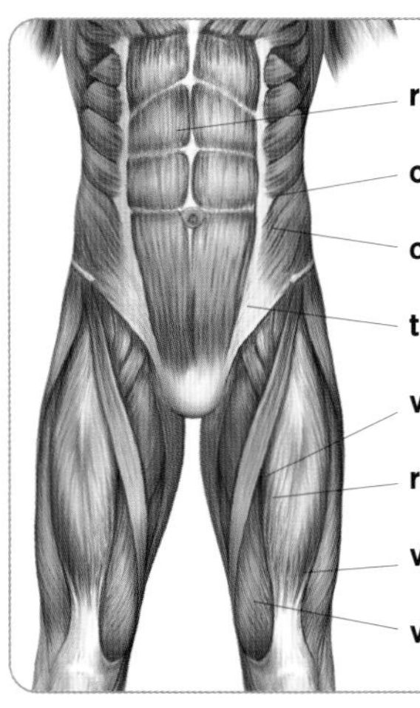

Annotation Key

Bold text indicates target muscles

Light text indicates other working muscles

* indicates deep muscles

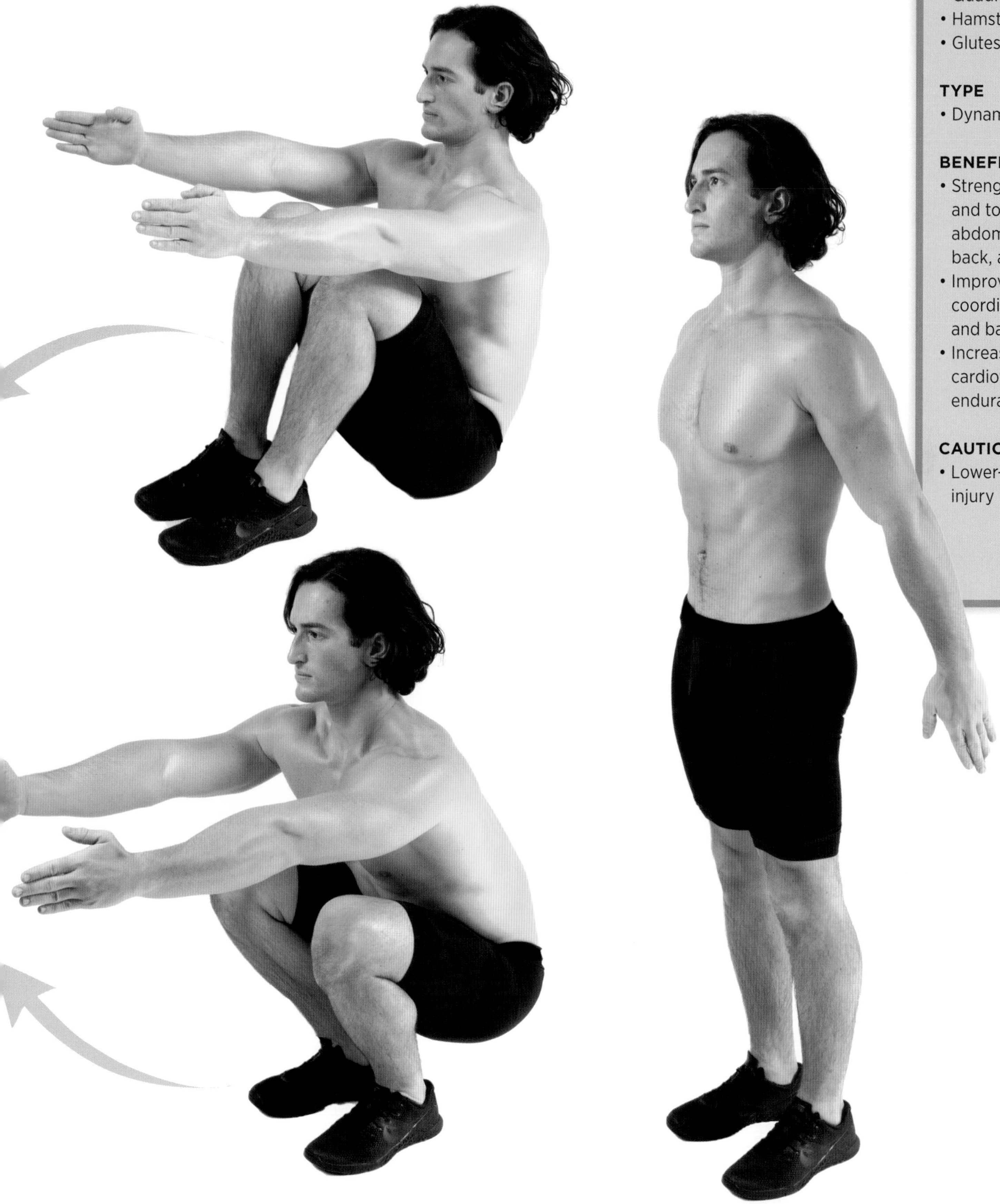

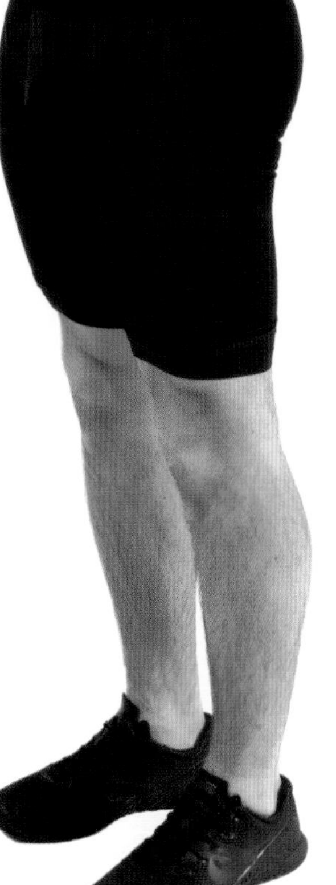

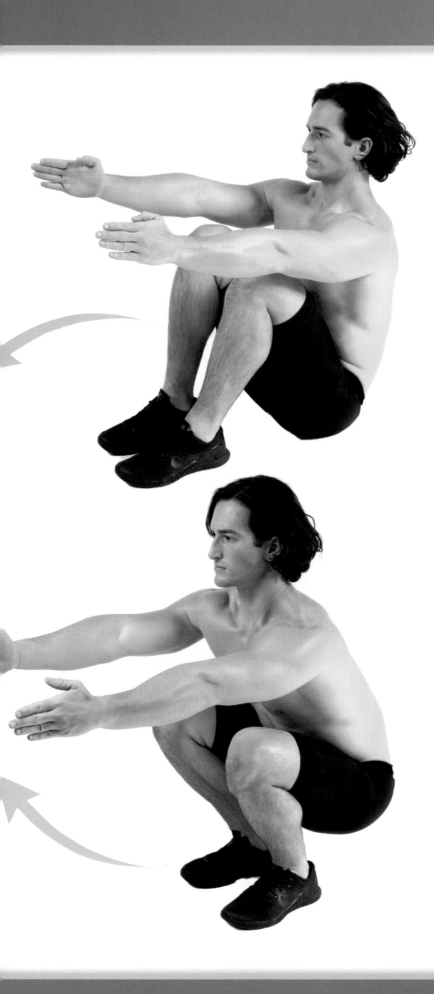

FACT FILE

TARGETS
- Abdominals
- Back
- Quadriceps
- Hamstrings
- Glutes

TYPE
- Dynamic

BENEFITS
- Strengthens and tones abdominals, back, and legs
- Improves coordination and balance
- Increases cardiovascular endurance

CAUTIONS
- Lower-back injury

Handstand Walk

The Handstand Walk is an advanced exercise that hits your entire body, demanding upper-body strength, as well as midline core and lower-extremity stability. Remember, just one hand after the other!

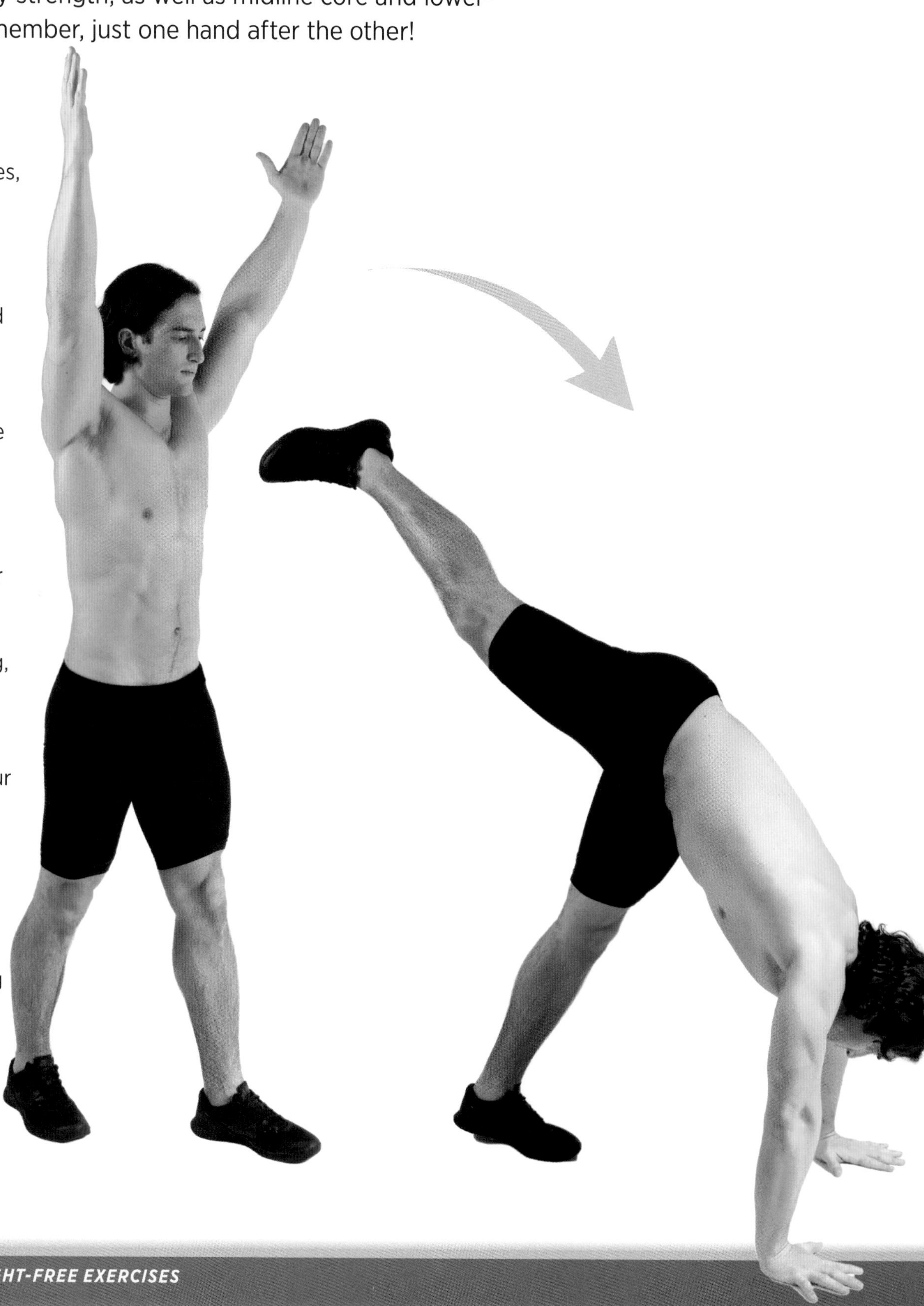

HOW TO DO IT

- Making sure you have plenty of space on all sides, stand with your feet hip-width apart.
- Raise your hands above your head, and then bend forward to place your hands on the floor in front of you just outside shoulders' width. Stabilize your palms on the floor with your fingers facing away from you.
- When ready, engage your core, and kick up into a handstand by extending one leg toward the ceiling, followed quickly by the other.
- Once in position, shift your body weight toward one side enough to be able to lift one hand and place in front of you.
- Repeat the step above, alternating hands, shifting your body weight over the planting arm. Repeat for the recommended repetitions, or for as long as you can maintain your form and balance.

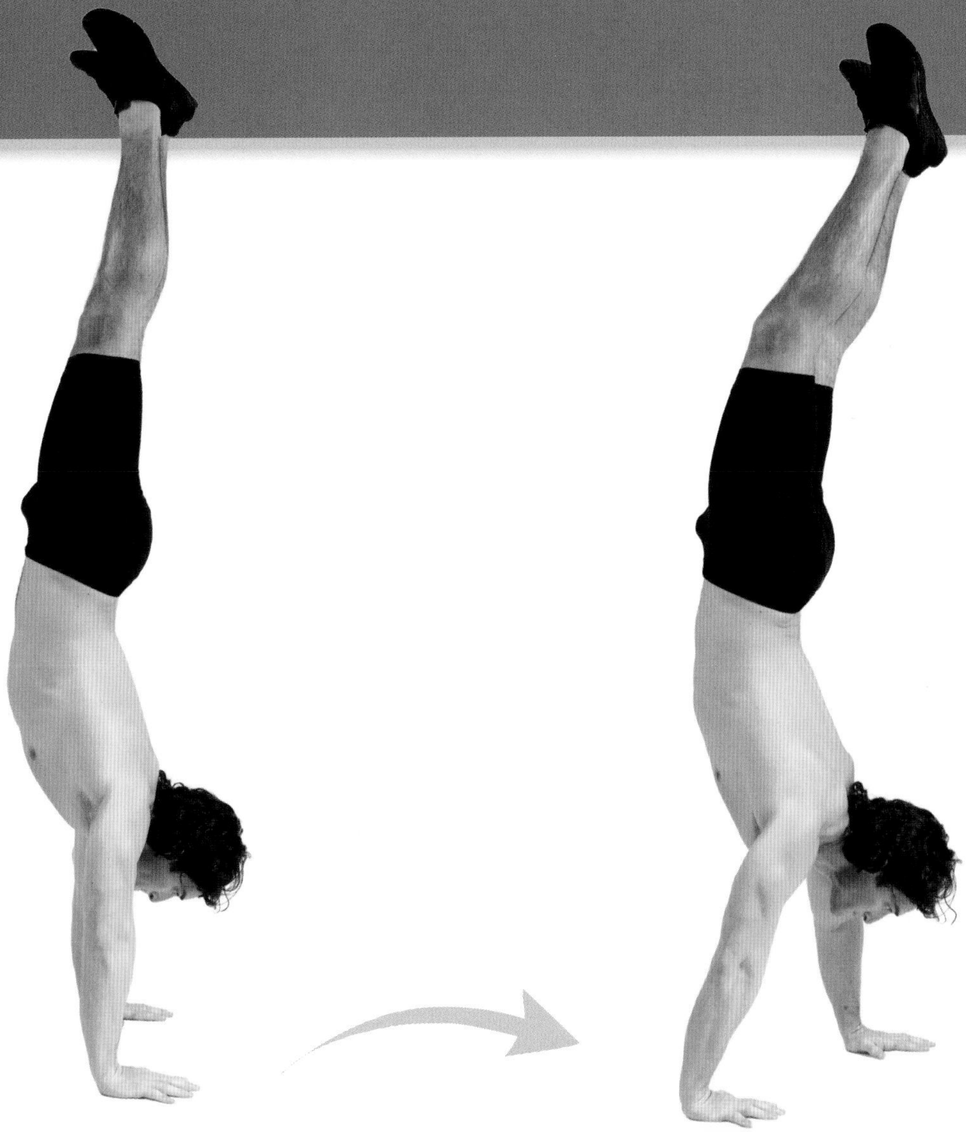

FACT FILE

TARGETS
- Quadriceps
- Glutes
- Triceps
- Deltoids
- Abdominals

TYPE
- Dynamic

BENEFITS
- Strengthens and tones arms, chest, and abdominals
- Improves balance and coordination

CAUTIONS
- Shoulder issues
- Wrist issues

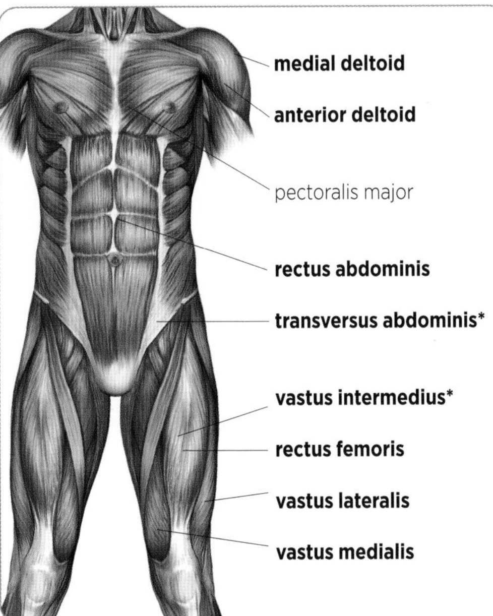

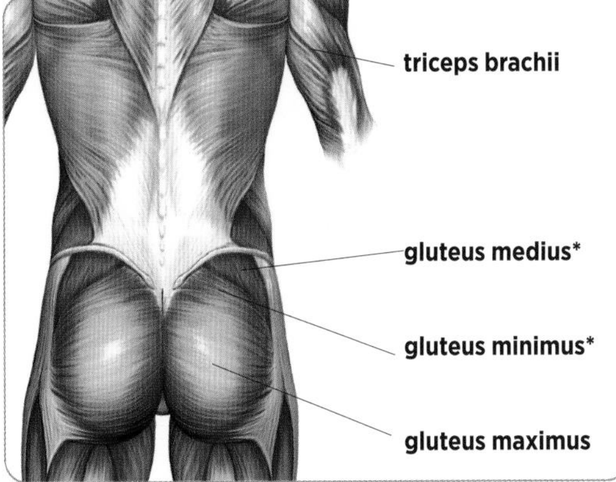

Annotation Key

Bold text indicates target muscles
Light text indicates other working muscles
* indicates deep muscles

DO IT RIGHT
- Keep your core engaged.
- Avoid excessive arching of your spine.
- Keep your shoulders shrugged and activated.
- Perfect the Handstand Push-Up (pages 192–93) before attempting this exercise, and use a spotter for safety.

Turkish Get-Up

A simple but powerful exercise, the Turkish Get-Up targets multiple muscles throughout your body, including those in the shoulders, core, thighs, back, glutes, and arms. It also increases hip stability and improves balance and coordination.

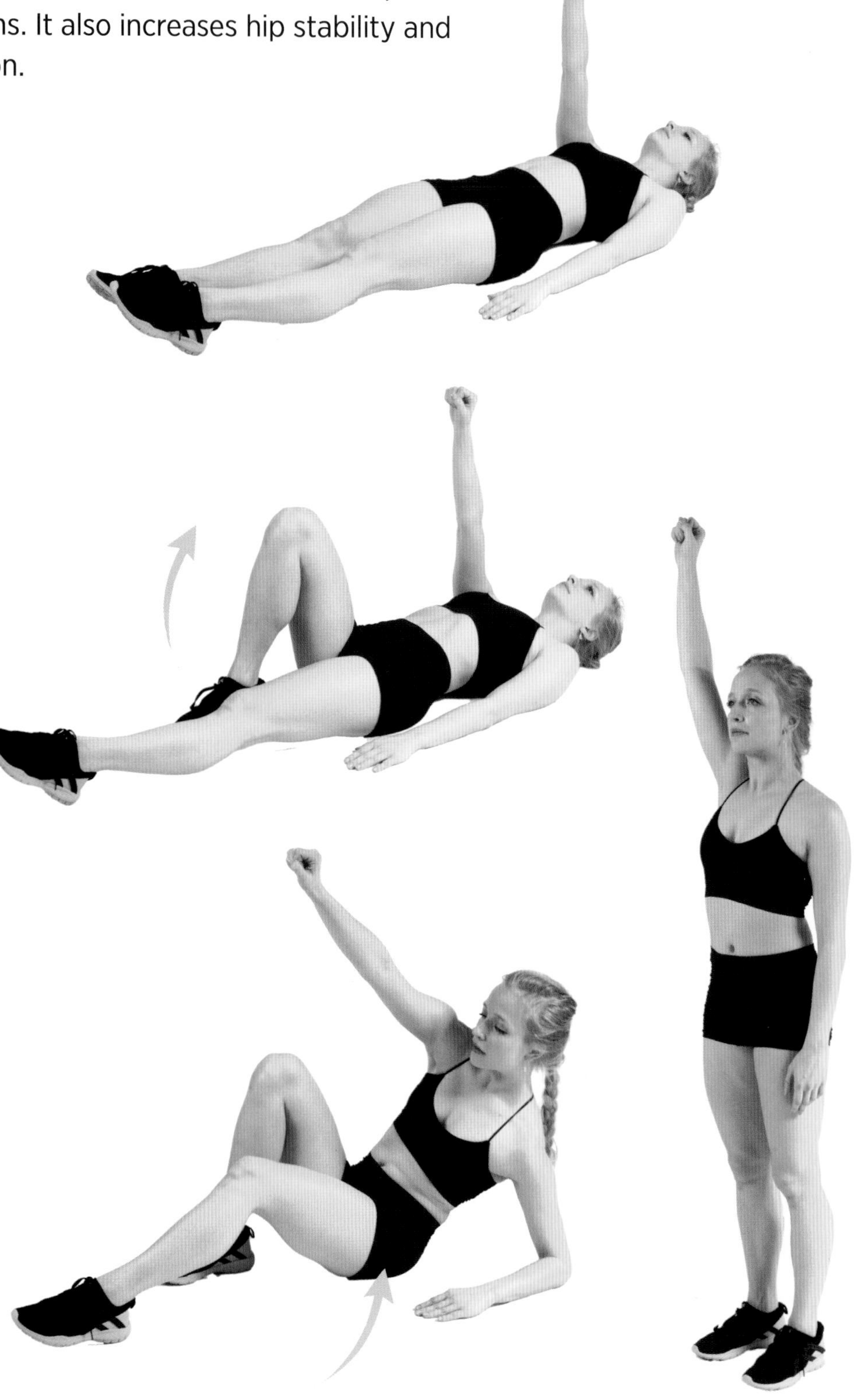

HOW TO DO IT

- Lie faceup with your legs together. Raise your right arm straight up above your chest and extend your left arm along your side.
- Flex your right knee, and place your right foot flat on the floor next to your left knee.
- Rotate your torso slightly to the left, and lift your shoulders off the floor. Plant your left hand on the floor, and lift yourself up to a sitting position.
- Lift your hips upward, and tuck your left leg under your body to support yourself on your left knee.
- Lift your left hand off the floor, and push through your right foot to rise to a standing position, keeping your right arm stretched over your head throughout the exercise.
- Return to the starting position, and then repeat on the other side. Repeat for the recommended repetitions.

DO IT RIGHT

- Keep your abs engaged throughout the movement.
- Avoid performing the exercise at excessive speed.

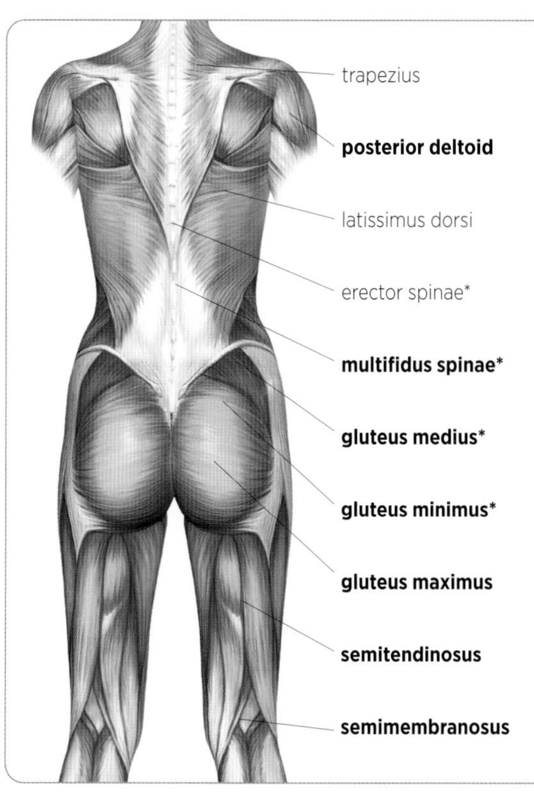

MODIFICATION

HARDER: Perform holding a hand weight or dumbbell in your raised hand.

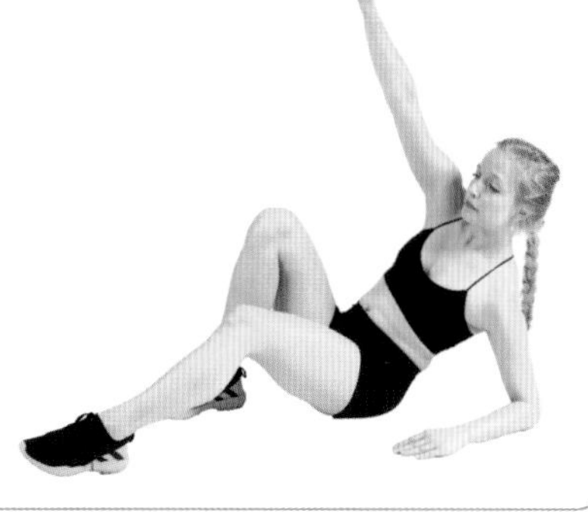

Annotation Key

Bold text indicates target muscles
Light text indicates other working muscles
* indicates deep muscles

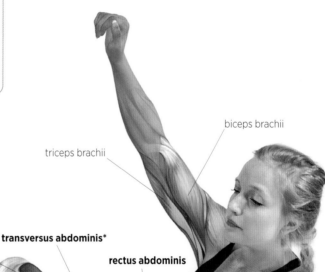

biceps brachii
triceps brachii
vastus medialis
transversus abdominis*
rectus abdominis
anterior deltoid
rectus femoris
sartorius
medial deltoid
vastus lateralis
obliquus externus
brachialis
obliquus internus*
biceps femoris
vastus intermedius*
tensor fasciae latae

FACT FILE

TARGETS
- Shoulders
- Core
- Thighs
- Glutes
- Upper back
- Triceps

TYPE
- Dynamic

BENEFITS
- Strengthens entire body
- Increases hip stability
- Improves balance and coordination

CAUTIONS
- Back pain

EQUIPMENT
- Optional: Hand weight or dumbbell for modification.

Forearm Plank

This form of the Plank-Up (pages 180-81) is a classic choice for the core, strengthening and stabilizing all of its muscles. It also builds extra strength into your lower back.

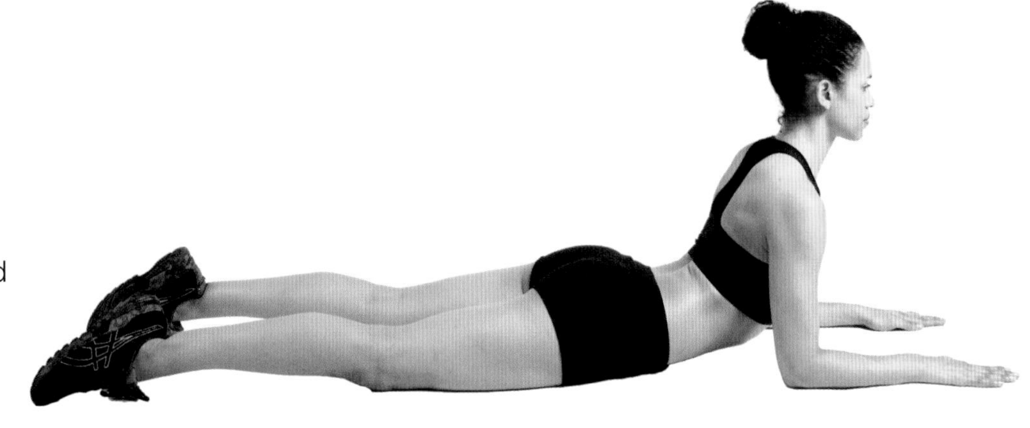

HOW TO DO IT

- Lie on your stomach on the floor, with your legs extended behind you and your torso raised off the floor. Bend your arms so that your forearms and palms rest flat on the floor.
- Bend your knees, supporting your weight between your knees and your forearms, and then push through with your forearms to bring your shoulders up toward the ceiling as you straighten your legs. Your toes are curled under.

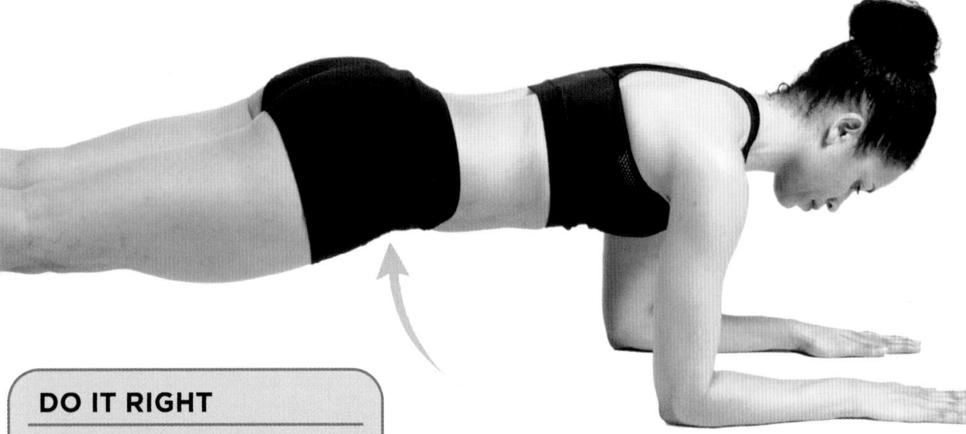

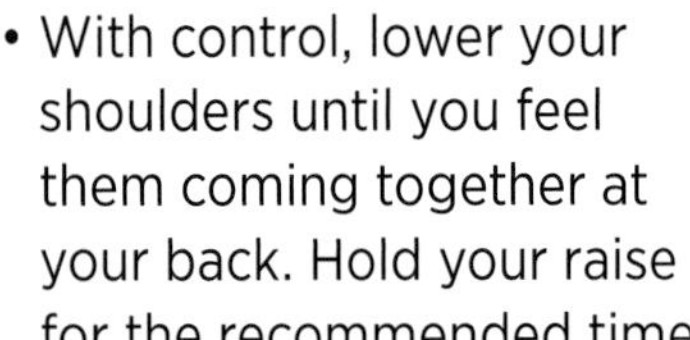

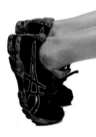

- With control, lower your shoulders until you feel them coming together at your back. Hold your raise for the recommended time.

DO IT RIGHT

- Keep your abs tight.
- Keep your body in a straight line.
- Keep your neck lengthened.
- Avoid allowing your shoulders to collapse into your shoulder joints.
- Avoid arching your neck.
- Avoid allowing your back to sag.

FACT FILE

TARGETS
- Abdominals
- Core
- Back

TYPE
- Static

BENEFITS
- Strengthens and stabilizes core

CAUTIONS
- Shoulder injury
- Severe back pain

MODIFICATION

HARDER: While in the plank position, lift and lower your legs one at a time. Keep the rest of your body still and your abs engaged throughout.

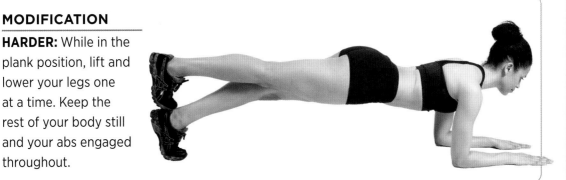

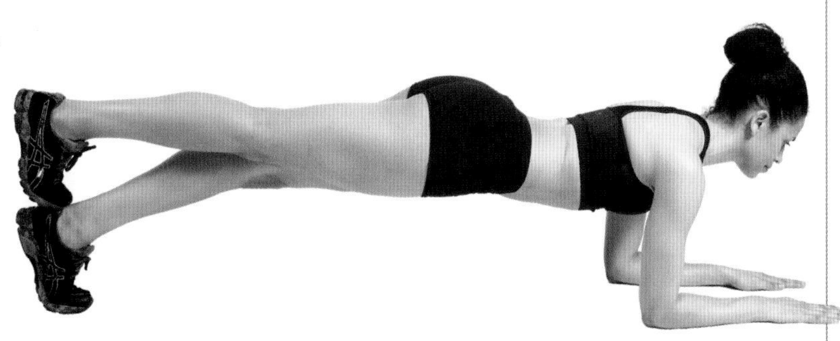

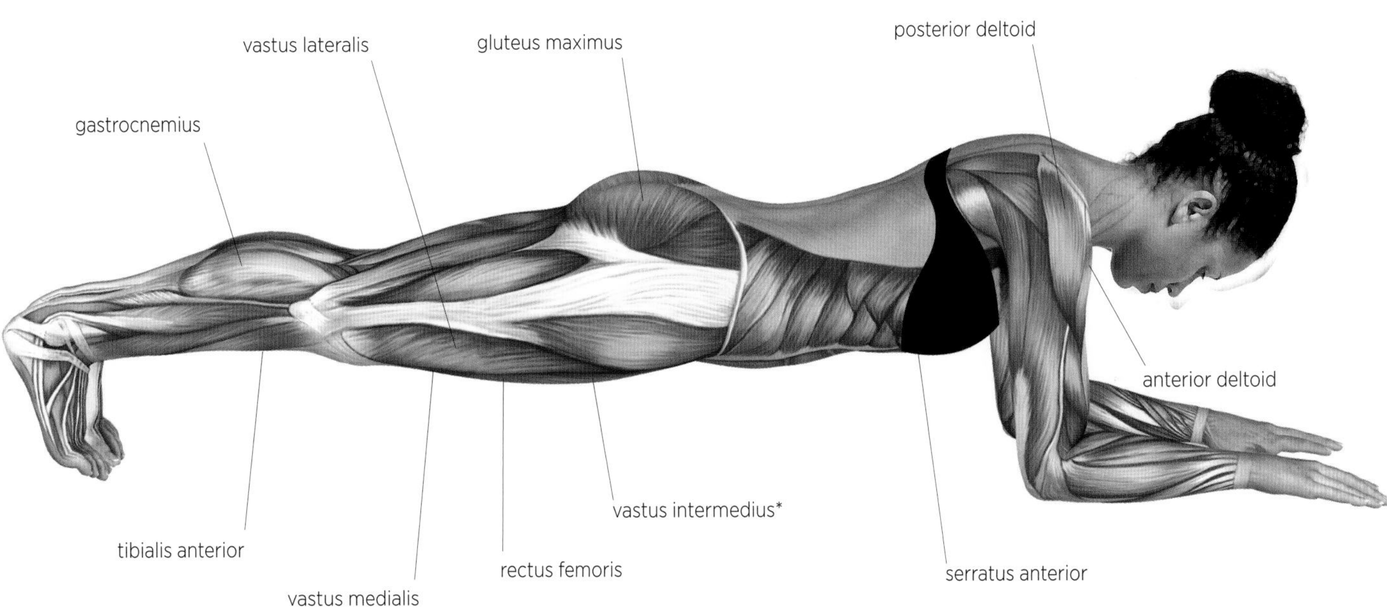

Annotation Key

Bold text indicates target muscles
Light text indicates other working muscles
* indicates deep muscles

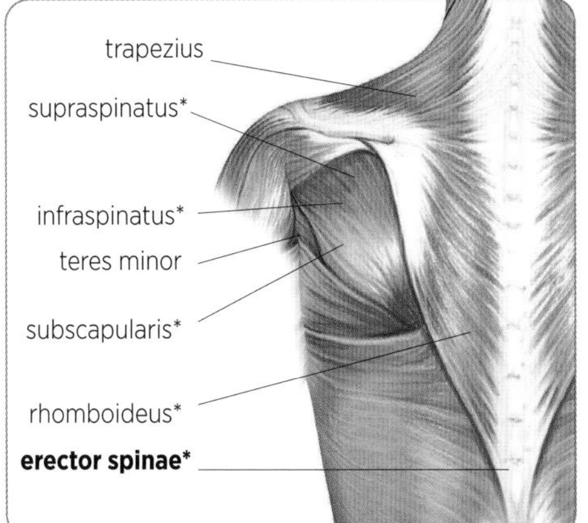

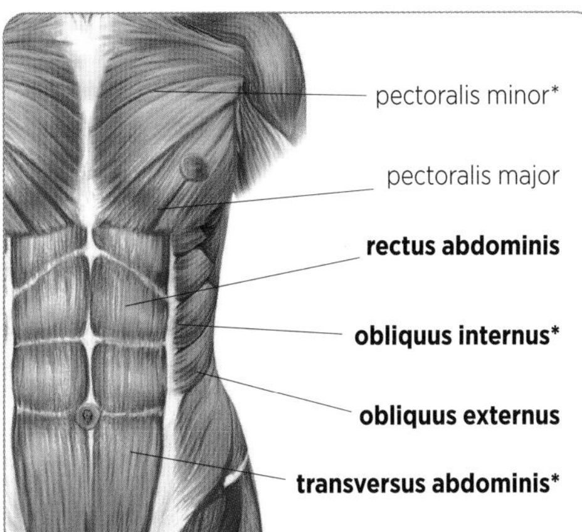

Up-Down

The Up-Down is a multiphase exercise designed to tax your cardiovascular system by using almost all of your muscles. It has the added benefit of increasing your coordination and agility.

HOW TO DO IT

- Run in place, bringing your knees waist-high with each step.
- Drop down and touch your chest to the floor.
- Immediately stand back up and continue running with high knees as quickly as possible.
- Repeat for the recommended repetitions.

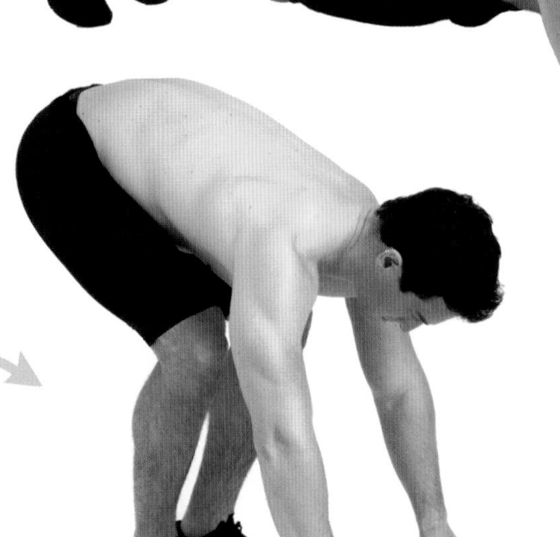

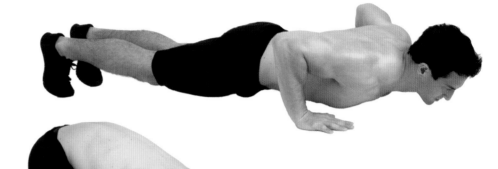

DO IT RIGHT

- Keep your knees at waist level while running in place.
- Avoid landing on your chest—allow your hands to contact the floor first, and then lower onto your chest.
- Avoid flopping onto the ground—move with control.

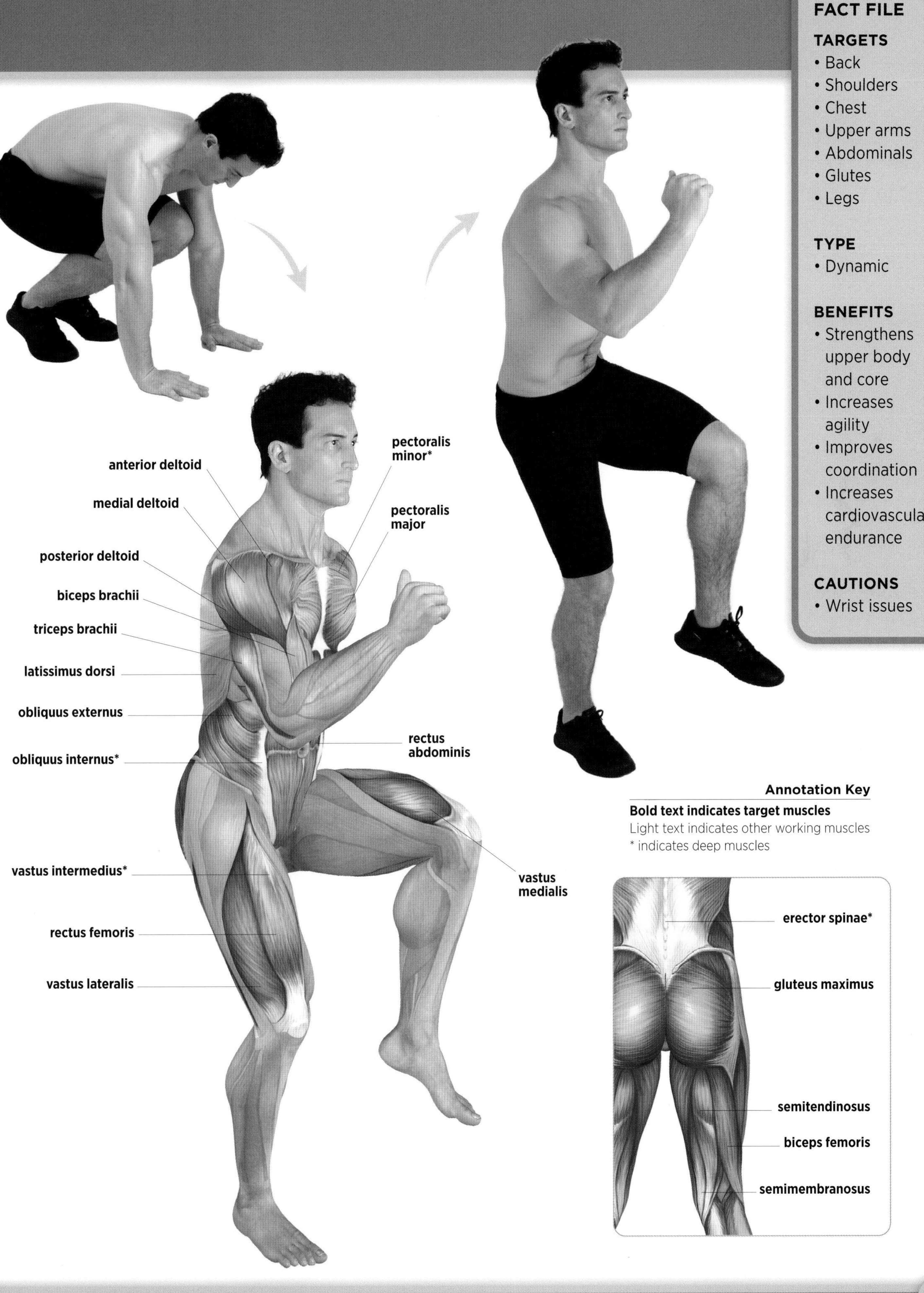

FACT FILE

TARGETS
- Back
- Shoulders
- Chest
- Upper arms
- Abdominals
- Glutes
- Legs

TYPE
- Dynamic

BENEFITS
- Strengthens upper body and core
- Increases agility
- Improves coordination
- Increases cardiovascular endurance

CAUTIONS
- Wrist issues

Annotation Key

Bold text indicates target muscles
Light text indicates other working muscles
* indicates deep muscles

T-Stabilization

T-Stabilization, another advanced variation on the traditional Plank, is a proven exercise for targeting your abdominals, including your obliques, as well as your hips and lower back.

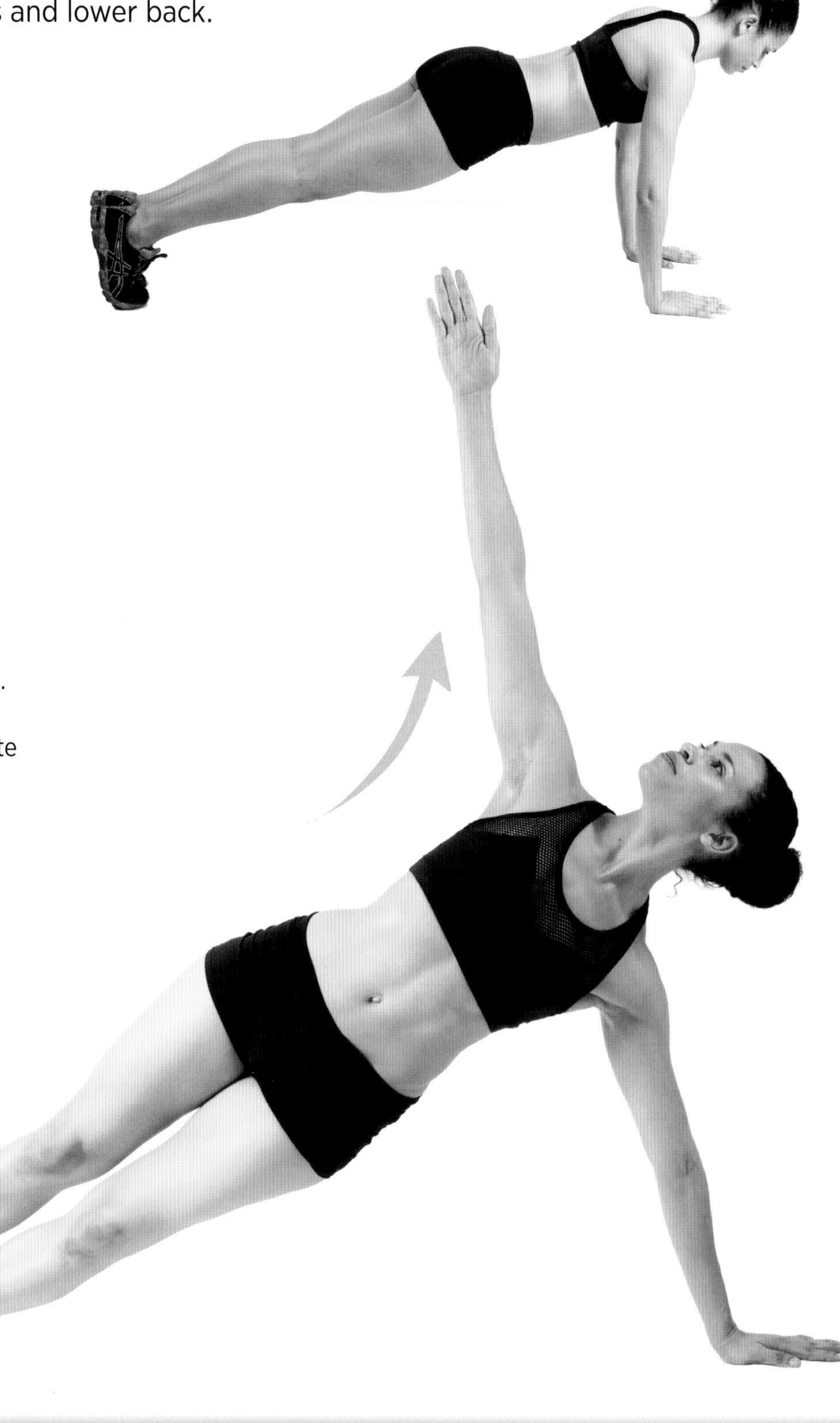

HOW TO DO IT

- Begin in a raised Plank position (pages 180–81). Your hands should be shoulder-width apart, palms on the floor with fingers pointing forward, feet together with toes tucked under, and your back straight.
- Turn your right-hand hip to one side, stacking your right foot on top of the left and raising your right arm across your body until you are pointing toward the ceiling. If you feel stable, look up toward your raised hand.
- Hold for the recommended time. Lower, returning to your raised plank, and repeat on the opposite side for the recommended repetitions.

DO IT RIGHT

- Keep your body in one straight line.
- Avoid arching or bridging your back.

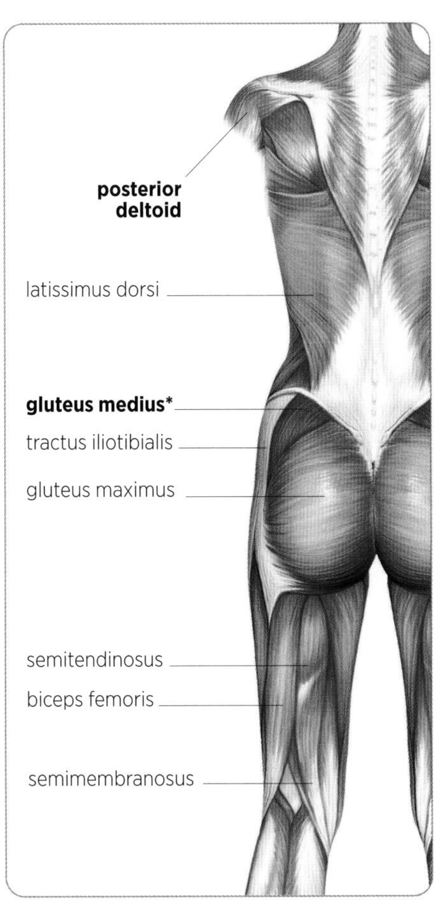

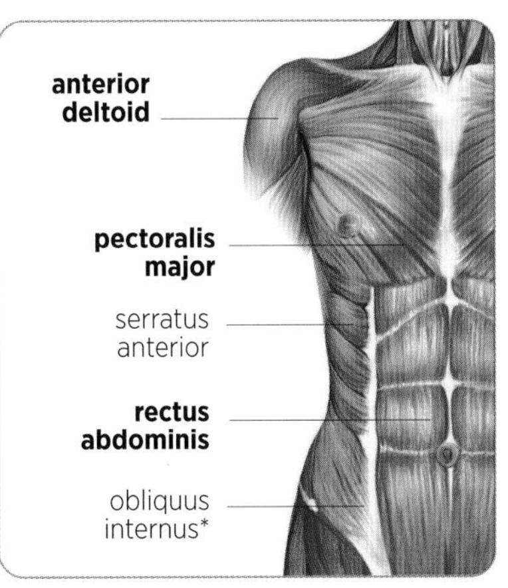

Annotation Key

Bold text indicates target muscles

Light text indicates other working muscles

* indicates deep muscles

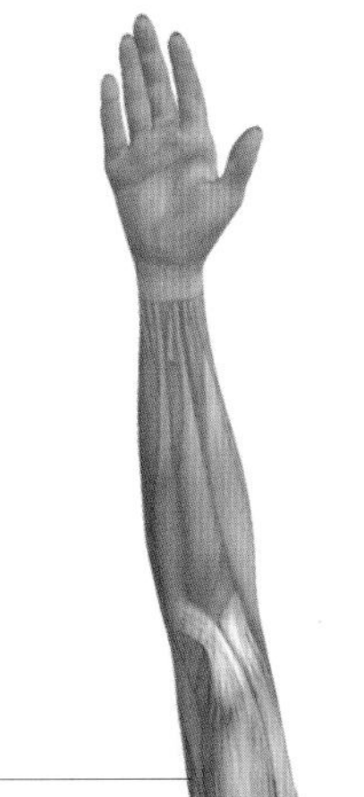

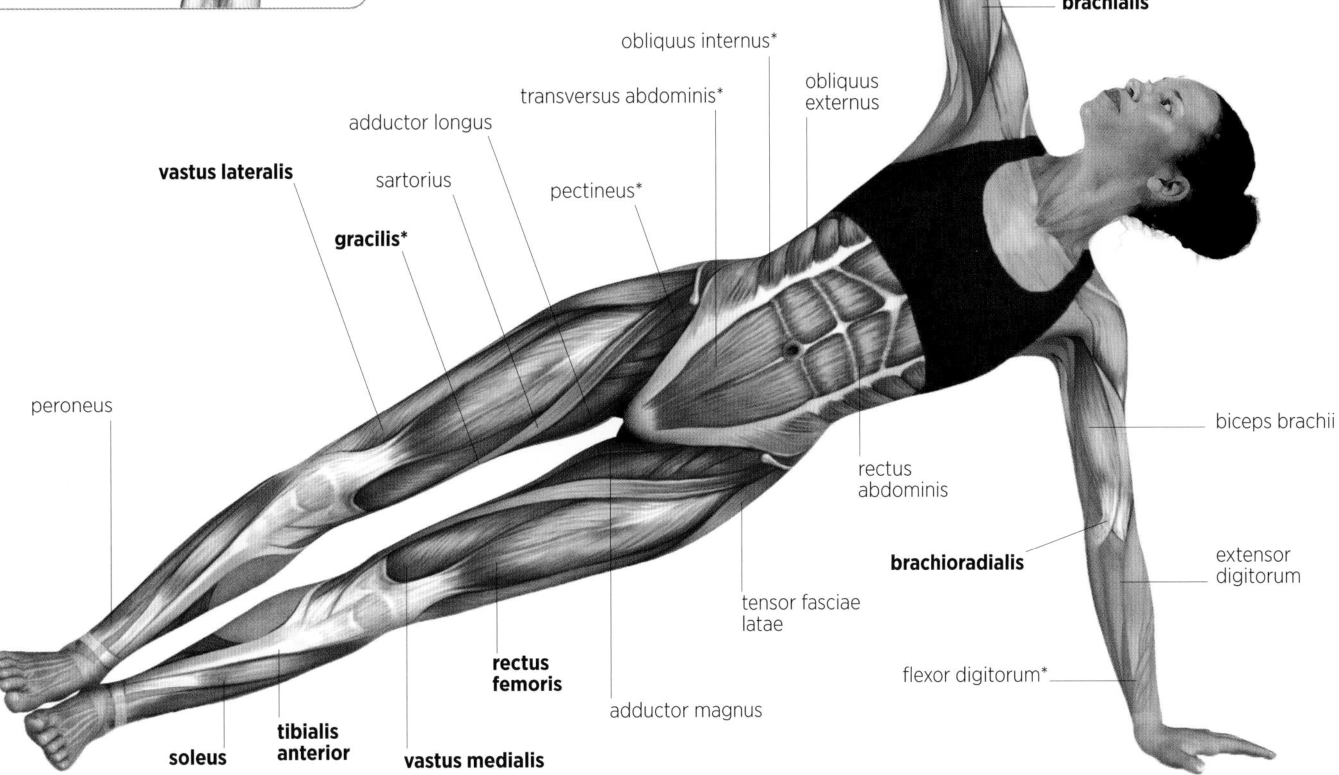

FACT FILE

TARGETS

- Shoulders and chest
- Triceps and elbow flexors
- Back
- Abdominals
- Glutes
- Legs

TYPE

- Dynamic

BENEFITS

- Stabilizes spine and core
- Strengthens leg abductors and adductors
- Strengthens back

CAUTIONS

- Shoulder issues
- Neck issues
- Wrist pain

Side Plank with Reach-Under

In Side Plank with Reach-Under, strength lies in stillness rather than in motion. As you maintain the static position of your torso and legs while moving one of your arms, you are effectively strengthening your abs, lower back, and shoulders.

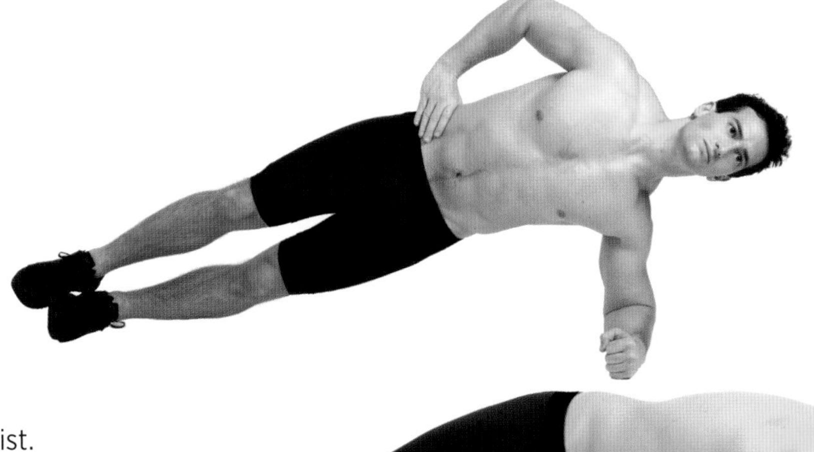

HOW TO DO IT

- Lie on your left side, with your legs extended and your right leg stacked on top of your left.
- Bend your left arm to a 90-degree angle with your fist on the floor, knuckles pointing forward. Rest your right arm along the side of your body or put your right hand on your waist.
- Push into the floor with your left hand and forearm, and raise your hips off the floor until your body forms a straight line.
- Twist your upper torso toward the floor as you reach your right arm under your chest as far as you can stretch.
- Twist your upper torso back to the front as you extend your right arm toward the ceiling.
- Repeat for the recommended repetitions, and then repeat on the opposite side for the recommended repetitions.

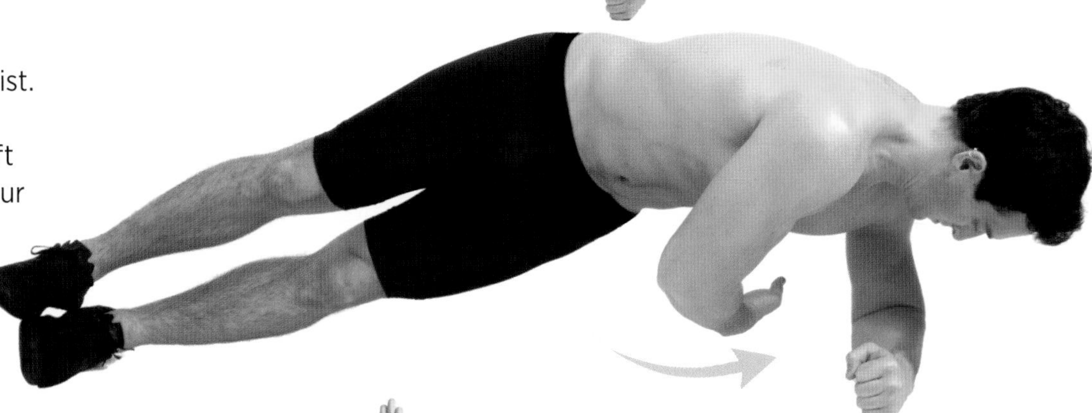

DO IT RIGHT

- Push equally from your forearm and hip as you raise your body.
- Allow your head and neck to follow the movement of your torso, so you look toward the floor during the reach-under and straight ahead in the finished position with your top arm extended.
- Keep your feet flexed and stacked.
- Avoid placing too much strain on your shoulders.
- Avoid losing your alignment when your top arm is extended.

FACT FILE

TARGETS
- Abdominals
- Back
- ITB
- Elbow flexors

TYPE
- Dynamic

BENEFITS
- Strengthens and stabilizes core
- Builds endurance
- Strengthens shoulders

CAUTIONS
- Neck issues
- Rotator cuff injury

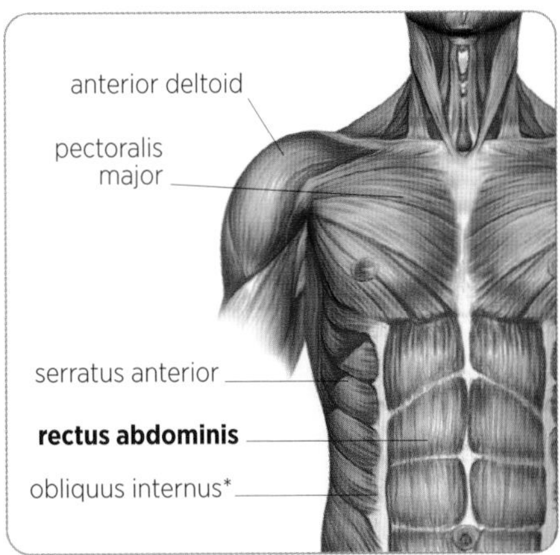

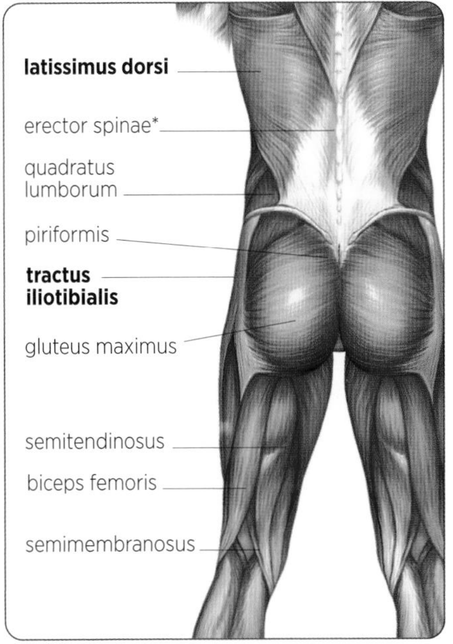

Annotation Key

Bold text indicates target muscles
Light text indicates other working muscles
* indicates deep muscles

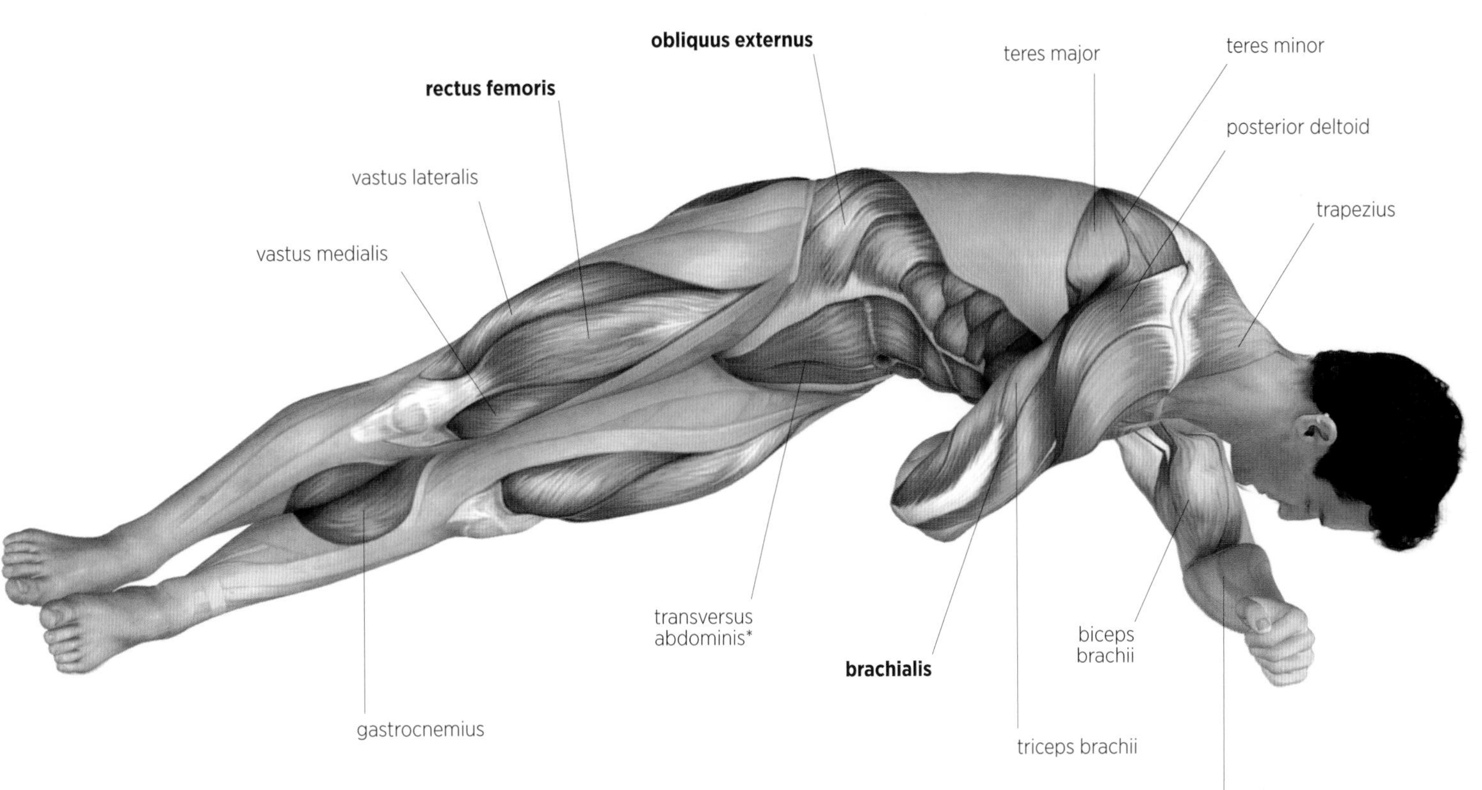

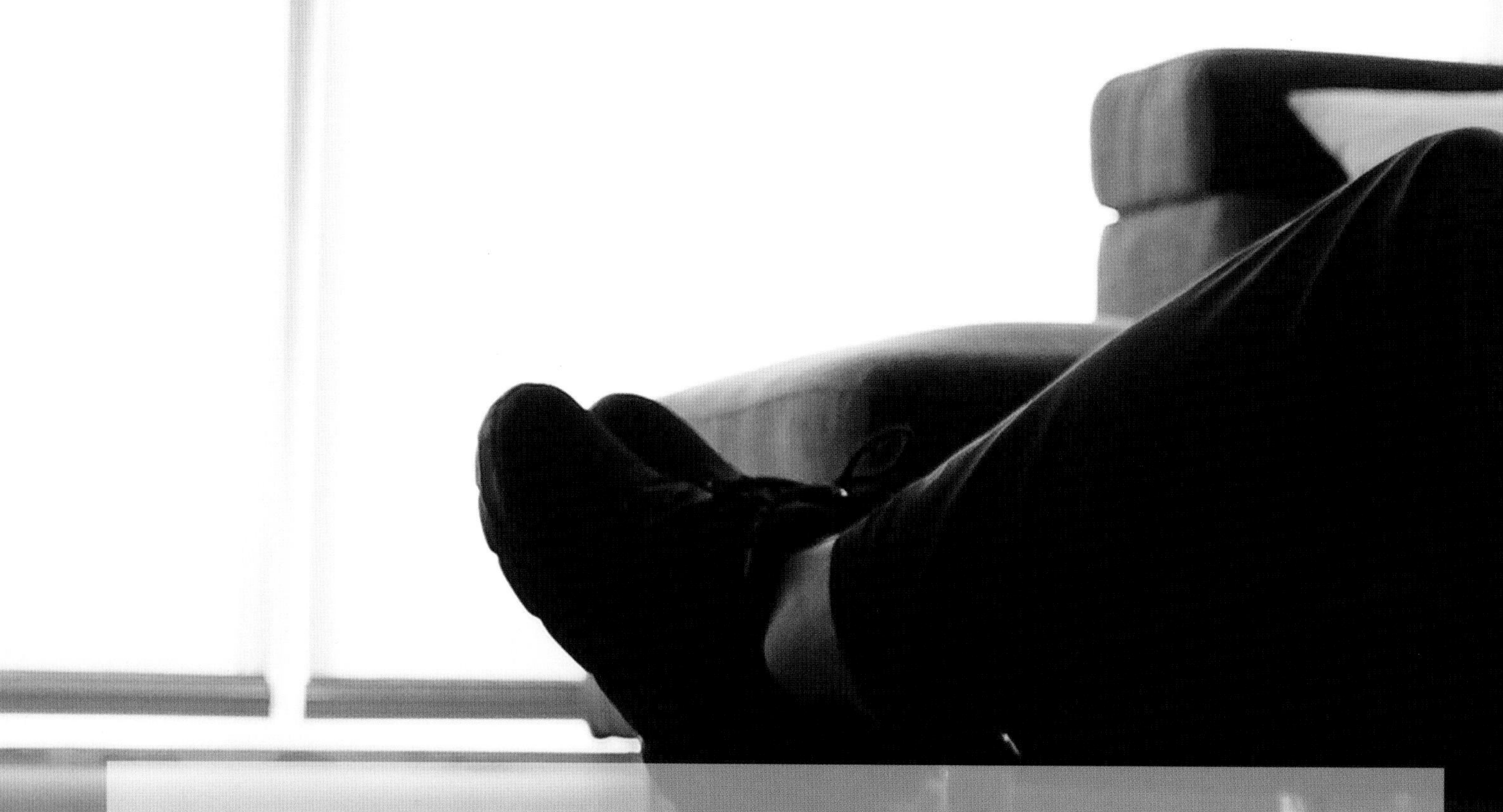

CHAPTER TEN

WORKOUT ROUTINES

Once you've familiarized yourself with the featured exercises, turn to this chapter to learn how to put them together in targeted Weight-Free routines. Each routine has a specific purpose, but all offer benefits beyond that. There's something here for all levels of fitness and experience, and remember that you can switch things down or up by changing repetitions or times, or by following the modifications suggested in the book.

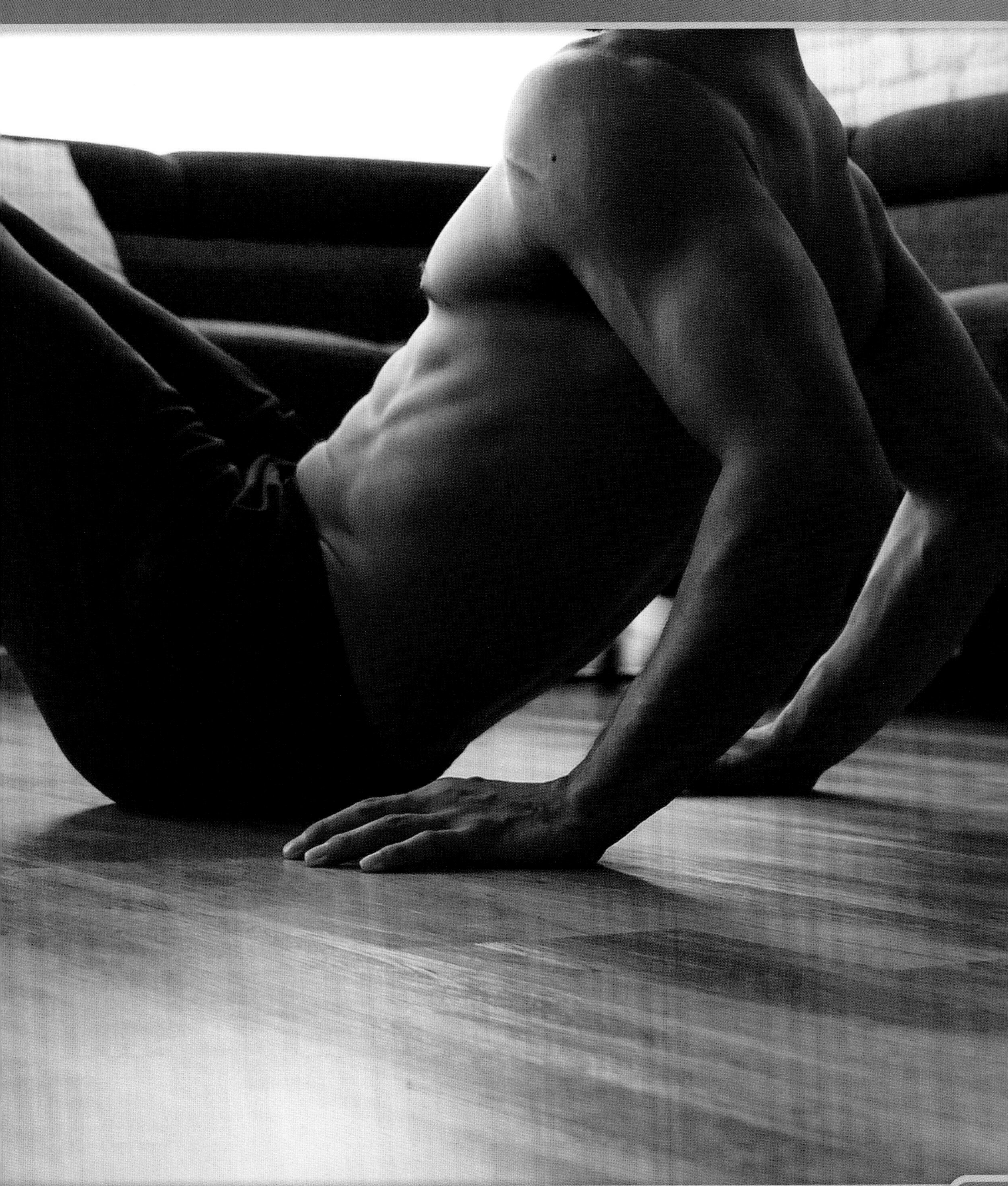

New Day Routine

Designed to get you moving and loose in order to seize the day.

1 GOOD MORNING STRETCH

Pages 18–19

- Perform 30–45 seconds.

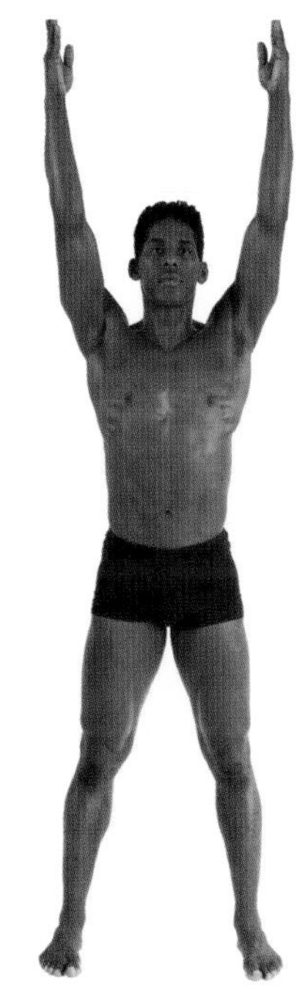

2 FLEXION STRETCH

Page 24

- Perform for 30 seconds.

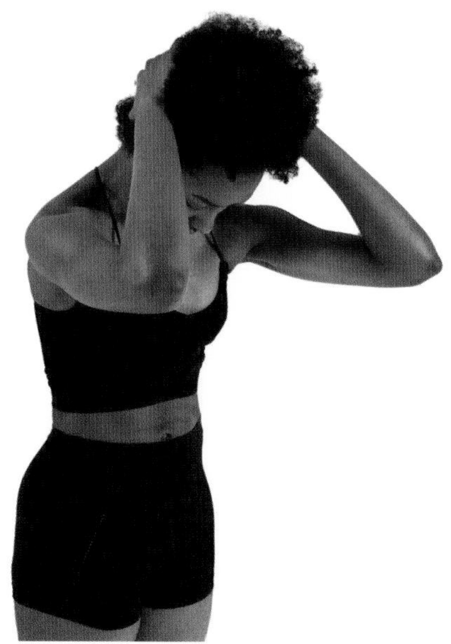

3 STANDING FORWARD BEND

Pages 68–69

- Perform 30–45 seconds.

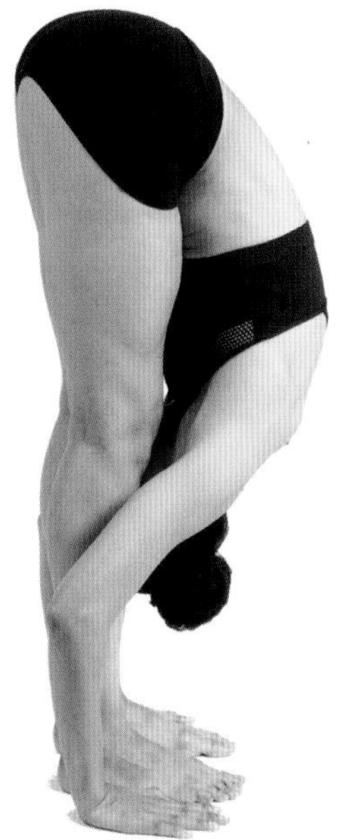

4 STANDING QUADRICEPS STRETCH

Page 40

- Perform for 30 seconds per leg.

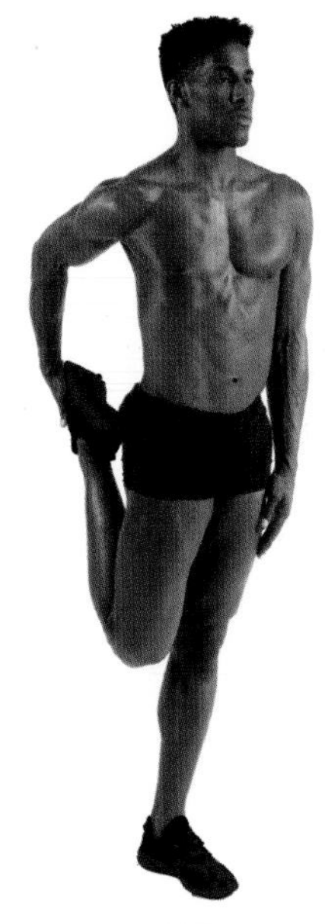

FACT FILE

TARGETS
- Whole Body

OBJECTIVE
- Pliability of muscle tissues

WORK/REST
- Approximately 30-45 seconds per exercise then onto the next

TOTAL TIME
- 8 minutes

TOTAL COMPLETED CIRCUIT SETS
- 1 set

5 HALF-KNEELING ROTATION

Pages 46–47

- Perform 10 repetitions per side.

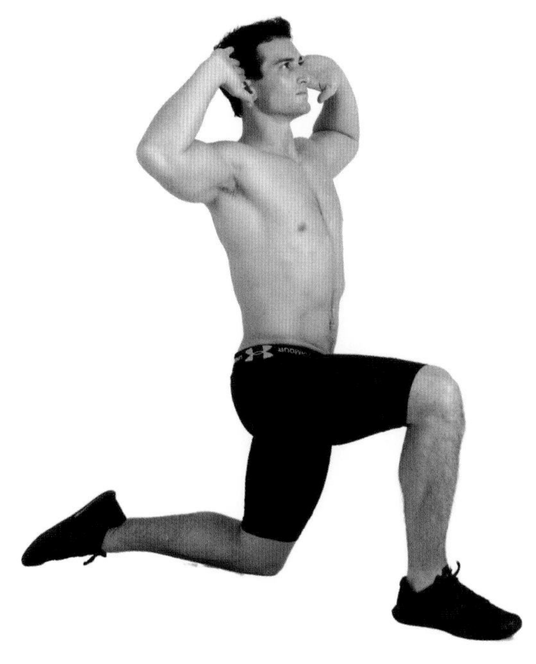

6 SAW STRETCH

Pages 32–33

- Perform 30-45 seconds.

7 COBRA STRETCH

Pages 50–51

- Perform for 15-30 seconds.

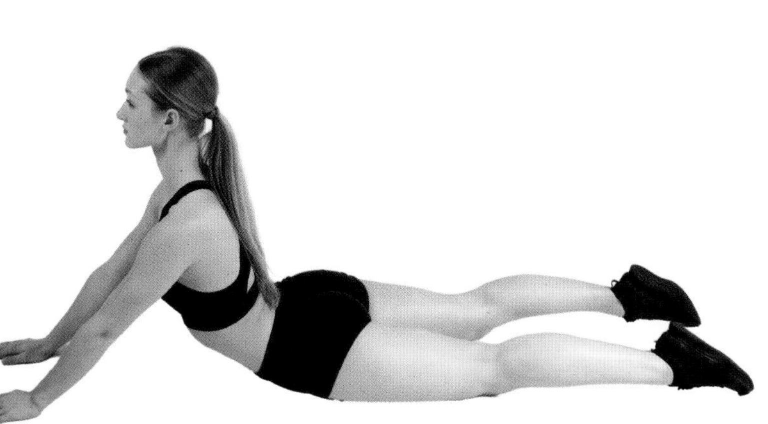

8 KNEE-TO-CHEST HUG

Pages 58–59

- Perform 30 seconds per side.

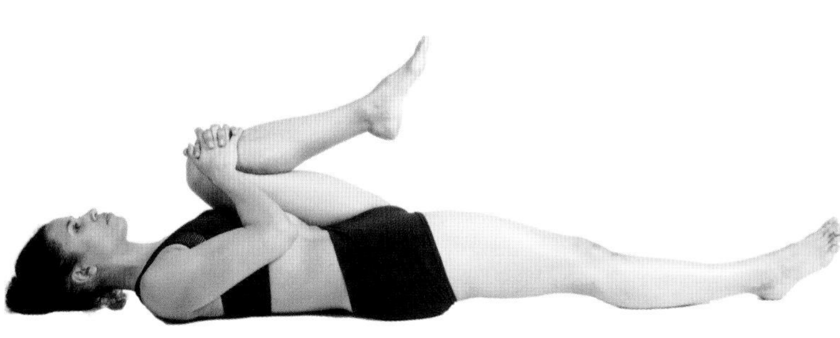

Off to the Game

Designed to prepare an immobile body for activity.

1 WALL-ASSISTED CHEST STRETCH

Pages 30–31

- Perform 30-45 seconds per side.

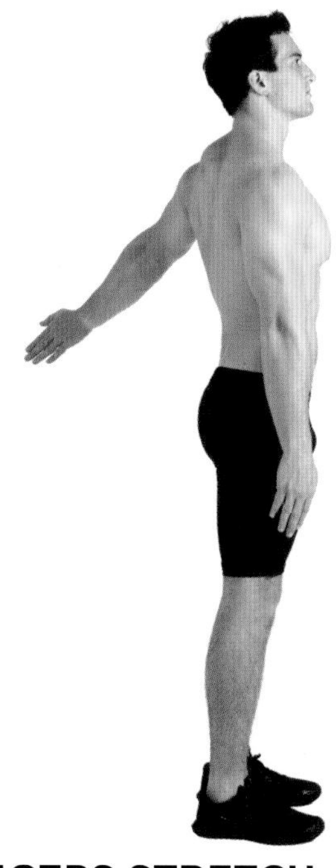

2 BICEPS-PECS STRETCH

Page 37

- Perform 30 seconds per side.

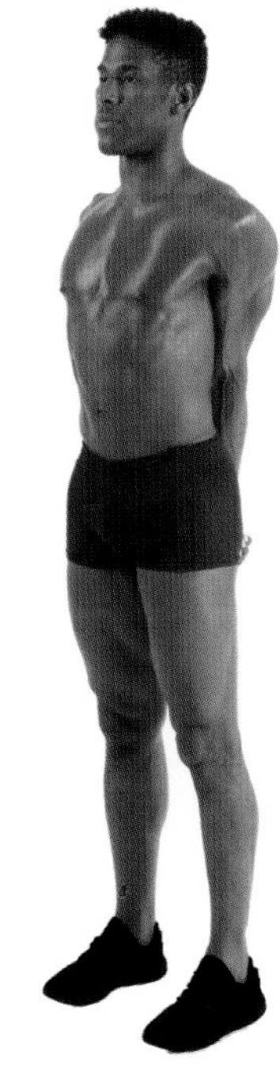

3 TRICEPS STRETCH

Page 36

- Perform 30 seconds per side.

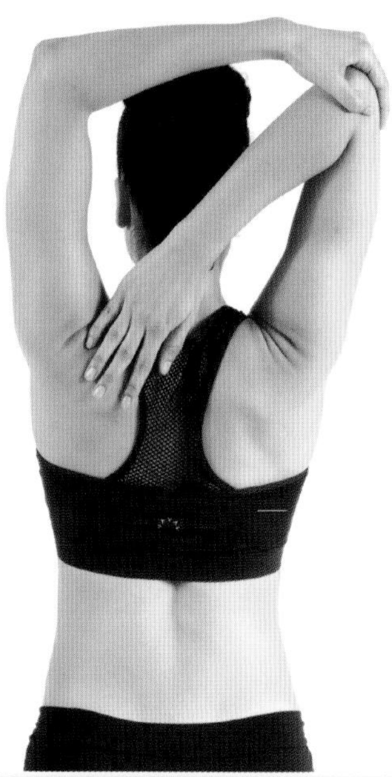

4 SPRAWL PUSH-UP

Pages 202–3

- Perform for 60 seconds, aim for 4-6 repetitions.

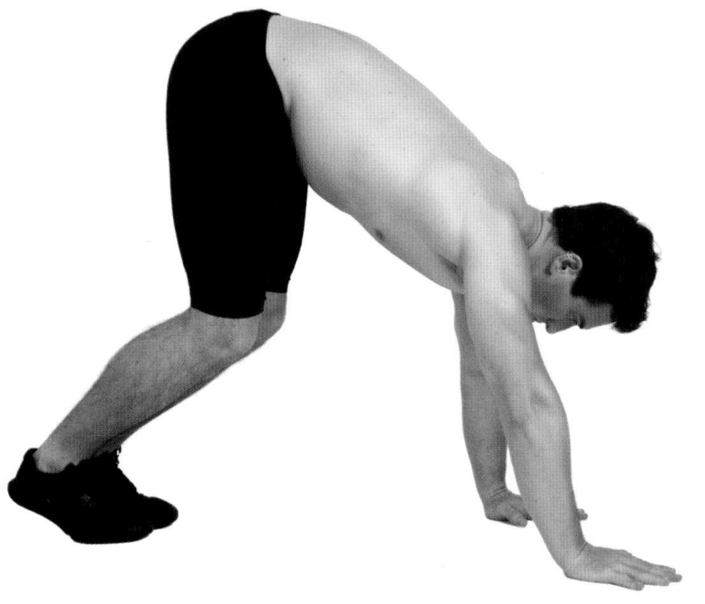

FACT FILE

TARGETS
- Whole Body

OBJECTIVE
- Pliability of muscle tissues

WORK/REST
- Approximately 30 seconds per exercise then onto the next

TOTAL TIME
- 8 minutes

TOTAL COMPLETED CIRCUIT SETS
- 1 set

5 SEATED RUSSIAN TWIST

Pages 64–65

- Perform 30 seconds per side.

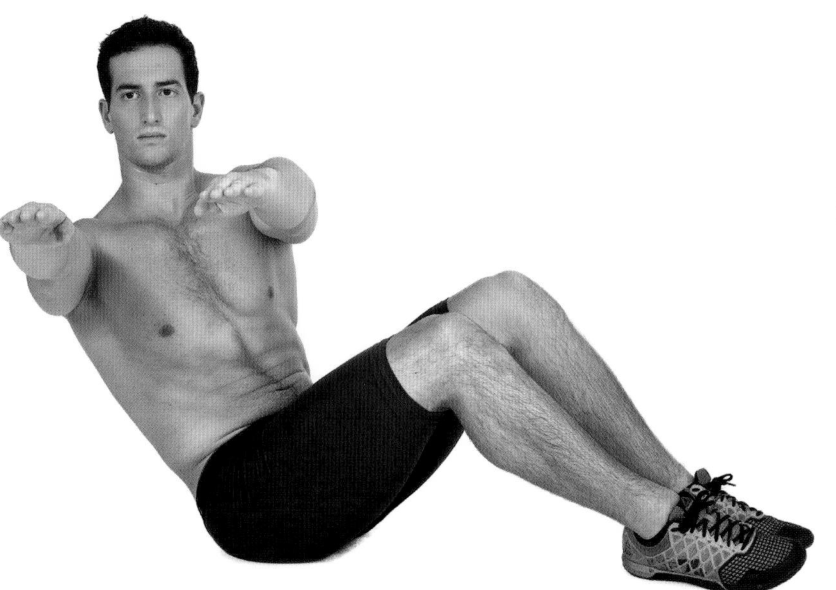

6 TWISTING CHAIR POSE

Pages 78–79

- Perform 30 seconds per side.

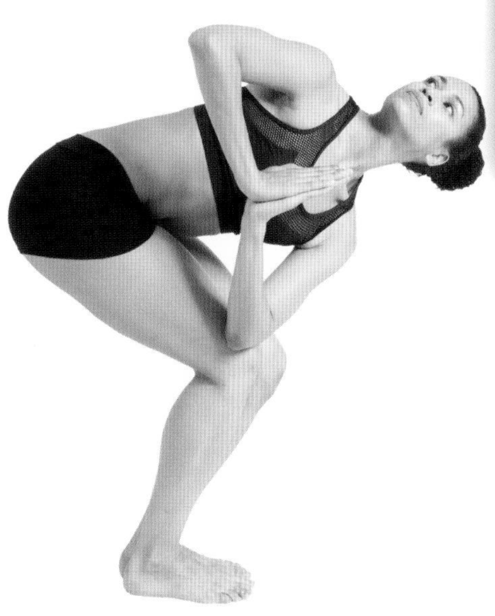

7 ILIOTIBIAL BAND STRETCH

Pages 44–45

- Perform 15 seconds per side.

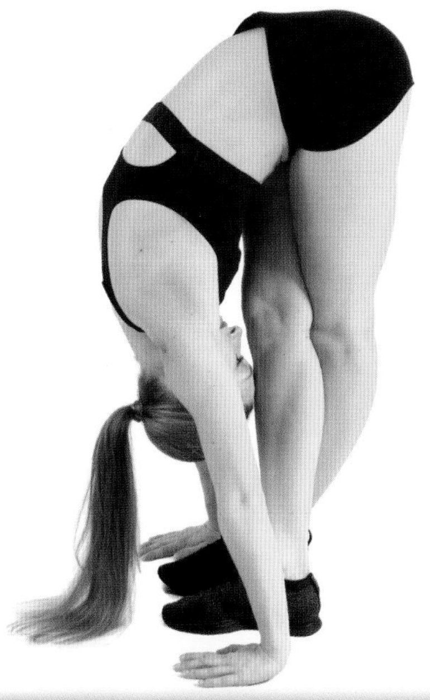

8 KNEELING SQUAT JUMP

Pages 138–39

- Perform for 60 seconds, aim for 4-6 repetitions.

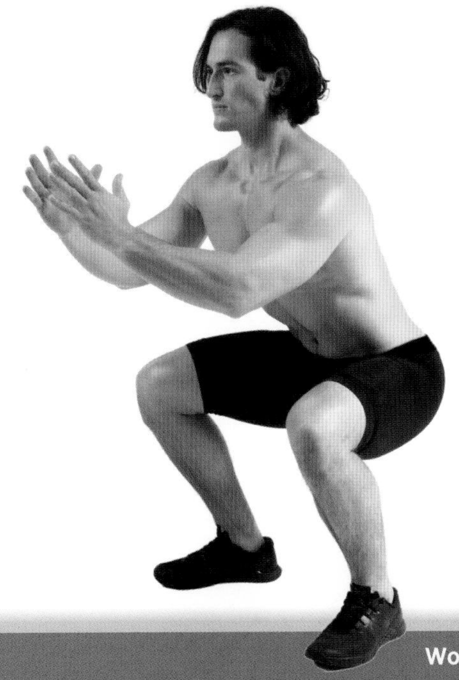

Parent Patrol

Designed to keep parents in motion while baby strolling.

1 MOUNTAIN POSE

Pages 74–75

- Hold for 3 to 6 breaths.

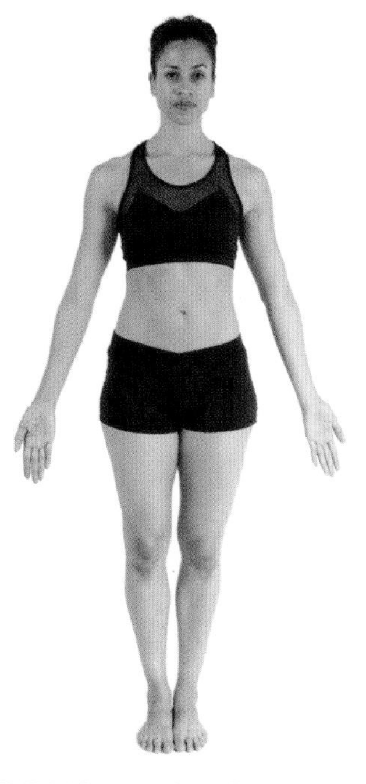

2 TREE POSE

Page 80–81

- Hold for 3 to 6 breaths.

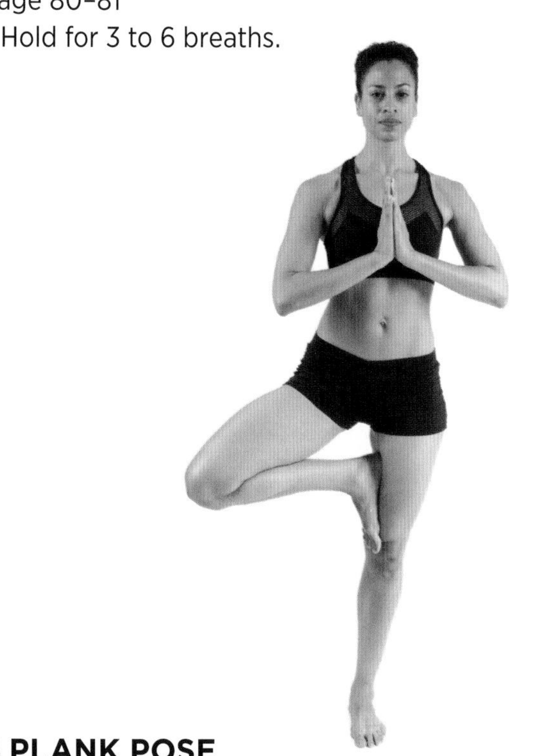

3 DOWNWARD-FACING DOG

Pages 84–85

- Hold for 3 to 6 breaths.

4 PLANK POSE

Pages 82–83

- Hold for 3 to 6 breaths.

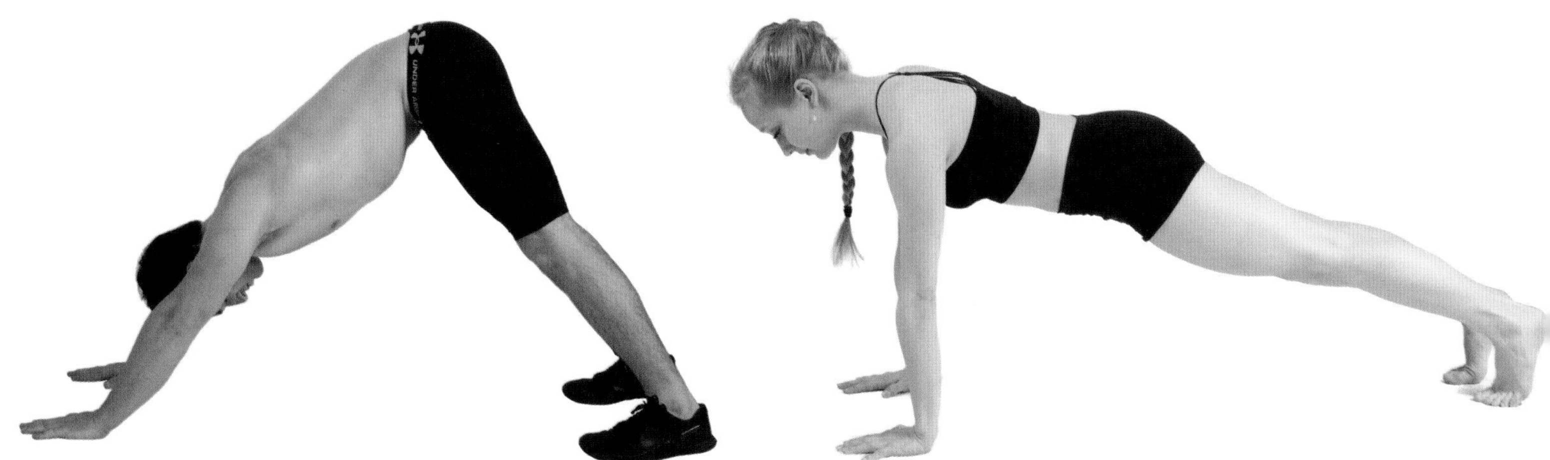

FACT FILE

TARGETS
- Whole Body

OBJECTIVE
- Functional stamina of muscle tissues

WORK/REST
- Approximately 3-6 breaths per exercise then onto the next

TOTAL TIME
- 8 minutes

TOTAL COMPLETED CIRCUIT SETS
- 1 set

5 FIRE-HYDRANT IN-OUT

Pages 242–43

- Perform 15 repetitions per side.

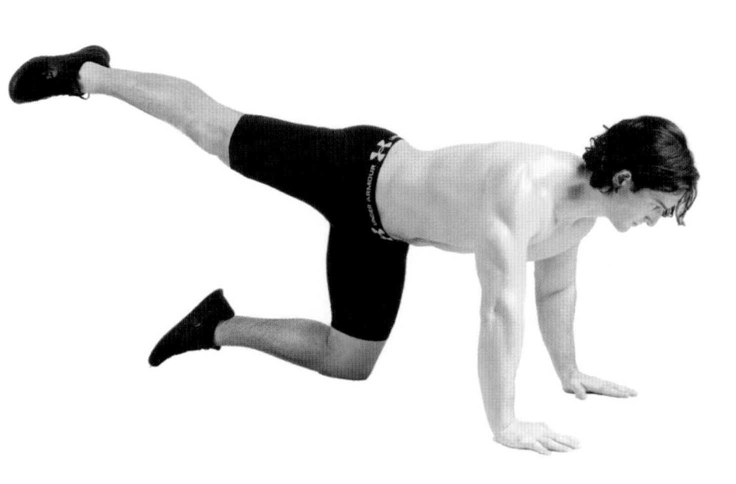

6 SQUAT

Pages 260–61

- Perform 15 repetitions.

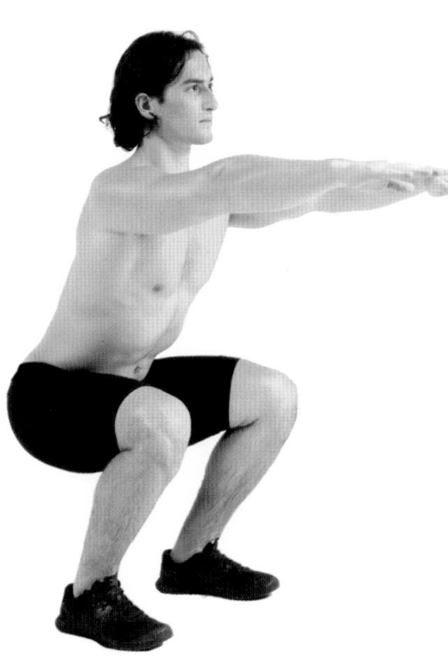

7 SINGLE-LEG GLUTEAL LIFT

Pages 262–63

- Perform 15 repetitions per leg.

8 EXTENSION HEEL BEATS

Pages 258–59

- Perform 5 sets of 10-count repetitions.

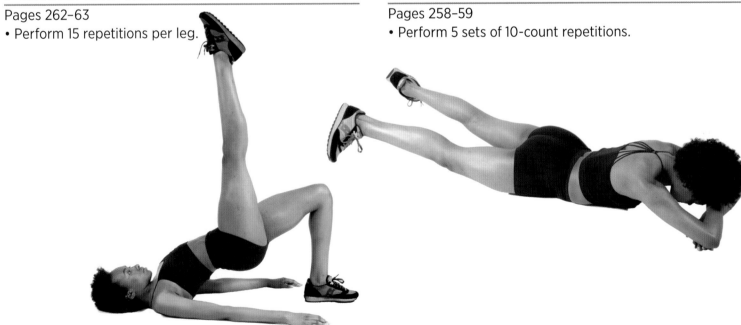

Post Lunch Break

Designed to relax an in-motion body prior to heading back to the office.

1 CERVICAL STARS

Pages 20–21

• Perform for 30 seconds per direction.

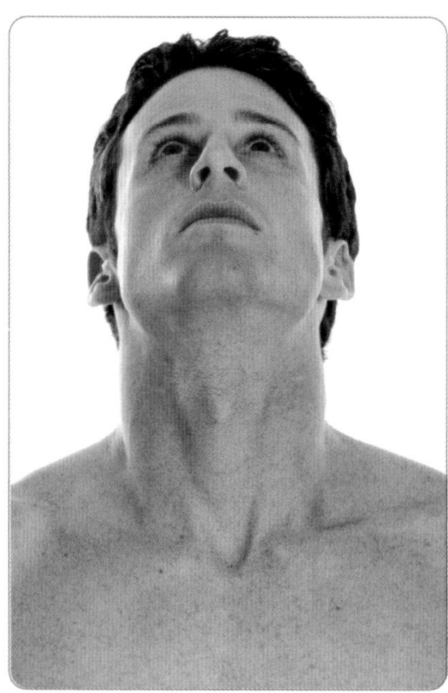

2 SHRUG

Page 23

• Perform for 30-45 seconds.

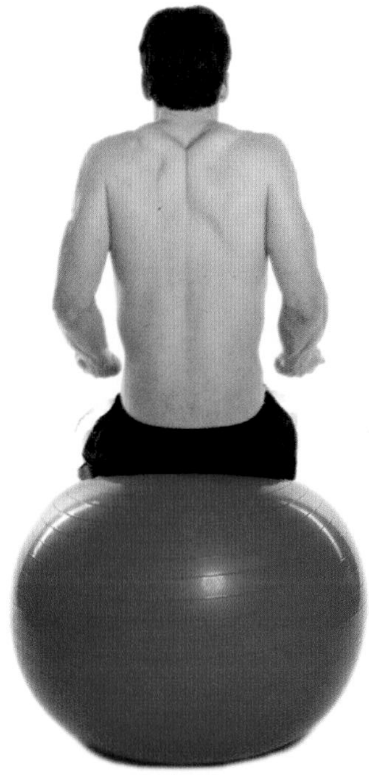

3 STANDING BACK ROLL

Page 52

• Perform for 30 seconds.

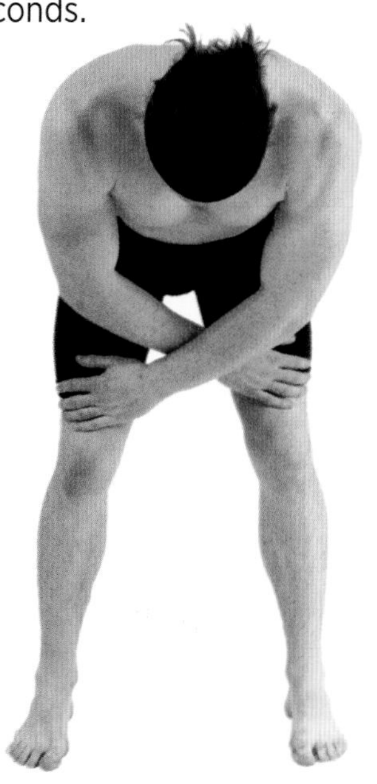

4 STANDING HAMSTRINGS STRETCH

Page 41

• Perform for 30 seconds per leg.

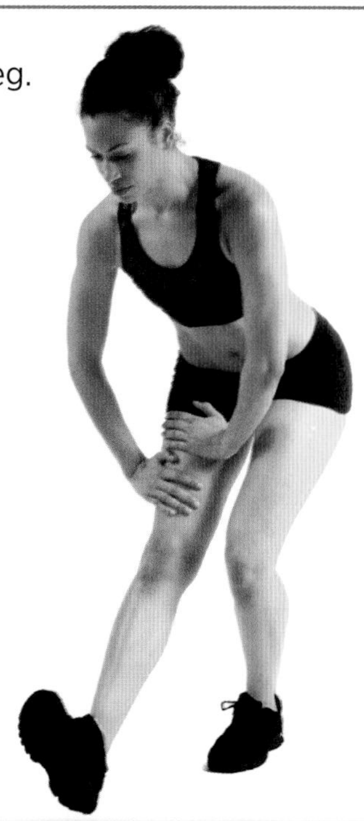

FACT FILE

TARGETS
- Whole Body

OBJECTIVE
- Relaxation/ Recovery of muscle tissues

WORK/REST
- Approximately 30 seconds per exercise then onto the next

TOTAL TIME
- 8 minutes

TOTAL COMPLETED CIRCUIT SETS
- 1 set

5 SPINE STRETCH FORWARD

Pages 54–55

- Perform for 30-45 seconds.

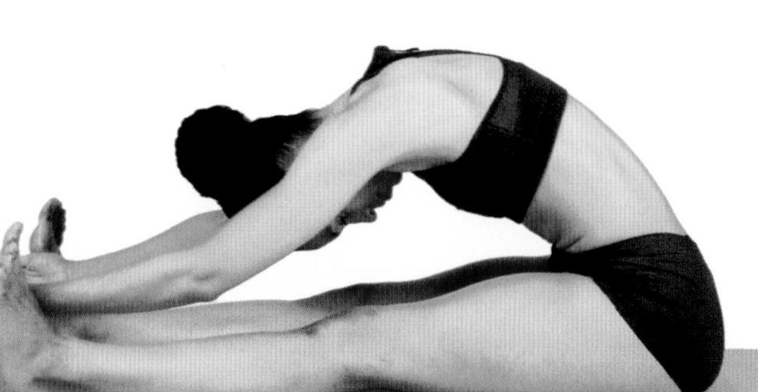

6 SIDE ANGLE POSE

Pages 110–11

- Hold for 3 to 6 breaths.

7 LYING-DOWN PRETZEL STRETCH

Pages 34–35

- Perform for 30 seconds per side.

8 HOLLOW HOLD TO SUPERMAN

Page 226–27

- Perform for 60 seconds, aim for 4-6 repetitions.

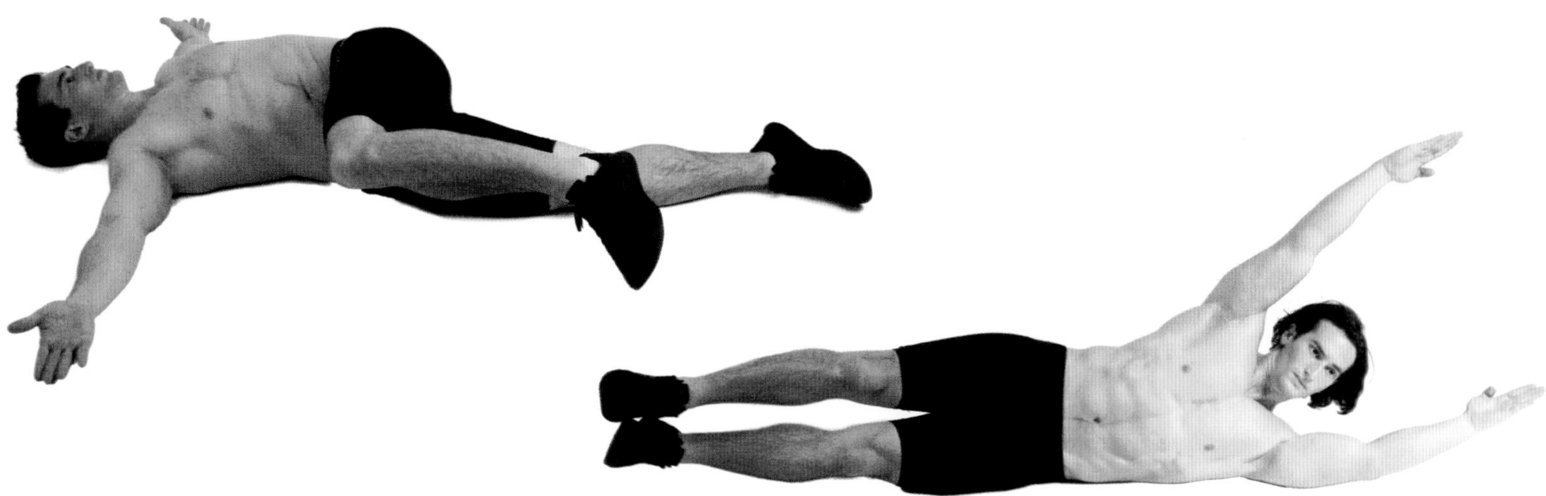

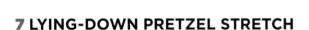

Gravity-free

Designed to help relieve stress from joints and make you feel nearly weightless.

1 WHEEL POSE

Pages 106-7

- Hold for 3 to 6 breaths.

2 METRONOME

Page 224–25

- Repetitions and time vary by objective.

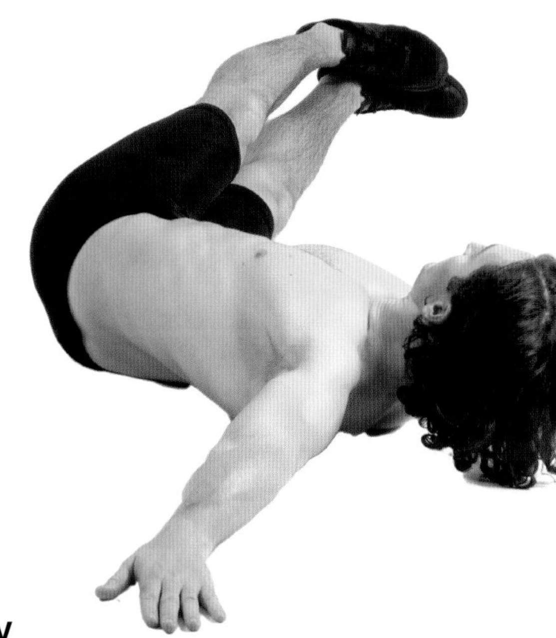

3 BRIDGE

Pages 256–57

- Perform 15 repetitions.

4 BODY SAW

Page 240–41

- Perform 20 repetitions.

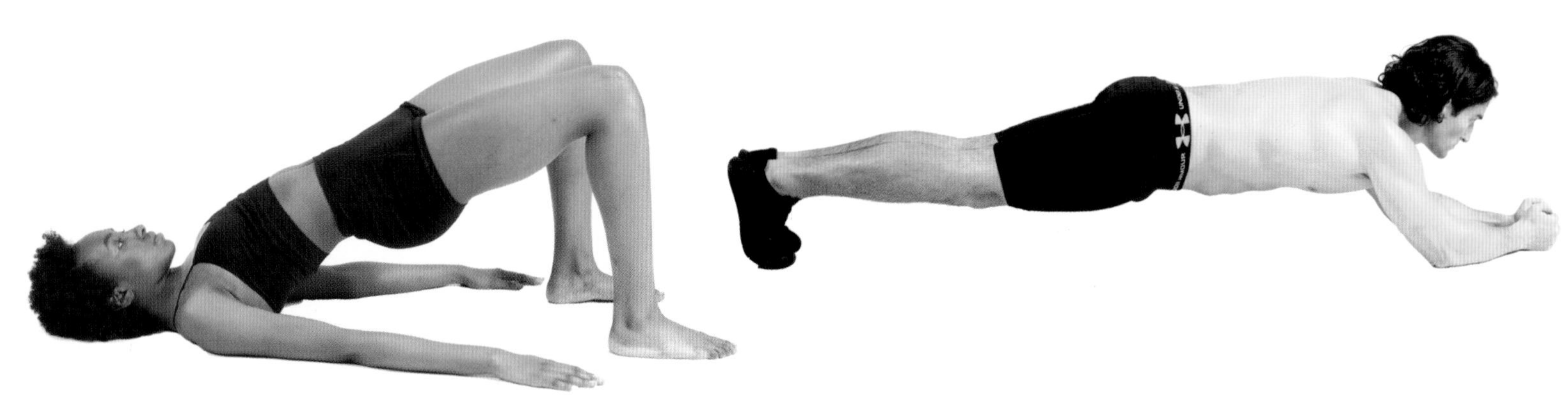

FACT FILE

TARGETS
• Whole Body

OBJECTIVE
• Relaxation/ Recovery of muscle tissues

WORK/REST
• Approximately 15 repetitions per side per exercise then onto the next

TOTAL TIME
• 8 minutes

TOTAL COMPLETED CIRCUIT SETS
• 1 set

5 ILIOTIBIAL BAND STRETCH

Pages 44–45
• Perform 15 seconds per side.

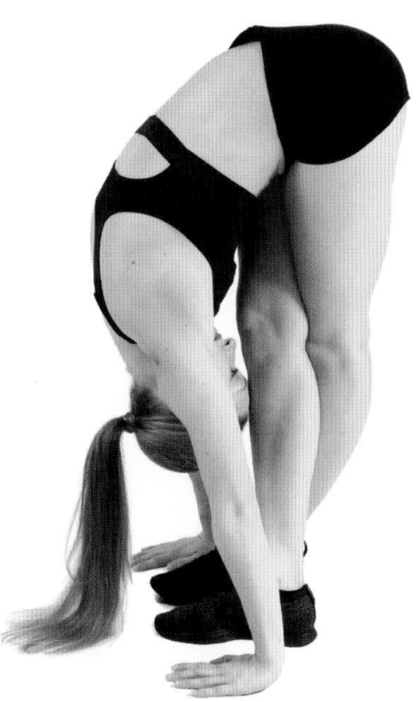

6 SQUAT

Pages 260–61
• Perform 15 repetitions.

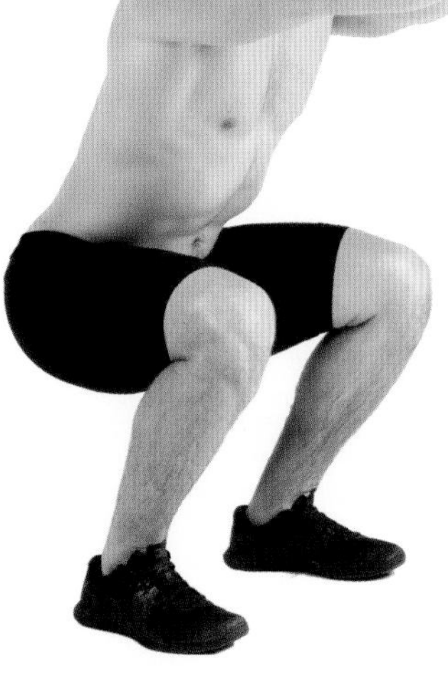

7 SPINE STRETCH FORWARD

Pages 54–55
• Perform for 30-45 seconds.

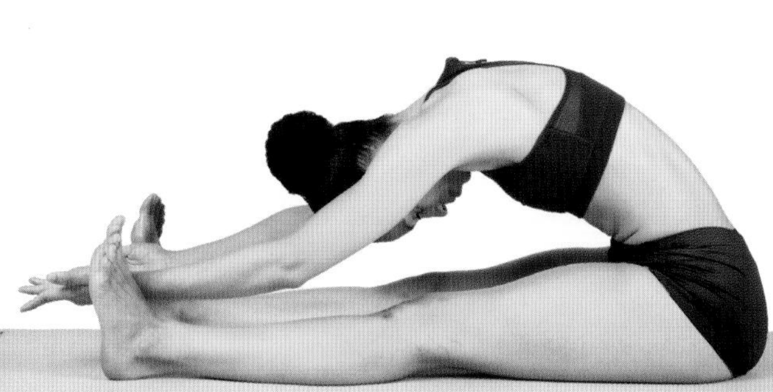

8 CLAMSHELLS

Pages 290–91
• Repetitions and time vary by objective.

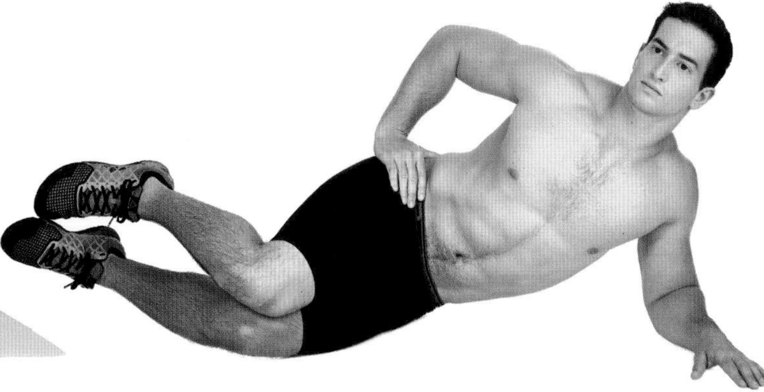

Down for the Count

Designed for a good ounce of relaxing energy before calling it a night.

1 DOLPHIN POSE

Page 94

- Hold for 3 to 6 breaths.

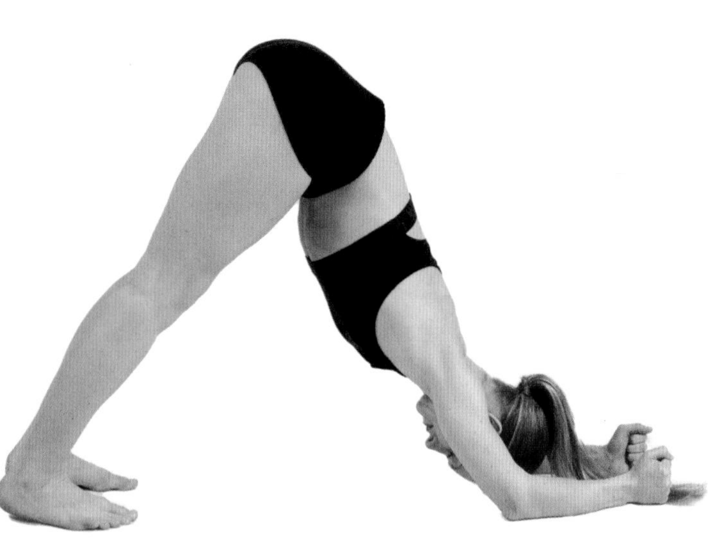

2 TRICEPS STRETCH

Page 36

- Perform for 30 seconds.

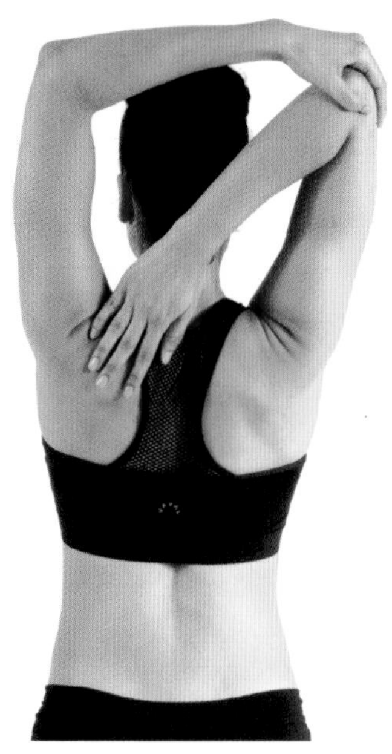

3 REVERSE CRUNCH

Pages 236–37

- Perform 20 repetitions.

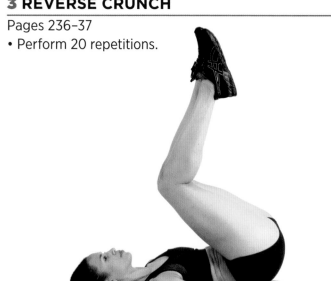

4 BODY SAW

Page 240–41

- Perform 20 repetitions.

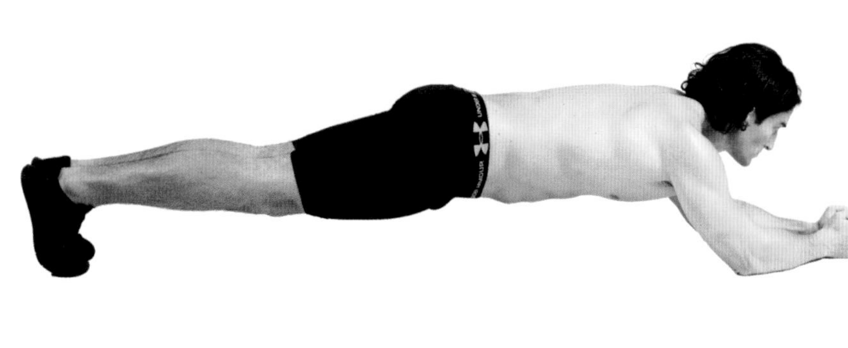

FACT FILE

TARGETS
- Whole Body

OBJECTIVE
- Relaxation/ Recovery of muscle tissues

WORK/REST
- Approximately 20 repetitions per side per exercise then onto the next

TOTAL TIME
- 8 minutes

TOTAL COMPLETED CIRCUIT SETS
- 1 set

5 SINGLE-LEG V-UP

Pages 244–45
- Perform 15 repetitions per leg.

6 WHEEL POSE

Pages 106–7
- Perform for 60 seconds. Aim for as many repetitions as you can perform.

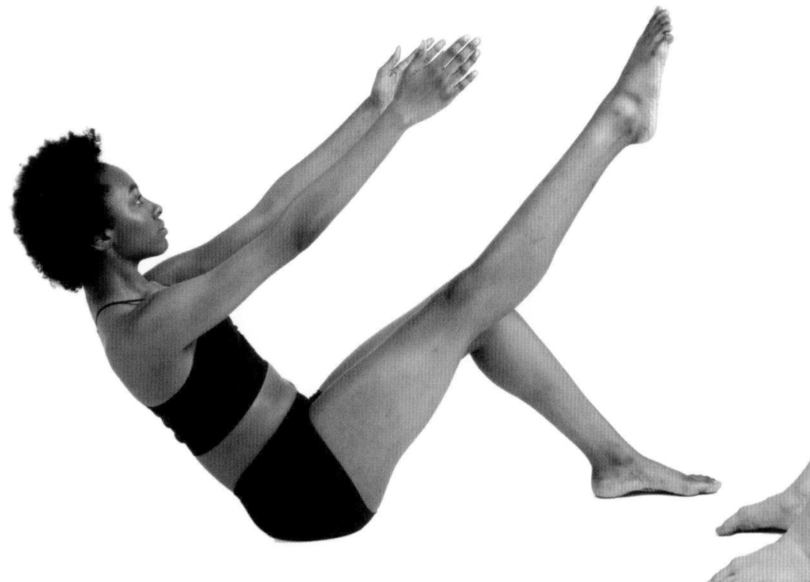

7 BRIDGE

Pages 256–57
- Perform 15 repetitions.

8 EXTENSION HEEL BEATS

Pages 258–59
- Perform 5 sets of 10-count repetitions.

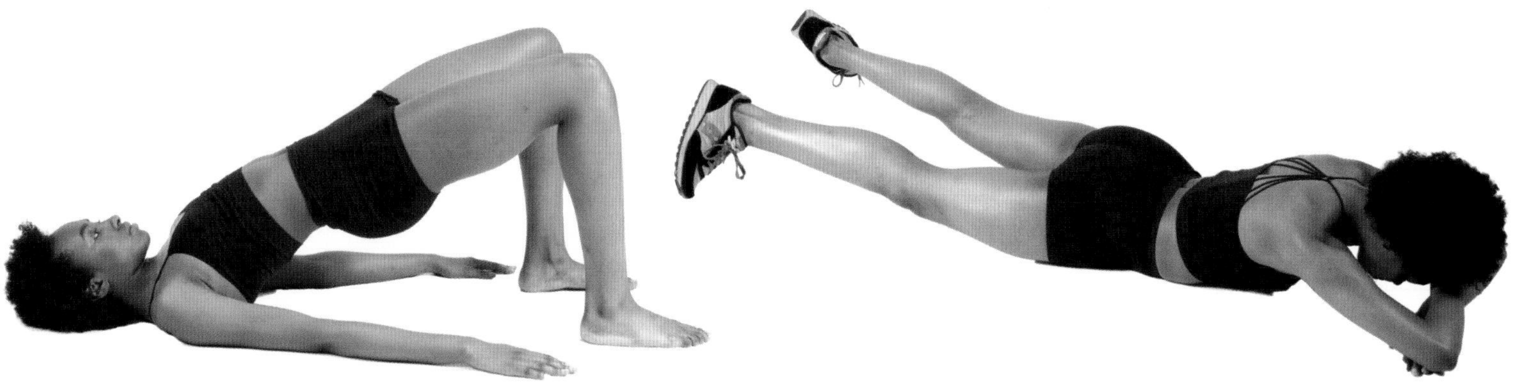

Upper Body Stretch

Designed to help lengthen, alleviate and provide better upper-body motion.

1 FRONT DELTOID TOWEL STRETCH

Page 56

- Perform for 30 seconds.

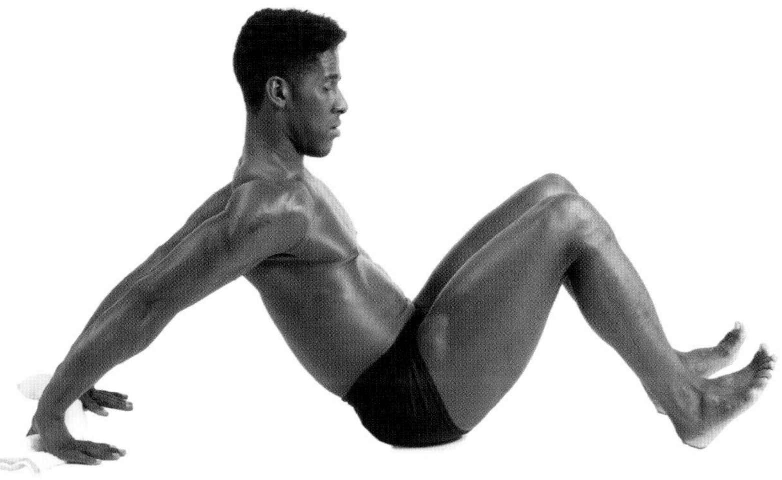

2 CERVICAL STARS

Page 20–21

- Perform 30 seconds per direction.

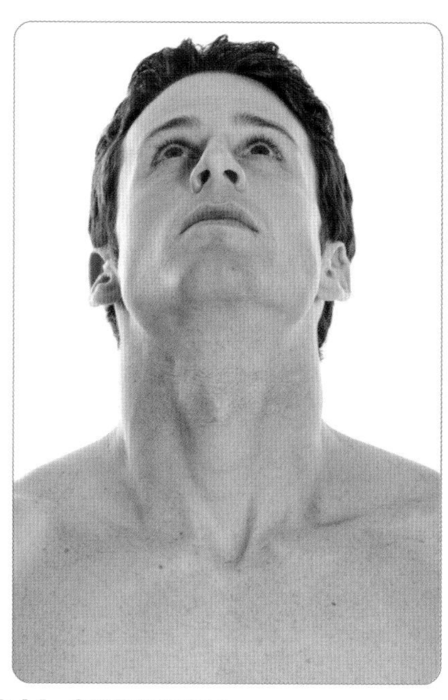

3 FLEXION STRETCH

Page 24

- Perform for 30 seconds.

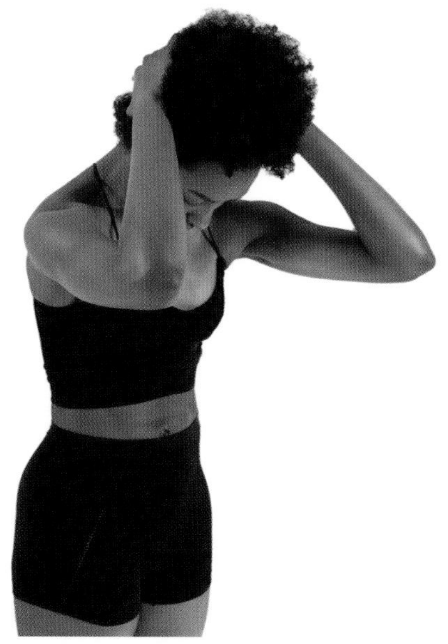

4 LATERAL STRETCH

Page 26

- Perform for 30 seconds per direction.

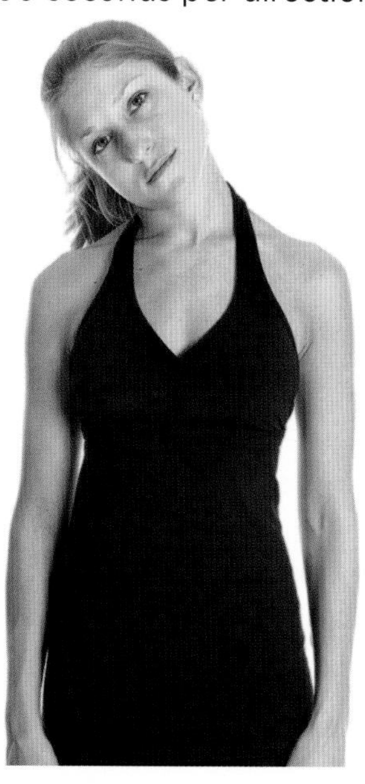

5 SHRUG

Page 23

- Perform for 30–45 seconds.

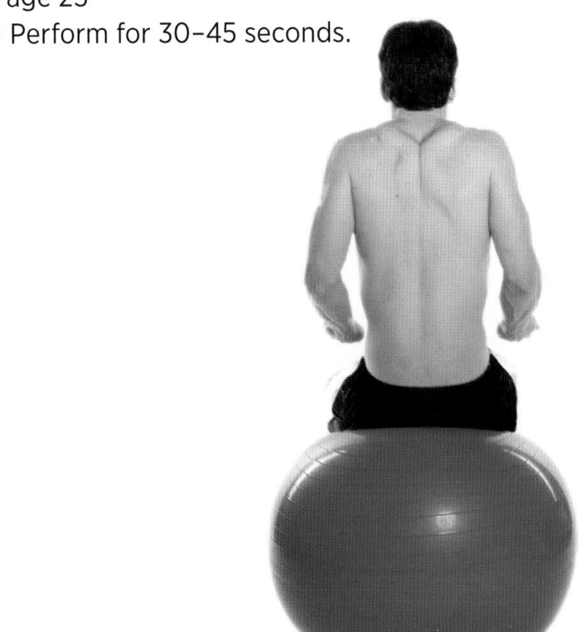

6 WALL-ASSISTED CHEST STRETCH

Pages 30–31

- Perform for 30-45 seconds per side.

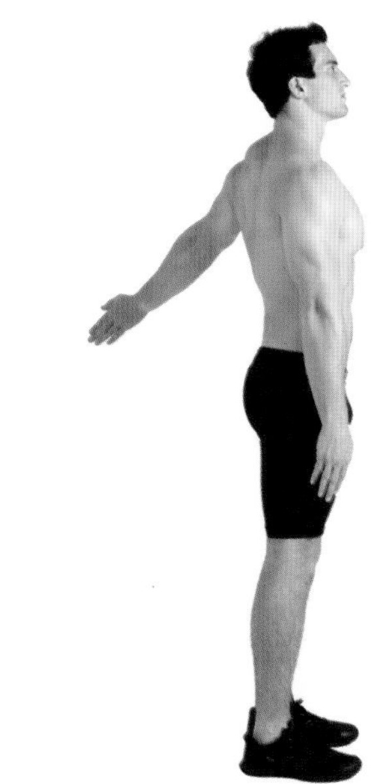

7 BICEPS-PECS STRETCH

Page 37

- Perform 30 seconds per side.

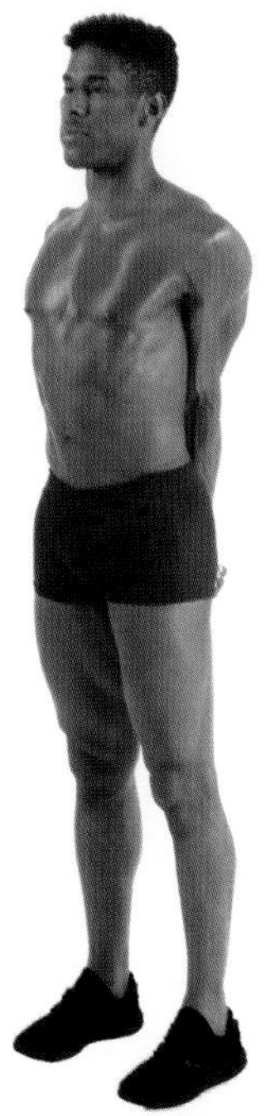

8 TRICEPS STRETCH

Page 36

- Perform for 30 seconds.

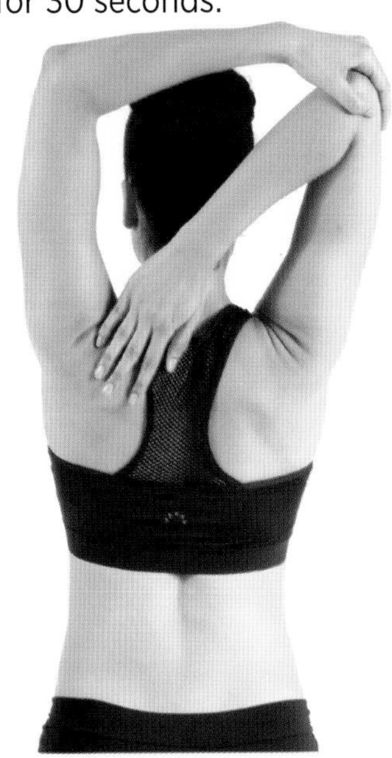

FACT FILE

TARGETS
- Upper Body

OBJECTIVE
- Pliability of upper body muscle tissues

WORK/REST
- Approximately 20 repetitions per side per exercise then onto the next

TOTAL TIME
- 6 minutes

TOTAL COMPLETED CIRCUIT SETS
- 1 set

Lower Body Stretch

Designed to help lengthen, alleviate and provide better lower-body motion.

1 STANDING QUADRICEPS STRETCH

Page 40

- Perform for 30 seconds per leg.

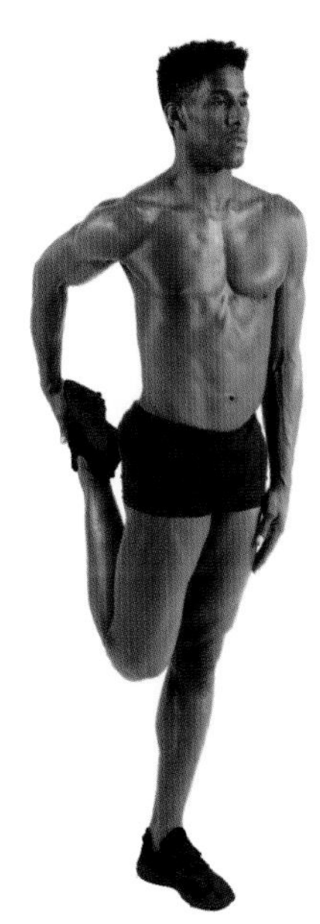

2 STANDING HAMSTRINGS STRETCH

Page 43

- Perform for 30 seconds per leg.

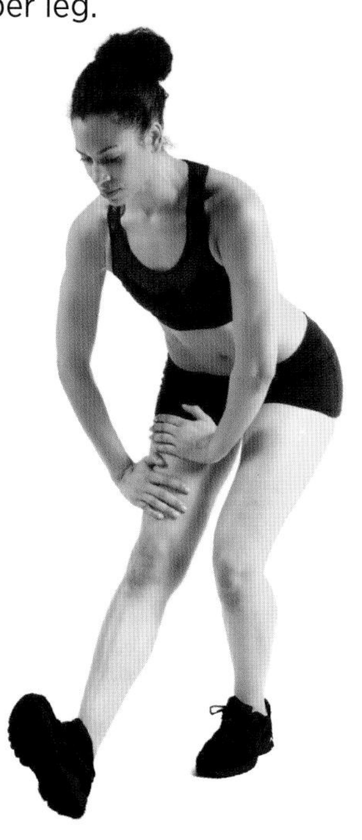

3 ILIOTIBIAL BAND STRETCH

Pages 44–45

- Perform for 15 seconds per side.

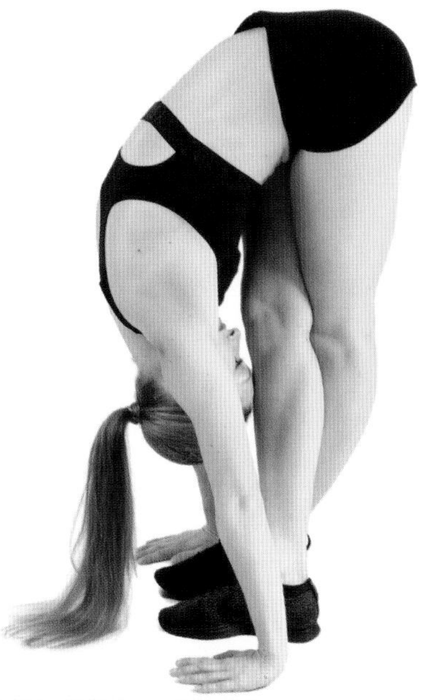

4 HALF-STRADDLE STRETCH

Pages 60–61

- Perform for 30 seconds per side.

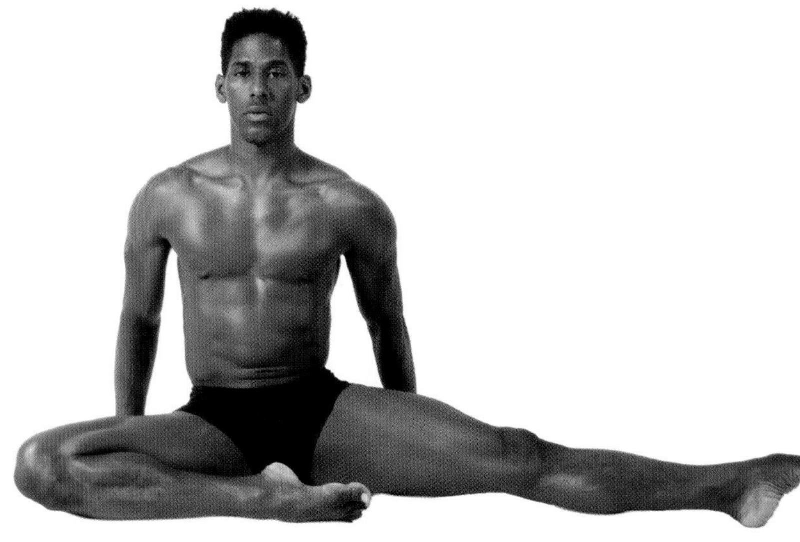

FACT FILE

TARGETS
- Lower Body

OBJECTIVE
- Pliability of lower body muscle tissues

WORK/REST
- Approximately 20 repetitions per side per exercise then onto the next

TOTAL TIME
- 6 minutes

TOTAL COMPLETED CIRCUIT SETS
- 1 set

5 ROLLOVER STRETCH

Pages 66–67

- Perform for 30–45 seconds.

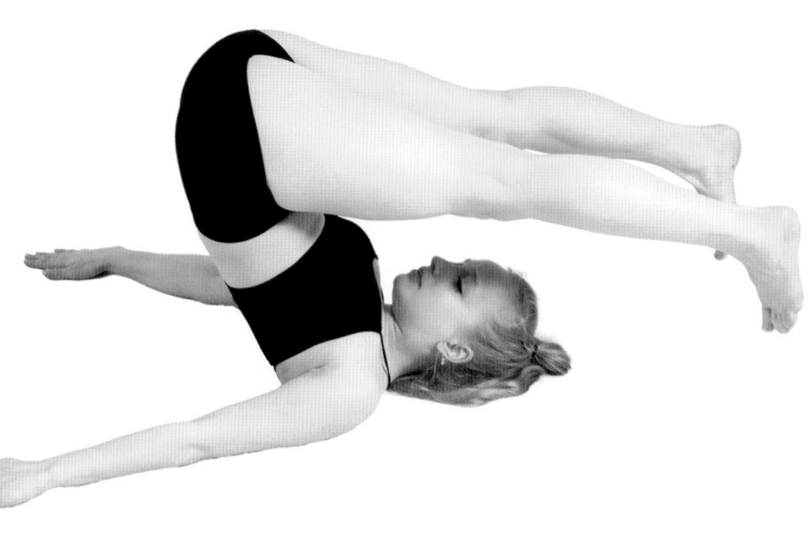

6 LATERAL LUNGE STRETCH

Pages 28–29

- Perform 3 x 30-second holds per leg.

7 STANDING FORWARD BEND

Pages 68–69

- Perform for 30–45 seconds.

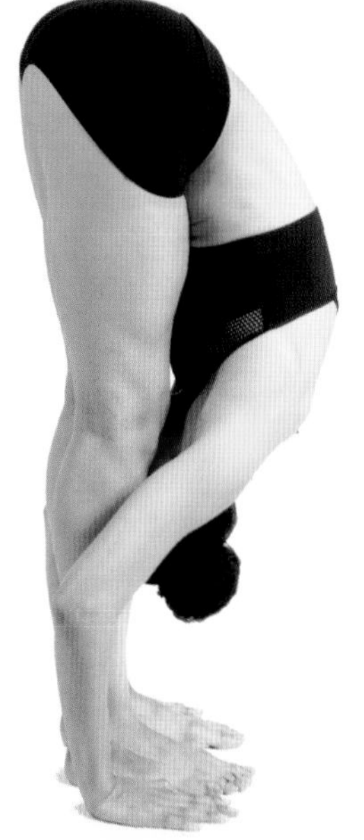

8 LORD OF THE DANCE POSE

Pages 118–19

- Hold for 3 to 6 breaths.

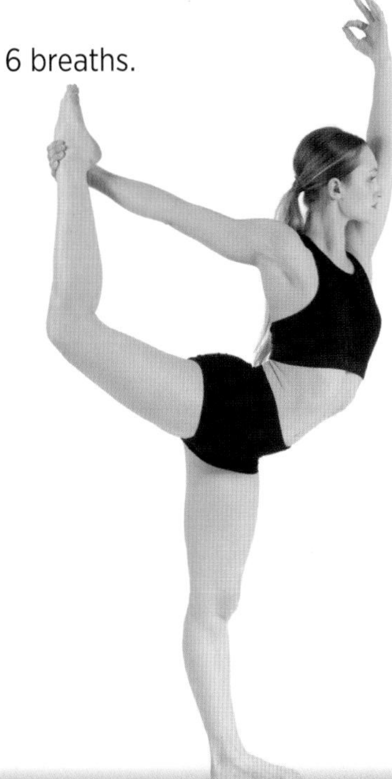

Upper Body Pump

Designed to keep working upper-body muscles primed, pumped, and ready.

1 SHOULDER-TAP PUSH-UP

Pages 208–9

- Repetitions and time vary by objective.

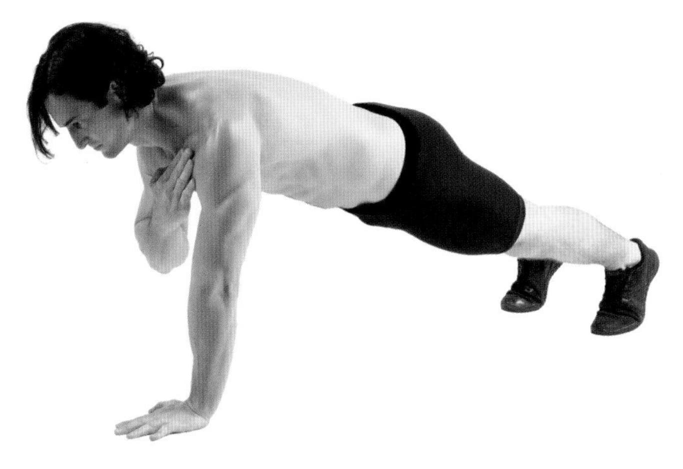

2 PUSH-UP HAND WALK-OVER

Page 210–11

- Perform for 30 seconds, 8–12 repetitions.

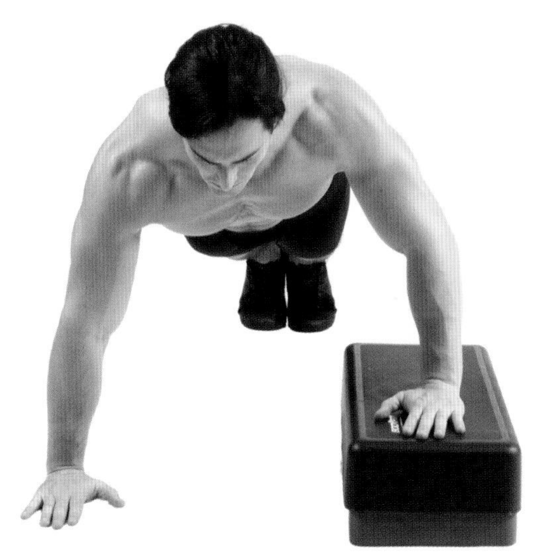

3 BEAR CRAWL

Pages 190

- Perform for 60 seconds.

4 BODY SAW

Page 240

- Perform for 30 seconds, 8–12 repetitions.

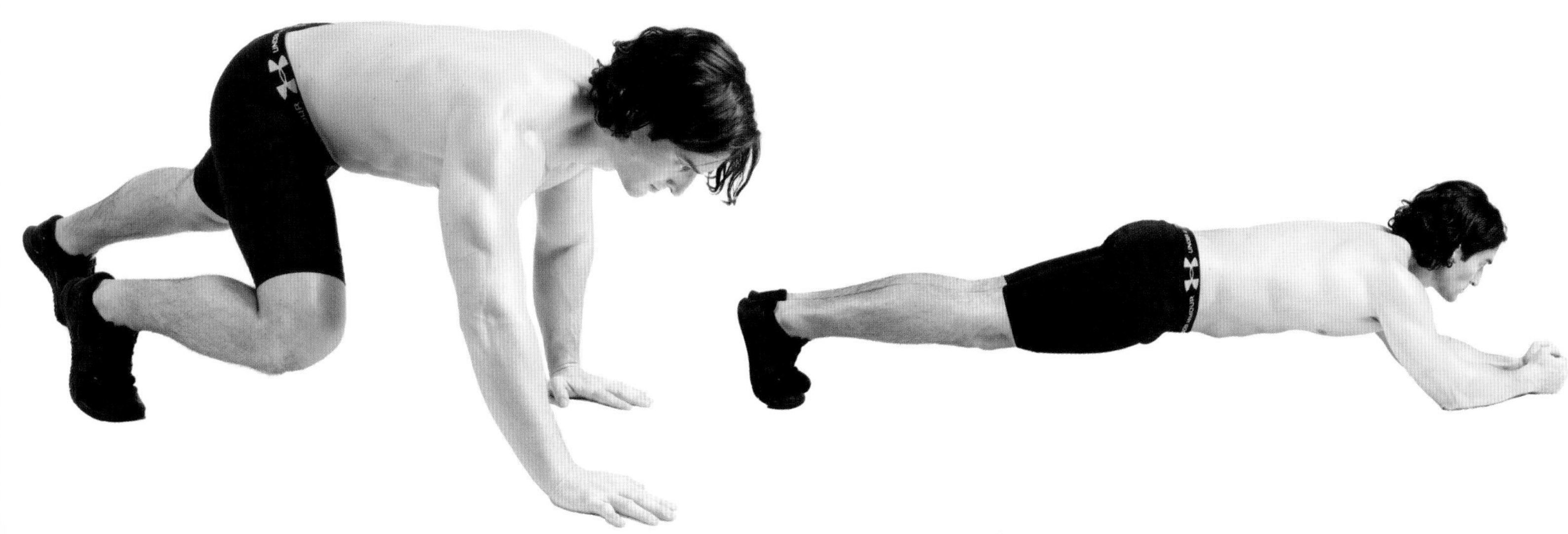

FACT FILE

TARGETS
- Upper Body

OBJECTIVE
- Increased strength of upper body muscle tissues

WORK/REST
- Approximately 30 seconds or 8-12 repetitions per exercise then onto the next

TOTAL TIME
- 7 minutes

TOTAL COMPLETED CIRCUIT SETS
- 1 set

5 TOWEL FLY

Pages 200–201

- Perform for 30 seconds, 8–12 repetitions.

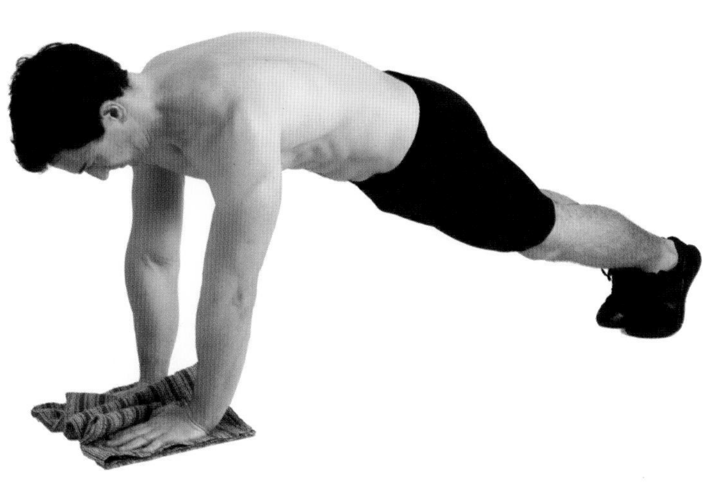

6 POWER PUNCH

Pages 182–83

- Perform for 30 seconds, 8–12 repetitions.

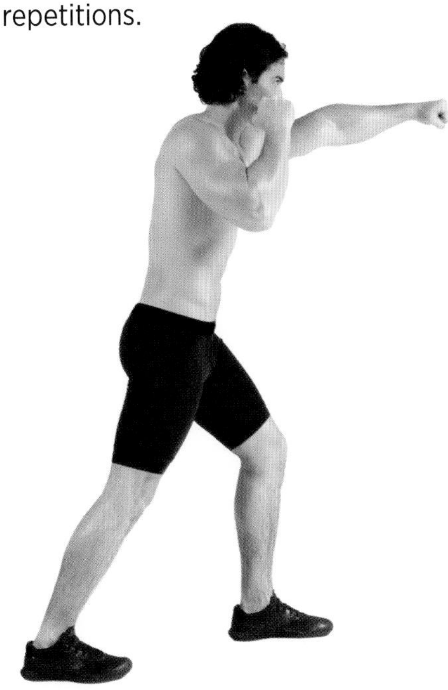

7 UPPERCUT

Pages 184–85

- Repetitions and time vary by objective.

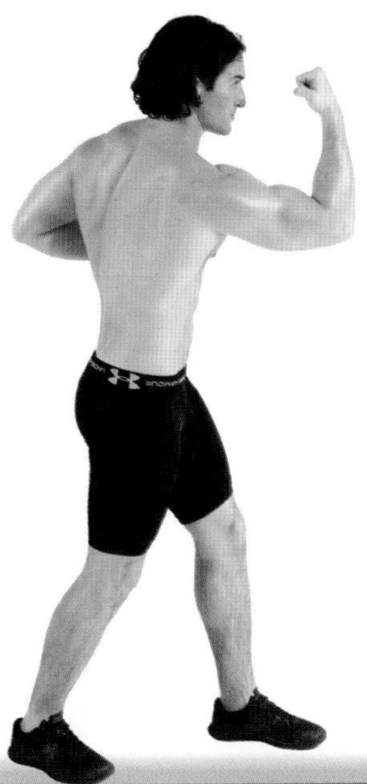

8 V-UP

Pages 26–27

- Repetitions and time vary by objective.

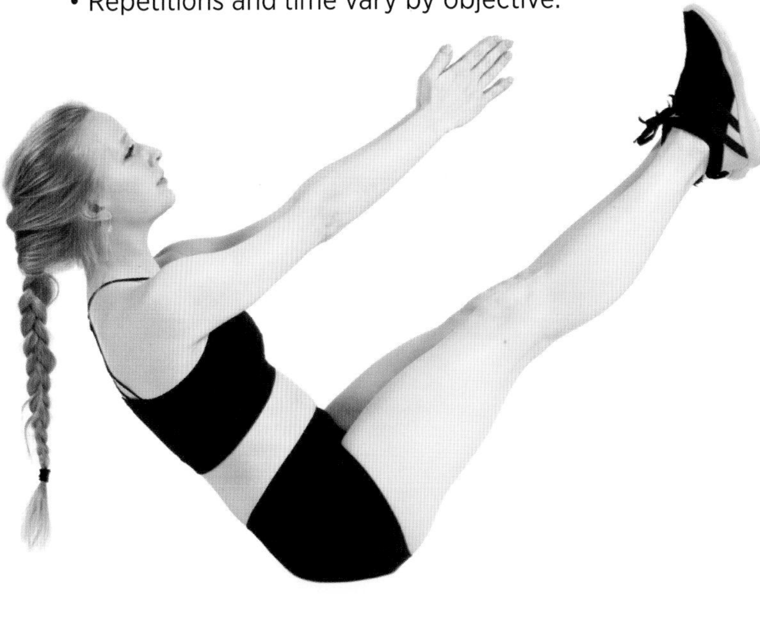

Lower Body Pump

Designed to keep working lower-body muscles primed, pumped, and ready.

1 BEAR CRAWL

Pages 190–91

- Perform for 60 seconds.

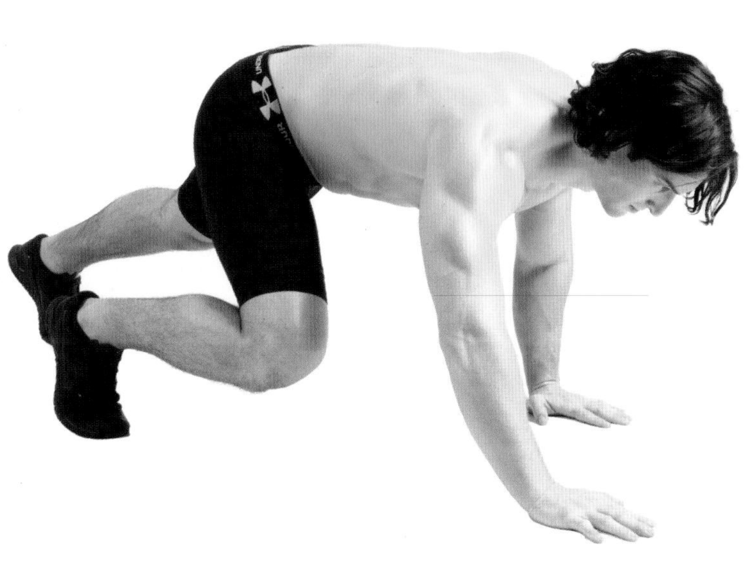

2 LATERAL LUNGE WITH SQUAT

Pages 266–67

- Perform for 30 seconds, 8-12 repetitions.

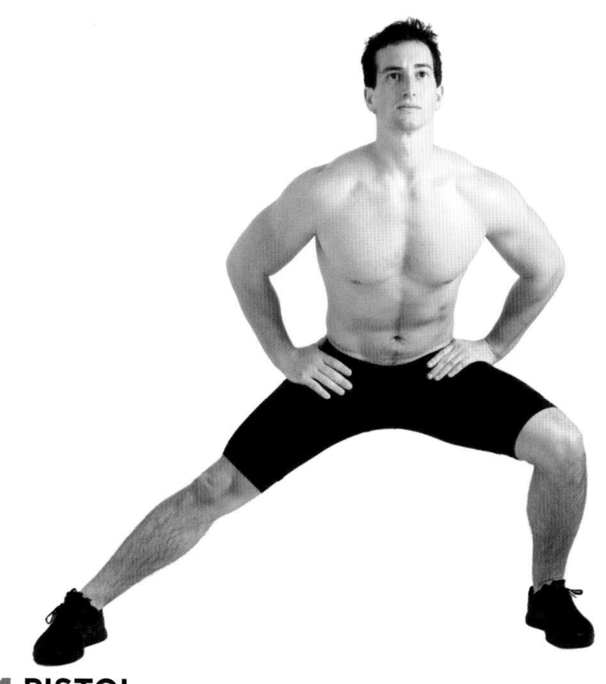

3 TOWEL HAMSTRINGS PULL

Page 274

- Perform for 20 seconds, 15+ repetitions.

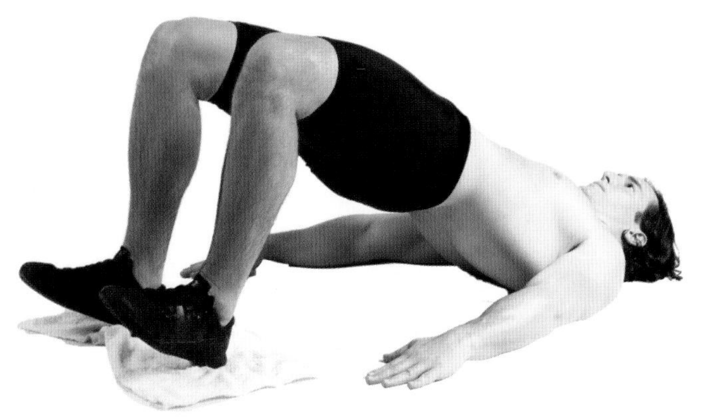

4 PISTOL

Page 137

- Perform for 60 seconds, 4-6 repetitions.

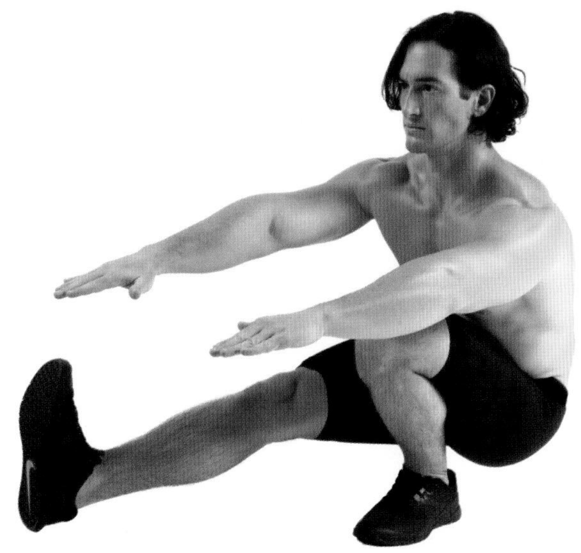

FACT FILE

TARGETS
- Lower Body

OBJECTIVE
- Increased strength of lower body muscle tissues

WORK/REST
- Approximately 30 seconds or 8-12 repetitions per exercise then onto the next

TOTAL TIME
- 7 minutes

TOTAL COMPLETED CIRCUIT SETS
- 1 set

5 SURRENDER

Page 276

- Perform for 30 seconds, 15+ repetitions.

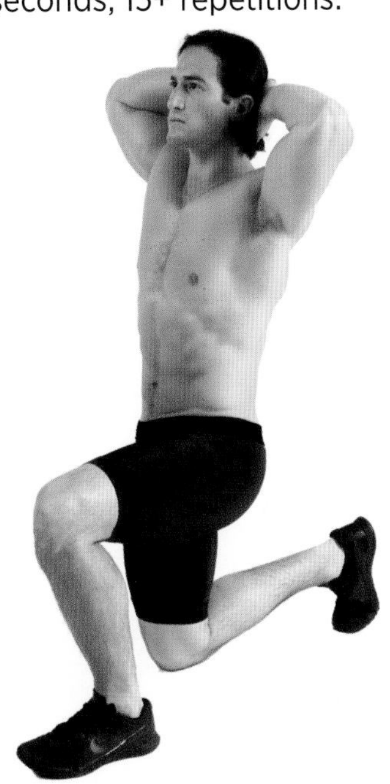

6 MOUNTAIN CLIMBER

Pages 298–99

- Repetitions and time vary by objective.

7 LATERAL-EXTENSION REVERSE LUNGE

Pages 280–81

- Perform 10 repetitions per side.

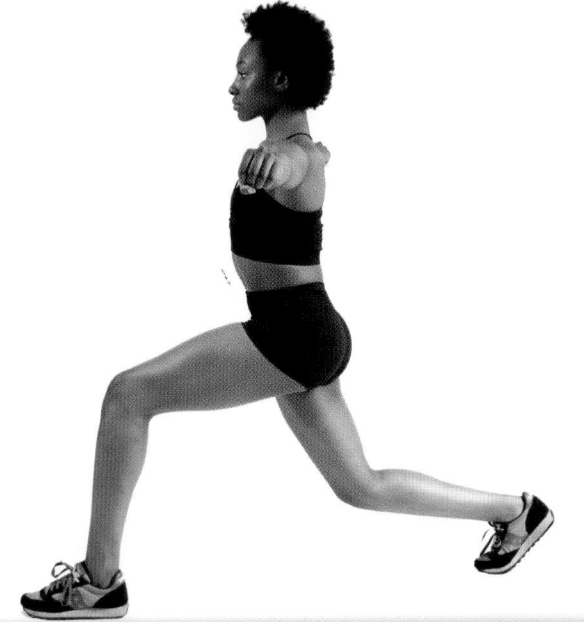

8 SKATER'S LUNGE

Pages 282–83

- Perform for 45-60 seconds.

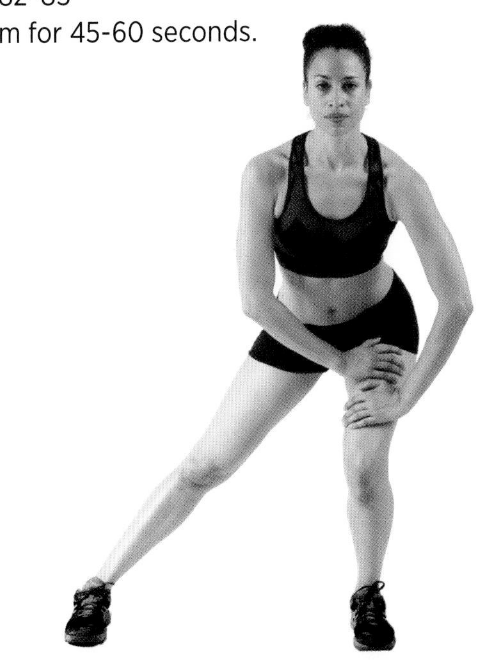

Mobility Workout

A functional routine designed to create more free, balanced, and agile movement in life.

1 DIVE-BOMBER PUSH-UP

Pages 206–7

- Repetitions and time vary by objective.

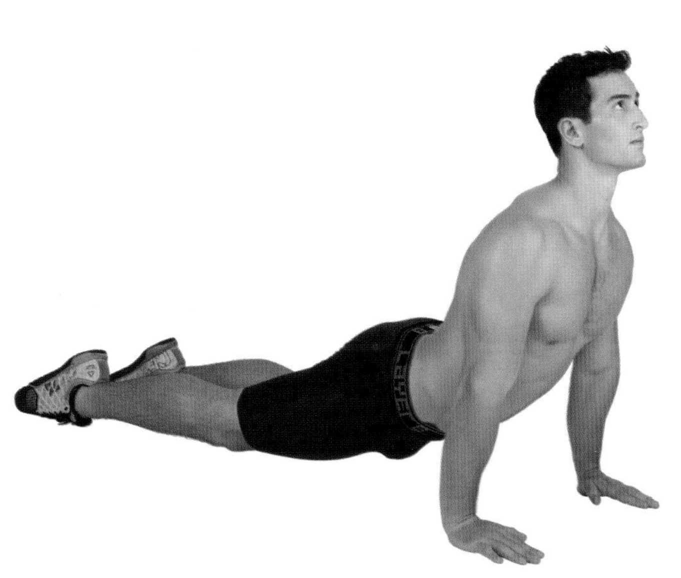

2 REVERSE CRUNCH

Pages 236–37

- Perform 20 repetitions.

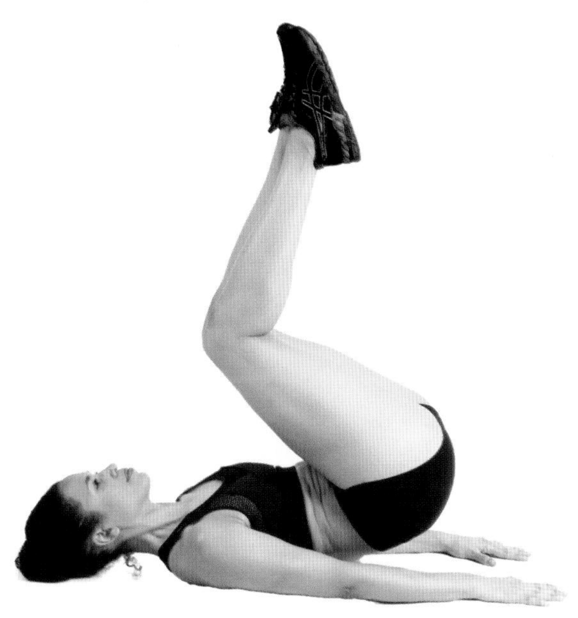

3 MOUNTAIN CLIMBER

Pages 298–99

- Repetitions and time vary by objective.

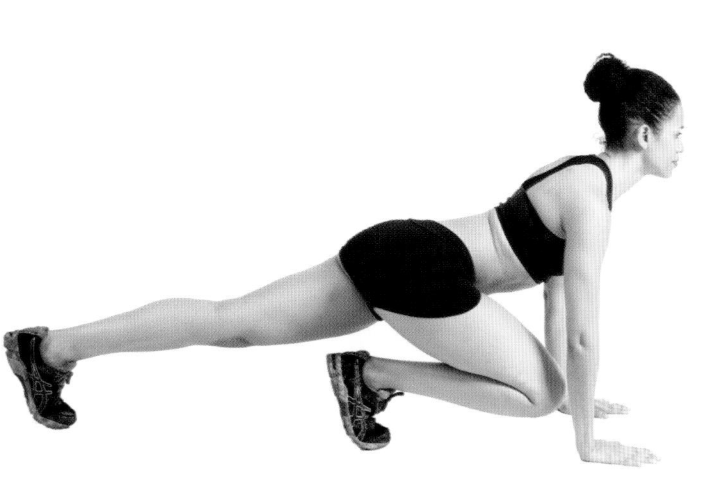

4 SPLIT SQUAT WITH OVERHEAD PRESS

Pages 278–79

- Perform for 30 seconds, 8-12 repetitions.

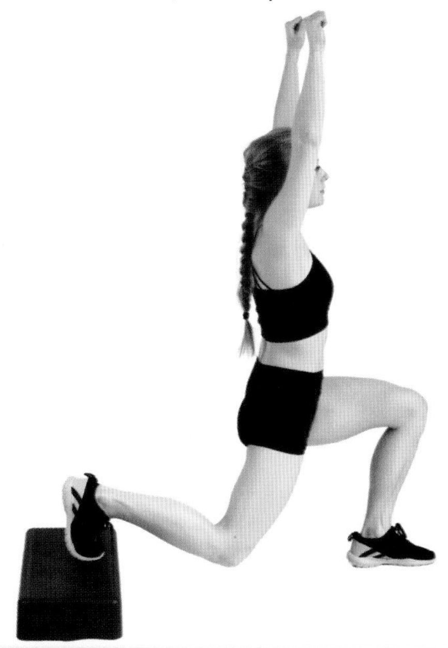

5 TURKISH GET-UP

Pages 304–5

• Repetitions and time vary by objective.

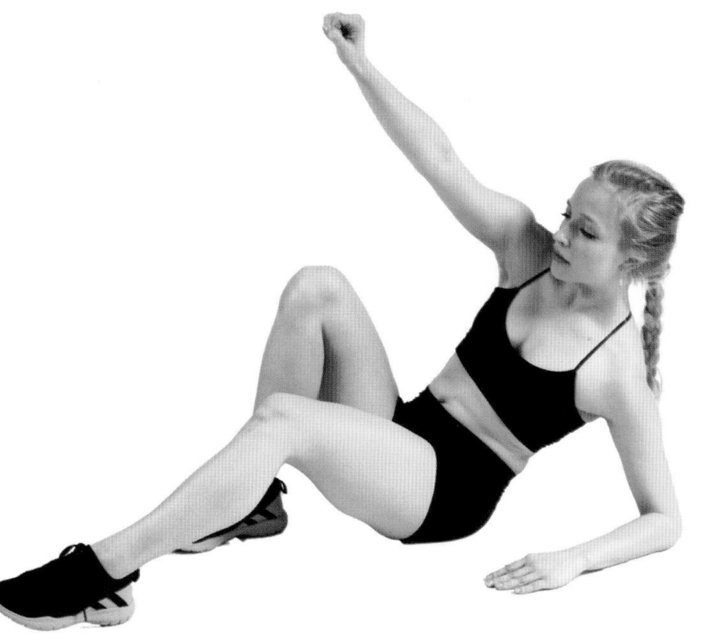

6 STEP-UP

Pages 286–87

• Perform 15 repetitions per side.

7 STEP-DOWN

Pages 284–85

• Perform 20 repetitions per leg.

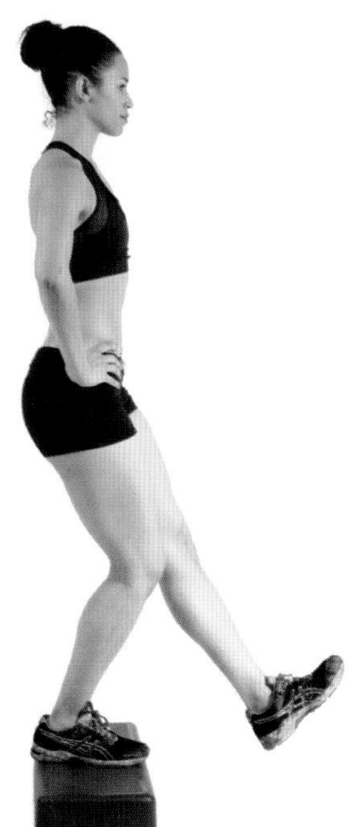

8 SKATER'S LUNGE

Pages 282–83

• Perform for 45-60 seconds.

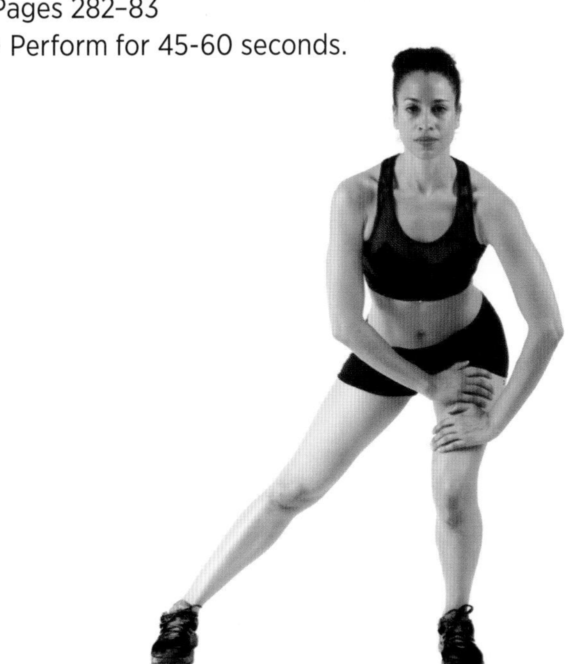

FACT FILE

TARGETS

• Whole Body / Cardio

OBJECTIVE

• Functional stamina of muscle tissues

WORK/REST

• 15-20 repetitions per exercise then onto the next

TOTAL TIME

• 8 minutes

TOTAL COMPLETED CIRCUIT SETS

• 1 set

Building Block Routine

Designed with the fundamentals in mind to give you the strength and flexibility needed to perform more advanced exercises.

1 PUSH-UP

Pages 198–99

- Repetitions and time vary by objective.

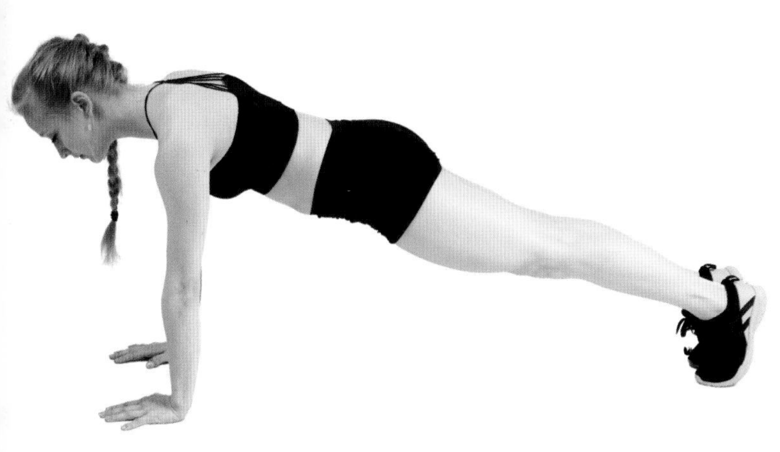

2 TRICEPS DIP

Page 190–91

- Perform 10-12 repetitions.

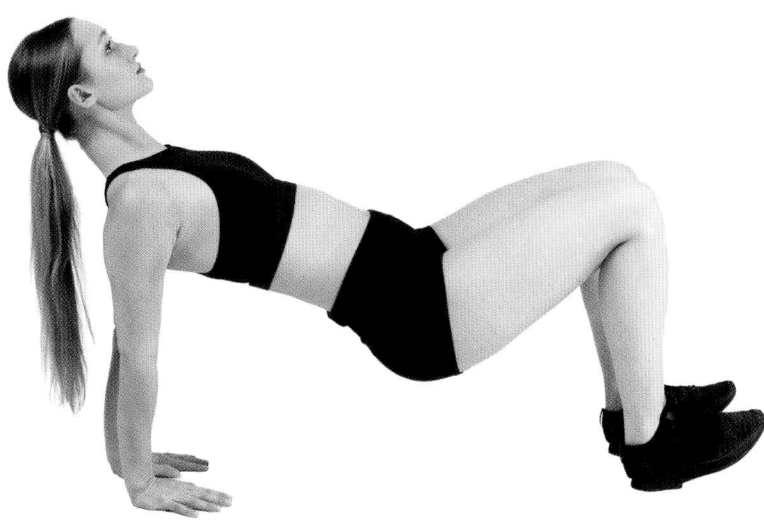

3 UP-DOWN

Pages 310–11

- Perform 10 repetitions.

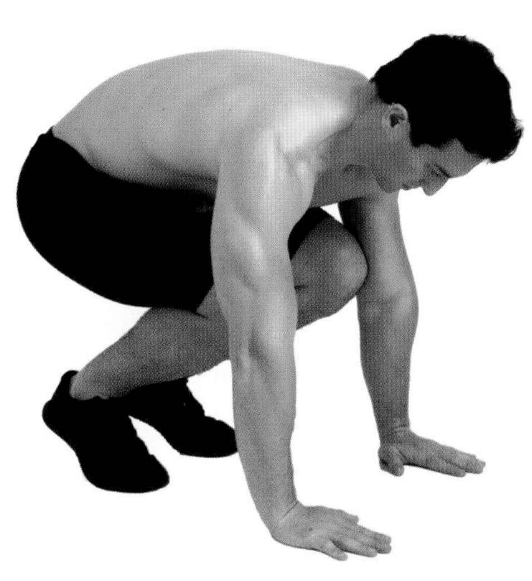

4 SQUAT

Pages 262–63

- Perform 15 repetitions.

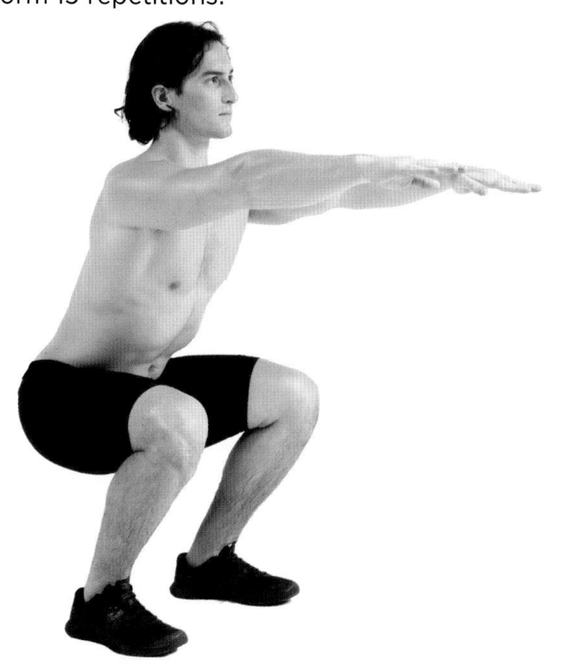

FACT FILE

TARGETS
- Lower Body

OBJECTIVE
- Overall strengthening of muscle tissues

WORK/REST
- 15 repetitions per exercise then onto the next

TOTAL TIME
- 8 minutes

TOTAL COMPLETED CIRCUIT SETS
- 1 set

5 LUNGE

Pages 266–67

- Perform 15 repetitions per leg.

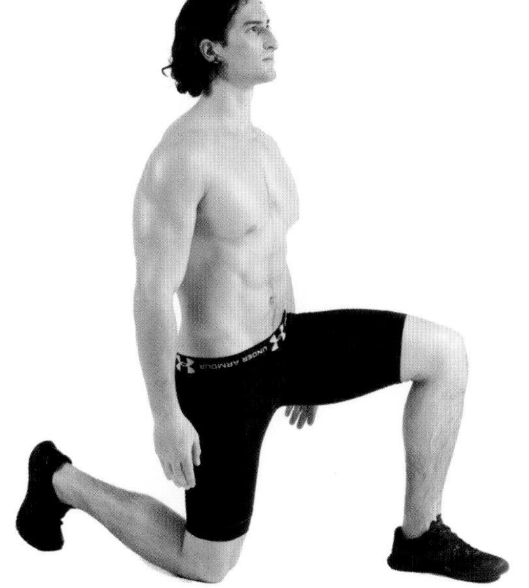

6 FOREARM PLANK

Pages 308–9

- Perform for 30 seconds to 2 minutes.

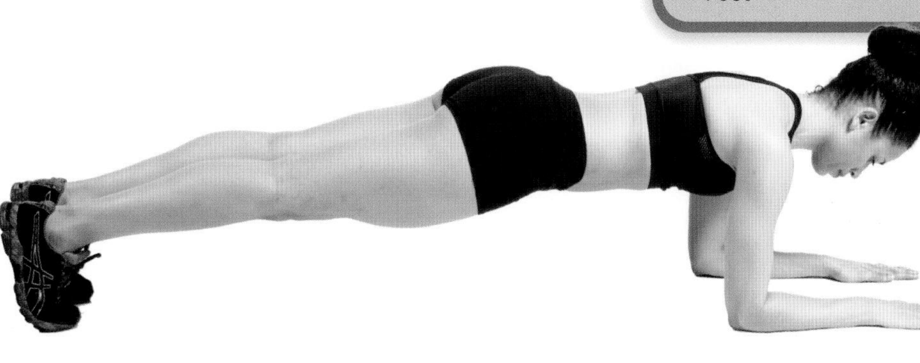

7 CRUNCH

Pages 230–31

- Repetitions and time vary by objective.

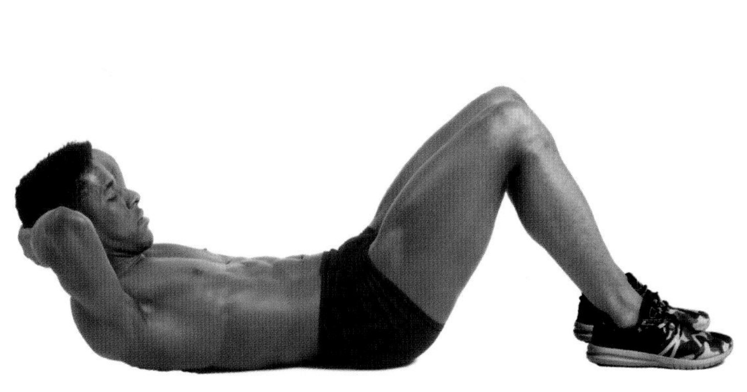

8 TWISTING KNEE RAISE

Pages 130–31

- Repetitions and time vary by objective.

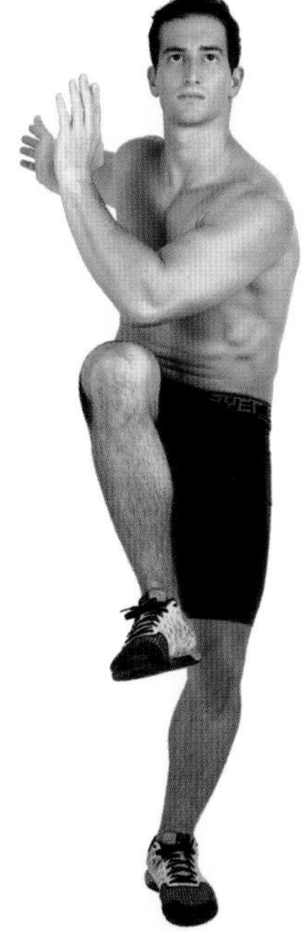

Navigation Routine

Designed with a focused assessment in mind to keep you on course.

1 SWIMMER

Pages 158–59

- Perform 6-8 repetitions per side.

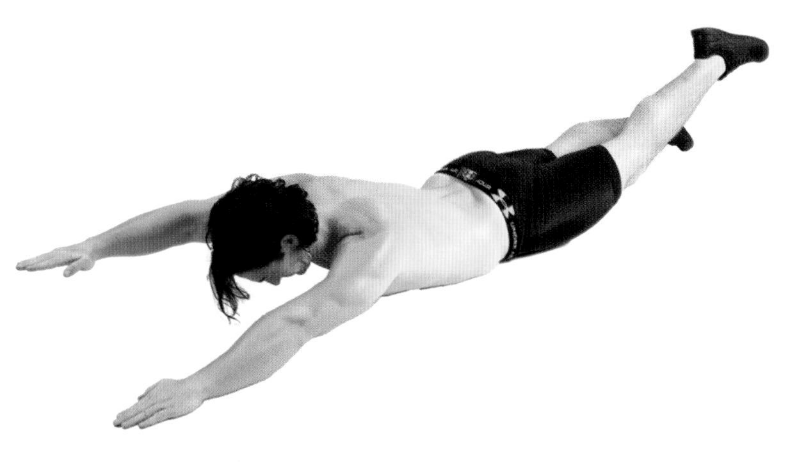

2 PUSH-UP HAND WALK-OVER

Pages 210–11

- Perform for 30 seconds, 8-12 repetitions.

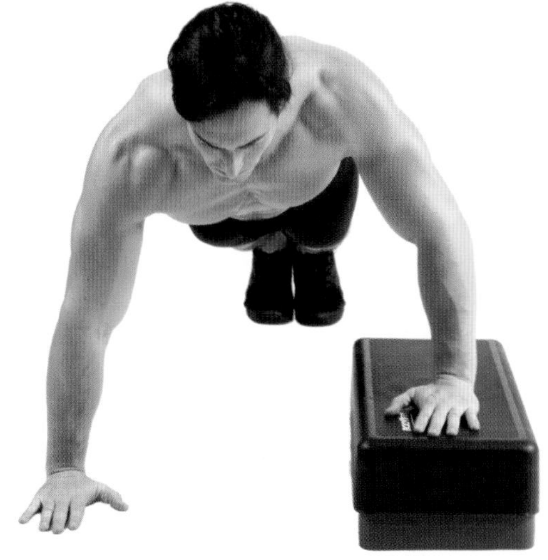

3 TWISTING KNEE RAISE

Pages 128–29

- Repetitions and time vary by objective.

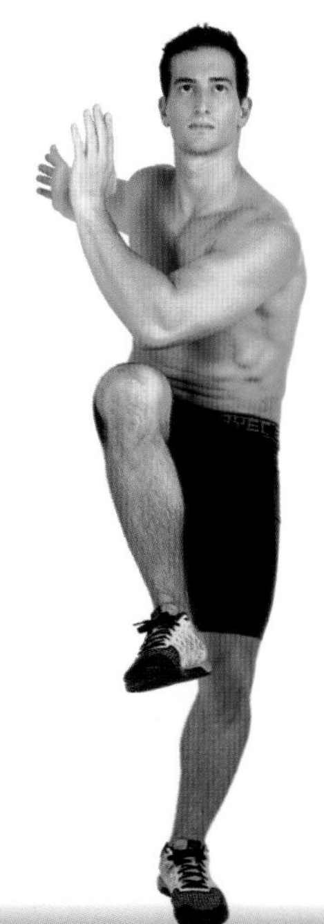

4 MOUNTAIN CLIMBER

Pages 298–99

- Repetitions and time vary by objective.

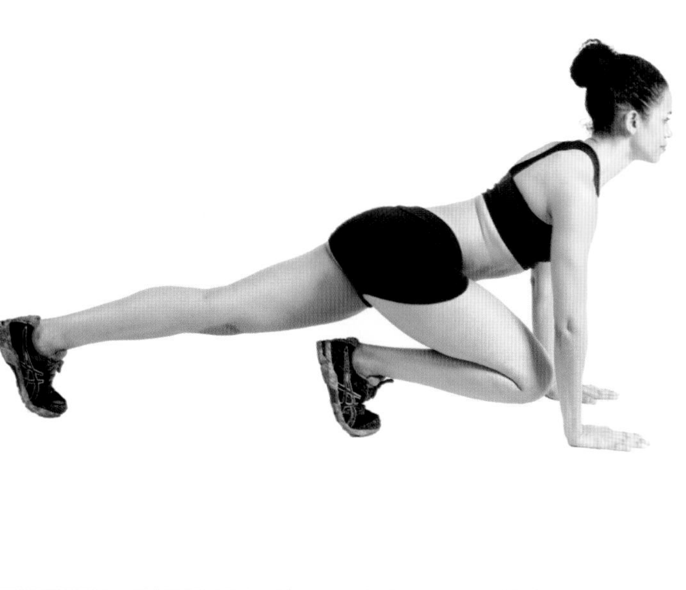

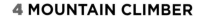

FACT FILE

TARGETS
- Upper and Lower Back

OBJECTIVE
- Precision movement of muscle tissues

WORK/REST
- 8-12 repetitions per exercise then onto the next

TOTAL TIME
- 8 minutes

TOTAL COMPLETED CIRCUIT SETS
- 1 set

5 SLALOM SKIER

Pages 296–97
- Perform for 30 seconds, 8-12 repetitions.

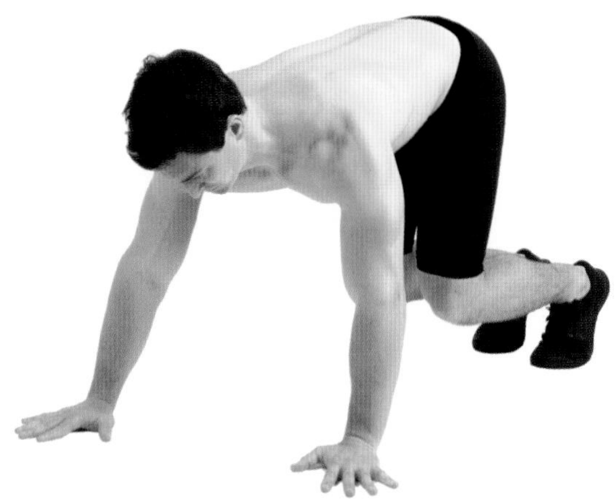

6 SIDE PLANK WITH REACH-UNDER

Pages 312–13
- Perform 15 repetitions per side.

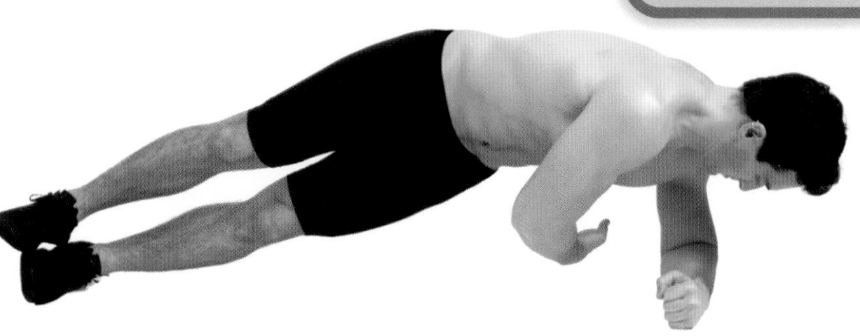

7 THE Y

Page 167
- Perform for 30 seconds, 15+ repetitions.

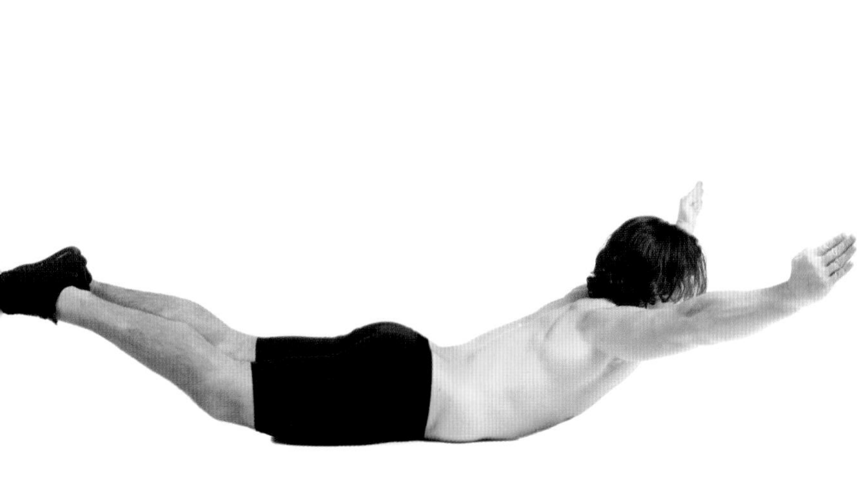

8 METRONOME

Pages 224–25
- Repetitions and time vary by objective.

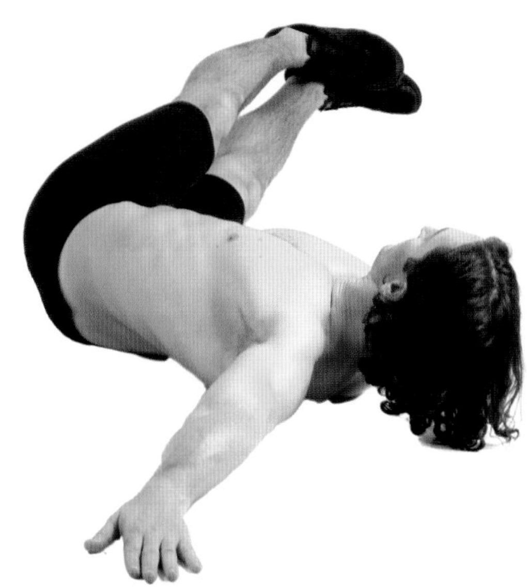

Mobility Routine

Designed to alleviate back pressure from a lengthy non-mobile posture.

1 CHAIR POSE

Pages 76–77

- Hold for 3 to 6 breaths.

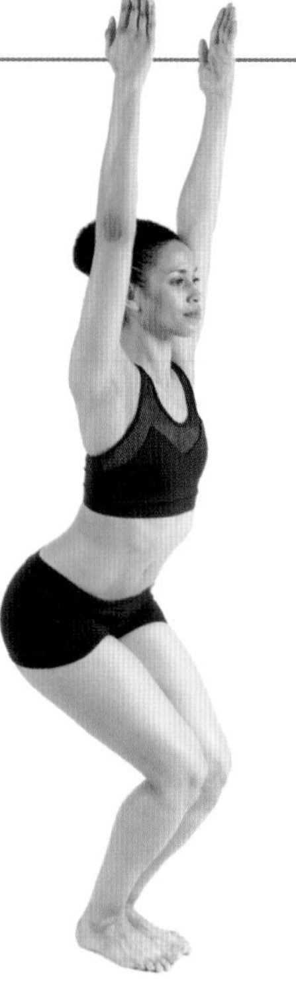

2 PUSH-UP

Pages 196–97

- Repetitions and time vary by objective.

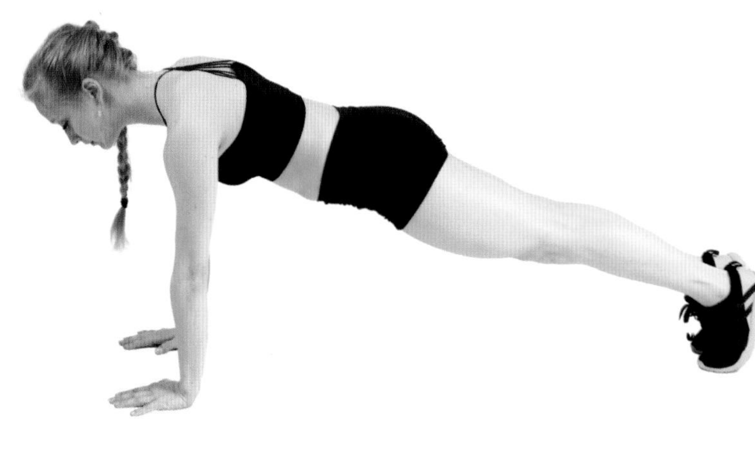

3 TRICEPS DIP

Pages 188–89

- Perform 10-12 repetitions.

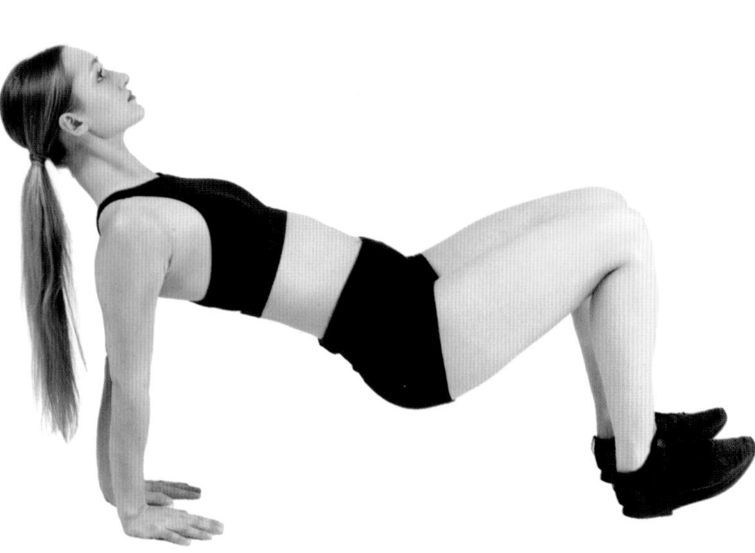

4 PISTOL

Page 137

- Repetitions and time vary by objective.

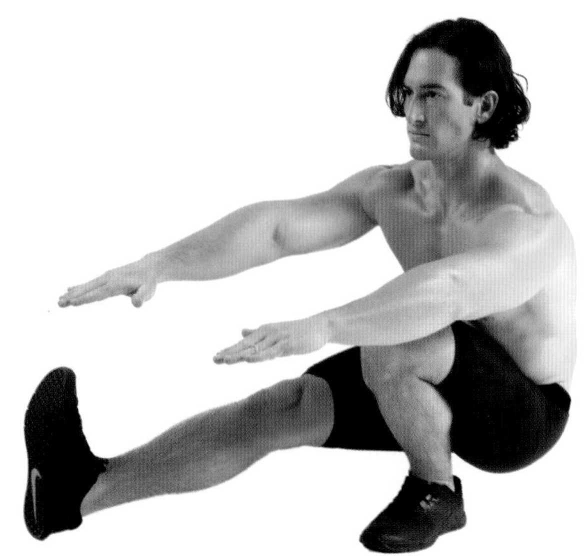

FACT FILE

TARGETS
• Whole Body

OBJECTIVE
• Relaxation of back muscles

WORK/REST
• 12-15 repetitions per exercise then onto the next

TOTAL TIME
• 8 minutes

TOTAL COMPLETED CIRCUIT SETS
• 1 set

5 REVERSE CRUNCH

Pages 236–37
• Perform 20 repetitions.

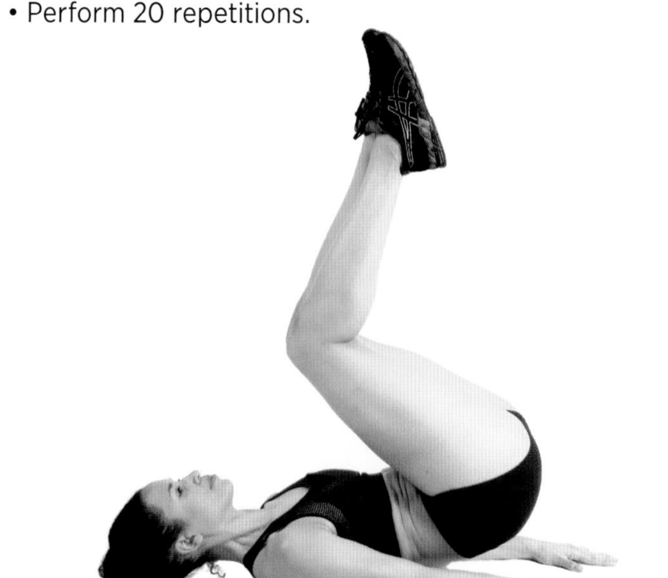

6 SQUAT

Pages 260–61
• Perform 15 repetitions.

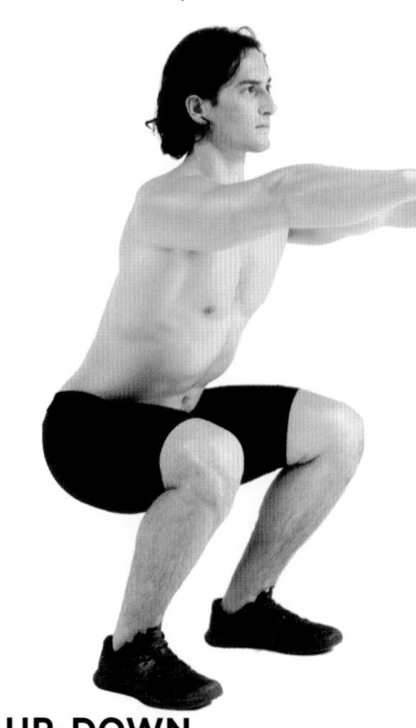

7 LUNGE

Pages 264–65
• Perform 15 repetitions per leg.

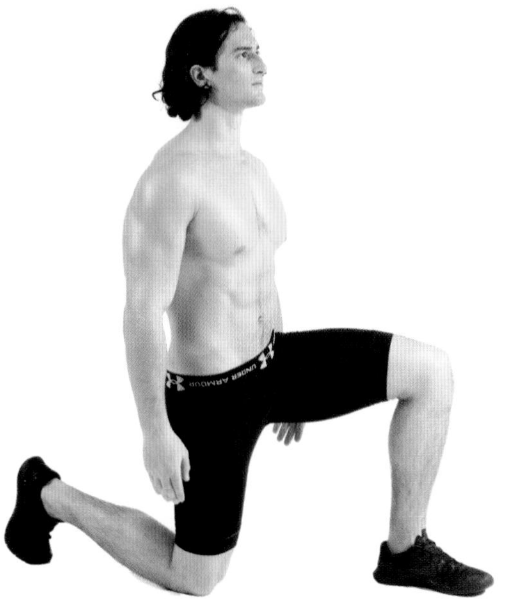

8 UP-DOWN

Pages 308–9
• Perform 10 repetitions.

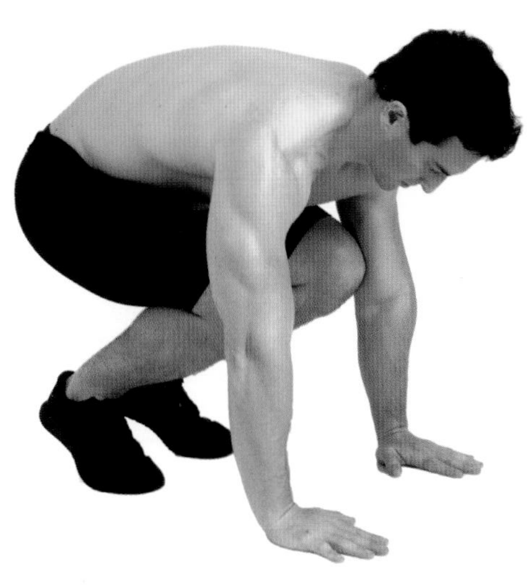

Dance Routine

Designed to warm-up and allow for more ease of movement through transitional movement.

1 TREE POSE

Pages 80–81

- Hold for 3 to 6 breaths.

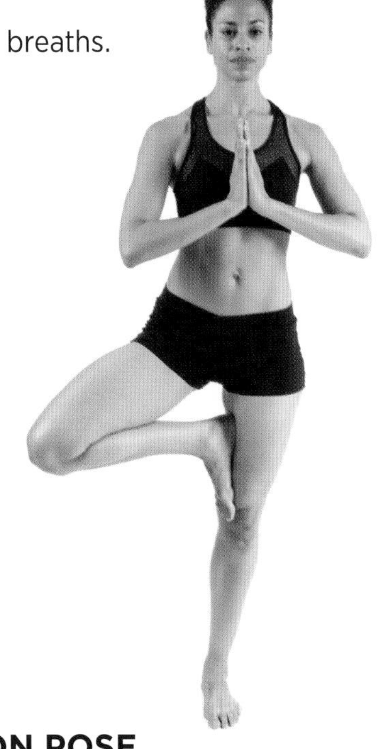

2 SIDE BENDING

Pages 48–49

- Perform 5 repetitions per side.

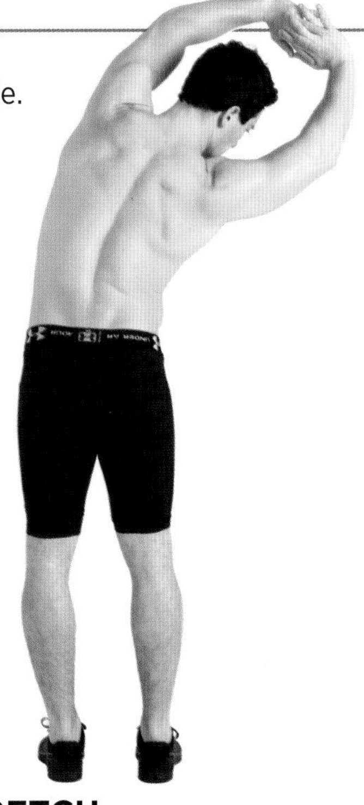

3 HALF MOON POSE

Pages 108–9

- Hold for 3 to 6 breaths.

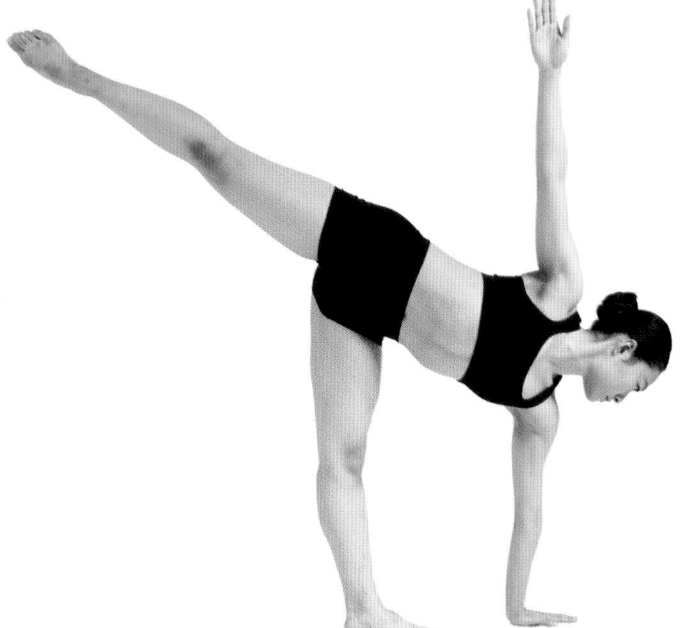

4 HALF STRADDLE STRETCH

Pages 60–61

- Perform for 30 seconds per side.

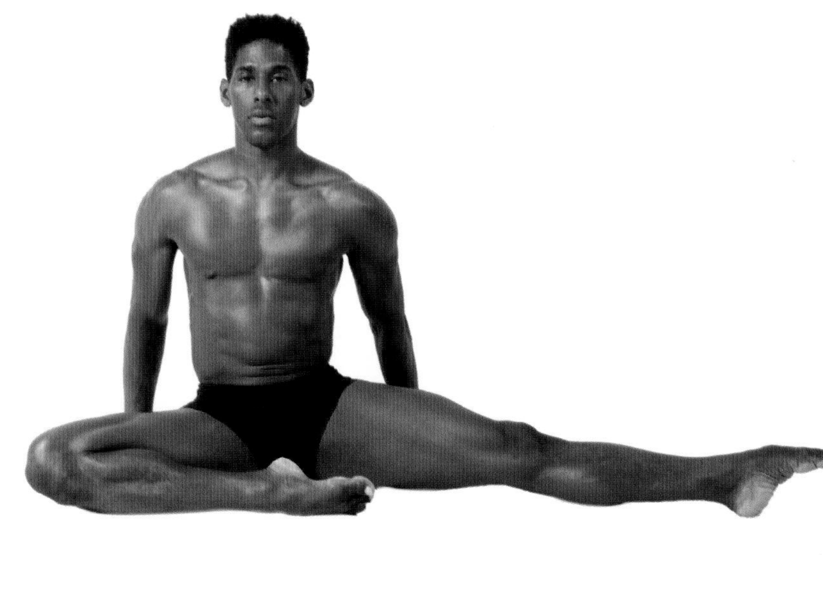

FACT FILE

TARGETS
- Whole Body

OBJECTIVE
- Pliability and functionality of muscle tissues

WORK/REST
- Approximately 3-6 breaths or 30 seconds per side per exercise then onto the next

TOTAL TIME
- 8 minutes

TOTAL COMPLETED CIRCUIT SETS
- 1 set

5 LATERAL LUNGE STRETCH

Pages 28–29

- Perform 3 x 30-second holds per leg.

6 ROLLOVER STRETCH

Pages 64–65

- Perform for 30-45 seconds.

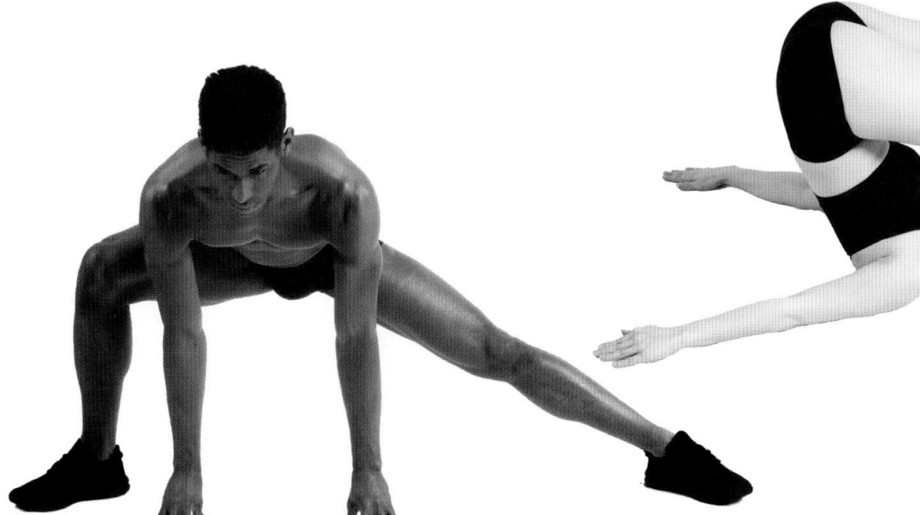

7 CROSSED-FOOT FORWARD BEND

Pages 112–13

- Hold for 3 to 6 breaths.

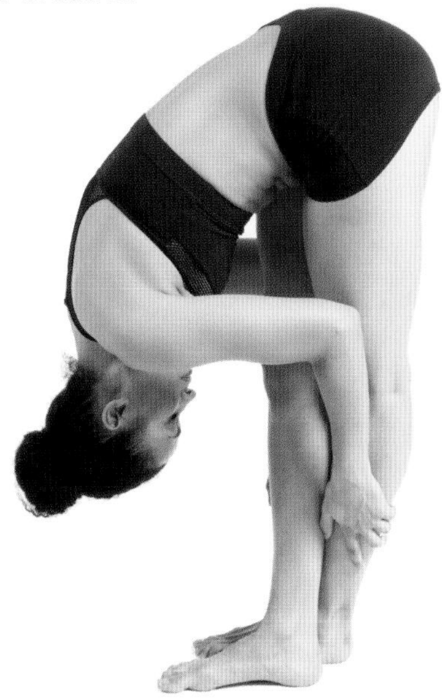

8 LORD OF THE DANCE POSE

Pages 118–19

- Hold for 3 to 6 breaths.

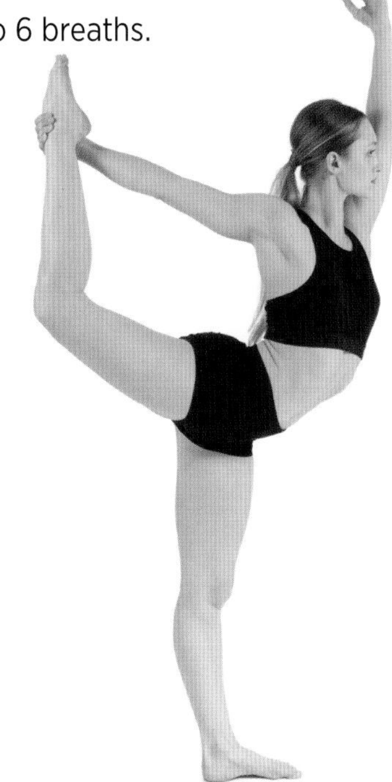

Gluteal Routine

Designed to enhance and tone the gluteal region.

1 SQUAT

Pages 260–61

- Perform 15 repetitions.

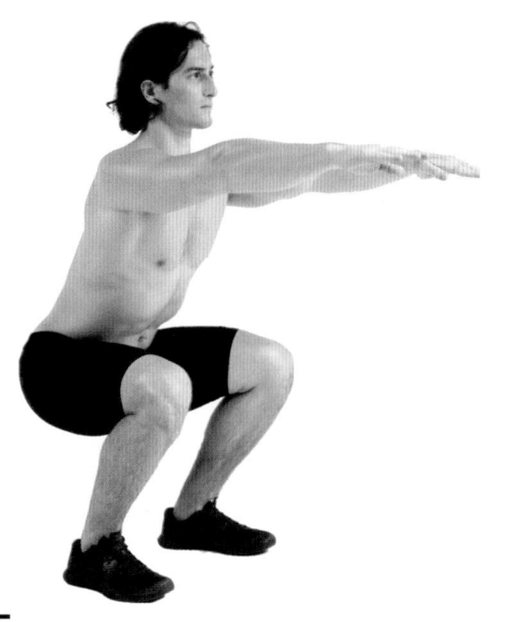

2 LUNGE

Page 264–65

- Perform 15 repetitions per leg.

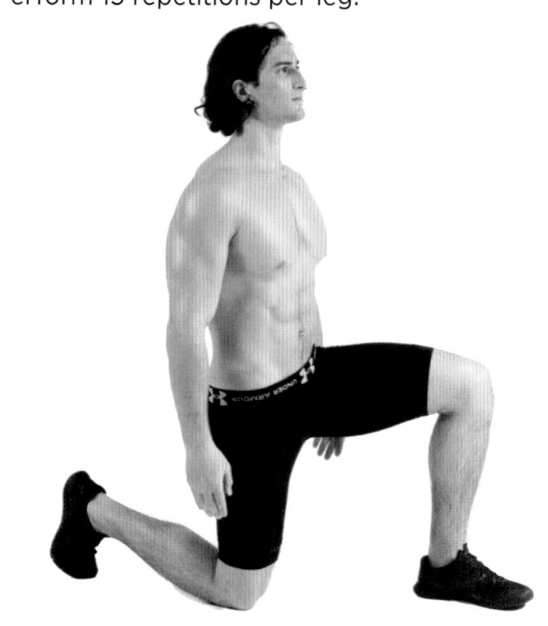

3 BRIDGE

Pages 256–57

- Perform 15 repetitions.

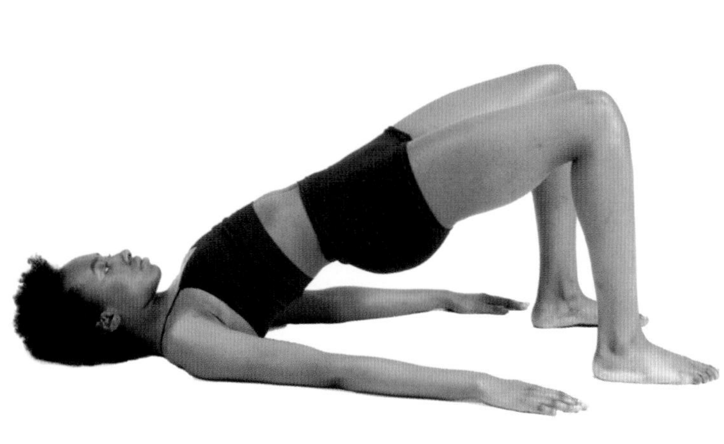

4 SWITCH LUNGE

Pages 144–45

- Repetitions and time vary by objective.

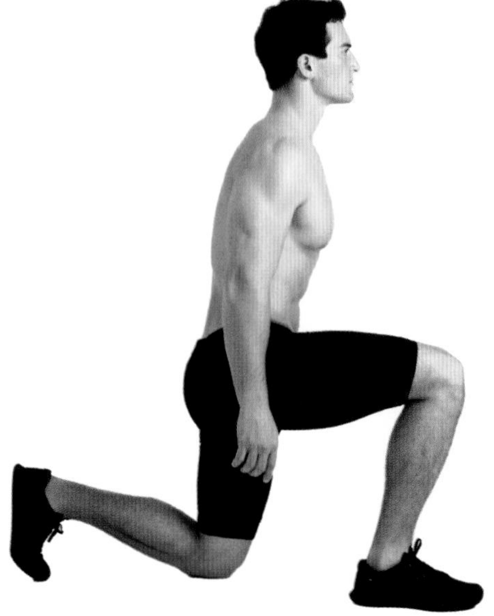

5 HALF MOON POSE

Pages 108–9

- Repetitions and time vary by objective.

6 HIGH LUNGE WITH TWIST

Pages 268–69

- Perform for 30 seconds, 15+ repetitions.

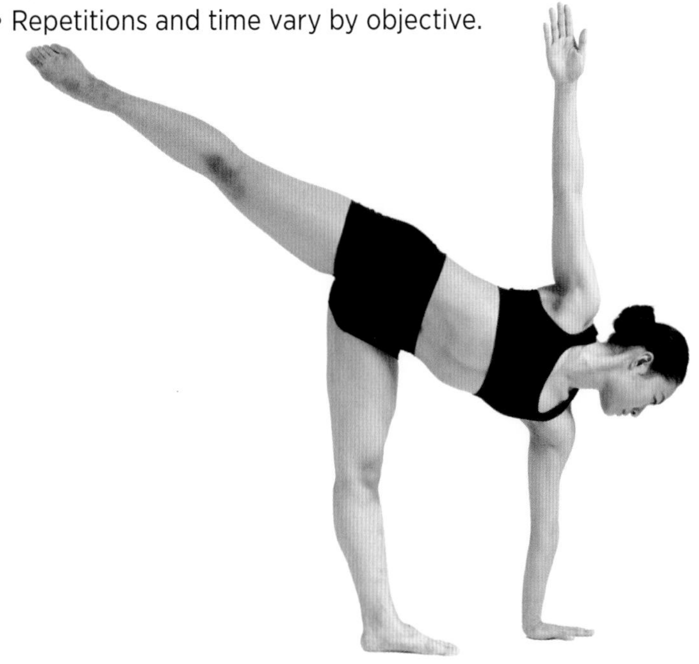

7 ALLIGATOR CRAWL

Pages 160–61

- Perform for 60 seconds.

8 MOUNTAIN CLIMBER

Pages 298–99

- Repetitions and time vary by objective.

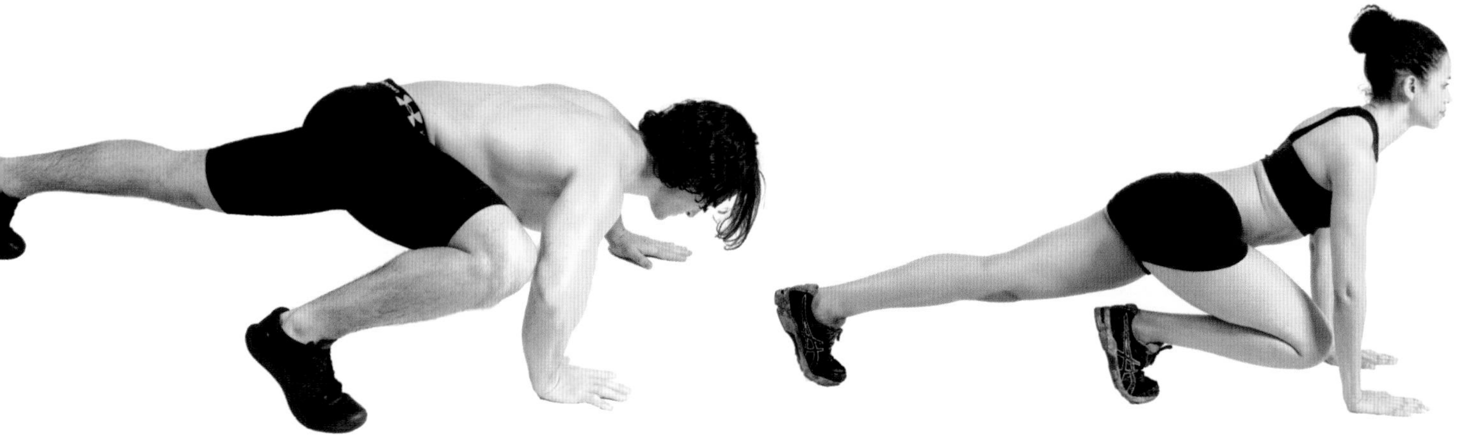

FACT FILE

TARGETS

- Gluteals and Thighs

OBJECTIVE

- Tone and aesthetic improvement of the gluteal muscle tissues

WORK/REST

- 15 repetitions per leg per exercise then onto the next

TOTAL TIME

- 8 minutes

TOTAL COMPLETED CIRCUIT SETS

- 1 set

Core Routine

Designed to enhance both power and control from the front and back muscles of the lower torso.

1 SIDE-LYING RIB STRETCH

Pages 62–63

- Perform for 30 seconds per side.

2 UPWARD PLANK POSE

Pages 90–91

- Hold for 3 to 6 breaths.

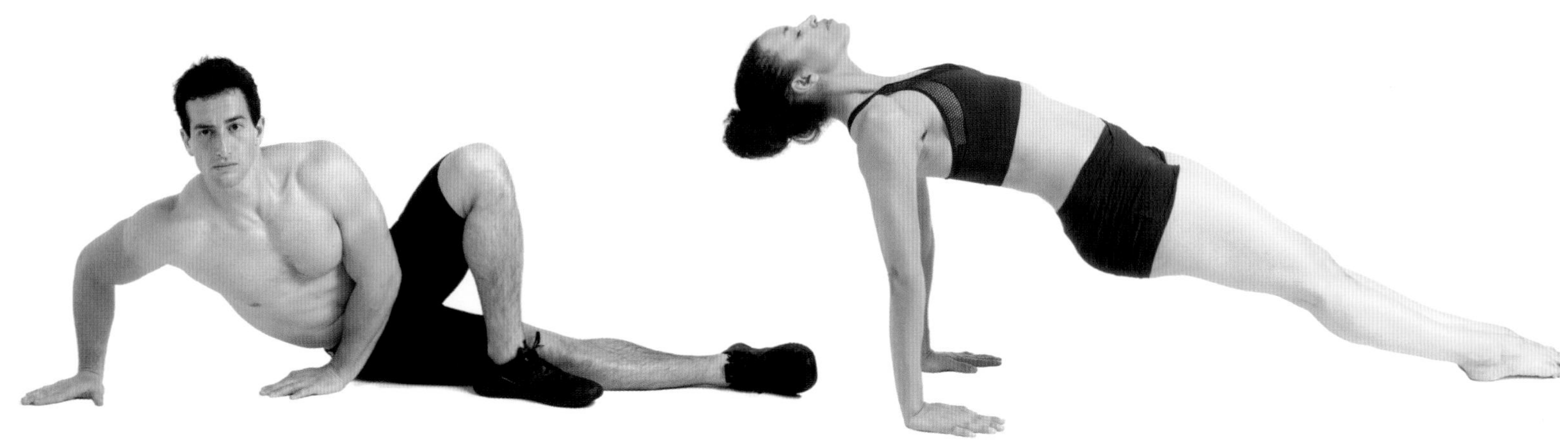

3 UPWARD PLANK WITH LIFTED LEG

Pages 92–93

- Hold for 3 to 6 breaths.

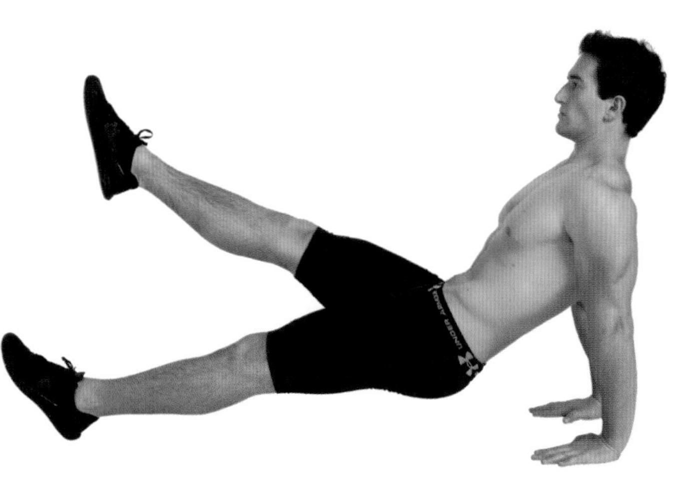

4 BENT-KNEE SIT-UP

Pages 214–15

- Repetitions and time vary by objective.

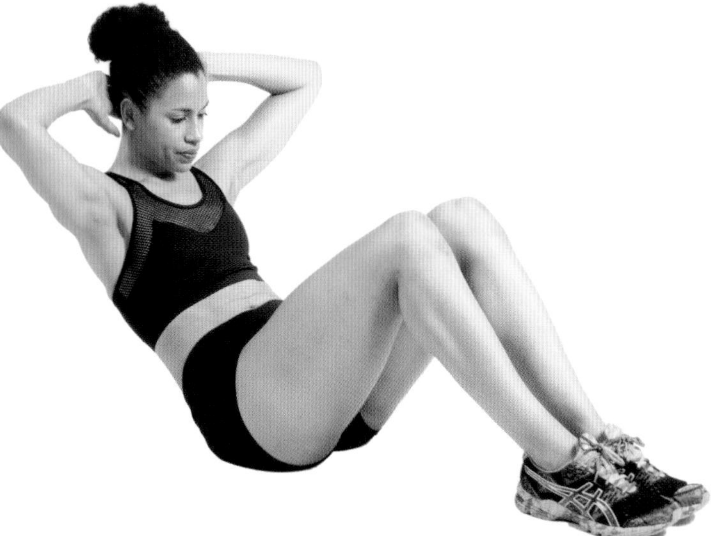

FACT FILE

TARGETS
- Core and lower back

OBJECTIVE
- Functionality of core muscle tissues

WORK/REST
- 20-25 repetitions per side per exercise then onto the next

TOTAL TIME
- 8 minutes

TOTAL COMPLETED CIRCUIT SETS
- 1 set

5 THIGH ROCK-BACK

Pages 234–35
- Perform 5 repetitions.

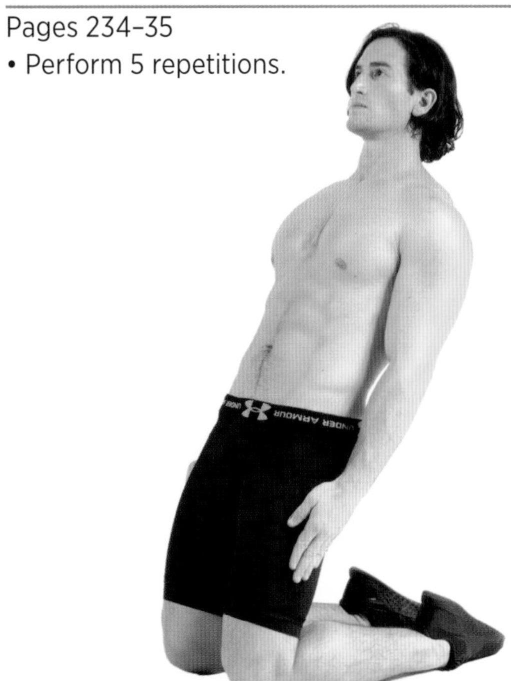

6 CRUNCH

Pages 228–29
- Repetitions and time vary by objective.

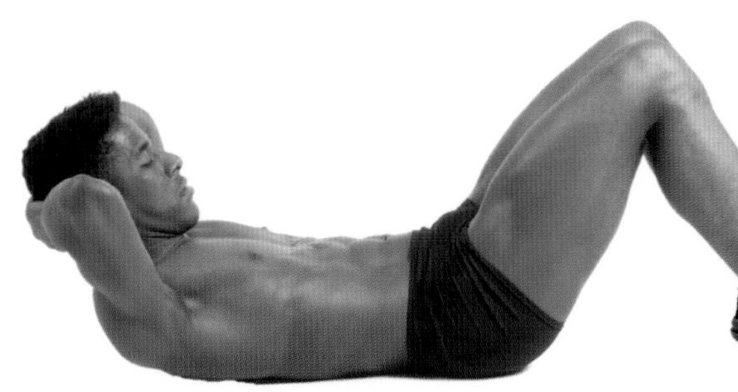

7 LEG LEVELERS

Pages 238–39
- Perform 25 repetitions.

8 BACK BURNER

Pages 162–63
- Perform 10 repetitions.

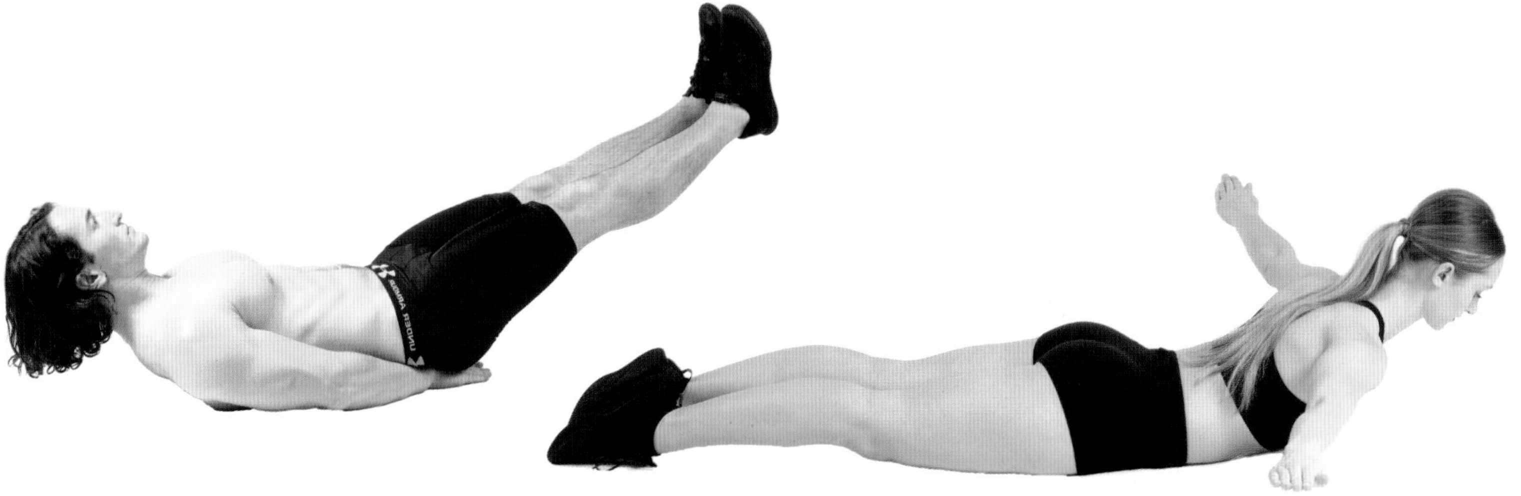

Back Routine

Designed to strengthen the back area to keep you moving and functioning.

1 ADVANCED SUPERMAN

Page 166

- Perform for 30 seconds, 8-12 repetitions.

2 BACK BURNER

Pages 162–63

- Perform 10 repetitions.

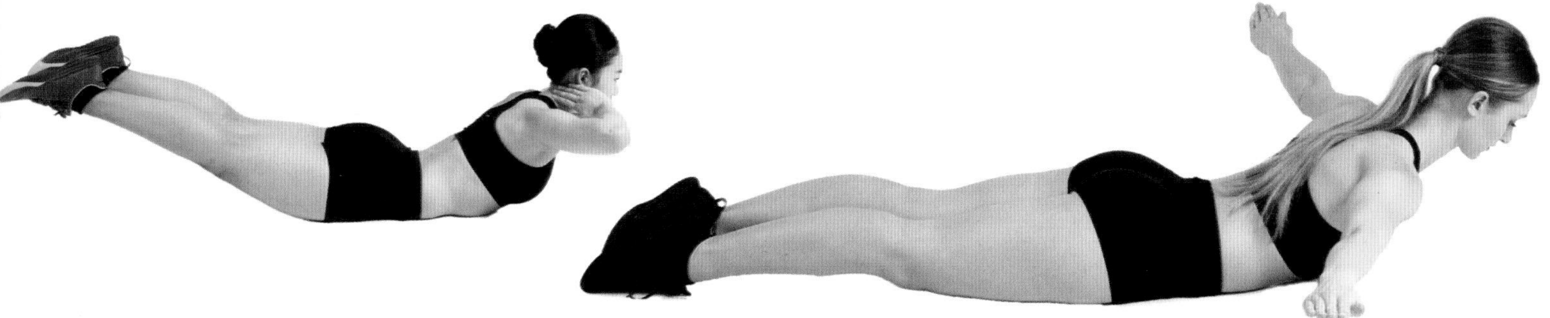

3 THE Y

Page 167

- Perform for 30 seconds, 15+ repetitions.

4 GOOD MORNING BOW

Pages 170–71

- Perform for 30 seconds, 15+ repetitions.

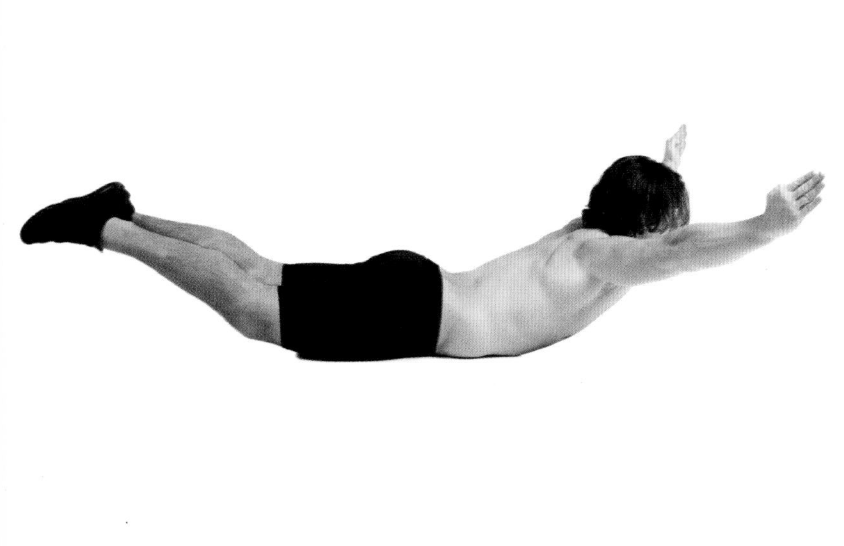

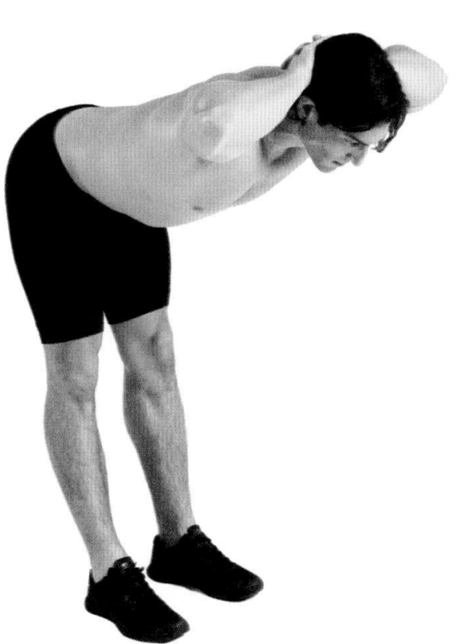

FACT FILE

TARGETS
- Upper and lower back

OBJECTIVE
- Strengthen the back muscle tissues

WORK/REST
- 15 repetitions per exercise then onto the next

TOTAL TIME
- 8 minutes

TOTAL COMPLETED CIRCUIT SETS
- 1 set

5 METRONOME

Pages 224–25

- Repetitions and time vary by objective.

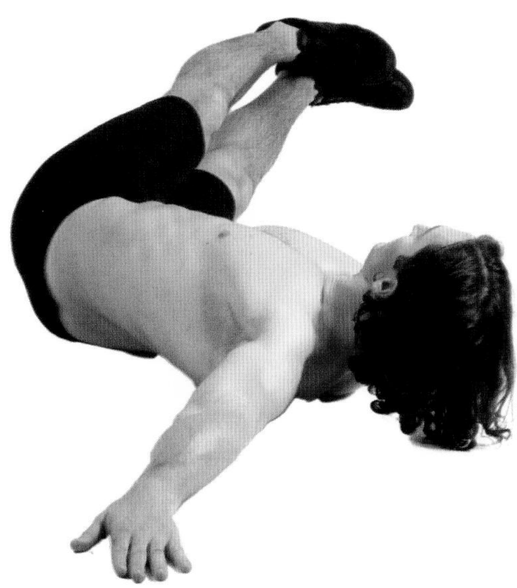

6 KNEES TO CHEST

Pages 220–21

- Repetitions and time vary by objective.

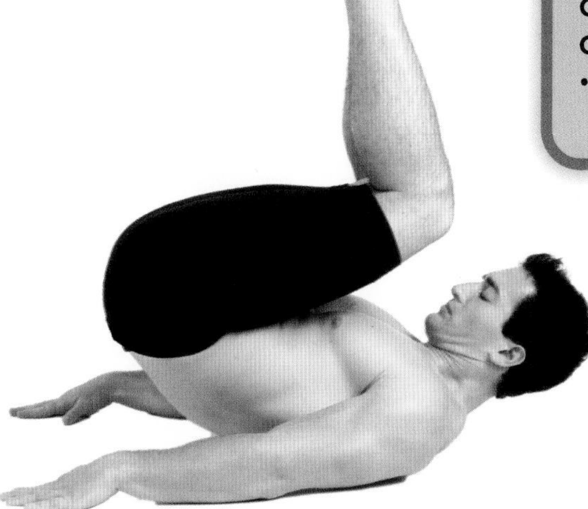

7 HIP CROSSOVER

Pages 156–57

- Perform 15 repetitions per side.

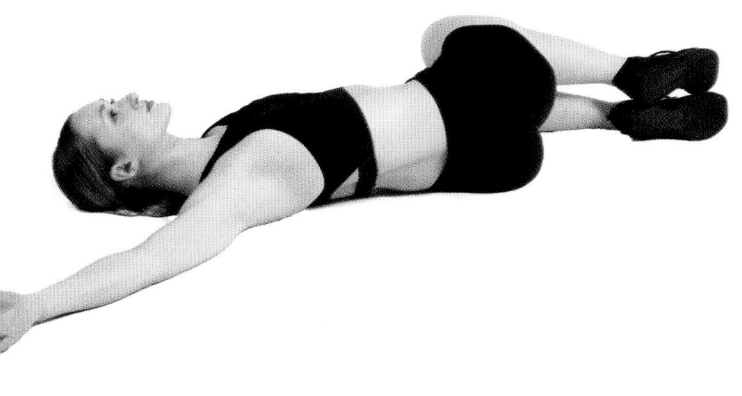

8 BRIDGE

Pages 256–57

- Perform 15 repetitions.

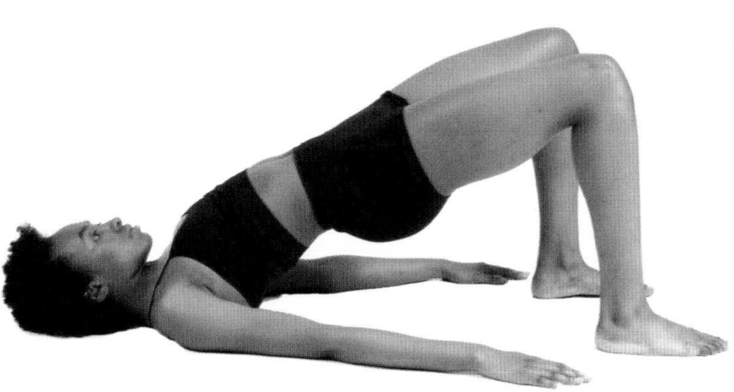

Cycling Routine

Designed for enhanced power and endurance at times when you're on two wheels.

1 HIP CROSSOVER

Pages 156–57

- Perform 15 repetitions per side.

2 SWIMMER

Page 158–59

- Perform 6-8 repetitions per side.

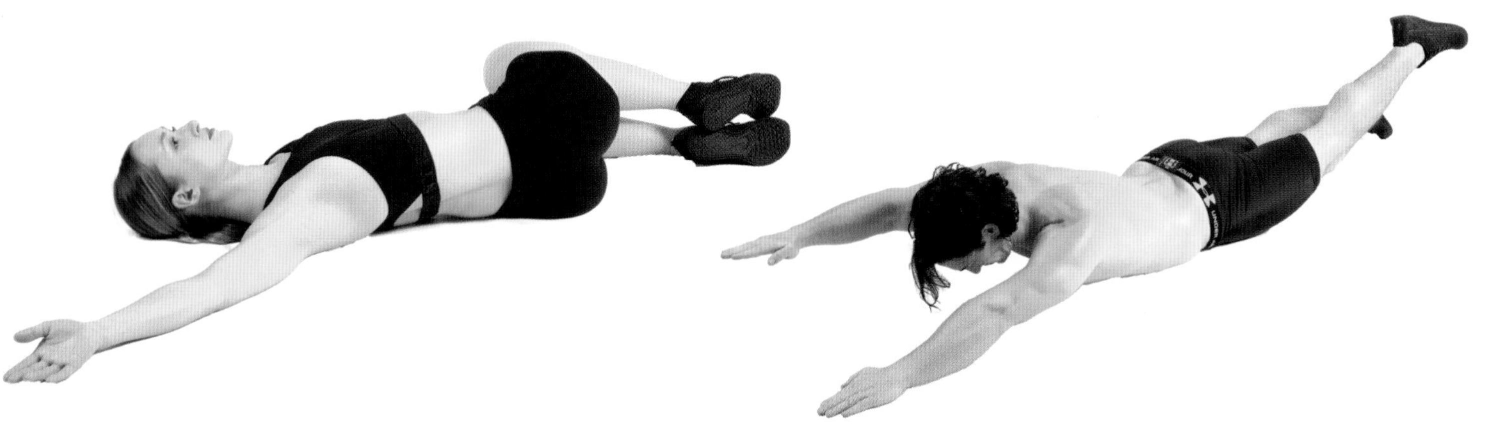

3 ALLIGATOR CRAWL

Pages 160–61

- Perform for 60 seconds.

4 BICYCLE CRUNCH

Pages 216–17

- Repetitions and time vary by objective.

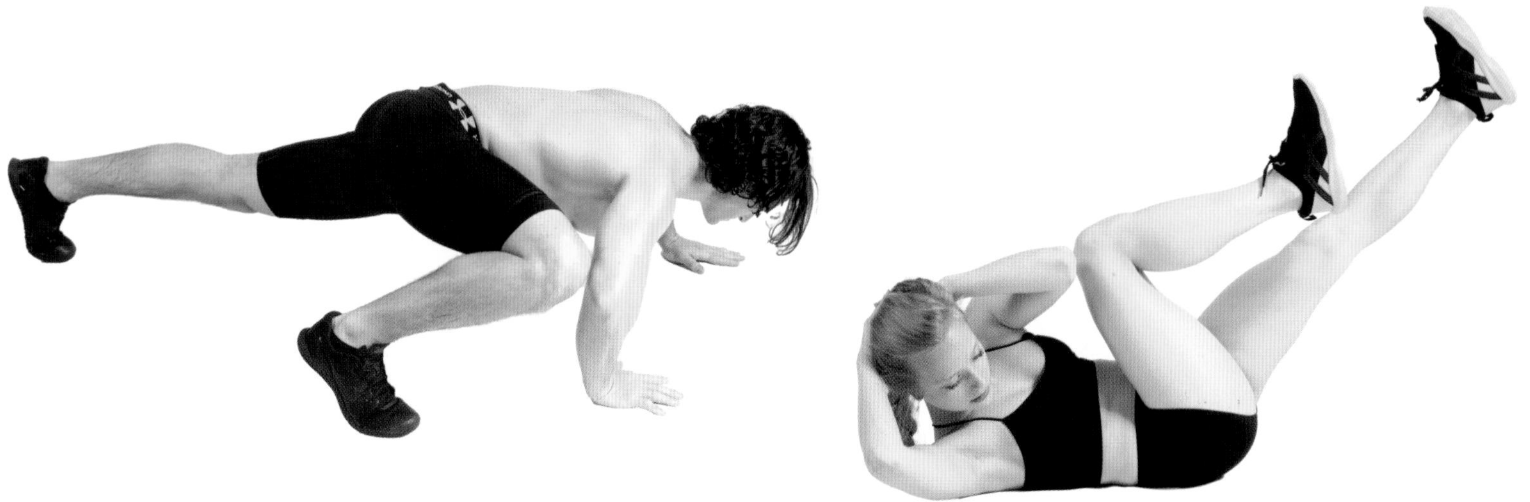

FACT FILE

TARGETS
- Legs and lower back

OBJECTIVE
- Power and stamina of lower body muscle tissues

WORK/REST
- 60 seconds per exercise

TOTAL TIME
- 8 minutes

TOTAL COMPLETED CIRCUIT SETS
- 1 set

5 DOUBLE LEG LIFT

Pages 222–23
- Repetitions and time vary by objective.

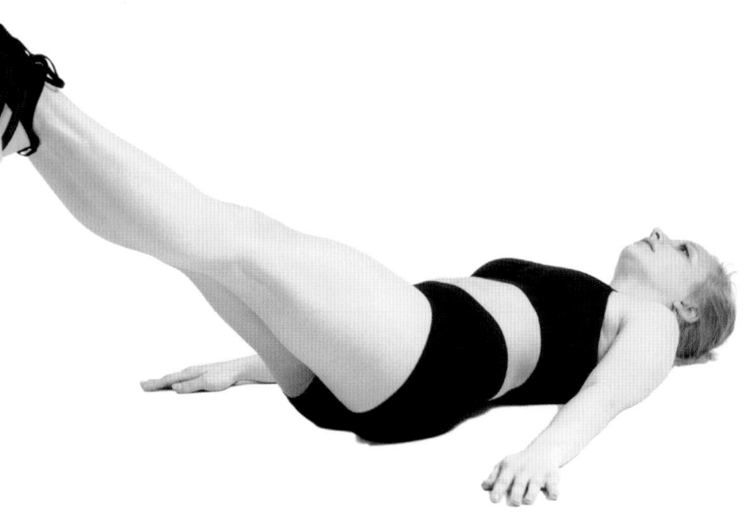

6 BEAR CRAWL

Pages 190–91
- Perform for 60 seconds.

7 ROLL-UP

Pages 300–301
- Perform for 30 seconds, 8-12 repetitions.

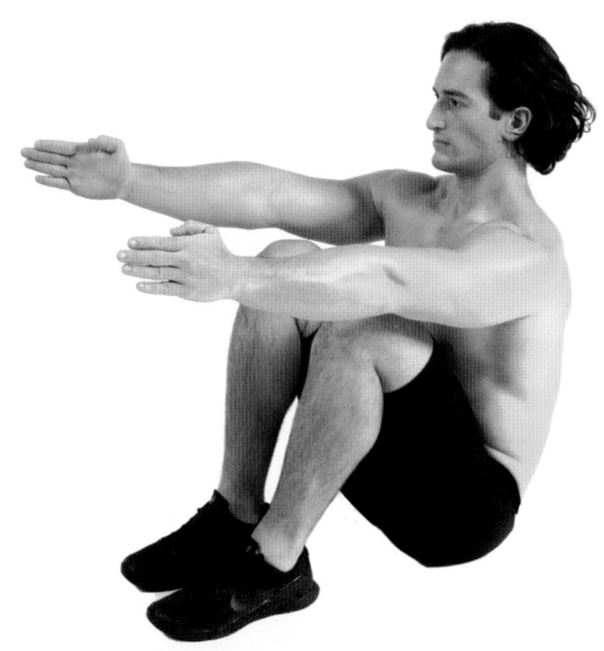

8 SLALOM SKIER

Pages 296–97
- Perform for 30 seconds, 8-12 repetitions.

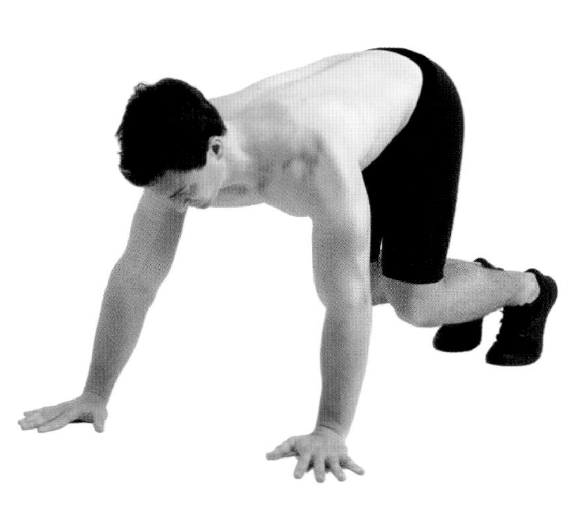

Half-Marathon Routine

Designed to keep you mobile and active for a challenge ahead.

1 WIDE-LEGGED FORWARD BEND

Pages 114–15

- Hold for 3 to 6 breaths.

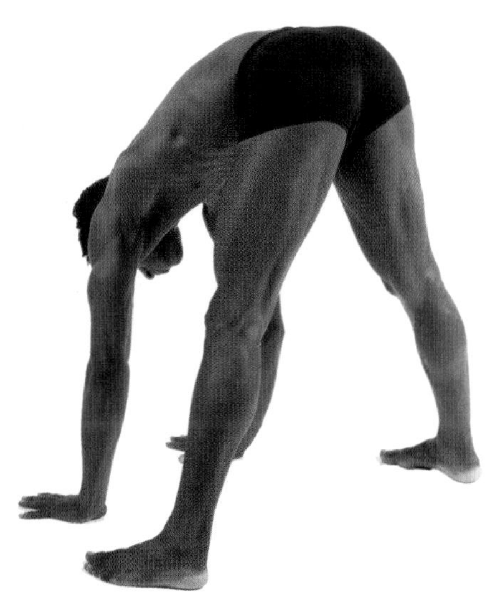

2 BUTT KICKS

Pages 124–25

- Repetitions and time vary by objective.

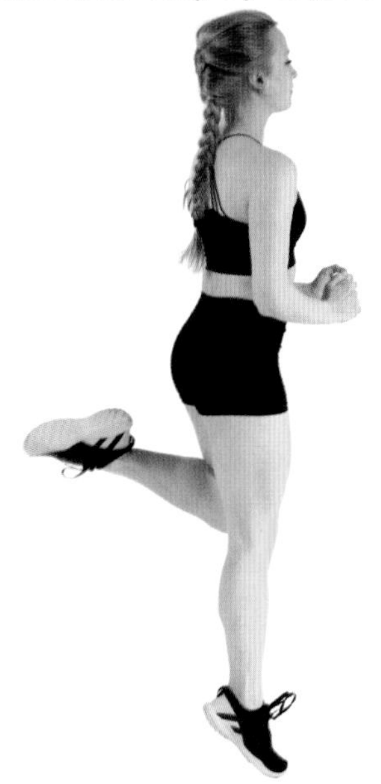

3 HIGH KNEES

Pages 142–43

- Repetitions and time vary by objective.

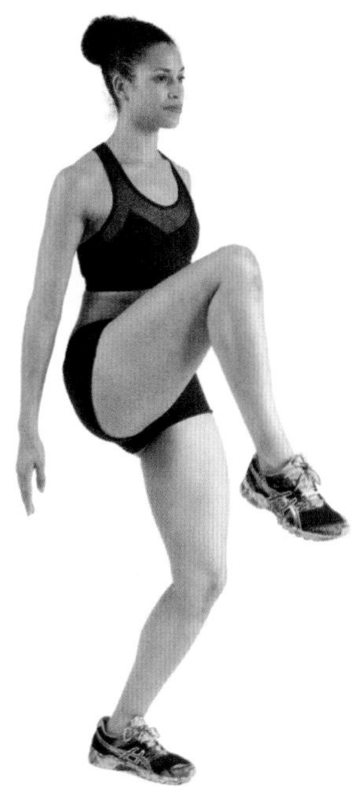

4 TWISTING KNEE RAISE

Pages 128–29

- Repetitions and time vary by objective.

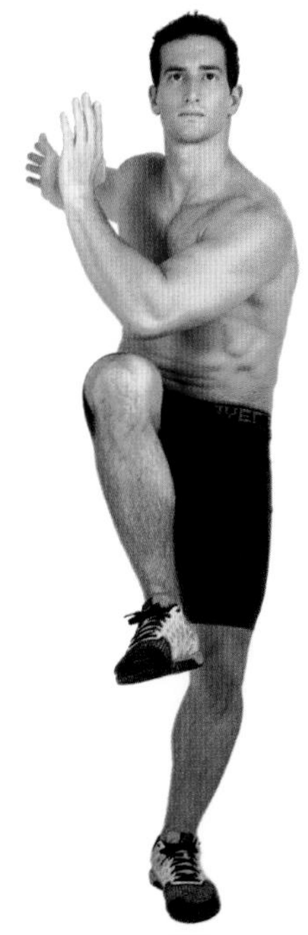

FACT FILE

TARGETS
- Legs and gluteals

OBJECTIVE
- Power and stamina of lower body muscle tissues

WORK/REST
- 15-20 repetitions per leg per exercise then onto the next

TOTAL TIME
- 8 minutes

TOTAL COMPLETED CIRCUIT SETS
- 1 set

5 SPEED SKATER

Pages 134–35
- Repetitions and time vary by objective.

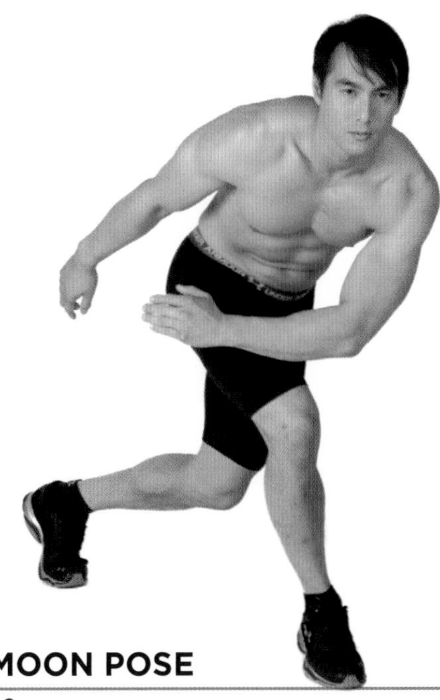

6 ALLIGATOR CRAWL

Pages 160–61
- Perform for 60 seconds.

7 HALF MOON POSE

Pages 108–9
- Repetitions and time vary by objective.

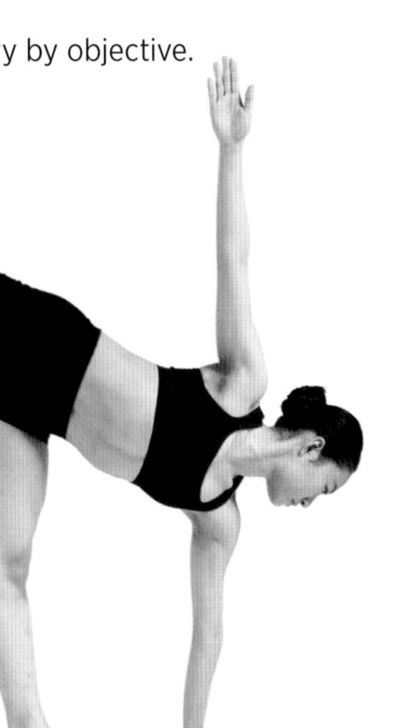

8 BEAR CRAWL

Pages 190–91
- Perform for 60 seconds.

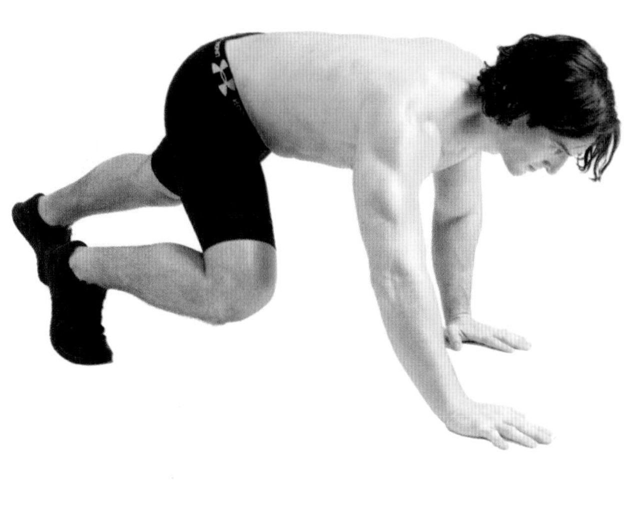

Marathon Routine

Designed to keep you increasingly mobile and active for a broader challenge ahead.

1 WIDE-LEGGED FORWARD BEND

Pages 114–15

- Hold for 3 to 6 breaths.

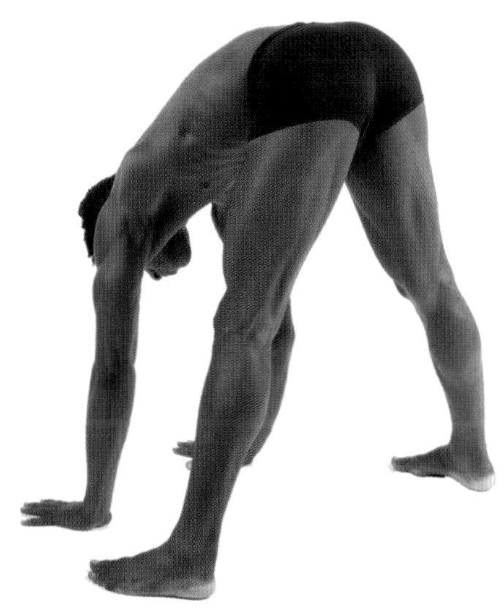

2 BUTT KICKS

Pages 124–25

- Repetitions and time vary by objective.

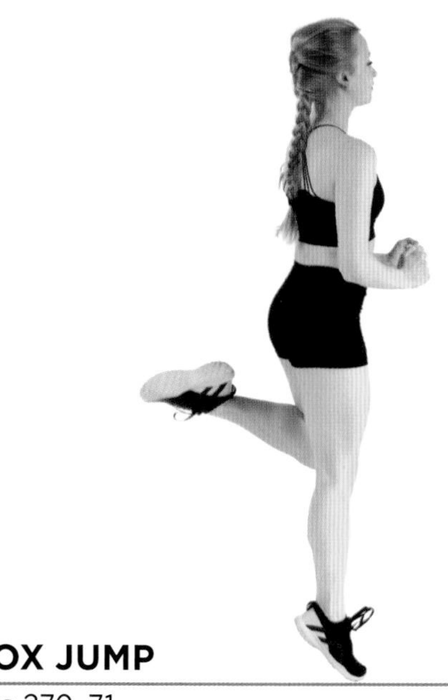

3 TWISTING KNEE RAISE

Pages 128–29

- Repetitions and time vary by objective.

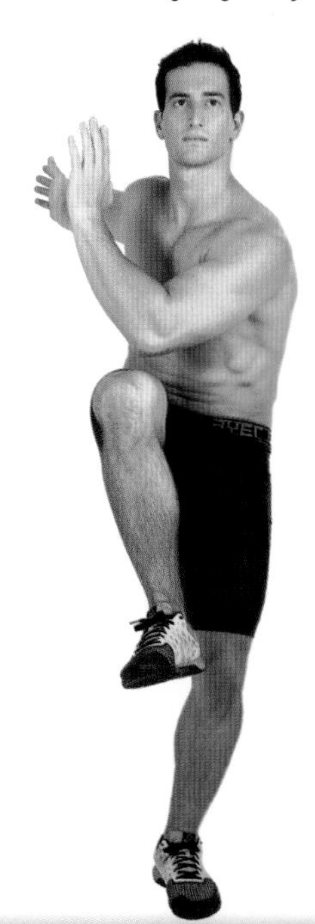

4 BOX JUMP

Pages 270–71

- Perform for 30 seconds or 8-12 repetitions.

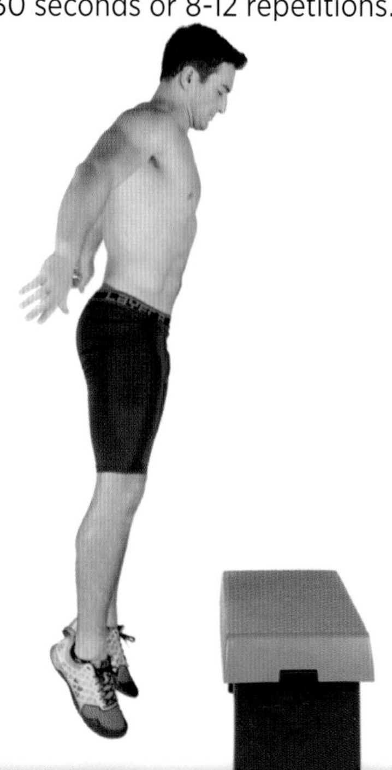

FACT FILE

TARGETS
- Legs and gluteals

OBJECTIVE
- Optimal power and stamina of lower body muscle tissues

WORK/REST
- 8-12 repetitions per leg per exercise then onto the next

TOTAL TIME
- 8 minutes

TOTAL COMPLETED CIRCUIT SETS
- 1 set

5 SWITCH LUNGE

Pages 144–45
- Repetitions and time vary by objective.

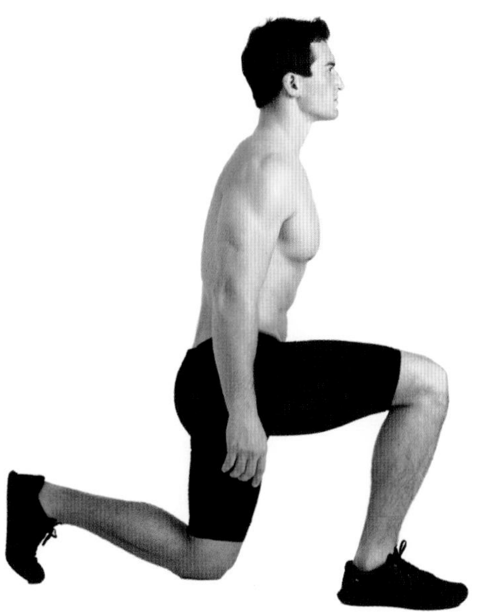

6 SINGLE-LEG GLUTEAL LIFT

Pages 262–63
- Repetitions and time vary by objective.

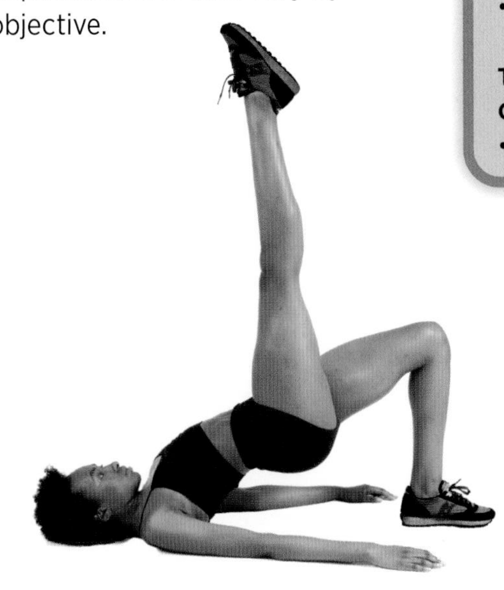

7 JUMP ROPE

Pages 150–51
- Repetitions and time vary by objective.

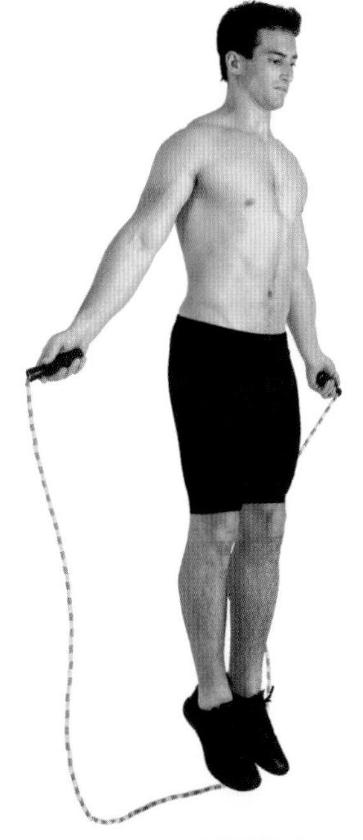

8 HIGH KNEES

Pages 142–43
- Repetitions and time vary by objective.

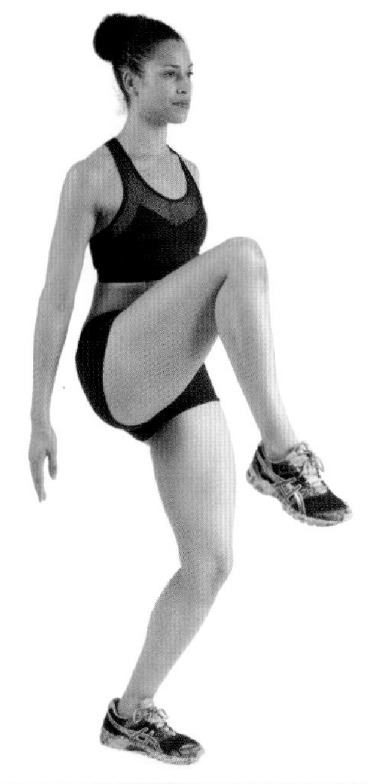

Kitchen Sink Routine

Designed for a medley of the majority of workout modalities.

1 BURPEE

Pages 122–23

- Repetitions and time vary by objective.

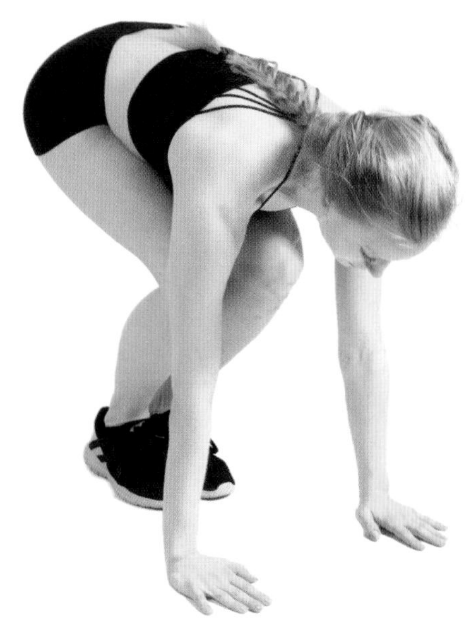

2 WARM-UP OBSTACLE COURSE

Page 126–27

- Repetitions and time vary by objective.

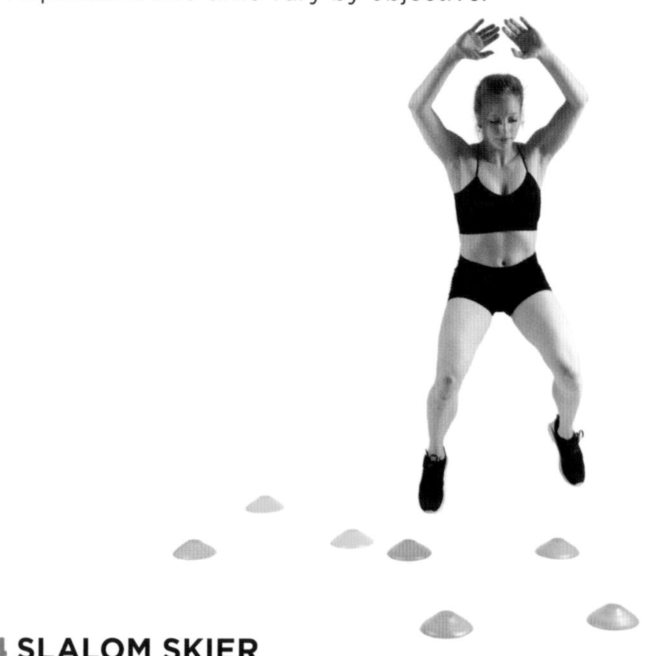

3 STAR JUMP

Pages 130–31

- Repetitions and time vary by objective.

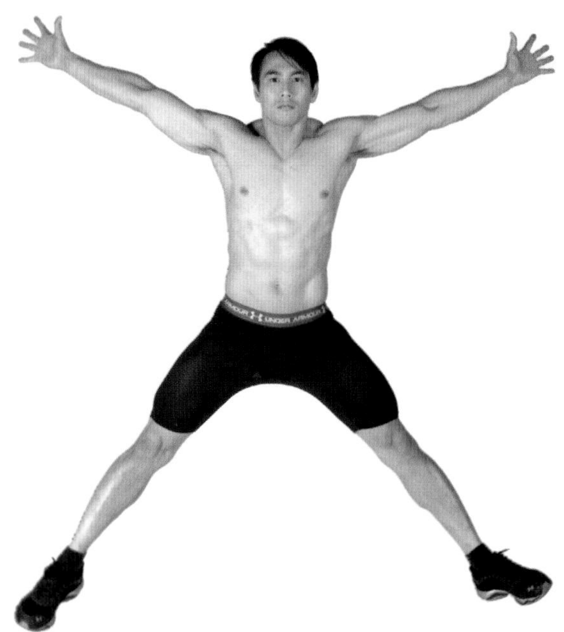

4 SLALOM SKIER

Pages 296–97

- Perform for 30 seconds, 8-12 repetitions.

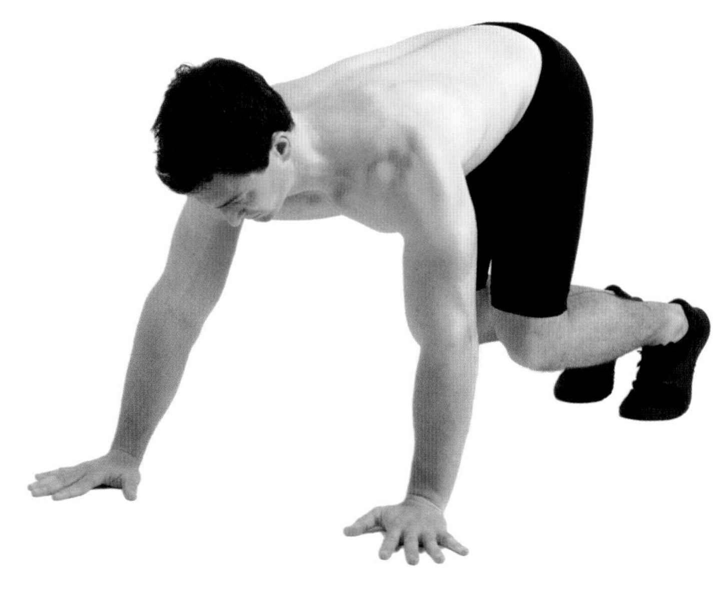

FACT FILE

TARGETS
- Cardio and whole body

OBJECTIVE
- Overall functionality of muscle tissues

WORK/REST
- 12-15 repetitions per exercise then onto the next

TOTAL TIME
- 8 minutes

TOTAL COMPLETED CIRCUIT SETS
- 1 set

5 BEAR CRAWL

Pages 190–91

- Perform for 60 seconds.

6 HIGH PLANK KICK-THROUGH

Pages 146–47

- Repetitions and time vary by objective.

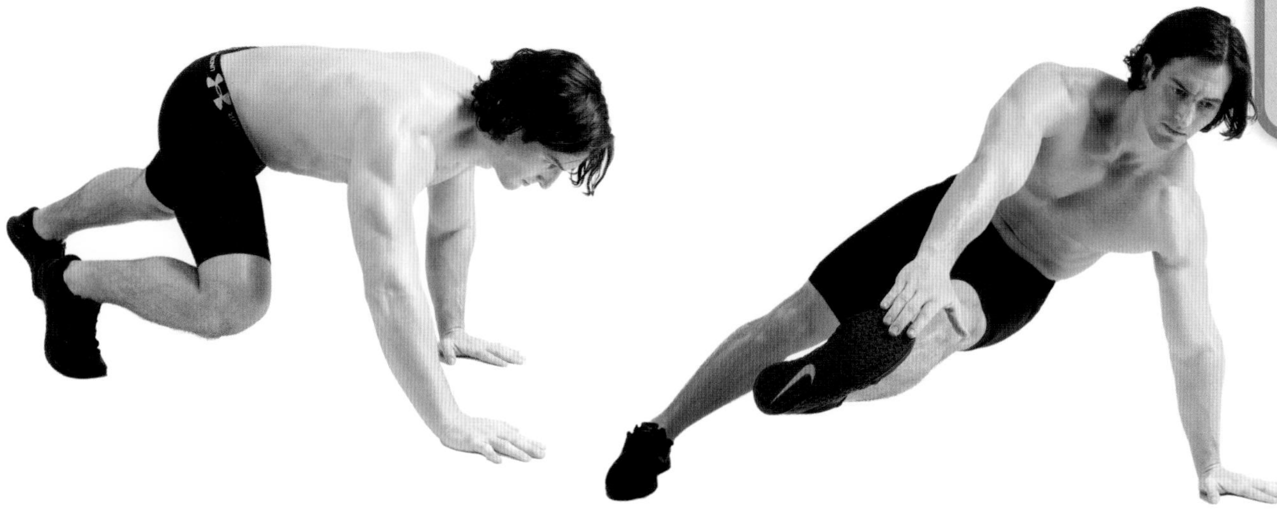

7 PUSH-UP HAND WALK-OVER

Pages 210–11

- Perform for 30 seconds, 8-12 repetitions.

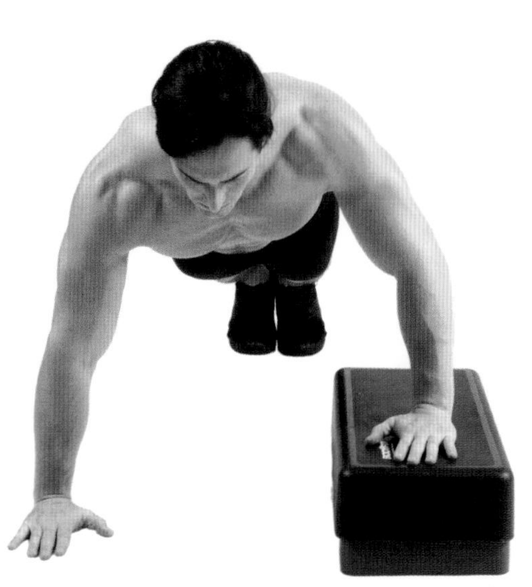

8 V-UP

Pages 26–27

- Repetitions and time vary by objective.

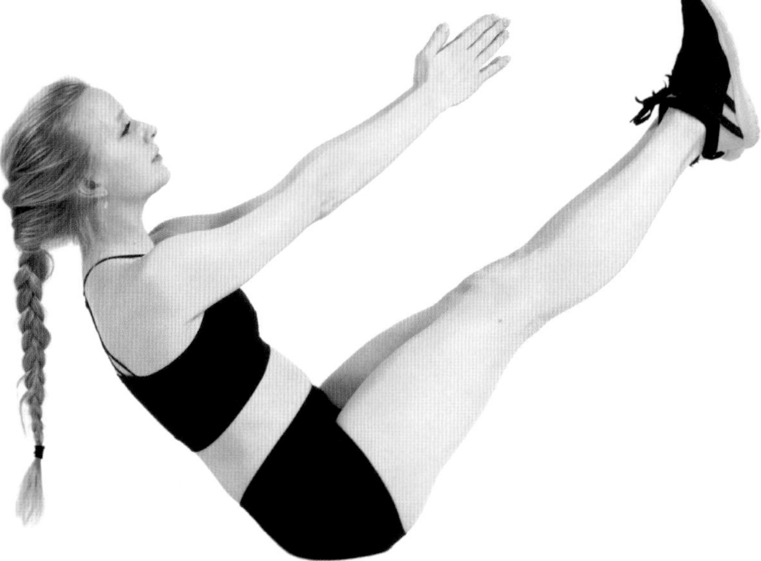

Advanced Flexibility Routine

Designed for ease of movement and the limbs from which activity springs.

1 REVERSE TABLETOP POSE

Pages 98–99

- Hold for 3 to 6 breaths.

2 HALF MOON POSE

Pages 108–10

- Hold for 3 to 6 breaths.

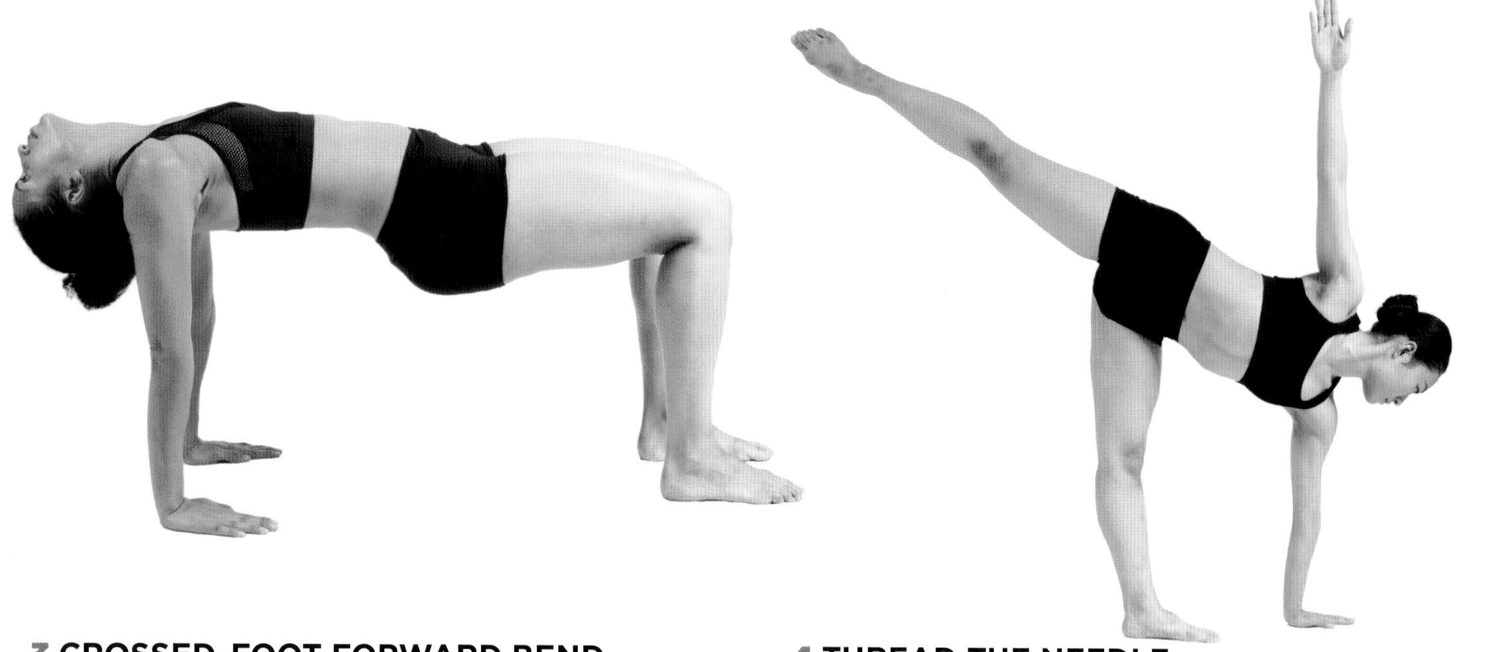

3 CROSSED-FOOT FORWARD BEND

Pages 112–13

- Hold for 3 to 6 breaths.

4 THREAD THE NEEDLE

Pages 154–55

- Perform 15 repetitions per side.

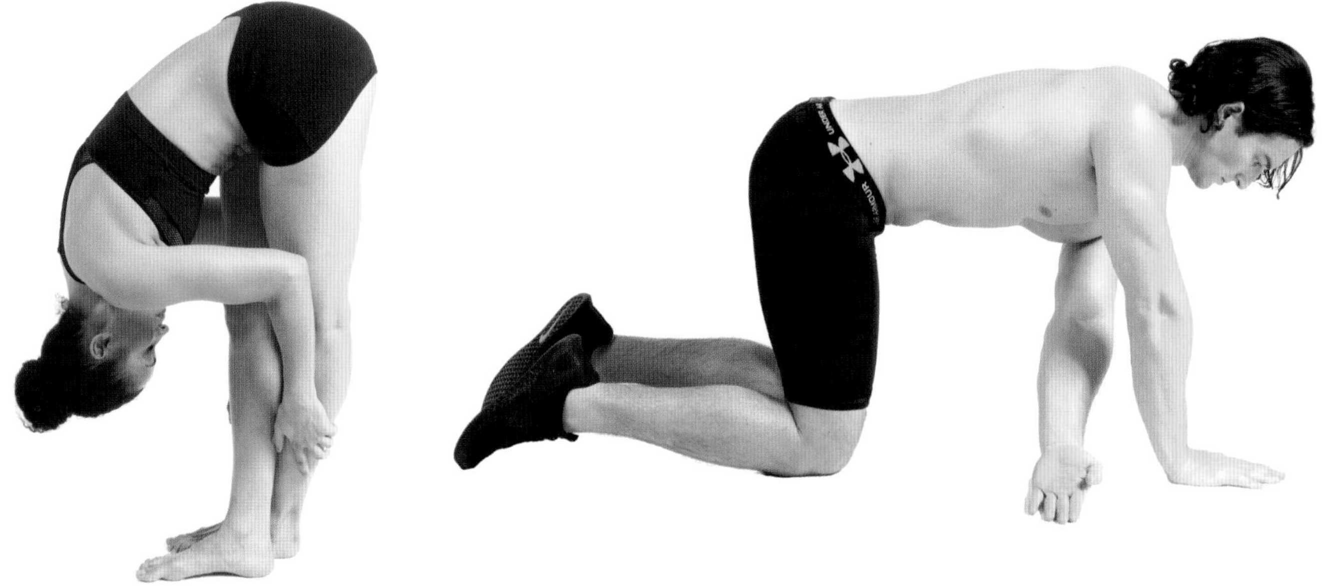

FACT FILE

TARGETS
- Whole body

OBJECTIVE
- Optimal pliability of muscle tissues

WORK/REST
- 12-15 repetitions per exercise then onto the next

TOTAL TIME
- 8 minutes

TOTAL COMPLETED CIRCUIT SETS
- 1 set

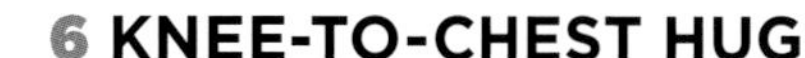

5 SCISSORS

Pages 232–33

- Perform 12-15 repetitions per leg.

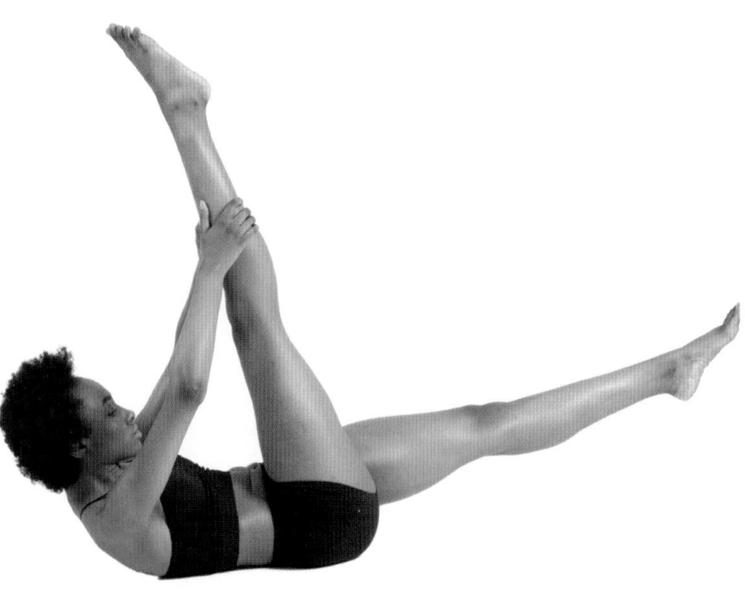

6 KNEE-TO-CHEST HUG

Pages 58–59

- Perform for 30 seconds per side.

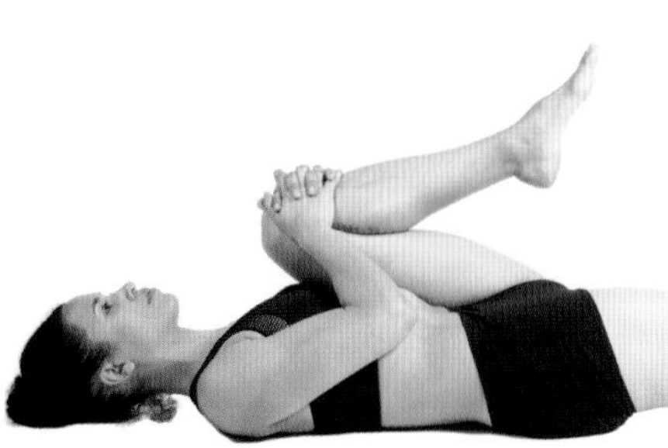

7 SAW STRETCH

Pages 32–33

- Perform for 30-45 seconds.

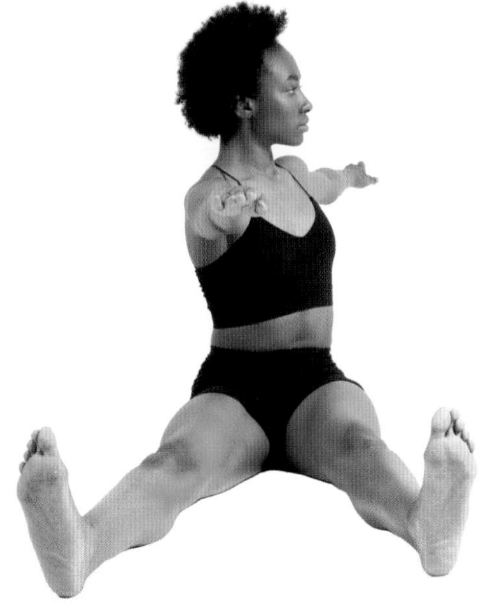

8 LYING-DOWN PRETZEL STRETCH

Pages 34–35

- Perform for 30 seconds per side.

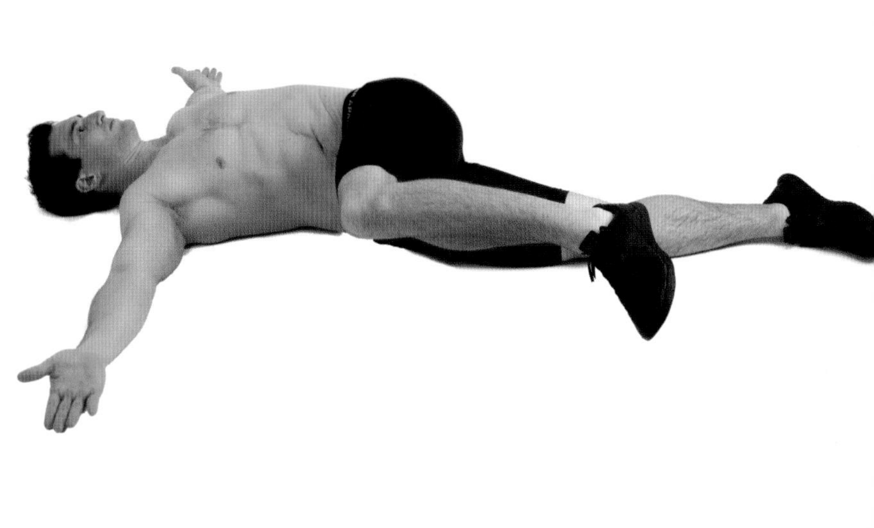

Endurance Routine

Designed to keep you going so you can keep on going.

1 TWISTING KNEE RAISE

Pages 128–29

- Repetitions and time vary by objective.

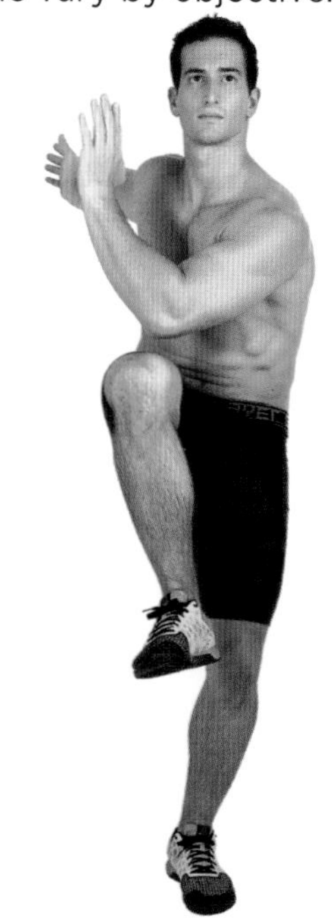

2 SPEED SKATER

Pages 134–35

- Repetitions and time vary by objective.

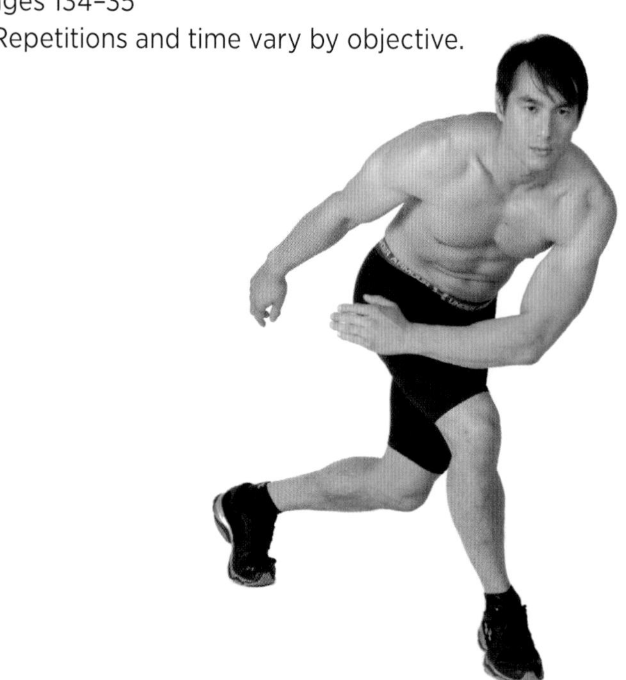

3 JUMP ROPE

Pages 150–51

- Repetitions and time vary by objective.

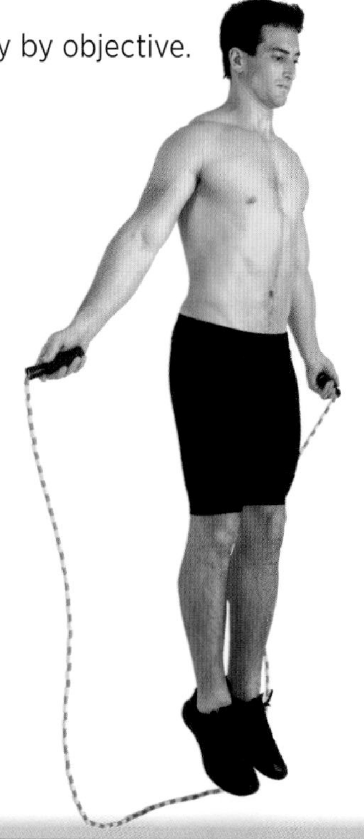

4 HIGH KNEES

Pages 142–43

- Repetitions and time vary by objective.

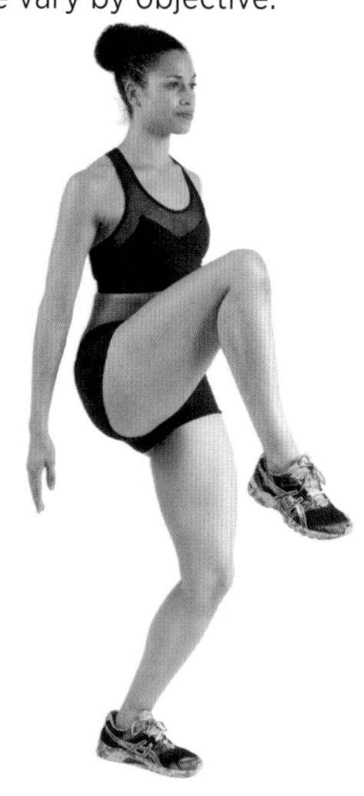

5 HALF MOON POSE

Pages 108–9

- Repetitions and time vary by objective.

6 SINGLE-LEG GLUTEAL LIFT

Pages 262–63

- Repetitions and time vary by objective.

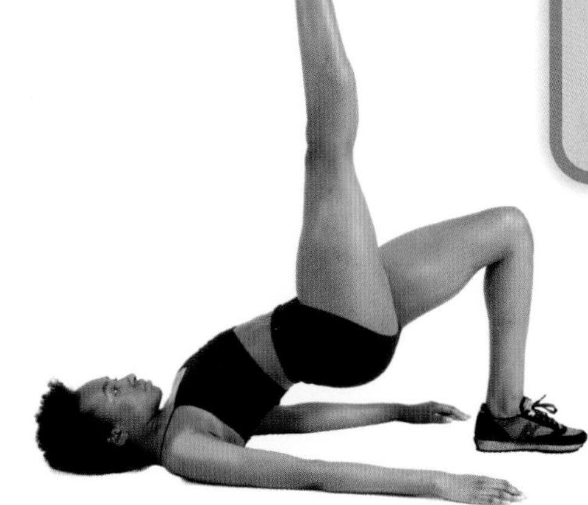

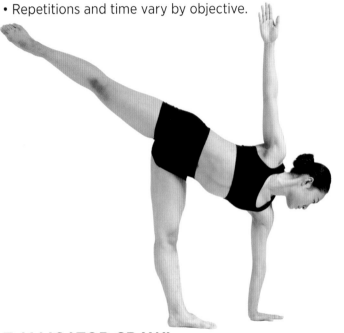

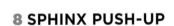

7 ALLIGATOR CRAWL

Pages 160–61

- Perform for 60 seconds.

8 SPHINX PUSH-UP

Page 140

- Perform for 30 seconds, 8-12 repetitions.

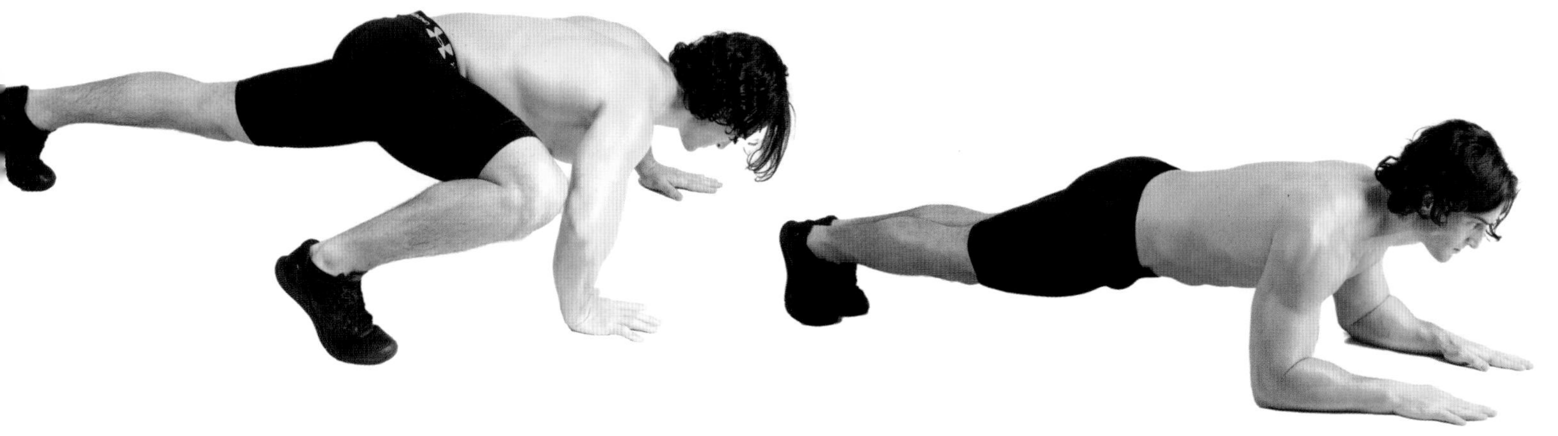

FACT FILE

TARGETS
- Cardio and whole body

OBJECTIVE
- Optimal stability of muscle tissues

WORK/REST
- 20-40 seconds per exercise then onto the next

TOTAL TIME
- 8 minutes

TOTAL COMPLETED CIRCUIT SETS
- 1 set

Power Routine

Designed for good old-fashioned enhanced strength.

1 PUSH UP

Pages 196–97

• Repetitions and time vary by objective.

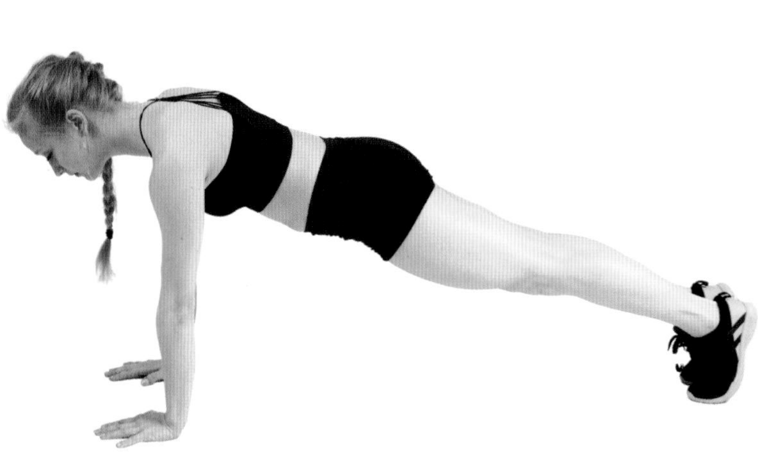

2 TWO-LEVEL PUSH-UP

Page 148–49

• Repetitions and time vary by objective.

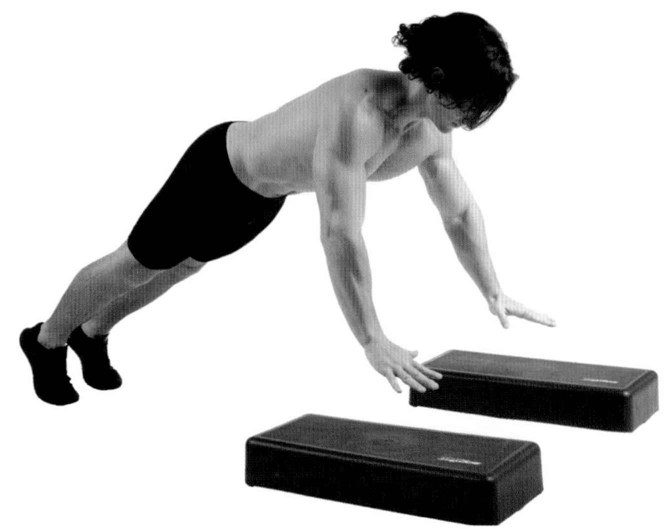

3 POWER PUNCH

Pages 182–83

• Perform for 30 seconds, 8-12 repetitions.

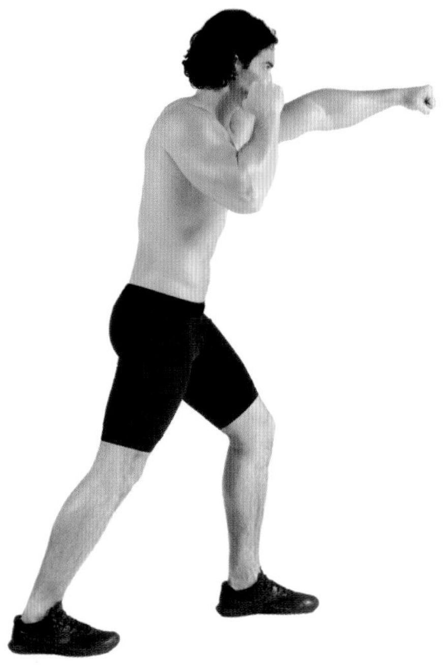

4 UPPERCUT

Pages 184–85

• Repetitions and time vary by objective.

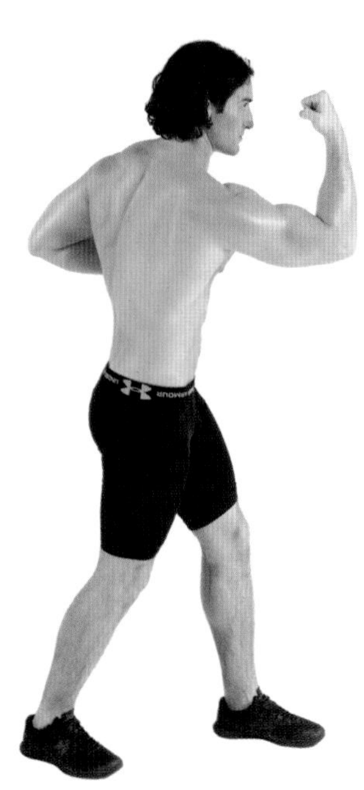

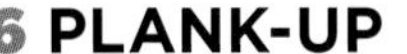

FACT FILE

TARGETS
- Cardio and whole body

OBJECTIVE
- Optimal pliability of muscle tissues

WORK/REST
- 12-15 repetitions per exercise then onto the next

TOTAL TIME
- 8 minutes

TOTAL COMPLETED CIRCUIT SETS
- 1 set

5 BENCH DIP

Pages 176–77
- Repetitions and time vary by objective.

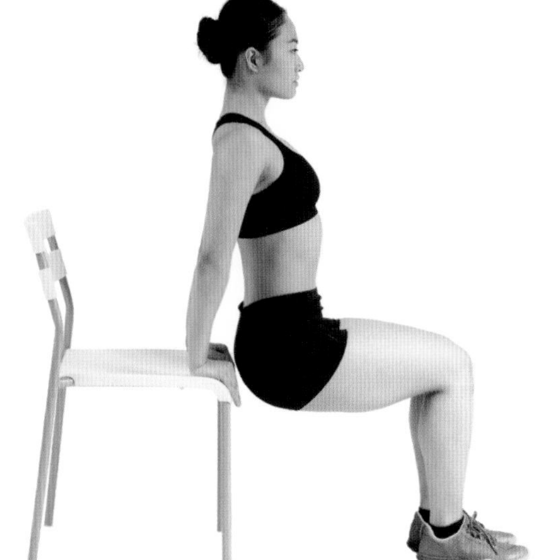

6 PLANK-UP

Pages 180–81
- Repetitions and time vary by objective.

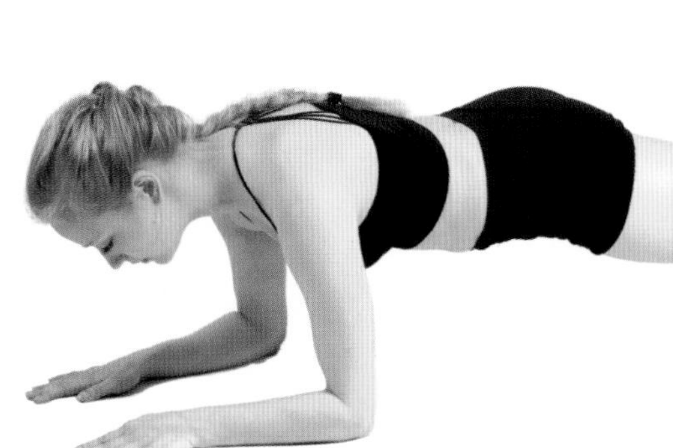

7 BICYCLE CRUNCH

Pages 216–17
- Repetitions and time vary by objective.

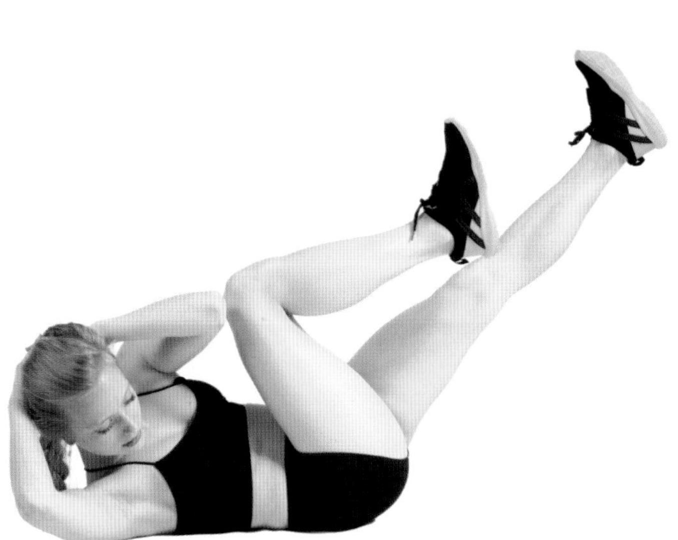

8 HALF MOON POSE

Pages 108–9
- Repetitions and time vary by objective.

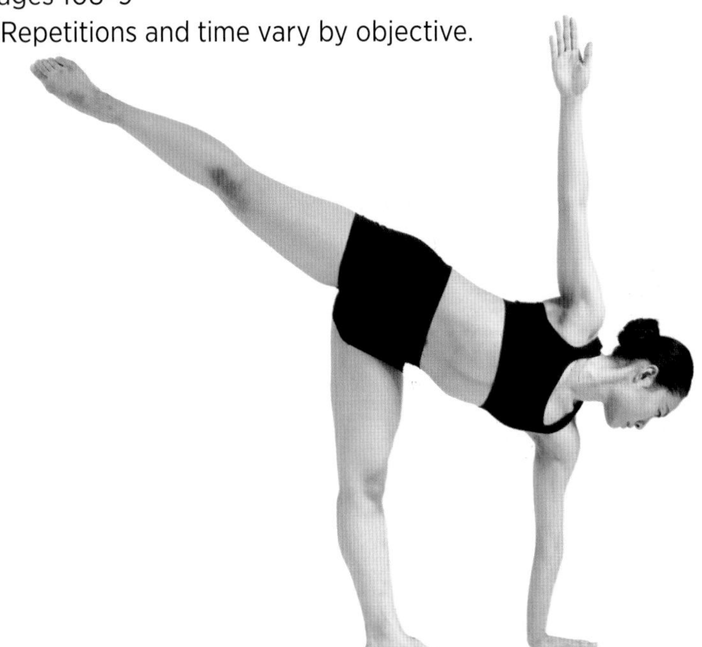

Balance Routine

Designed to create more control over the whole body for precise movement.

1 ONE-LEGGED PLANK

Pages 86–87

• Hold for 3 to 6 breaths.

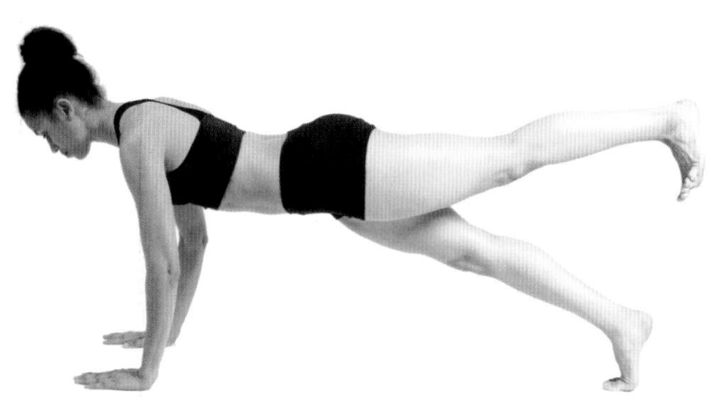

2 BIRD DOG POSE

Pages 88–89

• Hold for 3 to 6 breaths.

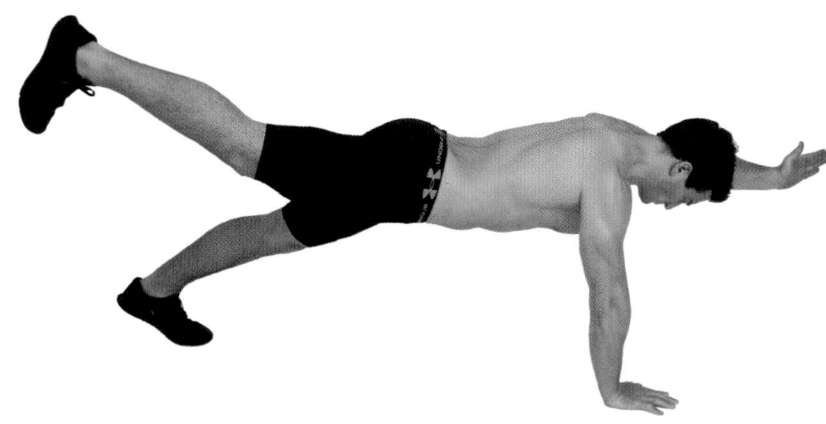

3 DOLPHIN PLANK WITH ARM REACH

Pages 96–97

• Hold for 3 to 6 breaths.

4 ONE-LEGGED BRIDGE

Page 116–17

• Hold for 3 to 6 breaths.

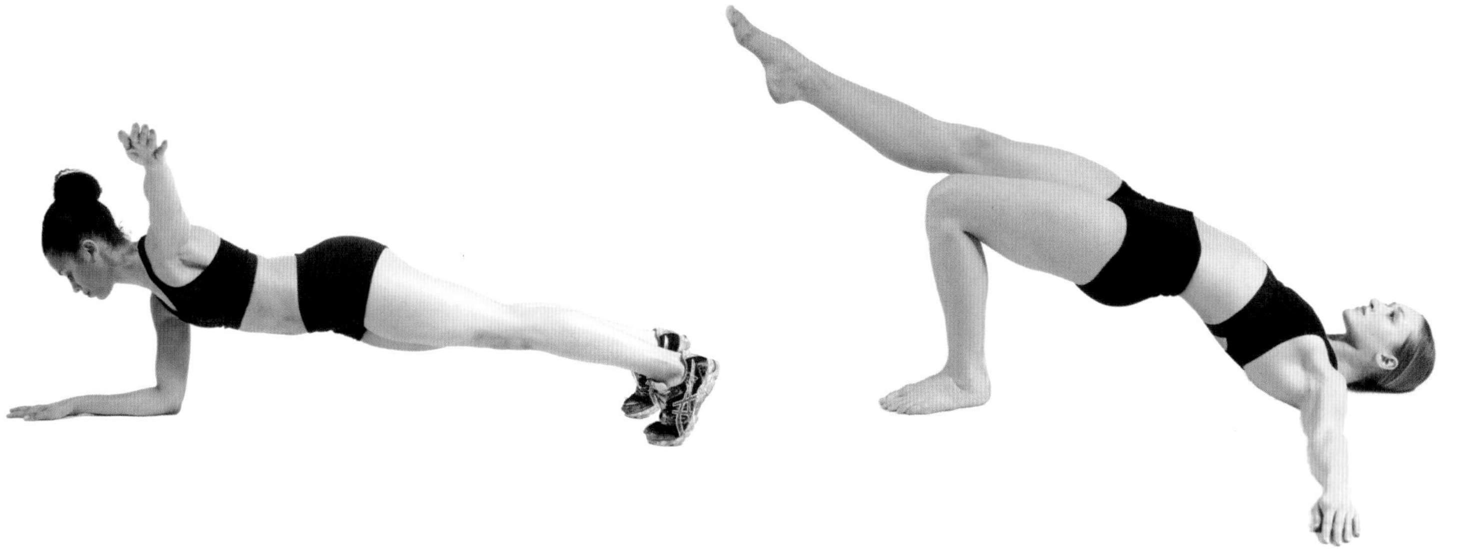

5 ABDOMINAL KICK

Pages 132–33

- Repetitions and time vary by objective.

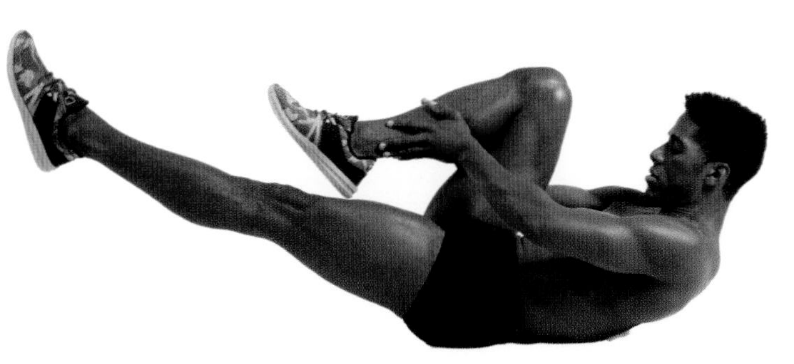

6 PLYO KNEE DRIVE

Pages 136

- Repetitions and time vary by objective.

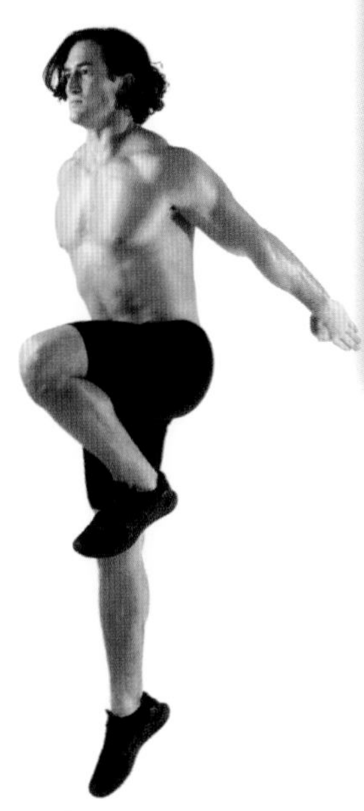

7 INCHWORM

Pages 186–87

- Repetitions and time vary by objective.

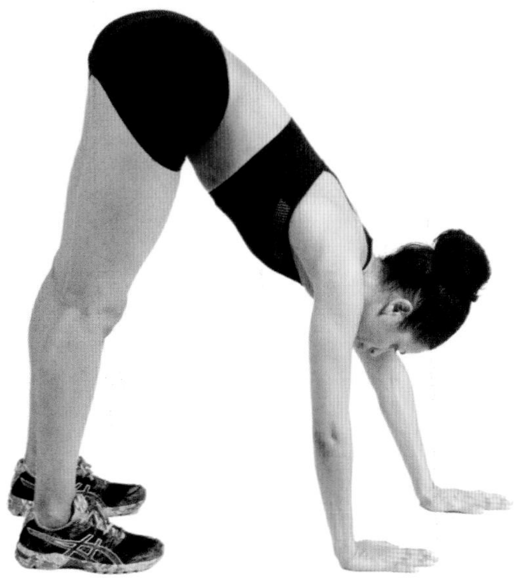

8 WIDE PUSH-UP

Pages 204–5

- Perform 10-12 repetitions.

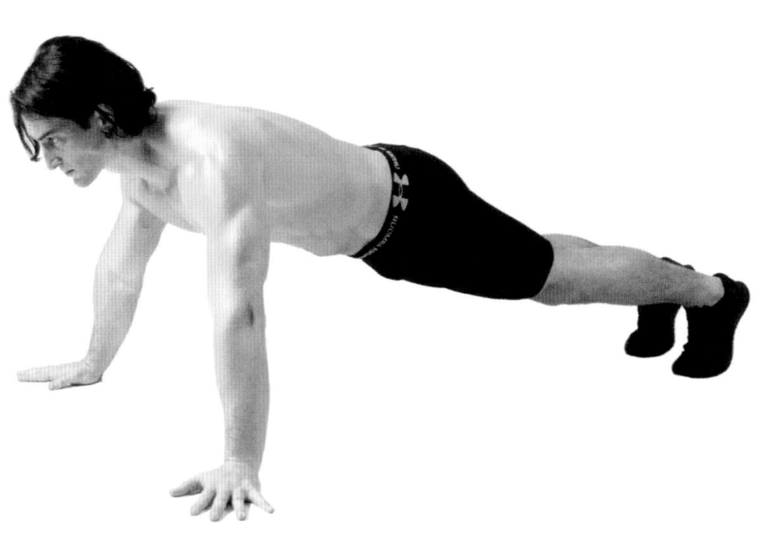

FACT FILE

TARGETS
- Whole body

OBJECTIVE
- Optimal precision movement of muscle tissues

WORK/REST
- 12-15 repetitions per exercise then onto the next

TOTAL TIME
- 8 minutes

TOTAL COMPLETED CIRCUIT SETS
- 1 set

Postural Routine

An advanced functional routine designed to create more free, balanced, and agile movement in life.

1 CELIBATE'S POSE

Pages 100–101

- Hold for 3 to 6 breaths.

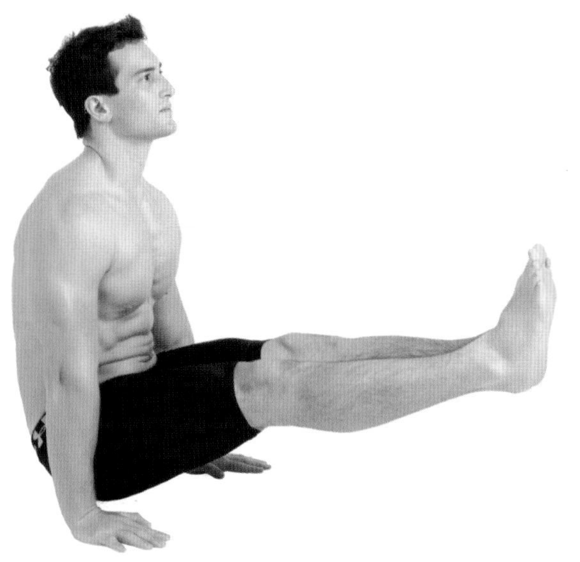

2 PLANK-UP

Pages 180–81

- Repetitions and time vary by objective.

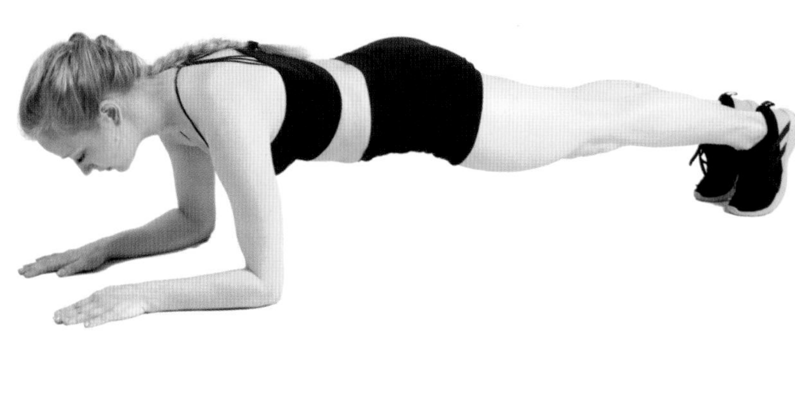

3 ADVANCED SUPERMAN

Page 166

- Perform for 30 seconds, 8-12 repetitions.

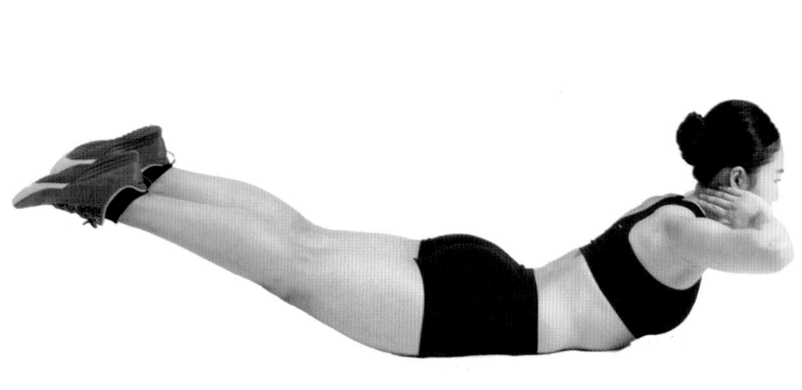

4 GOOD MORNING BOW

Pages 170–71

- Perform for 30 seconds, 15+ repetitions.

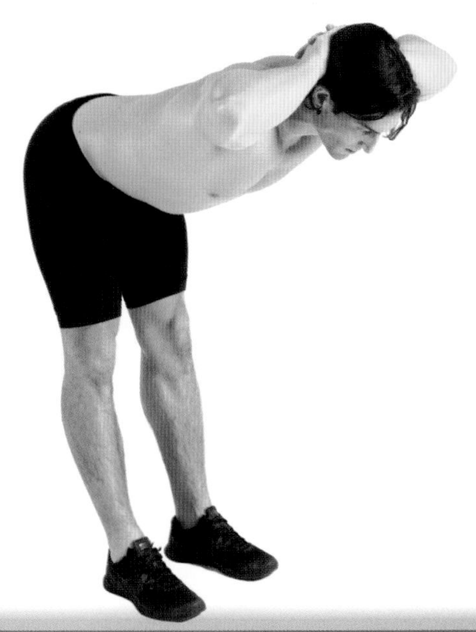

FACT FILE

TARGETS
- Whole body

OBJECTIVE
- Optimal stance and precision movement of muscle tissues

WORK/REST
- 12-15 repetitions per exercise then onto the next

TOTAL TIME
- 8 minutes

TOTAL COMPLETED CIRCUIT SETS
- 1 set

5 METRONOME

Pages 224–25

- Repetitions and time vary by objective.

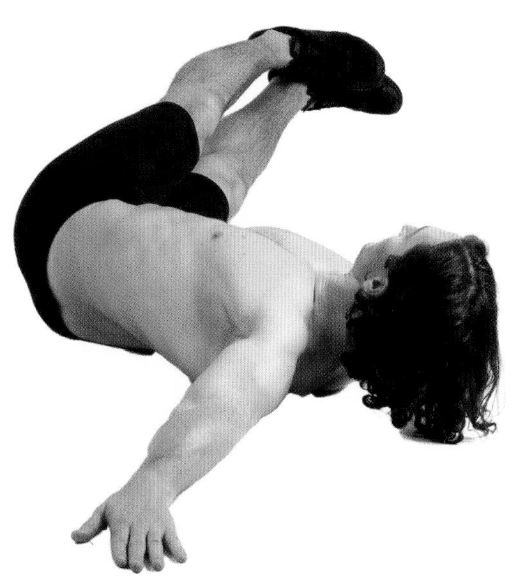

6 ARM HAULER

Pages 164–65

- Perform for 30 seconds, 15+ repetitions.

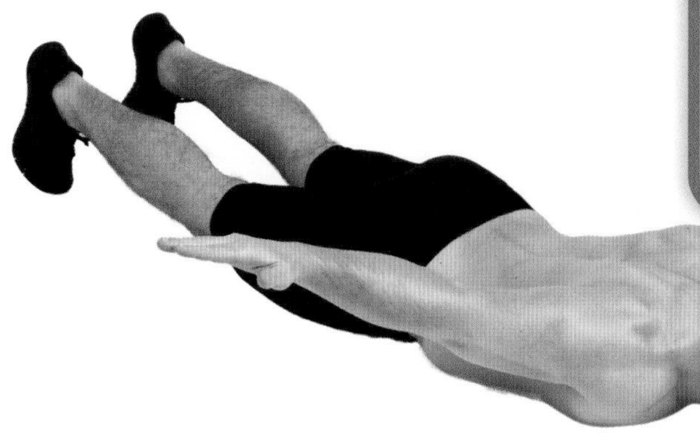

7 SWIMMER

Pages 158-59

- Perform 6–8 repetitions per side.

8 PENGUIN CRUNCH

Pages 230–31

- Perform 25 repetitions per side.

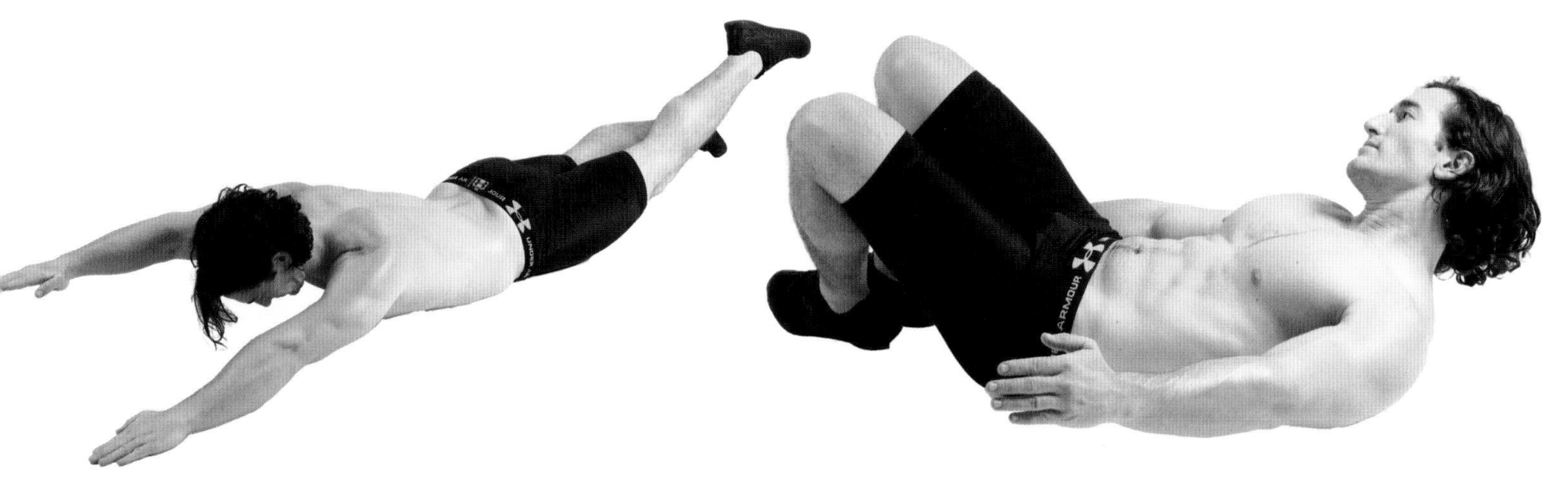

Master Routine

Designed for truly challenging oneself through multiple modalities.

1 CROW POSE

Pages 102–3

- Hold for 3 to 6 breaths.

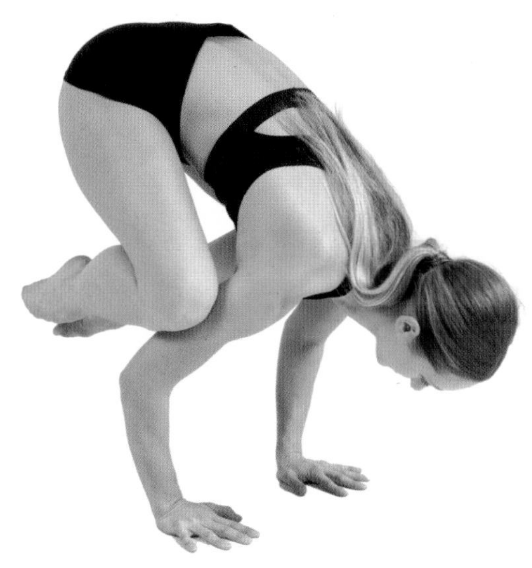

2 SUPPORTED HEADSTAND

Page 104–5

- Hold for 2 to 4 breaths.

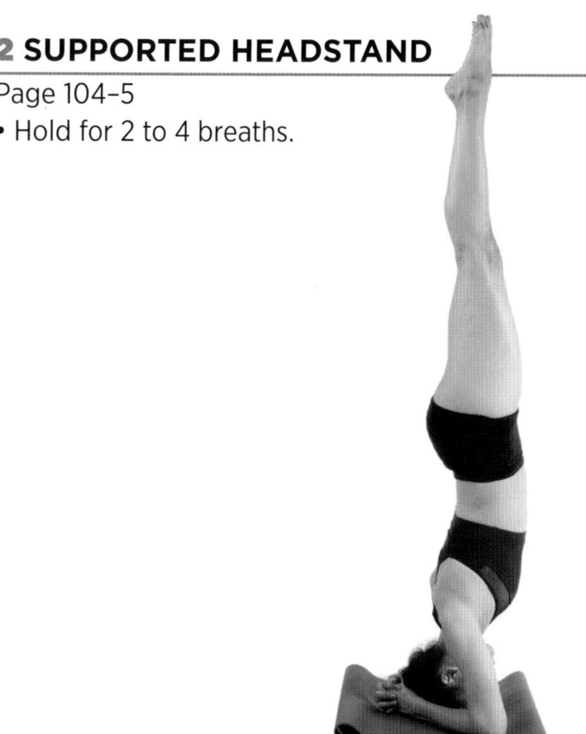

3 ALTERNATING SINGLE-ARM PUSH-UP

Page 198–99

- Perform for 60 seconds, 4-6 reps.

4 TRICEPS PUSH-UP

Pages 178–79

- Repetitions and time vary by objective.

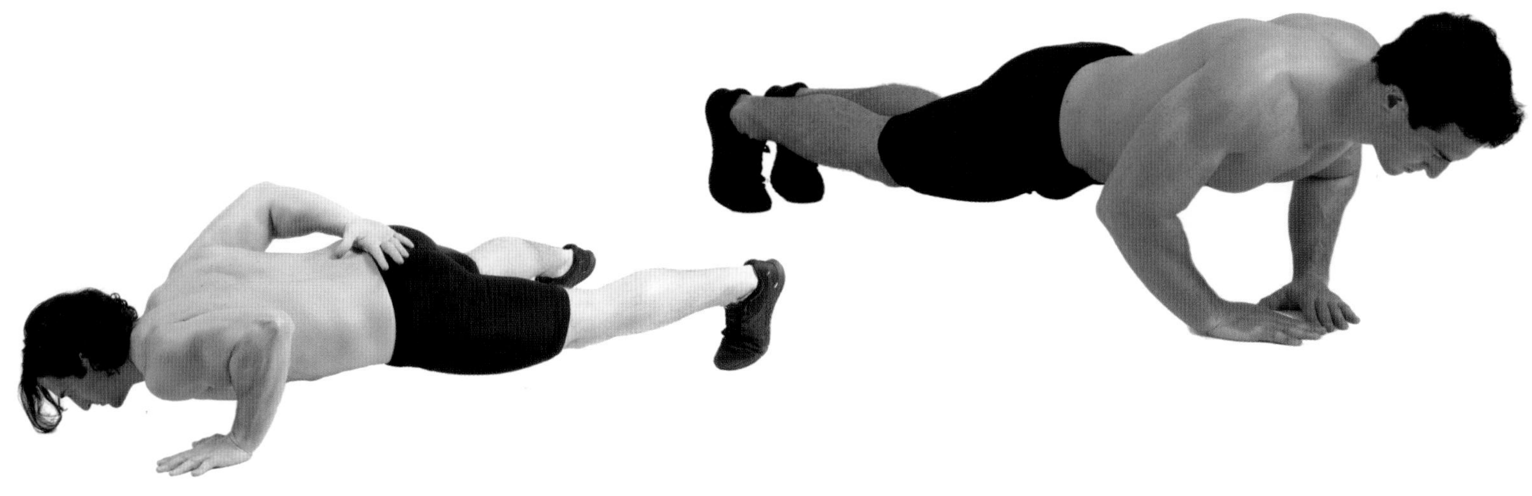

5 BURPEE

Pages 122–23

- Repetitions and time vary by objective.

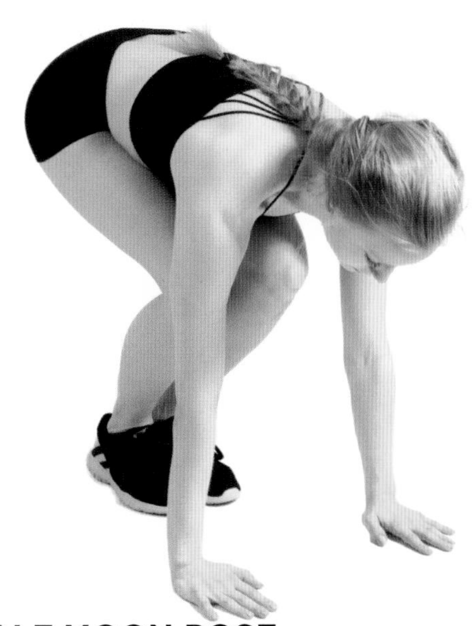

6 HIGH KNEES

Pages 142–43

- Repetitions and time vary by objective.

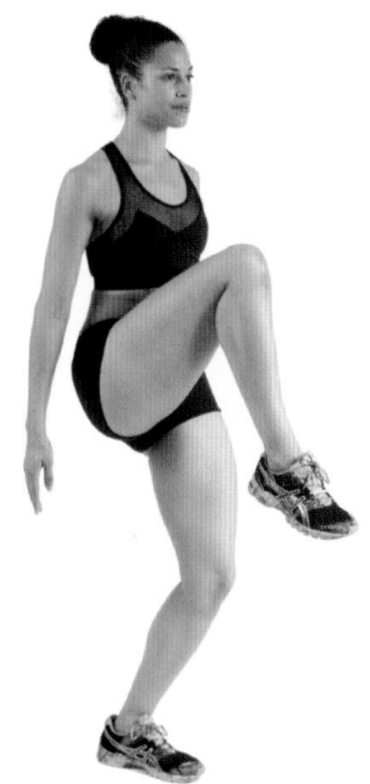

7 HALF MOON POSE

Pages 108–9

- Repetitions and time vary by objective.

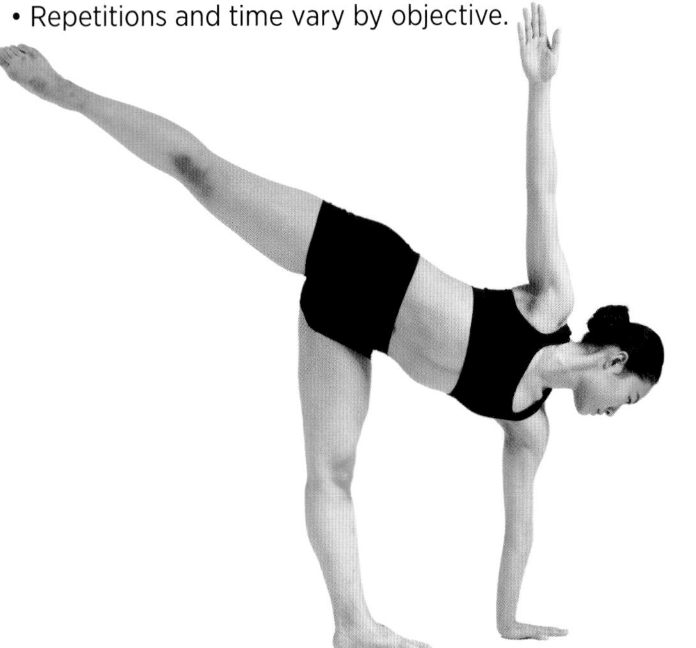

8 HANDSTAND PUSH-UP

Pages 192–93

- Perform for 60 seconds or as many as able.

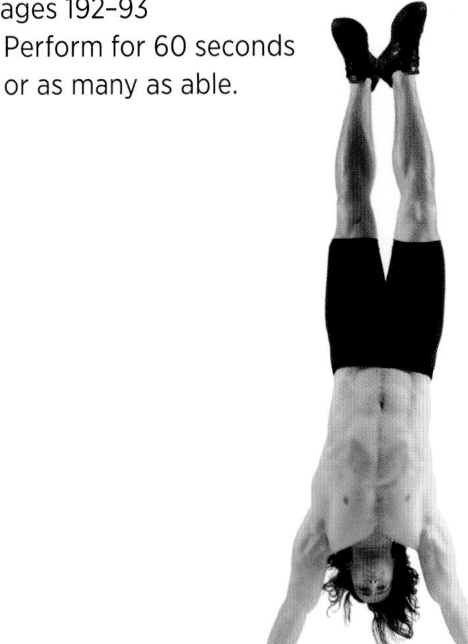

FACT FILE

TARGETS
- Whole body

OBJECTIVE
- Optimal strength, endurance, and flexibility of muscle tissues

WORK/REST
- 12-15 repetitions per exercise then onto the next

TOTAL TIME
- 8 minutes

TOTAL COMPLETED CIRCUIT SETS
- 1 set

Power Sport Routine

Designed to thoroughly prepare and improve the overall body for adaptive sport.

1 TRICEPS PUSH-UP

Pages 178–79

- Repetitions and time vary by objective.

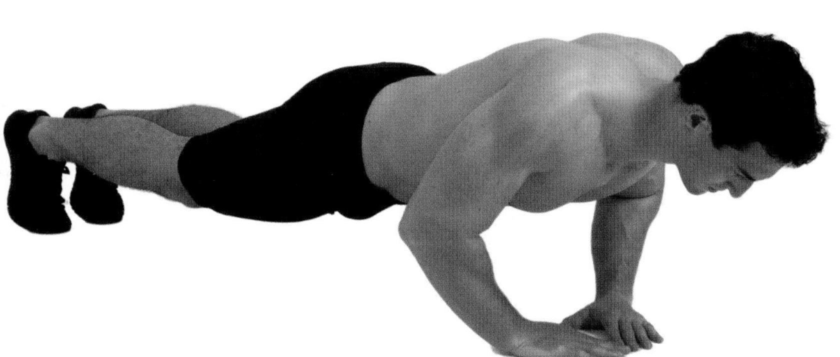

2 HANDSTAND WALK

Pages 302–3

- Perform for 60 seconds, 4-6 repetitions.

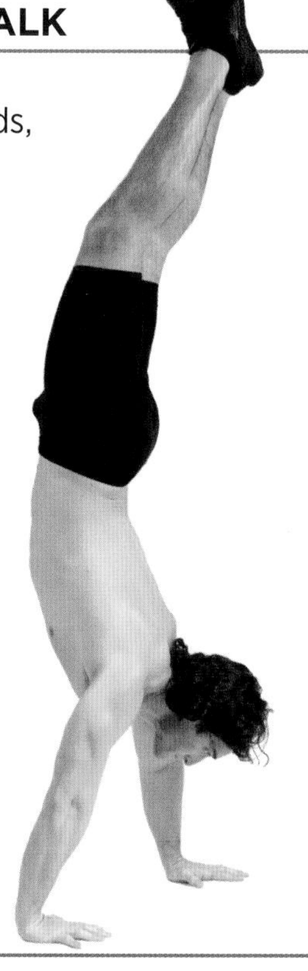

3 WIDE-LEGGED FORWARD BEND

Pages 114–15

- Hold for 3 to 6 breaths.

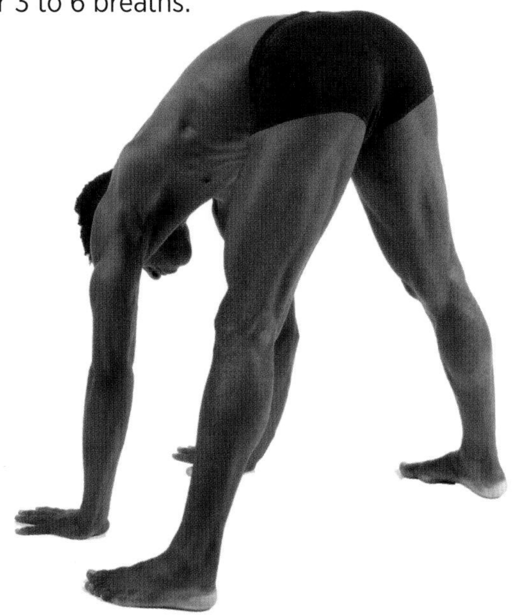

4 BURPEE

Pages 122–23

- Repetitions and time vary by objective.

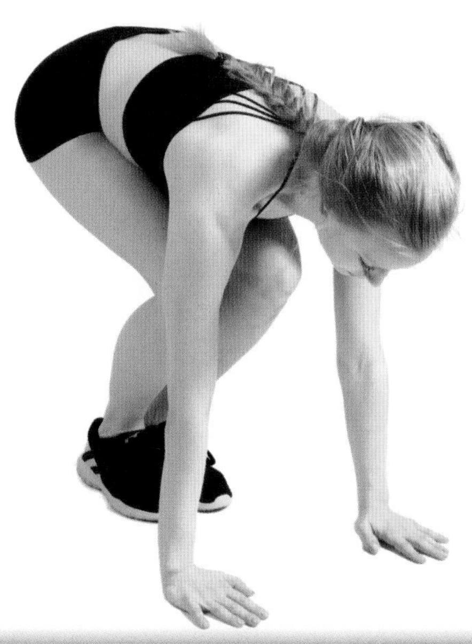

FACT FILE

TARGETS
- Whole body

OBJECTIVE
- Optimal preparation for sustained usage of muscle tissues

WORK/REST
- 12-15 repetitions per exercise then onto the next

TOTAL TIME
- 8 minutes

TOTAL COMPLETED CIRCUIT SETS
- 1 set

5 TWISTING KNEE RAISE

Pages 128–29
- Repetitions and time vary by objective.

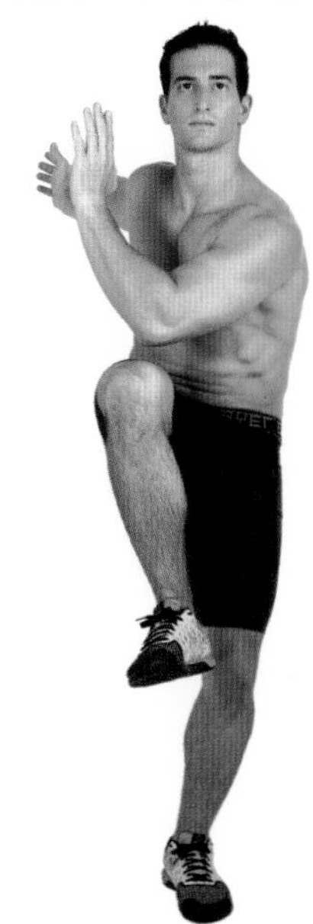

6 PLYO KNEE DRIVE

Pages 136–37
- Repetitions and time vary by objective.

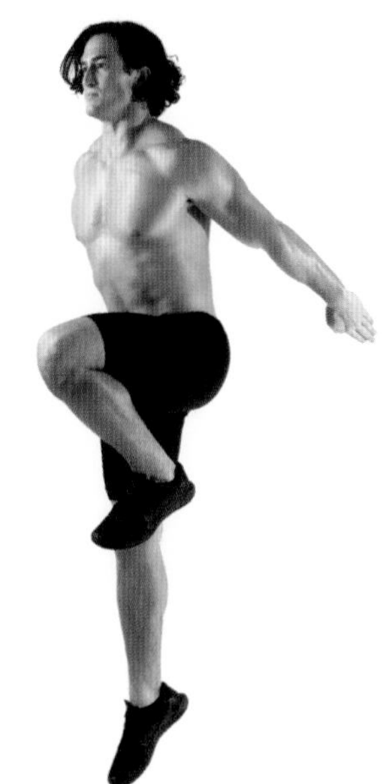

7 HALF MOON POSE

Pages 108–9
- Repetitions and time vary by objective.

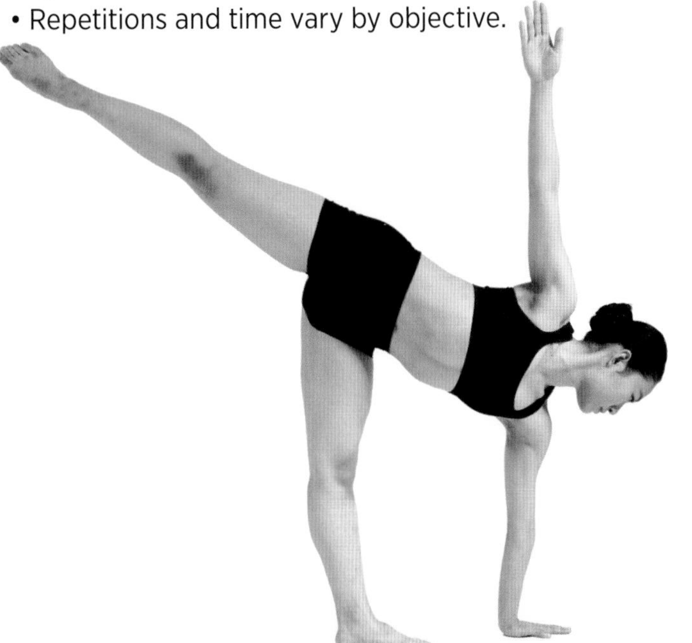

8 T-STABILIZATION

Pages 310–11
- Hold for 30-60 seconds per side.

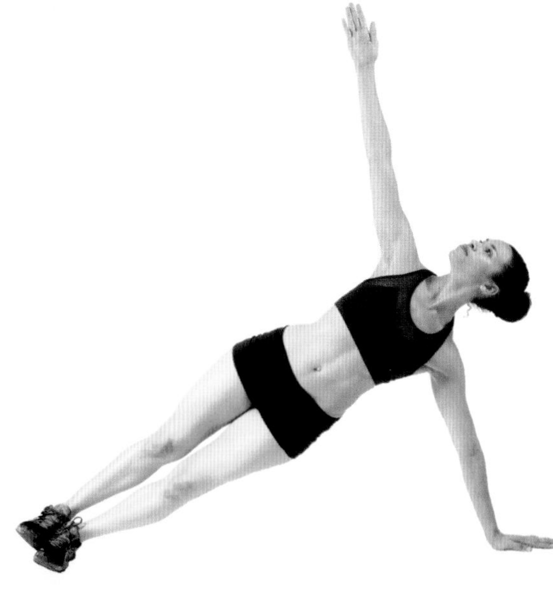

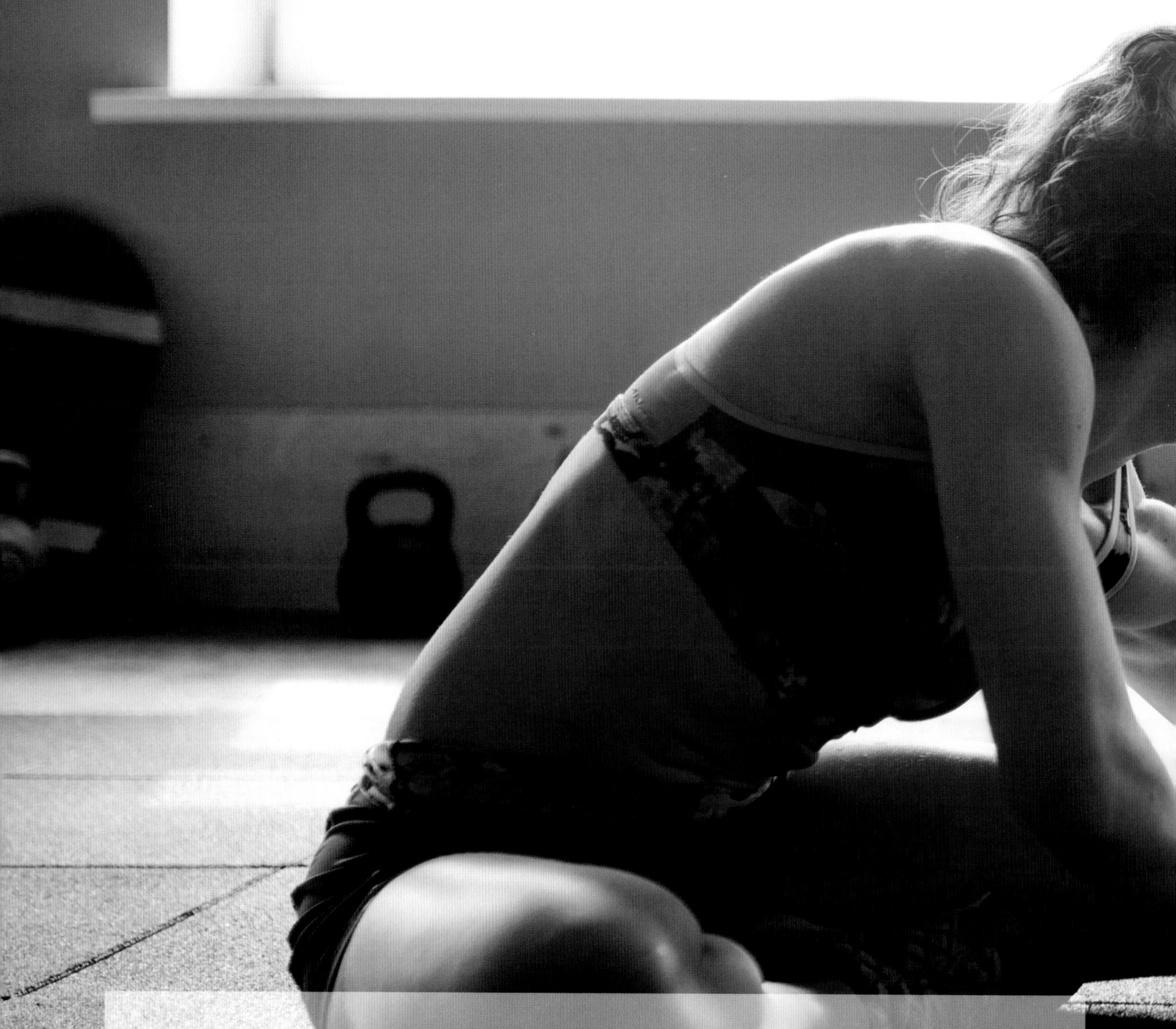

APPENDICES

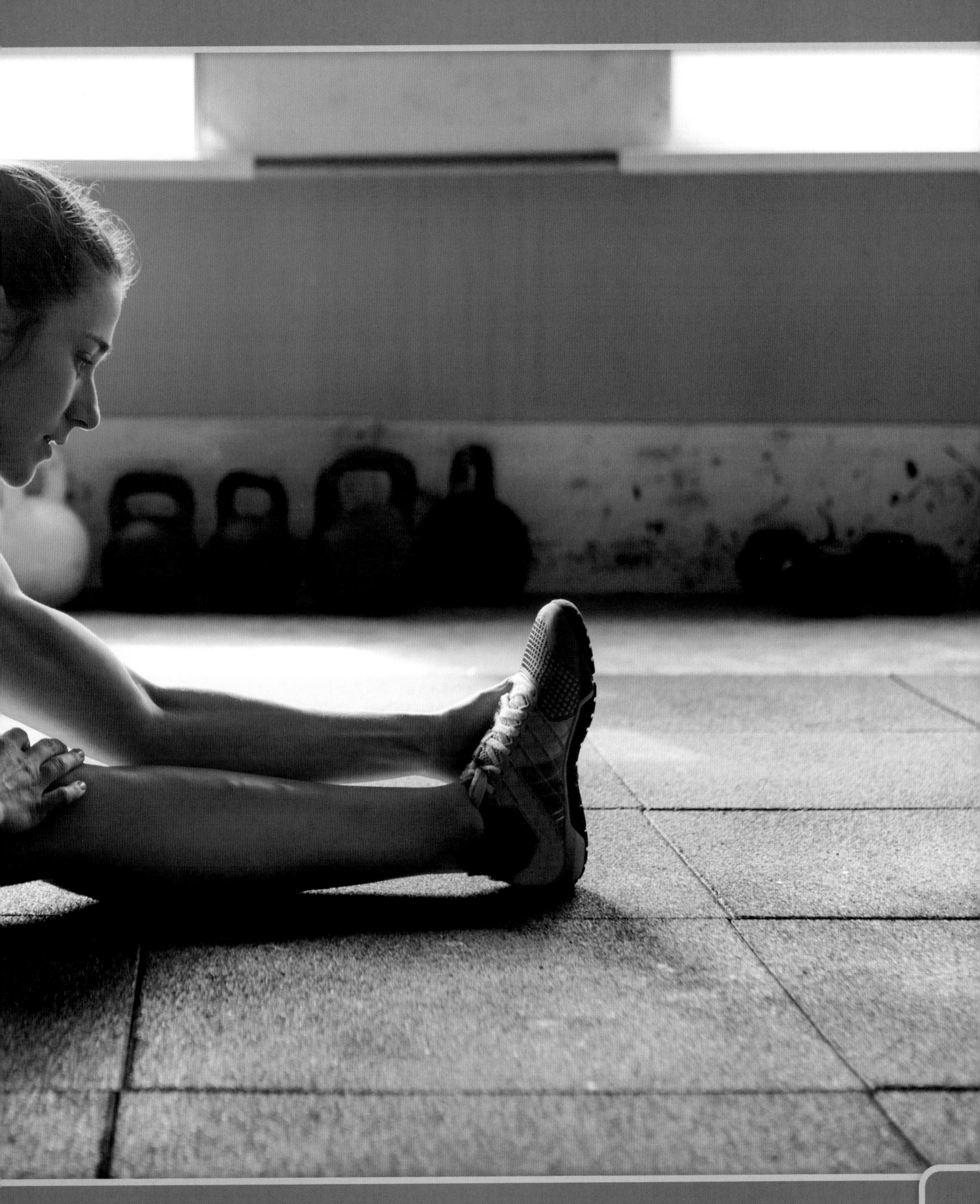

Glossary

GENERAL TERMS

abduction: Movement away from your body.

active isolated stretching (AIS): A stretching technique in which the stretch is held for a couple of seconds at a time and is performed in several repetitions, with the goal of exceeding the previous point of resistance by a few degrees in each ensuing repetition.

active stretching: A stretching technique in which added force is applied by the person stretching for greater intensity.

adduction: Movement toward your body.

aerobic exercise: A type of exercise involving aerobic metabolism in which your body uses oxygen to create energy; refers to sustained activity.

anaerobic exercise: A type of exercise involving anaerobic metabolism in which your muscles do not use oxygen to create energy; refers to short bursts of activity.

anterior: Located in the front of your body.

ballistic stretching: An active form of stretching that forces a part of your body to go beyond its normal range of motion by bouncing to a stretched position.

cardiovascular exercise: Any exercise that increases your heart rate, making oxygen and nutrient-rich blood available to working muscles.

cooldown: An exercise performed at the end of the workout session that works to cool and relax your body.

core: Refers to the deep muscle layers that lie close to your spine and provide structural support for your entire body. The core is divided into two groups: the major and the minor muscles. The major core muscles reside in the abdominal area and in the middle and lower back. This area encompasses the pelvic floor muscles (levator ani, pubococcygeus, iliococcygeus, puborectalis, and coccygeus), the abdominals (rectus abdominis, transversus abdominis, obliquus externus, and obliquus internus), the spinal extensors (multifidus spinae, erector spinae, splenius, longissimus thoracis, and semispinalis), and the diaphragm. The minor core muscles include the latissimus dorsi, gluteus maximus, and trapezius. The minor core muscles assist the major muscles when your body engages in activities or movements that require added stability.

core stabilizer: An exercise that calls for resisting motion along your lumbar spine through activation of your abdominal muscles and deep stabilizers; improves core strength and endurance.

core strengthener: An exercise that allows for motion in your lumbar spine, while working your abdominal muscles and deep stabilizers; improves core strength.

dynamic stretching: A stretching technique that requires the use of continuous movement patterns.

extension: The straightening of a joint.

extensor muscle: A muscle that extends a limb, or other body part, away from your body.

flexion: The bending of a joint.

flexor muscle: A muscle that decreases the angle between two bones, as when bending your elbow or raising your thigh toward your abdomen.

hamstrings: The three muscles at the back your thigh (semitendinosus, semimembranosus, and biceps femoris) that flexes your knee and extends your hip.

hyperextension: An exercise that works your lower back as well as your middle and upper back, specifically the erector spinae, which usually involves raising your torso and/or lower body from the floor while keeping your pelvis firmly anchored.

iliotibial band (ITB): A thick band of fibrous tissue that runs down the outside of your thigh, beginning at your hip and extending to the outer side of your tibia just below your knee joint. The band functions in concert with several of your thigh muscles to provide stability to the outside of your knee joint.

internal rotation: The act of moving a part of your body toward the center of your body.

interval: A period of activity or rest.

isolation exercise: A movement that focuses on only one muscle or muscle group.

lateral: Refers to the outer side of your body; the opposite of medial.

lunge: A lower-body exercise in which one leg is positioned forward with your knee bent and foot flat on the floor while your other leg is positioned behind you.

medial: Refers to the middle of your body; the opposite of lateral.

meditation: The focusing and calming of your mind, often through breath work to reach deeper levels of consciousness.

myofascial release stretching: A stretching technique that involves the use of applied force or an external stretching device to apply gentle, sustained pressure to specific points of muscle tightness or discomfort.

neutral: Describes the position of your legs, pelvis, hips, or other part of your body that is neither arched nor curved forward.

neutral position: A position in which the natural curve of your spine is maintained, typically adopted when lying on your back with one or both feet on the mat.

passive, or isometric, stretching: A stretching technique in which added force is applied by an external source (e.g., a partner or an assistive device) to increase intensity.

posterior: Refers to the back of your body.

posterior chain: Your gluteals, hamstrings, and back.

props: Tools such as mats, blocks, blankets, and straps used to extend your range of motion or facilitate achieving a pose.

pulling muscles: The primary muscle groups associated with pulling movements: abdominals, biceps, forearms, latissimus dorsi, hamstrings, obliques, and trapezius.

pushing muscles: The primary muscle groups associated with pushing movements: calves, deltoids, gluteals, pectorals, quadriceps, and triceps.

quadriceps: A large muscle group that includes the four prevailing muscles at the front of your thigh: rectus femoris, vastus intermedius, vastus lateralis, and vastus medialis; the main extensor muscles of your knee that surround the front and sides of your femur muscle.

range of motion: The distance and direction a joint can move between the flexed and the extended positions.

resistance: The weight your muscles are working against to complete a movement, whether your own body weight or added weight, such as dumbbells.

rotator muscle: One of a group of muscles that assists the rotation of a joint, such as your hip or shoulder.

scapula: The protrusion of bone in your middle to upper back known as your shoulder blade.

set: Refers to how many times you repeat a given number of repetitions of an exercise.

static stretching: A stretching technique in which the stretches are performed by extending the targeted muscle to its maximal point, and then holding that position for a particular length of time.

stretch: Refers to the straightening or extending of your body, or a part of your body, to full length.

ventral aspect: The front of your body.

warm-up: Any form of light exercise of short duration that prepares your body for more intense exercises.

yoga: From the Sanskrit *yug* ("yoke"), meaning "union." Yoga is an ancient discipline in which physical postures, breath practice, meditation, and philosophical study are used as tools for achieving liberation.

yogi: A male/female practitioner of yoga.

LATIN TERMS

The following glossary explains the Latin scientific terminology used to describe the muscles of the human body. Certain words are derived from Greek, which is indicated in each instance.

ABDOMEN

obliquus (externus and internus): *obliquus*, "slanting"

rectus abdominis: *rego,* "straight, upright," and *abdomen,* "belly"

serratus anterior: *serra*, "saw," and *ante*, "before"

transversus abdominis: *transversus*, "athwart," and *abdomen*, "belly"

BACK

erector spinae: *erectus*, "straight," and *spina*, "thorn"

latissimus dorsi: *latus*, "wide," and *dorsum*, "back"

multifidus spinae: *multifid*, "to cut into divisions," and *spinae*, "spine"

quadratus lumborum: *quadratus*, "square, rectangular," and *lumbus*, "loin"

rhomboideus: Greek *rhembesthai*, "to spin"

trapezius: Greek *trapezion*, "small table"

CHEST

coracobrachialis: Greek *korakoeidés*, "ravenlike," and *brachium*, "arm"

pectoralis (major and minor): *pectus*, "breast"

HIPS

gemellus (inferior and superior): *geminus*, "twin"

gluteus maximus: Greek *gloutós*, "rump," and *maximus*, "largest"

gluteus medius: Greek *gloutós*, "rump" and *medialis*, "middle"

gluteus minimus: Greek *gloutós*, "rump" and *minimus*, "smallest"

iliopsoas: *ilium,* "groin," and Greek *psoa*, "groin muscle"

obturator externus: *obturare,* "to block" and *externus,* "outward"

obturator internus: *obturare*, "to block," and *internus*, "within"

pectineus: *pectin*, "comb"

piriformis: *pirum*, "pear," and *forma,* "shape"

quadratus femoris: *quadratus*, "square, rectangular," and *femur*, "thigh"

LOWER ARM

anconeus: Greek *anconad*, "elbow"

brachioradialis: *brachium*, "arm," and *radius*, "spoke"

extensor carpi radialis: *extendere*, "to extend," Greek *karpós*, "wrist" and *radius*, "spoke"

extensor digitorum: *extendere*, "to extend," and *digitus*, "finger, toe"

flexor carpi pollicis longus: *flectere*, "to bend," Greek *karpós*, "wrist," *pollicis*, "thumb" and *longus*, "long"

flexor carpi radialis: *flectere*, "to bend," Greek *karpós*, "wrist" and *radius*, "spoke"

flexor carpi ulnaris: *flectere*, "to bend," Greek *karpós*, "wrist" and *ulnaris*, "forearm"

flexor digitorum: *flectere*, "to bend," and *digitus*, "finger, toe"

palmaris longus: *palmaris*, "palm," and *longus*, "long"

pronator teres: *pronate*, "to rotate," and *teres*, "rounded"

LOWER LEG

adductor digiti minimi: *adducere*, "to contract," *digitus*, "finger, toe" and *minimum* "smallest"

adductor hallucis: *adducere*, "to contract," and *hallex*, "big toe"

extensor digitorum longus: *extendere*, "to extend," *digitus*, "finger, toe" and *longus*, "long"

extensor hallucis longus: *extendere*, "to extend," *hallex*, "big toe," and *longus*, "long"

flexor digitorum longus: *flectere*, "to bend," *digitus*, "finger, toe" and *longus*, "long"

flexor hallucis longus: *flectere*, "to bend," and *hallex*, "big toe" and *longus*, "long"

gastrocnemius: Greek *gastroknémía*, "calf [of the leg]"

peroneus: *peronei*, "of the fibula"

plantaris: *planta*, "the sole"

soleus: *solea*, "sandal"

tibialis (anterior and posterior): *tibia*, "reed pipe"

NECK

scalenus: Greek *skalénós*, "unequal"

semispinalis: *semi*, "half," and *spinae*, "spine"

splenius: Greek *splénion*, "plaster, patch"

sternocleidomastoideus: Greek *stérnon,* "chest," Greek *kleís*, "key" and Greek *mastoeidés*, "breastlike"

SHOULDERS

deltoideus (anterior, medialis, and posterior): Greek *deltoeidés*, "delta-shaped"

infraspinatus: *infra*, "under," and *spina*, "thorn"

levator scapulae: *levare*, "to raise," and *scapulae*, "shoulder [blades]"

subscapularis: *sub*, "below," and *scapulae*, "shoulder [blades]"

supraspinatus: *supra,* "above," and *spina*, "thorn"

teres (major and minor): *teres*, "rounded"

UPPER ARM

biceps brachii: *biceps*, "two-headed," and *brachium*, "arm"

brachialis: *brachium*, "arm"

triceps brachii: *triceps*, "three-headed" and *brachium*, "arm"

UPPER LEG

adductor longus: *adducere*, "to contract," and *longus*, "long"

adductor magnus: *adducere*, "to contract," and *magnus*, "major"

biceps femoris: *biceps*, "two-headed," and *femur*, "thigh"

gracilis: *gracilis*, "slim, slender"

rectus femoris: *rego*, "straight, upright," and *femur*, "thigh"

sartorius: *sarcio*, "to patch" or "to repair"

semimembranosus: *semi*, "half," and *membrum*, "limb"

semitendinosus: *semi*, "half," and *tendo*, "tendon"

tensor fasciae latae: *tenere*, "to stretch," *fasciae*, "band," and *latae*, "laid down"

vastus intermedius: *vastus*, "immense, huge," and *intermedius*, "between"

vastus lateralis: *vastus*, "immense, huge," and lateralis, "side"

vastus medialis: *vastus*, "immense, huge," and *medialis*, "middle"

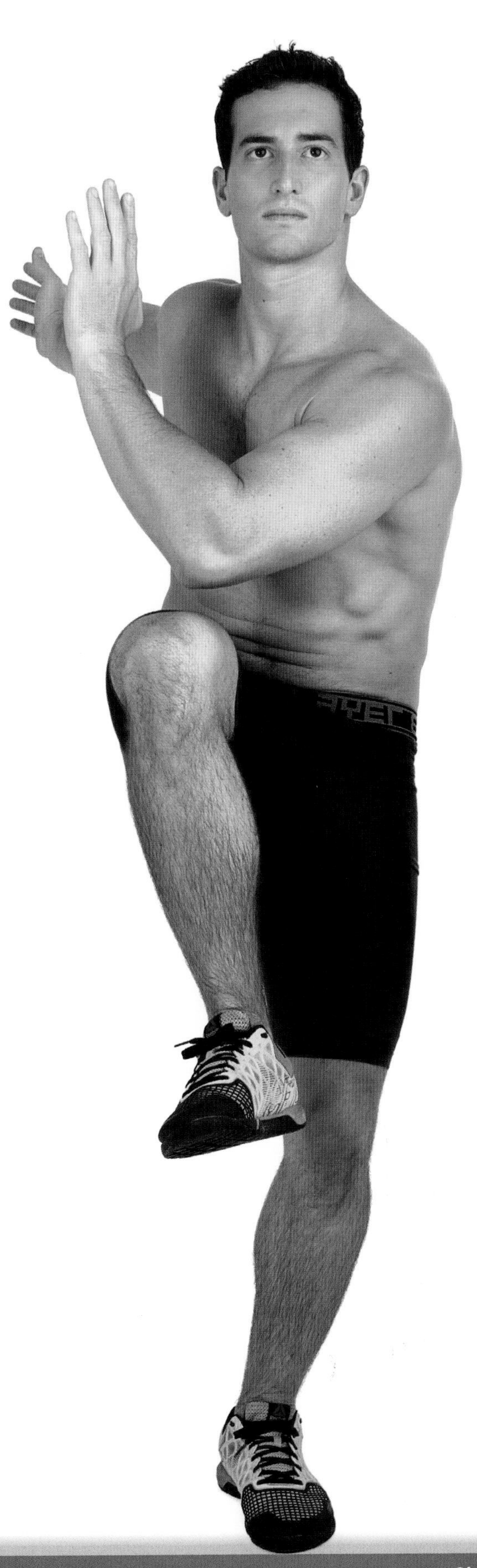

Icon Index

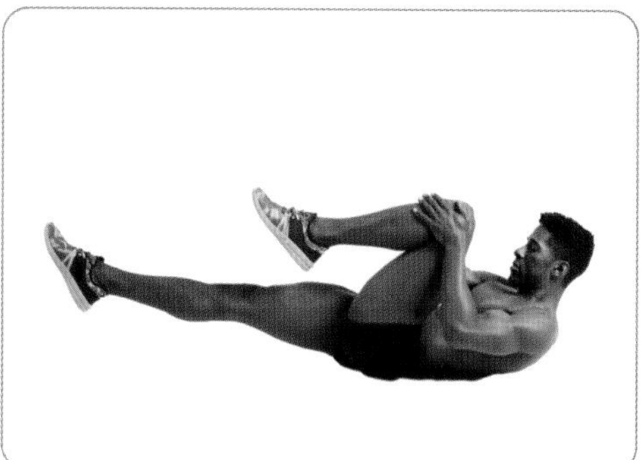

Abdominal Kick
pages 132-33

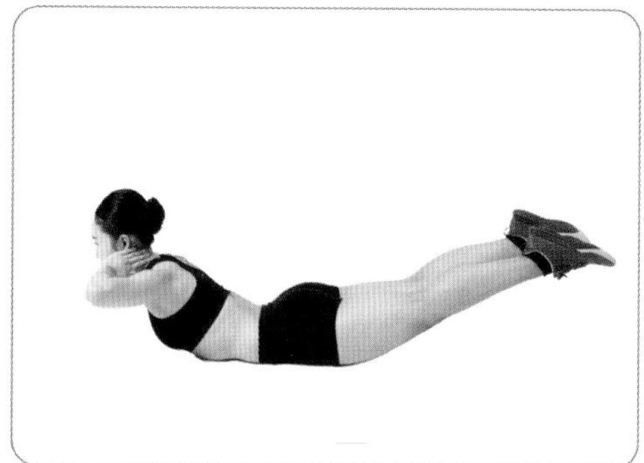

Advanced Superman
page 166

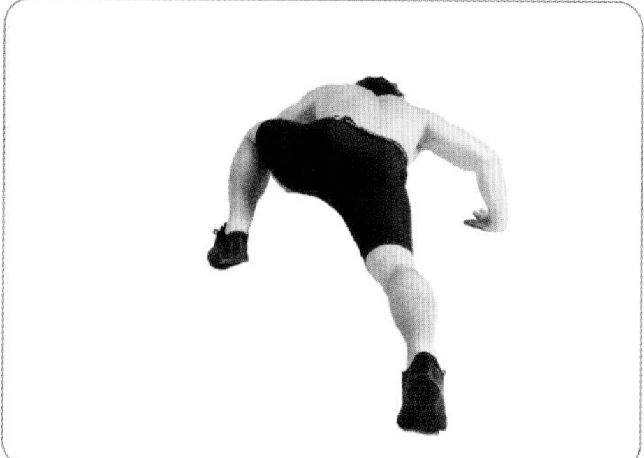

Alligator Crawl
pages 160-61

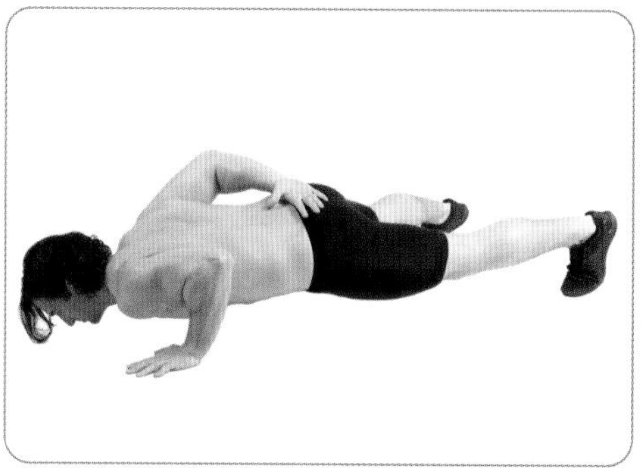

Alternating Single-Arm Push-Up
pages 198-99

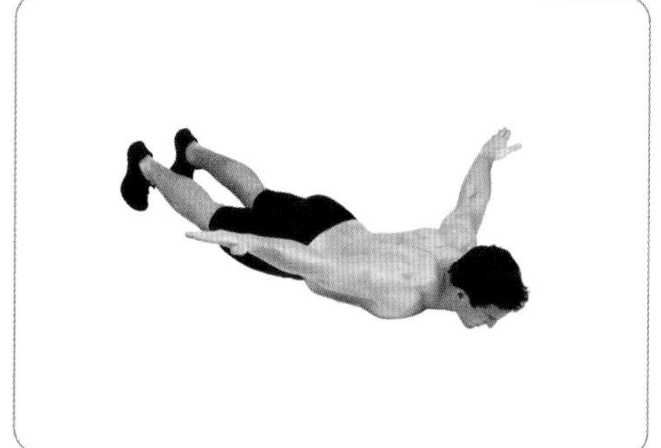

Arm Hauler
pages 164-65

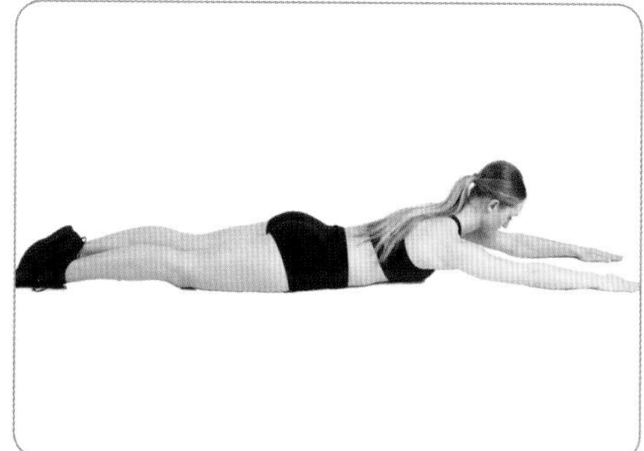

Back Burner
pages 162-63

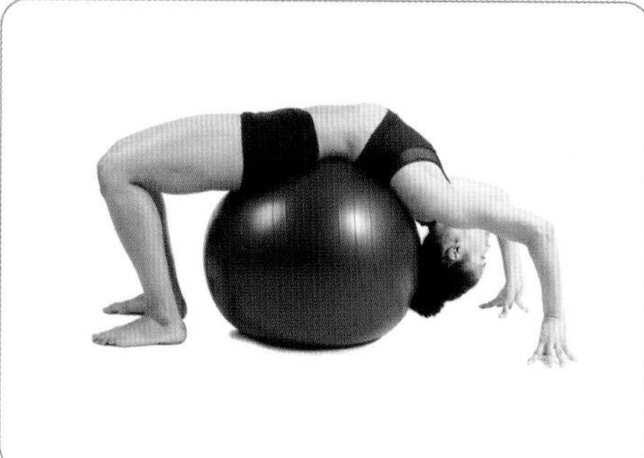

Backward Ball Stretch
pages 70-71

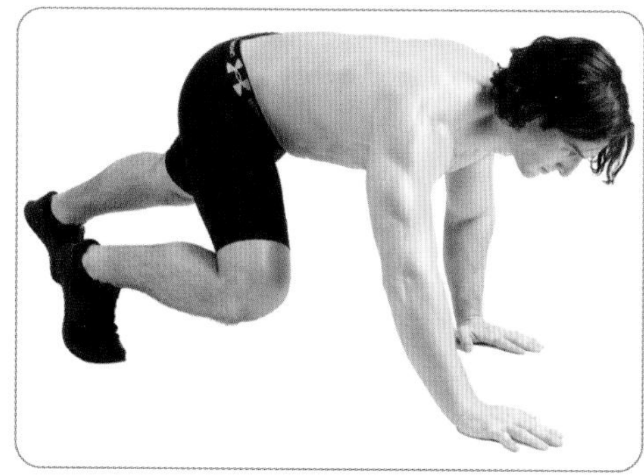

Bear Crawl
pages 190-91

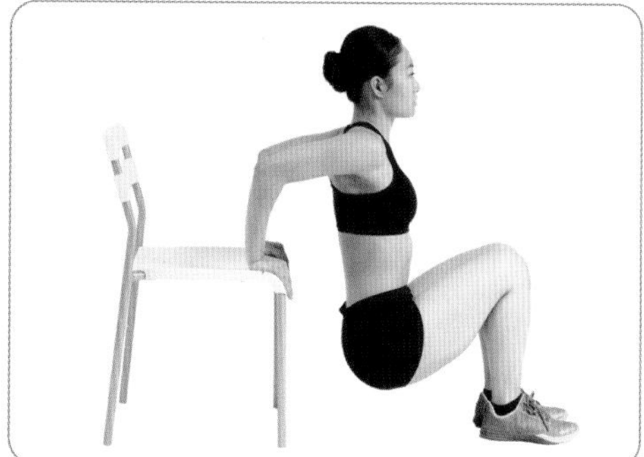

Bench Dip
pages 176-77

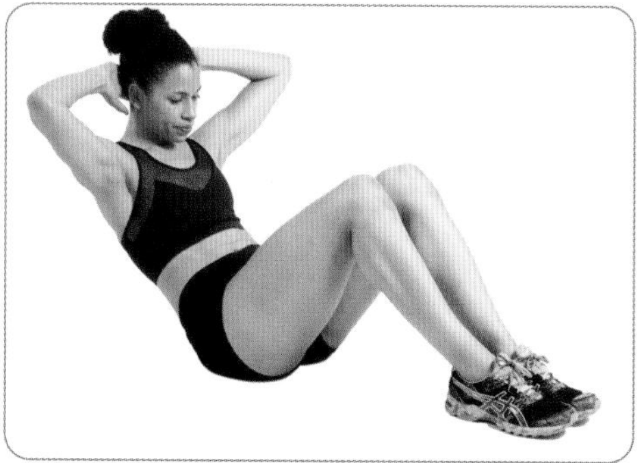

Bent-Knee Sit-Up
pages 214-15

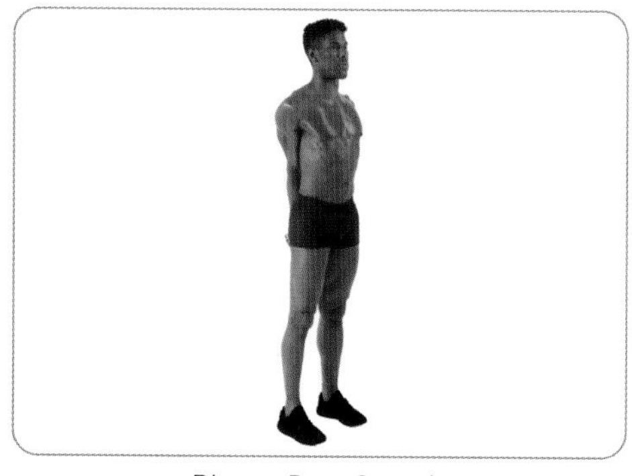

Biceps-Pecs Stretch
page 37

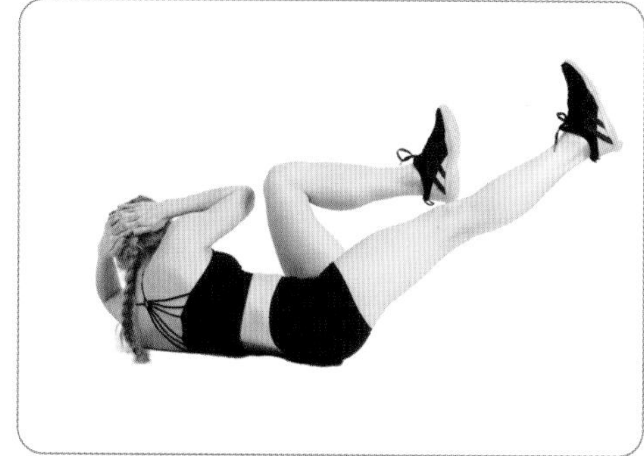

Bicycle Crunch
pages 216-17

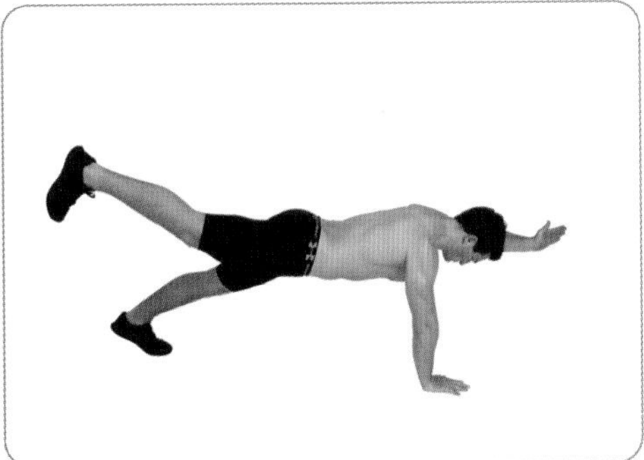
Bird Dog Pose
pages 88-89

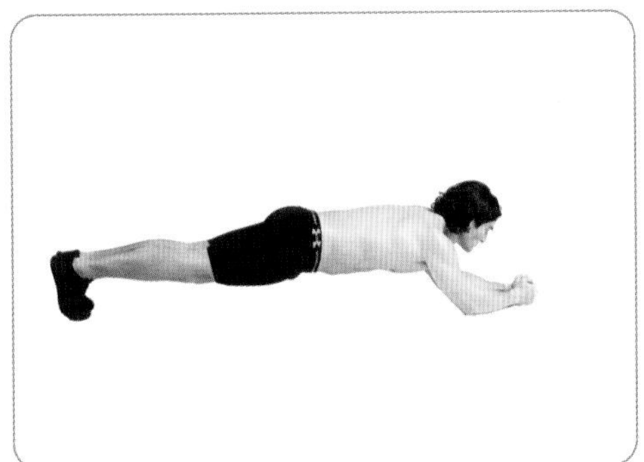
Body Saw
pages 240-41

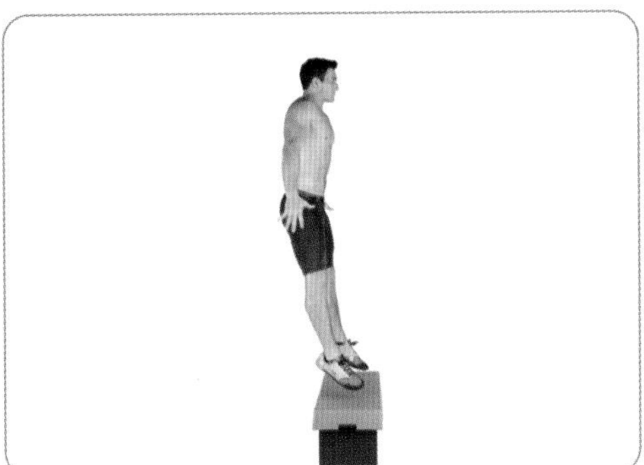
Box Jump
pages 270-71

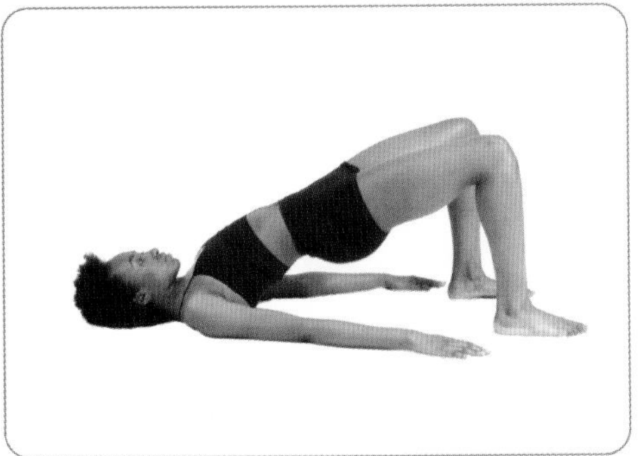
Bridge
pages 256-57

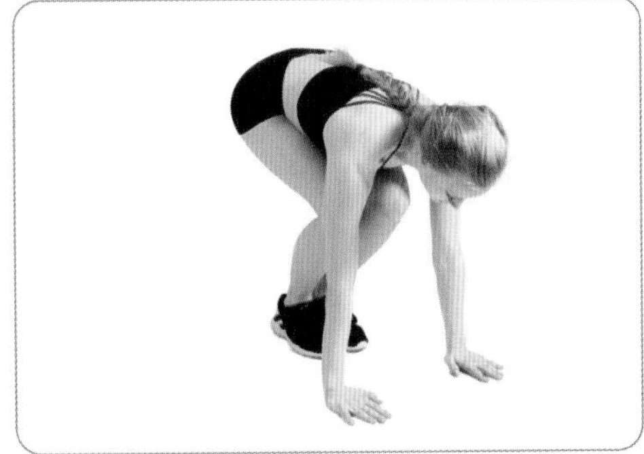
Burpee
pages 122-23

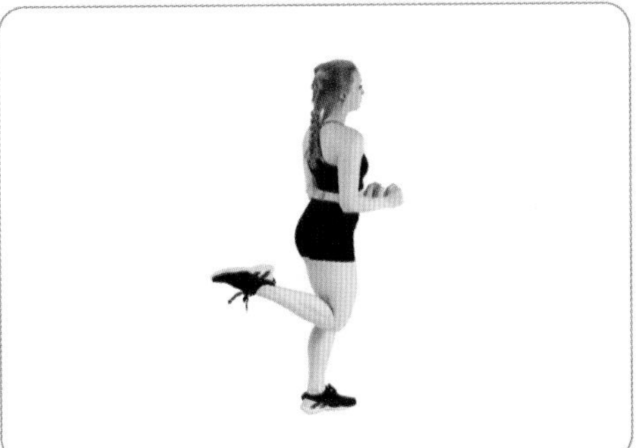
Butt Kick
pages 124-25

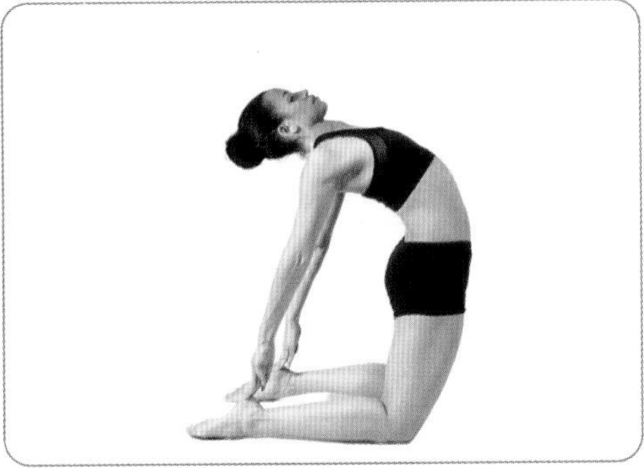
Camel Yoga Stretch
pages 172-73

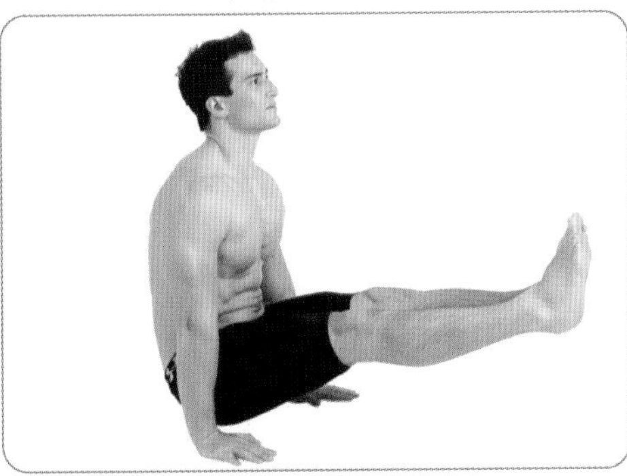
Celibate's Pose
pages 100-101

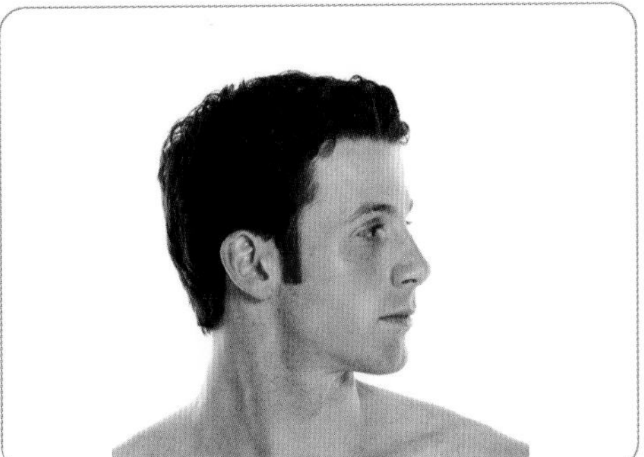
Cervical Stars
pages 20-21

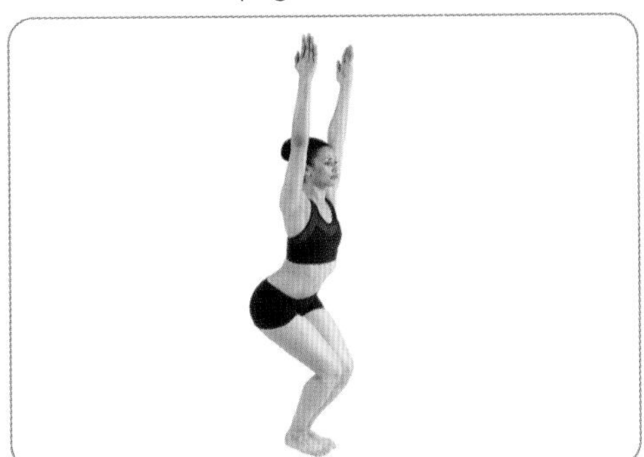
Chair Pose
pages 76-77

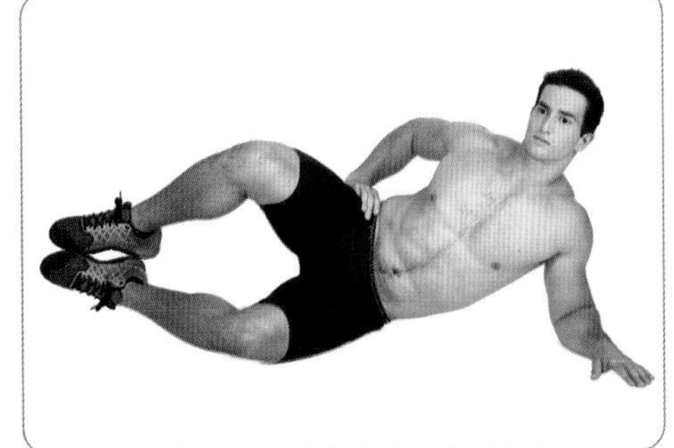
Clamshells
pages 290-91

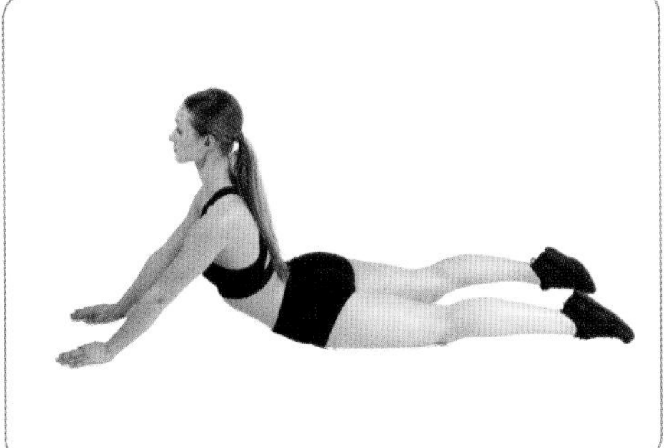
Cobra Stretch
pages 50-51

Icon Index

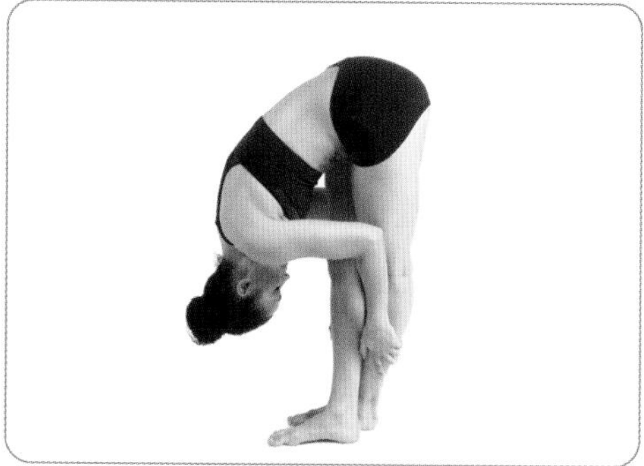
Crossed-Foot Forward Bend
pages 112-13

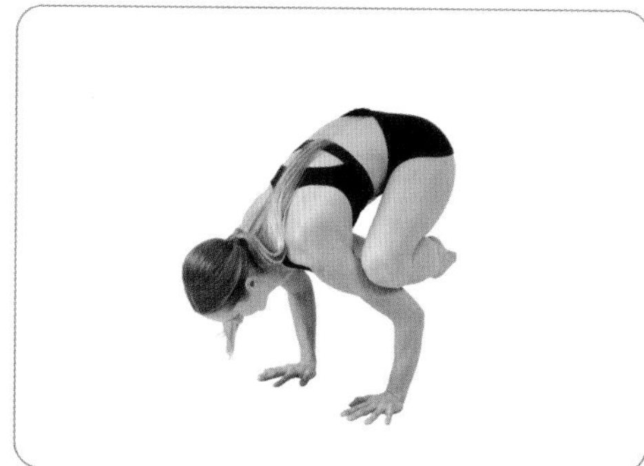
Crow Pose
pages 102-3

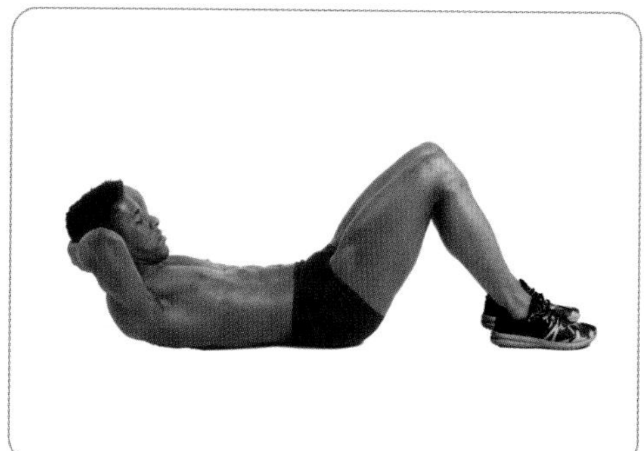
Crunch
pages 228-29

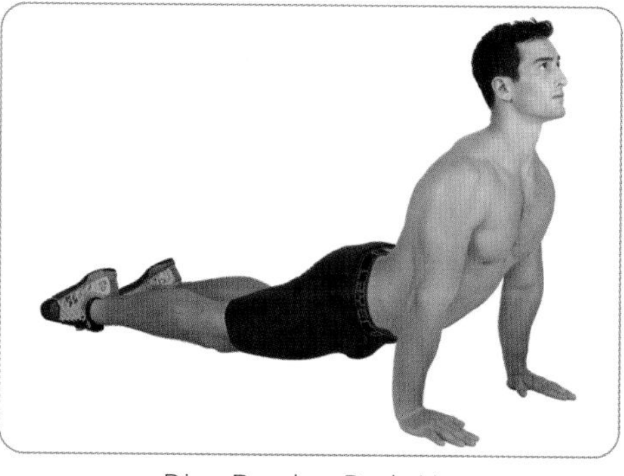
Dive-Bomber Push-Up
pages 206-7

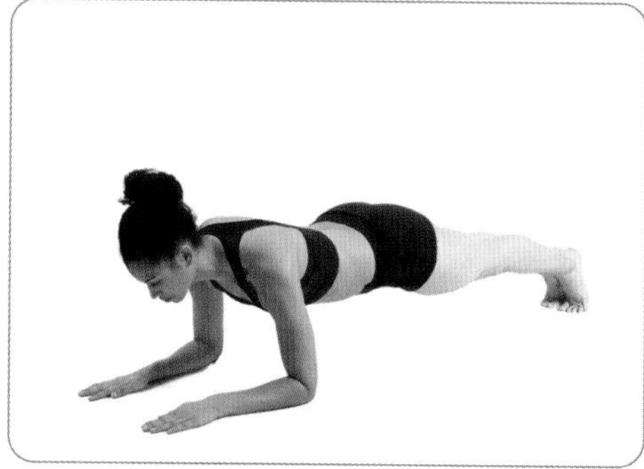
Dolphin Plank Pose
page 95

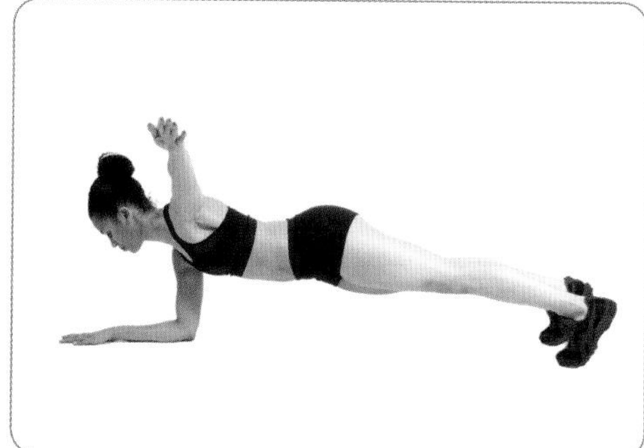
Dolphin Plank with Arm Reach
pages 96-97

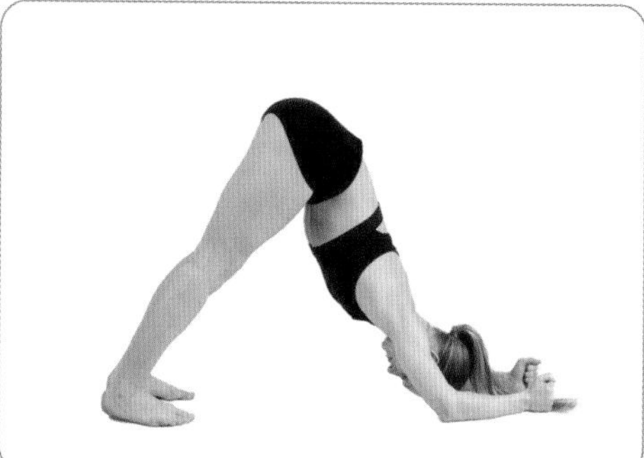
Dolphin Pose
page 94

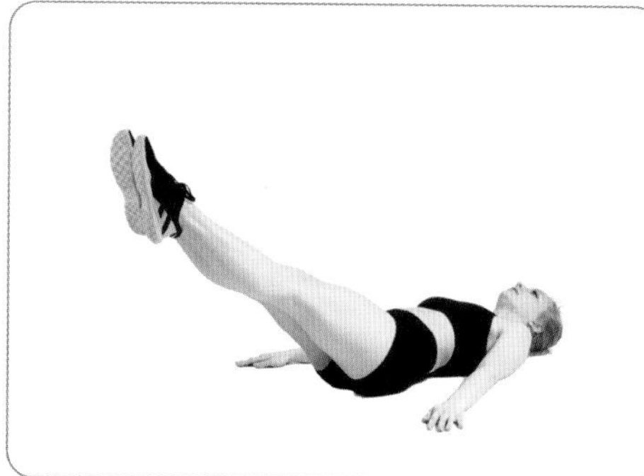
Double Leg Lift
pages 222-23

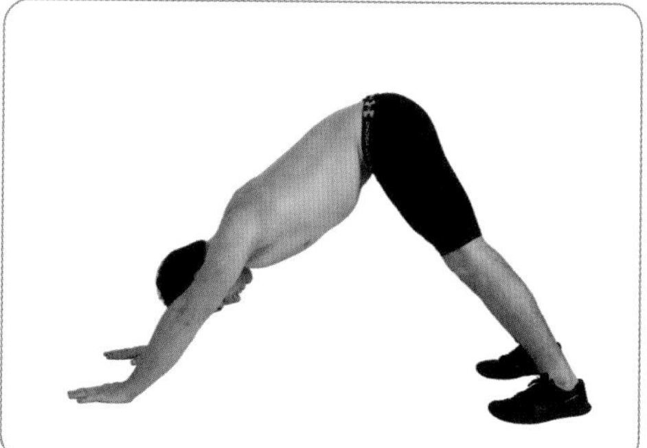
Downward-Facing Dog
pages 84-85

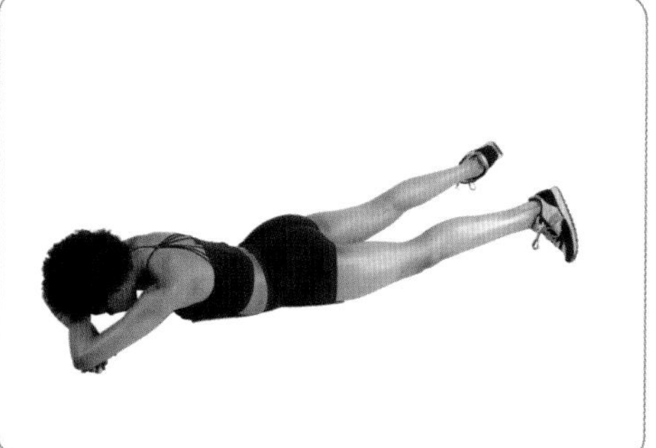
Extension Heel Beats
pages 258-59

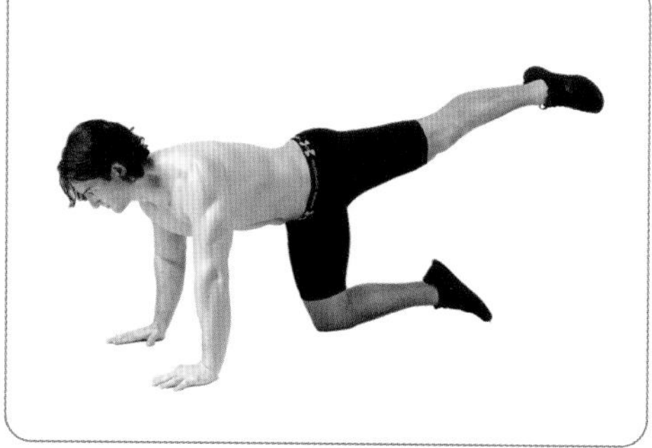
Fire-Hydrant In-Out
pages 242-43

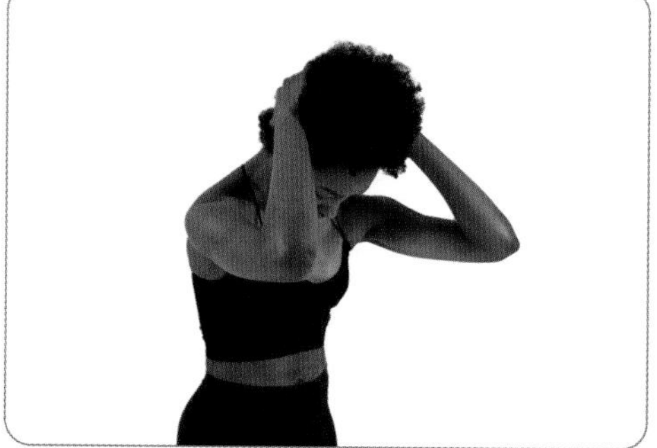
Flexion Stretch
page 24

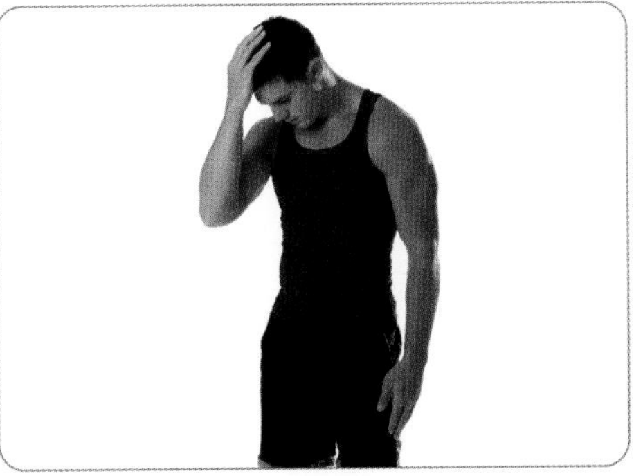
Flexion Isometric
page 25

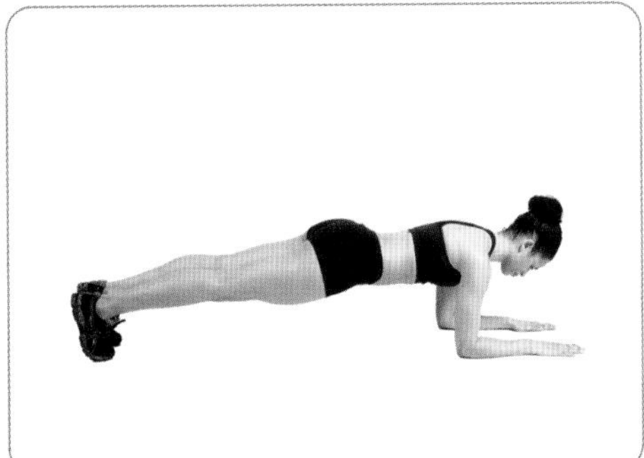
Forearm Plank
pages 306-7

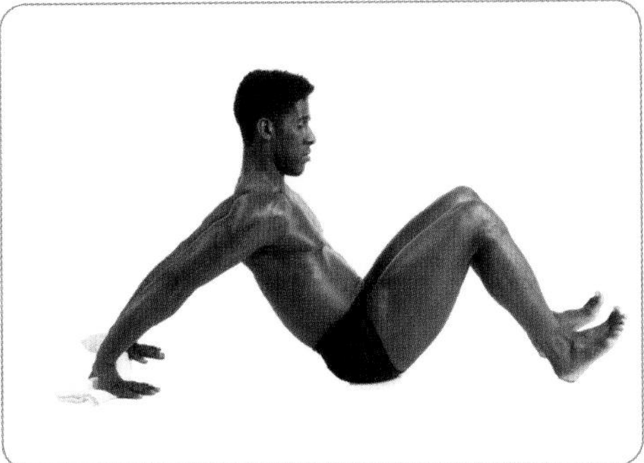
Front Deltoid Towel Stretch
page 56

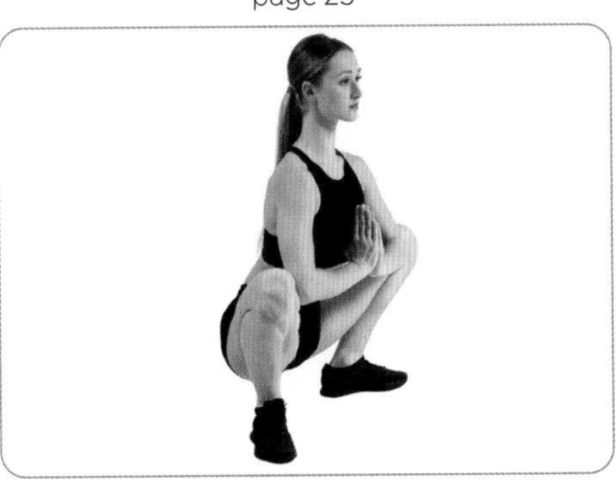
Garland Yoga Stretch
pages 42-43

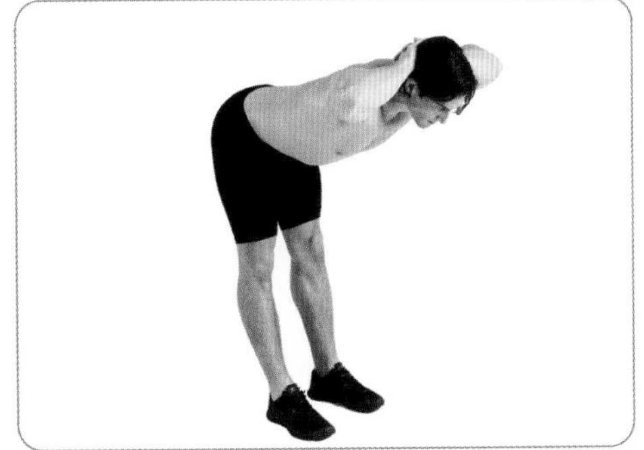
Good Morning Bow
page 170

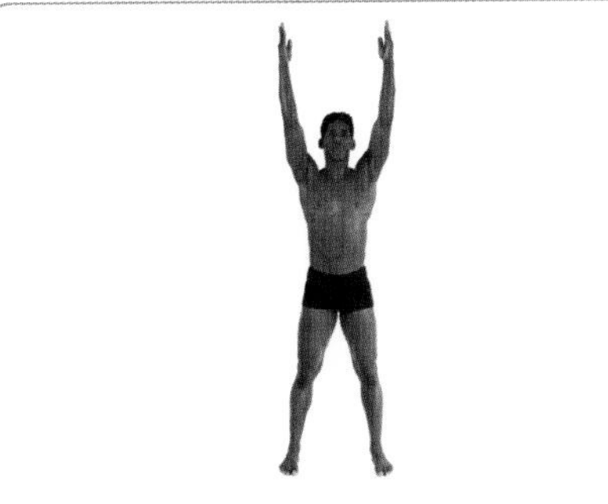
Good Morning Stretch
pages 18-19

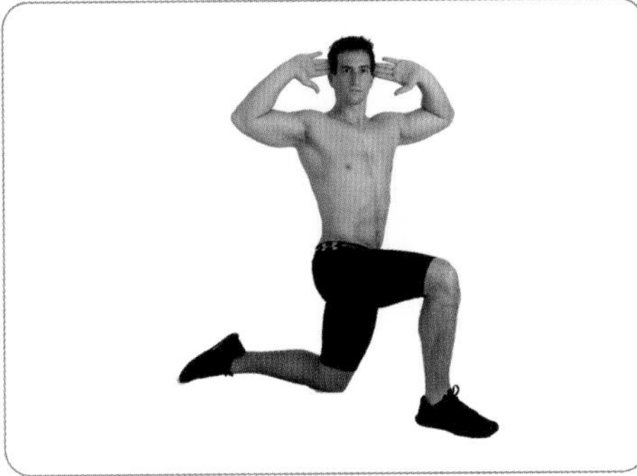
Half-Kneeling Rotation
pages 46-47

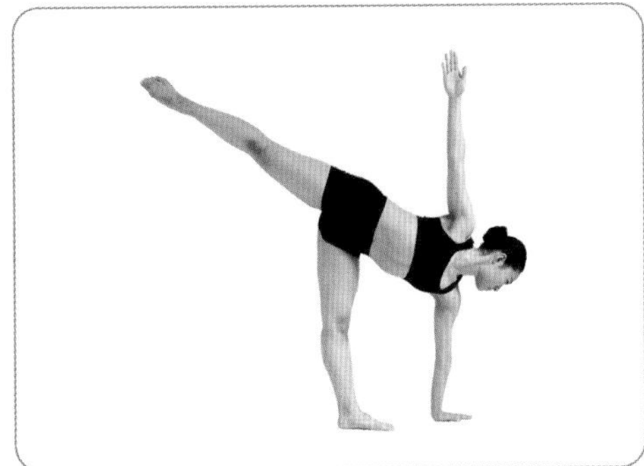
Half Moon Pose
pages 108-9

Half Straddle Stretch
pages 60-61

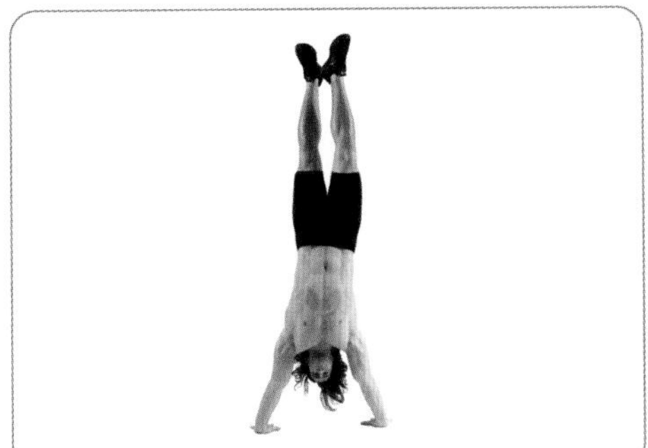
Handstand Push-Up
pages 192-93

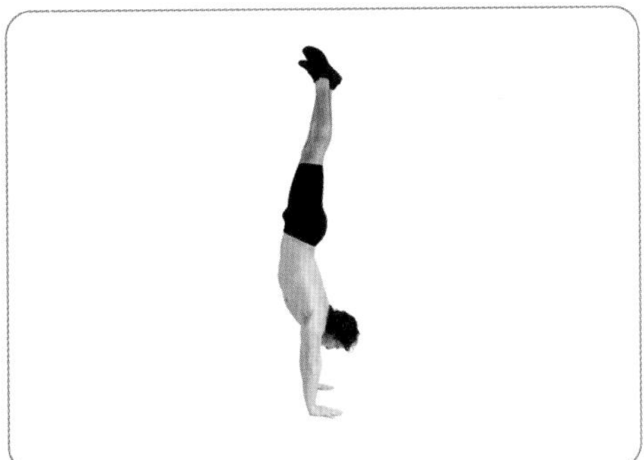
Handstand Walk
pages 302-3

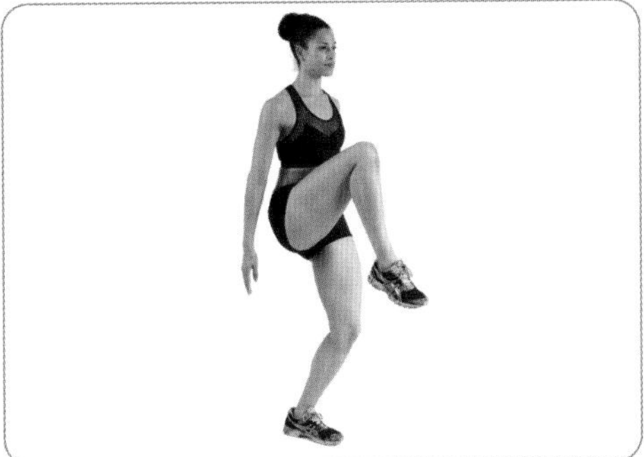

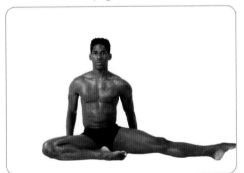
High Knees
pages 142-43

Icon Index

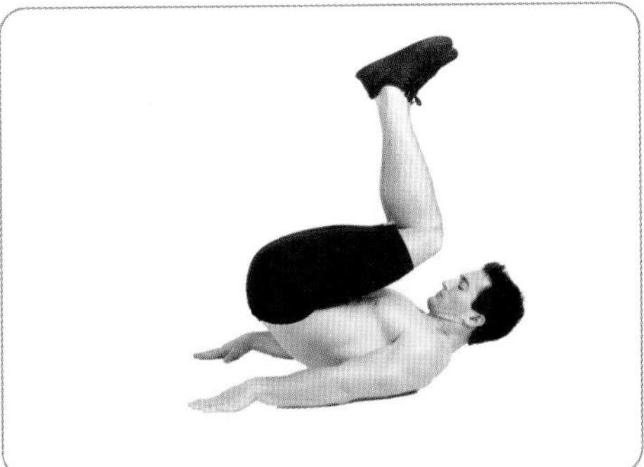

Knees to Chest
pages 220-21

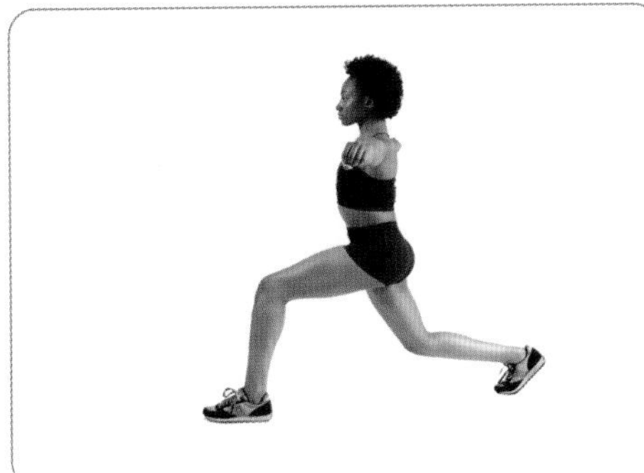

Lateral-Extension Reverse Lunge
pages 280-81

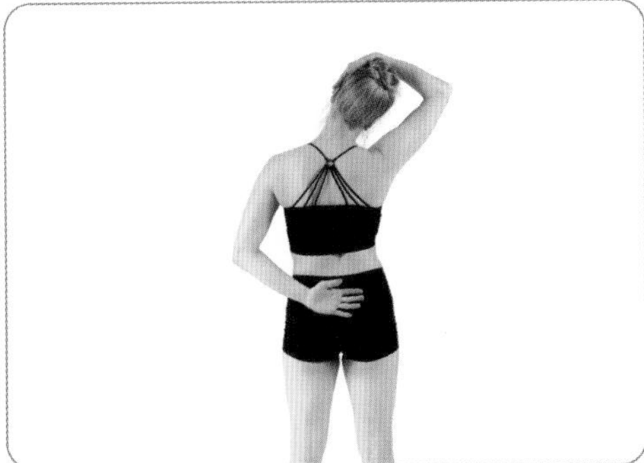

Lateral Isometric
page 27

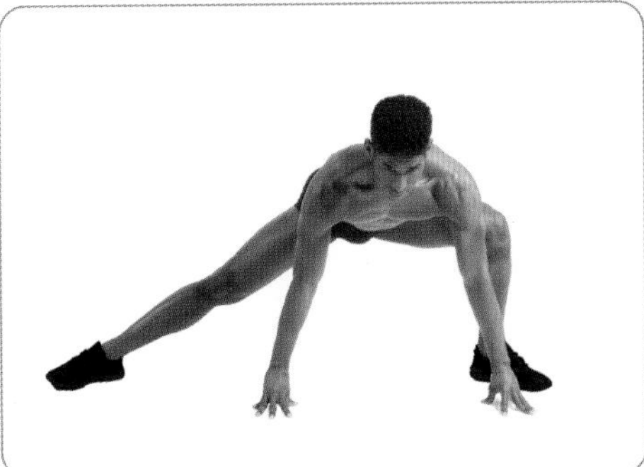

Lateral Lunge Stretch
pages 28-29

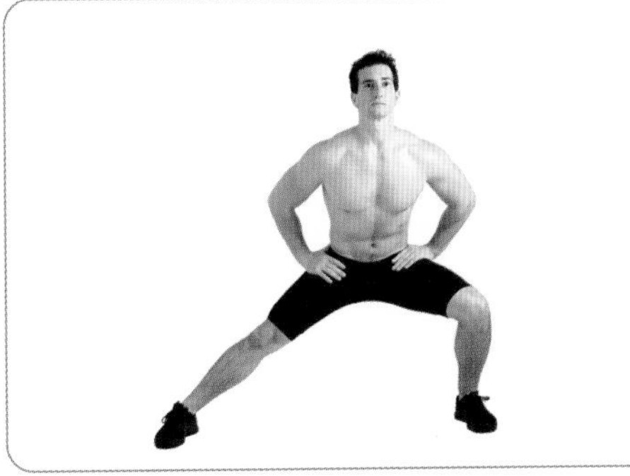

Lateral Lunge with Squat
pages 266-67

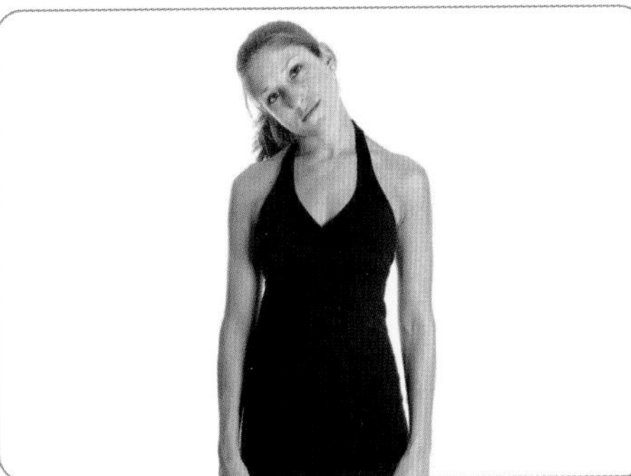

Lateral Stretch
page 26

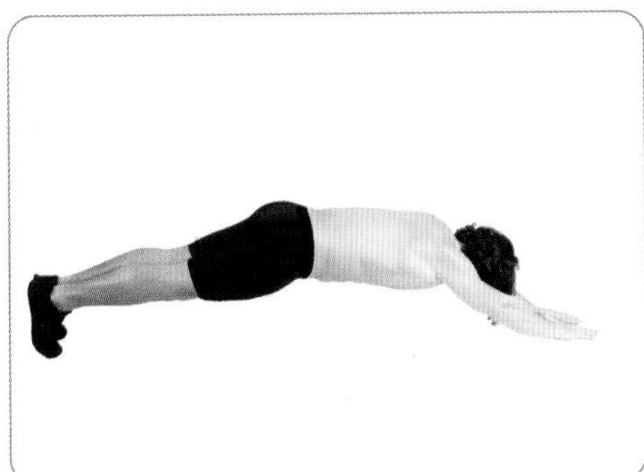

Layout Push-Up
page 171

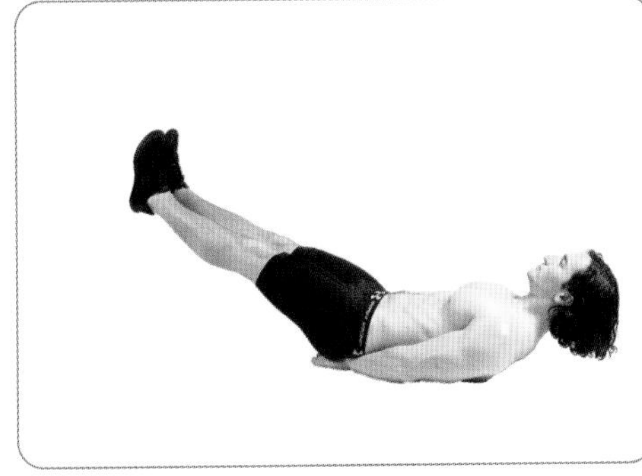

Leg Levelers
pages 238-39

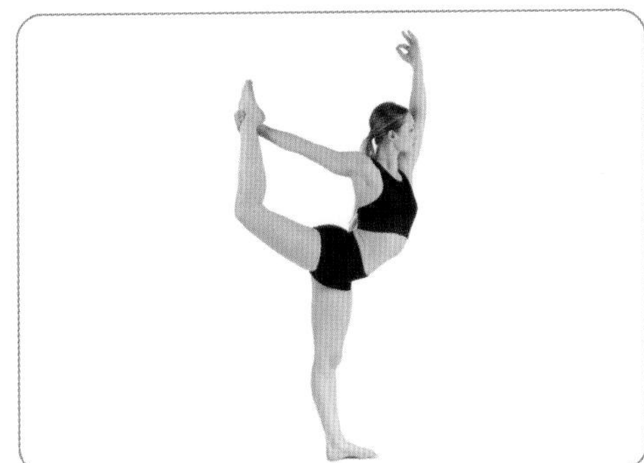

Lord of the Dance Pose
pages 118-19

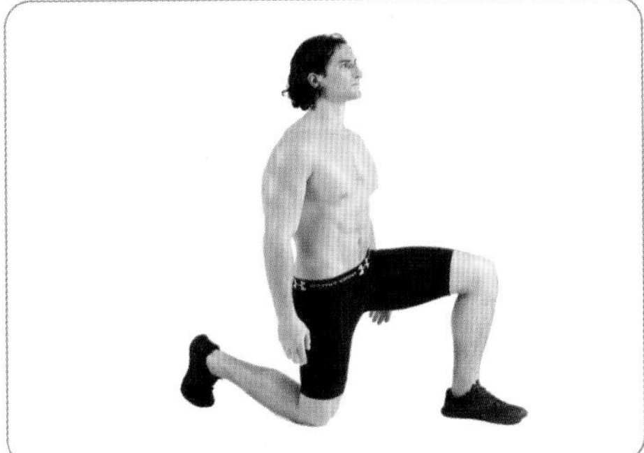

Lunge
pages 264-65

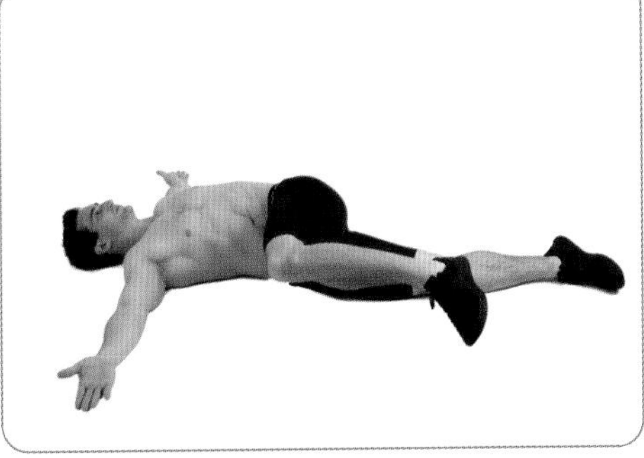

Lying-Down Pretzel Stretch
pages 34-35

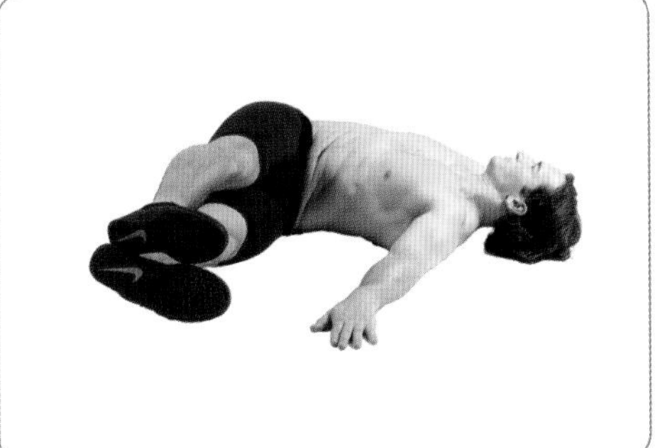

Metronome
pages 224-25

Icon Index

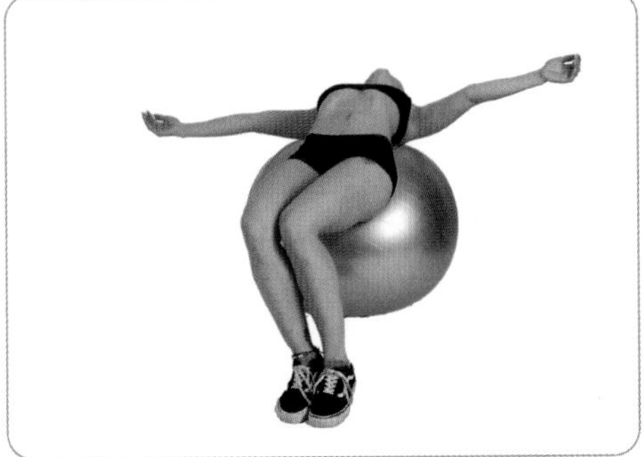
Reverse Bridge Ball Roll
pages 246-47

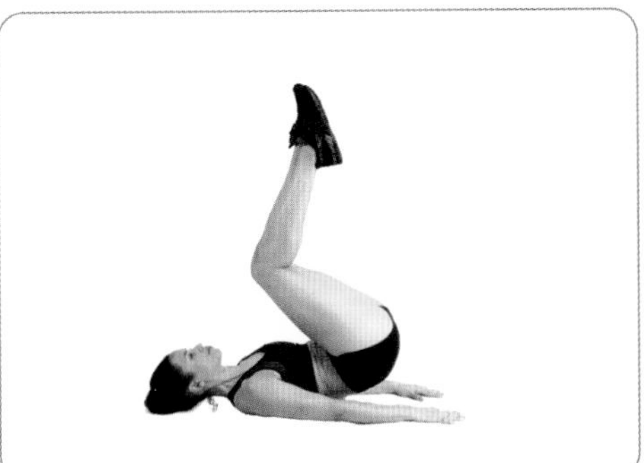
Reverse Crunch
pages 236-37

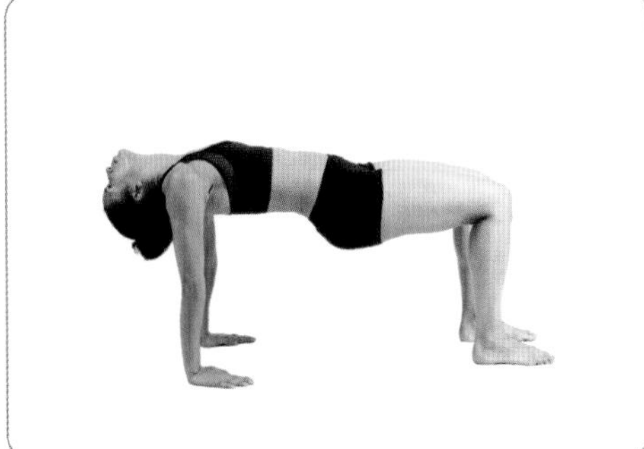
Reverse Tabletop Pose
pages 98-99

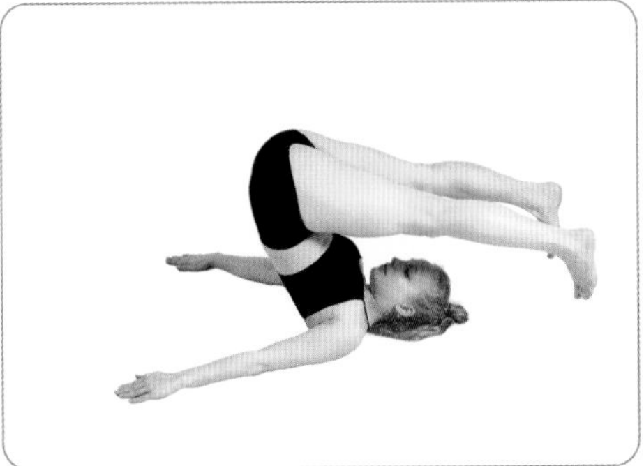
Rollover Stretch
pages 66-67

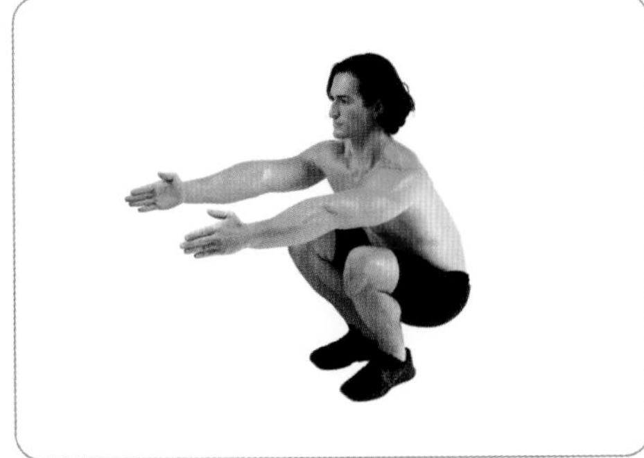
Roll-Up
pages 300-301

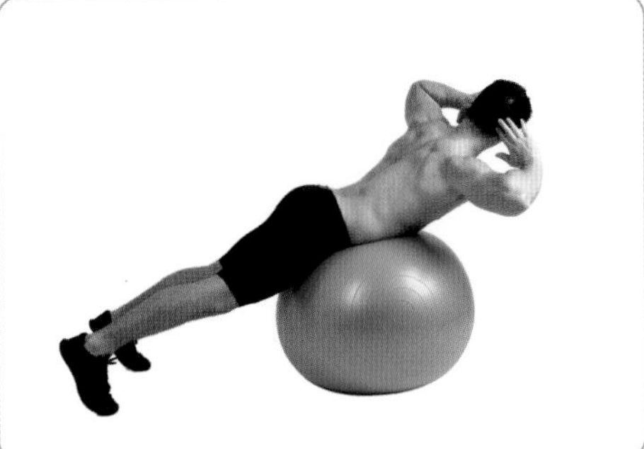
Rotated Back Extension
pages 168-69

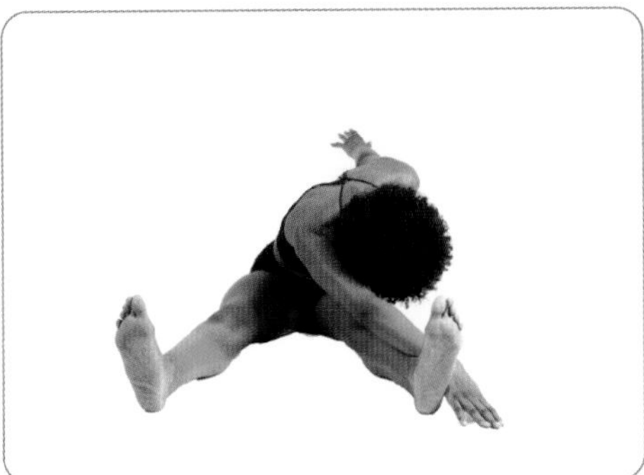
Saw Stretch
pages 32-33

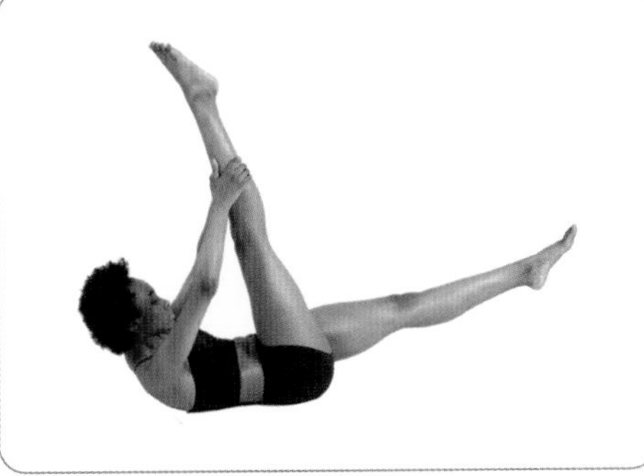
Scissors
pages 232-33

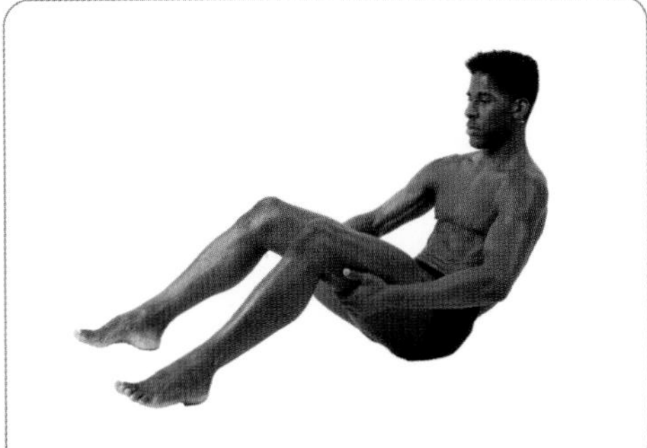
Scoop Rhomboids
page 53

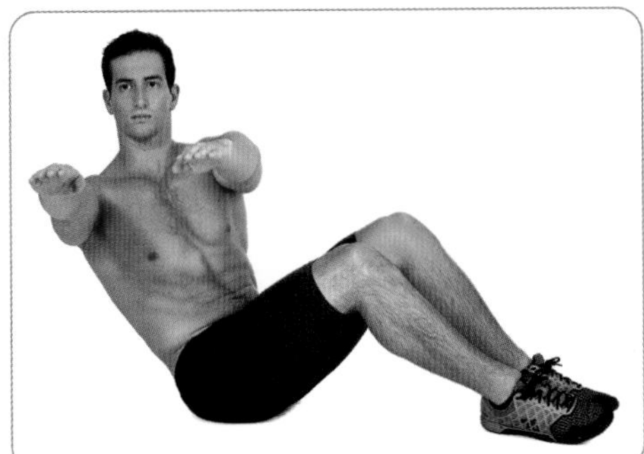
Seated Russian Twist
pages 64-65

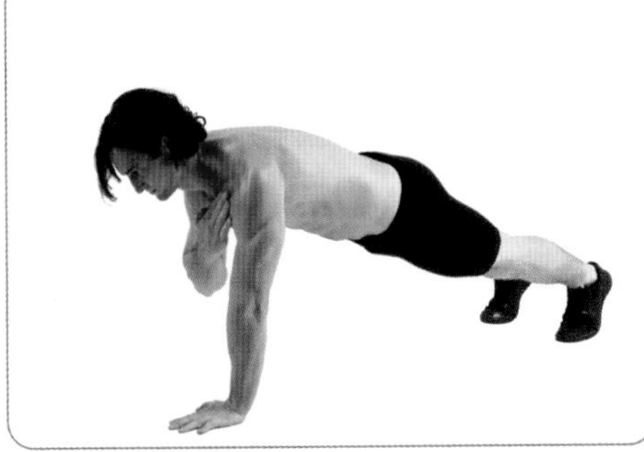
Shoulder-Tap Push-Up
pages 208-9

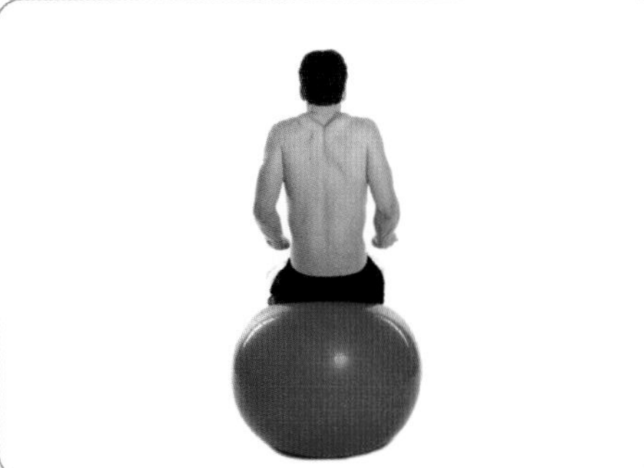
Shrug
page 23

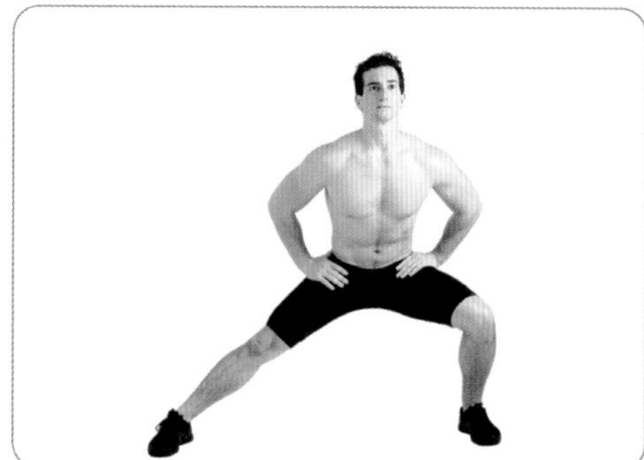

Side Adductor Stretch
pages 288-89

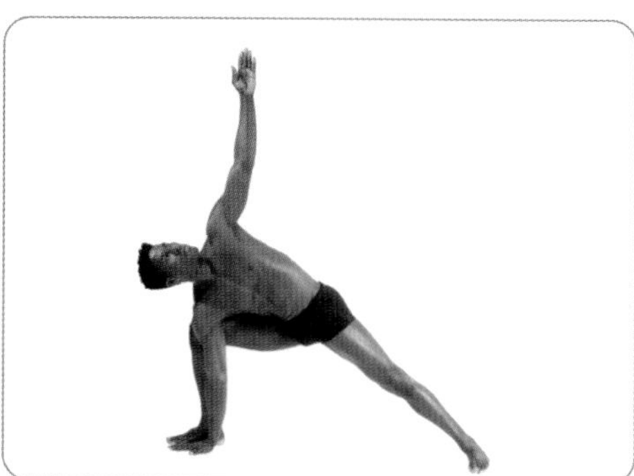

Side Angle Pose
pages 110-11

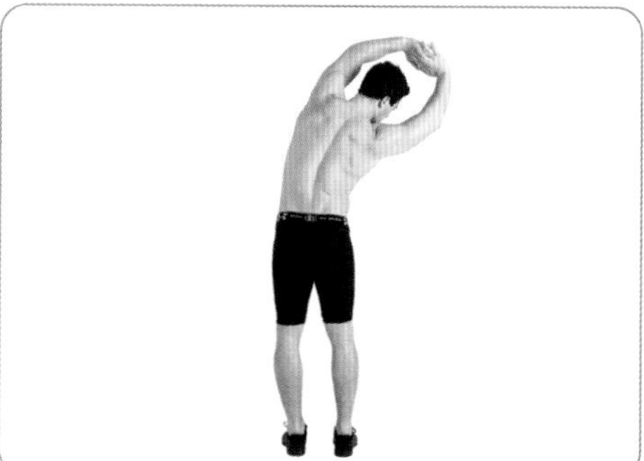

Side Bending
pages 48-49

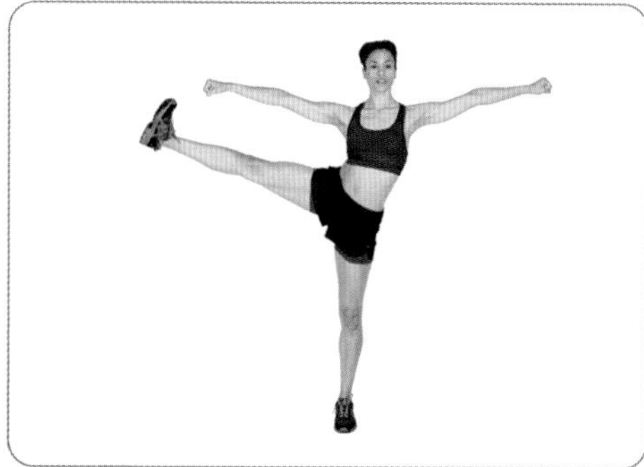

Side Kick
pages 272-73

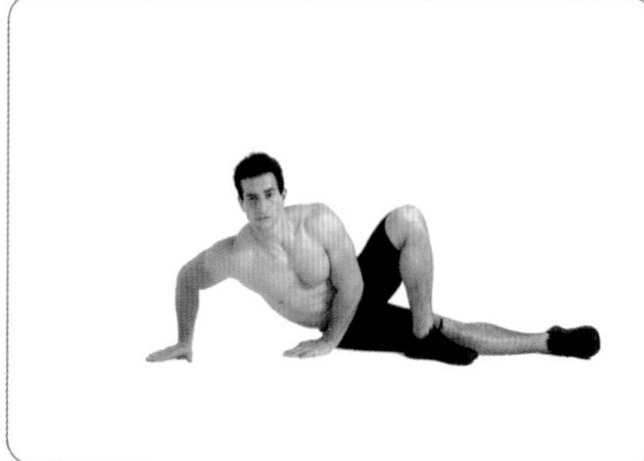

Side-Lying Rib Stretch
pages 62-63

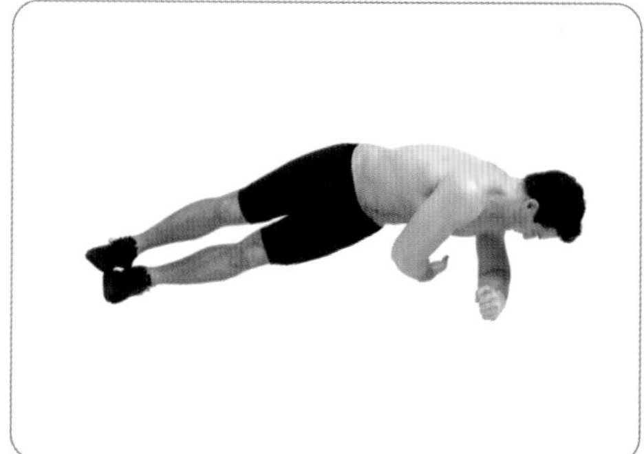

Side Plank with Reach-Under
pages 312-13

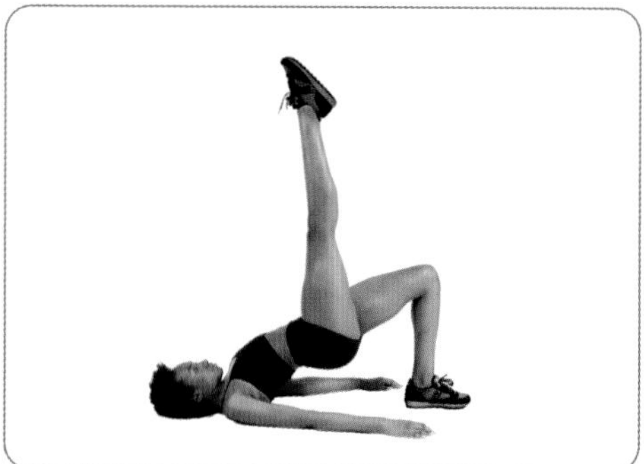

Single-Leg Gluteal Lift
pages 262-63

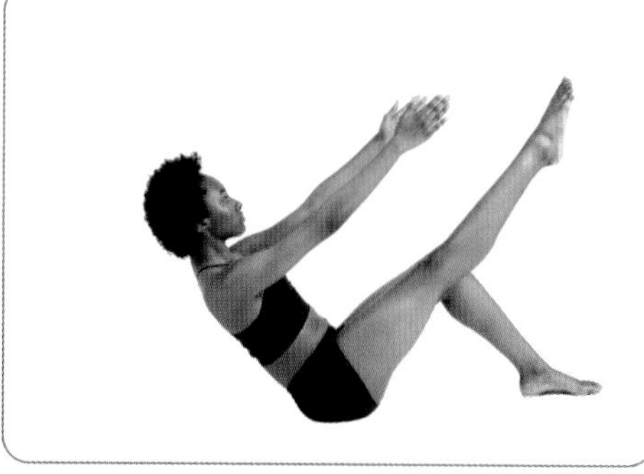

Single-Leg V-Up
pages 244-45

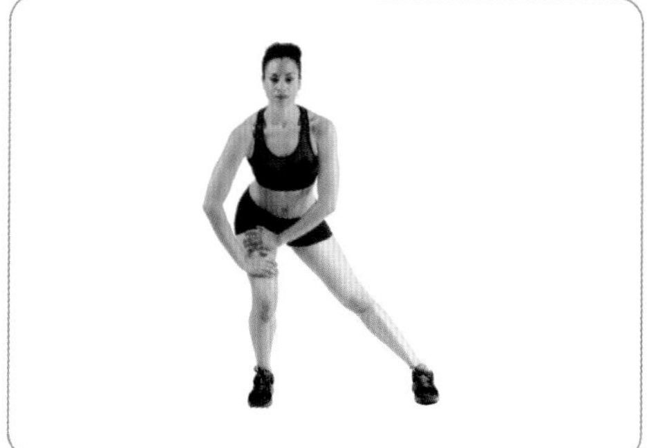

Skater's Lunge
pages 282-83

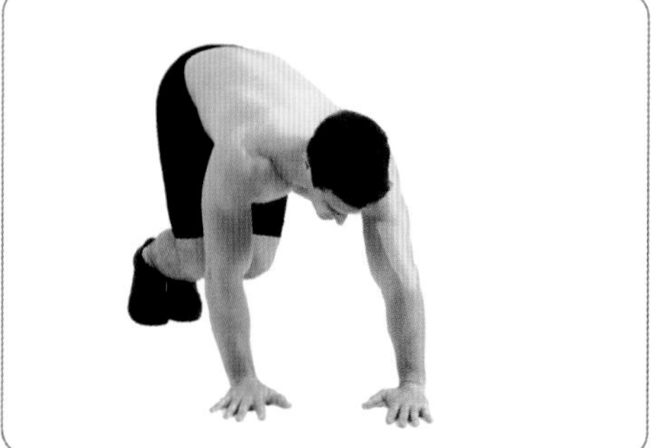

Slalom Skier
pages 296-97

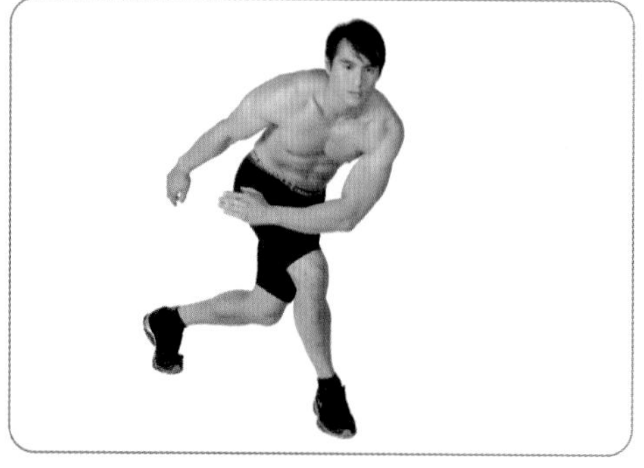

Speed Skater
pages 134-35

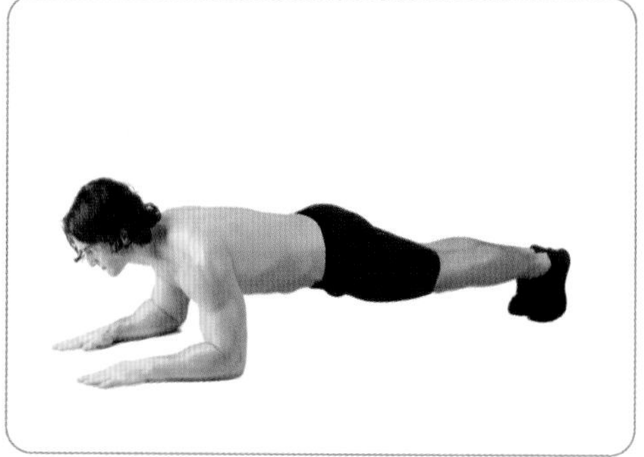

Sphinx Push-Up
page 140

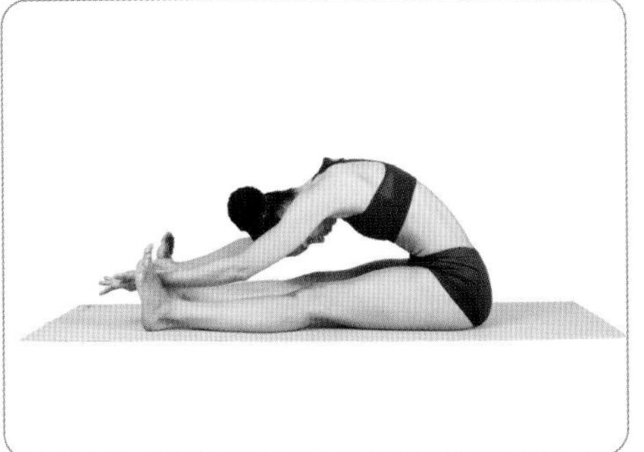
Spine Stretch Forward
pages 54-55

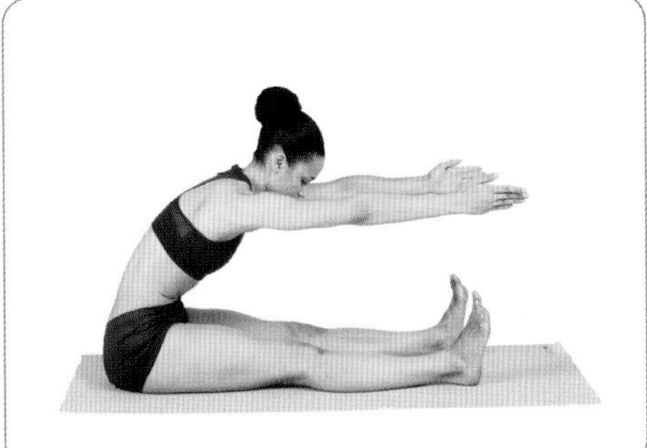
Spine Stretch Reaching
page 57

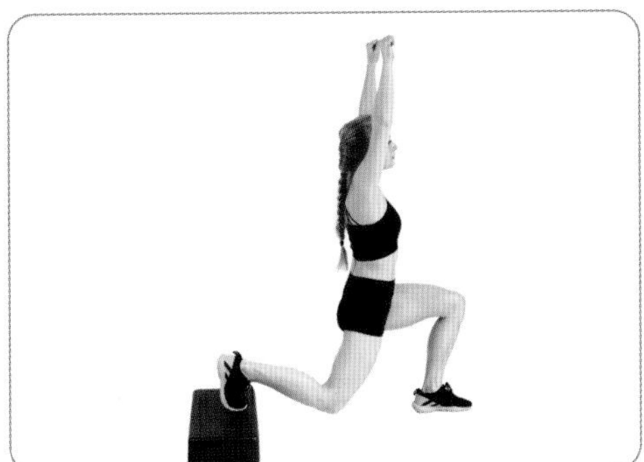
Split Squat with Overhead Press
pages 278-79

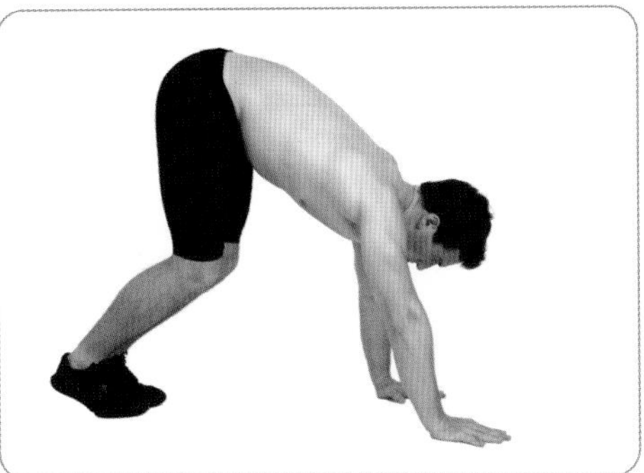
Sprawl Push-Up
pages 202-3

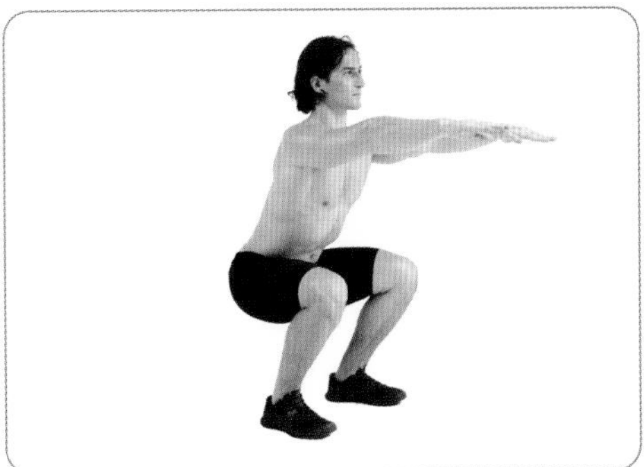
Squat
pages 260-61

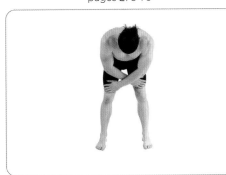
Standing Back Roll
pages 52-53

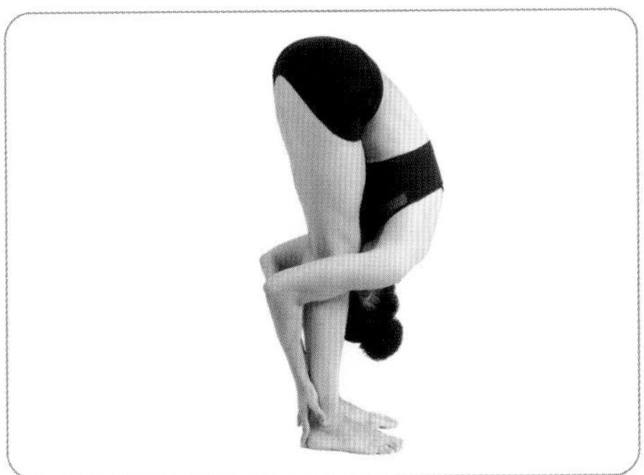
Standing Forward Bend
pages 68-69

Standing Hamstrings Stretch
page 41

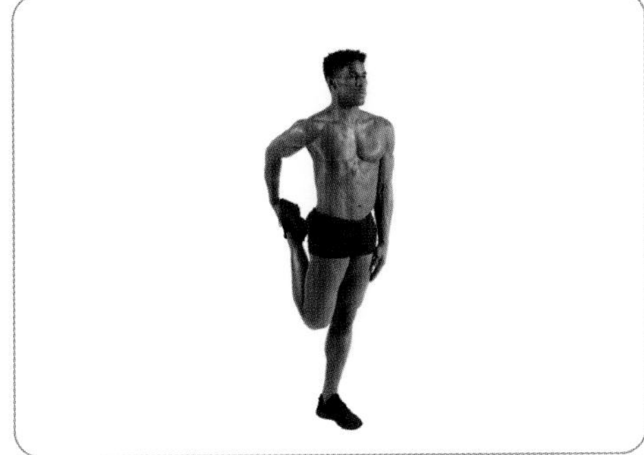
Standing Quadriceps Stretch
page 40

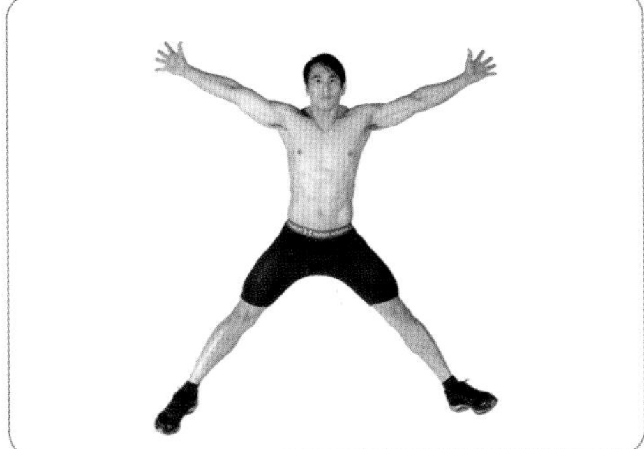
Star Jump
pages 130-31

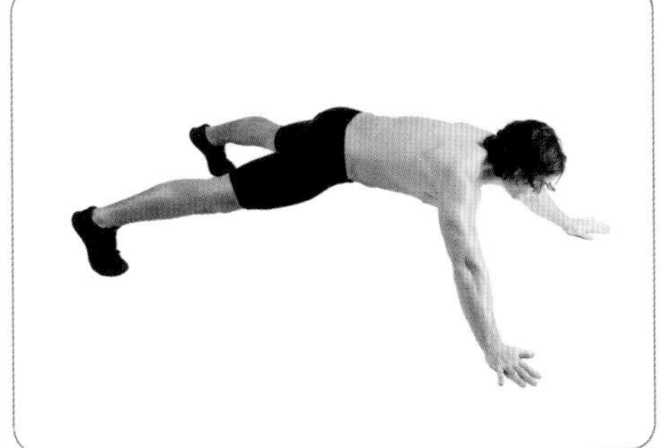
Star Push-Up
page 141

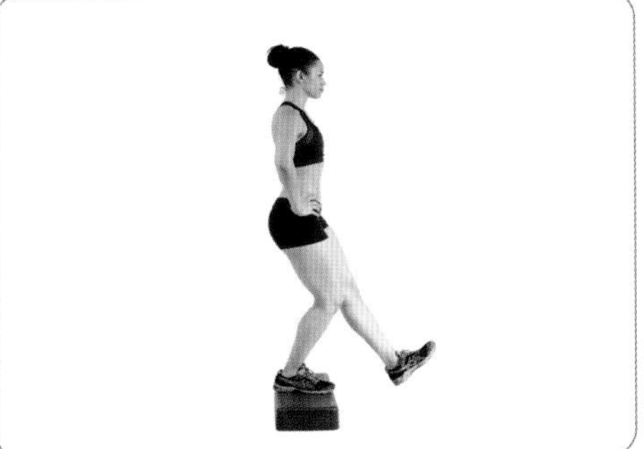

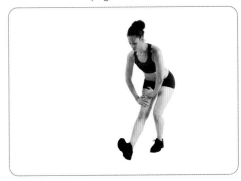
Step-Down
pages 284-85

Icon Index

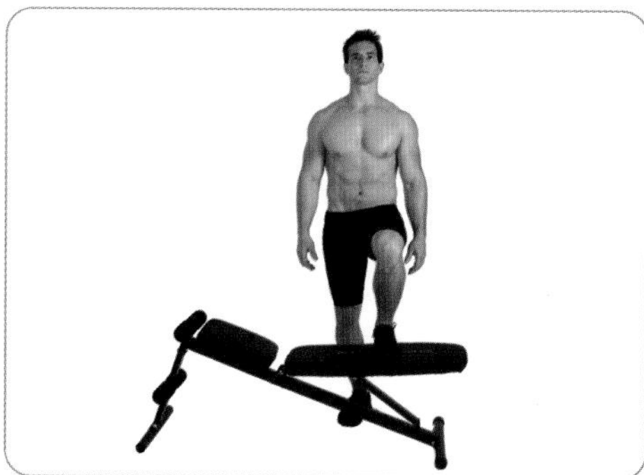
Step-Up
pages 286-87

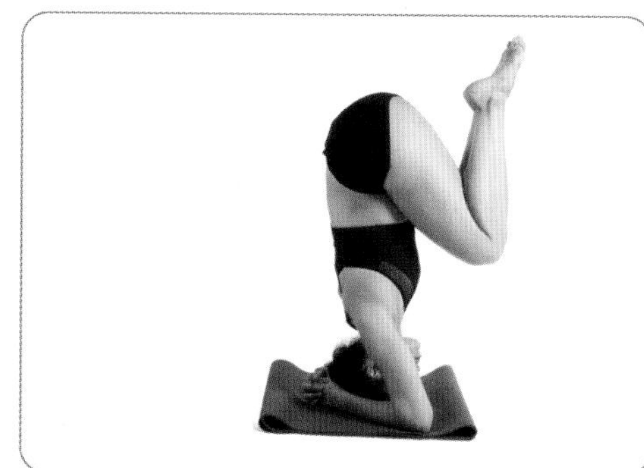
Supported Headstand
pages 104-5

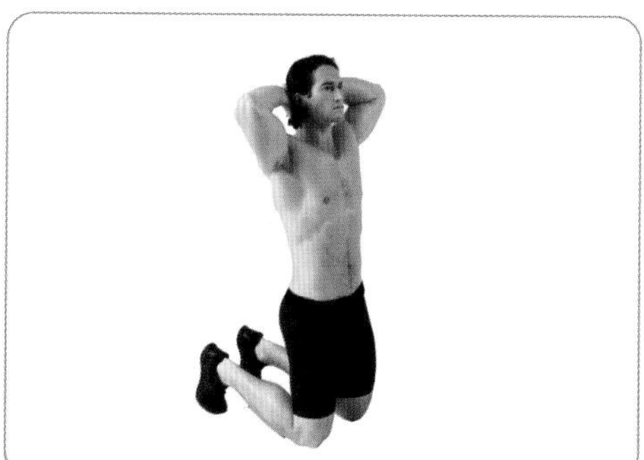
Surrender
page 276

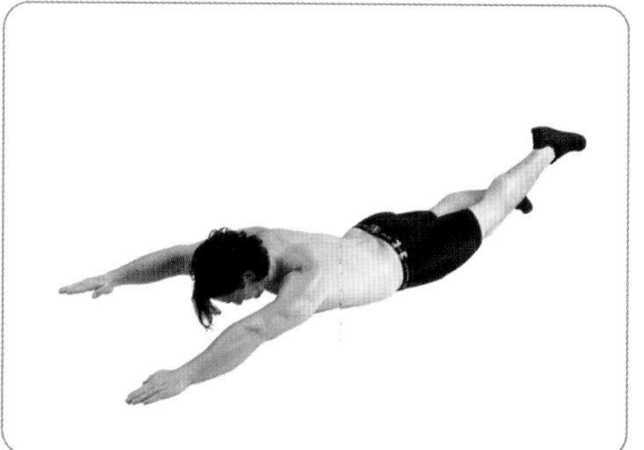
Swimmer
pages 158-59

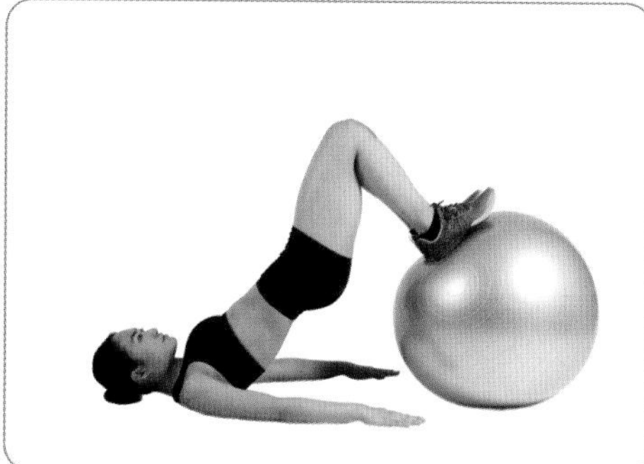

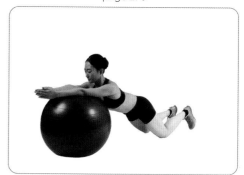
Swiss Ball Hamstrings Curl
pages 292-93

Swiss Ball Rollout
pages 252-53

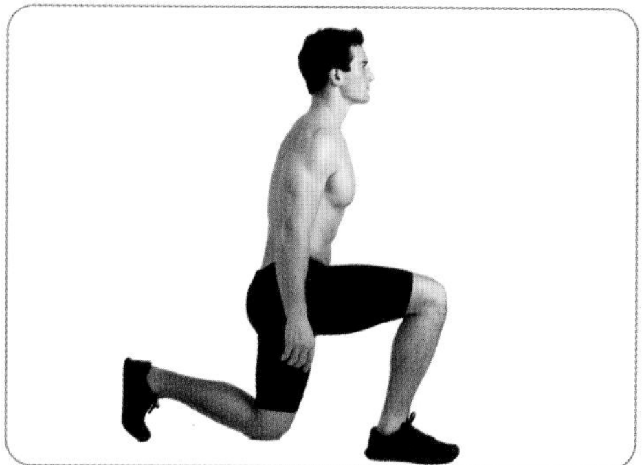
Switch Lunge
pages 144-45

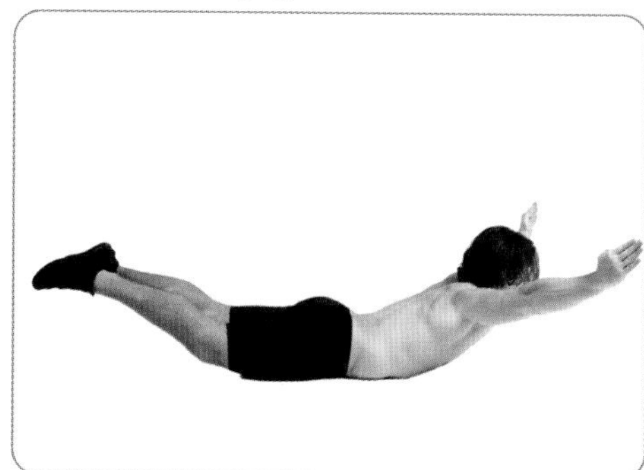
The Y
page 167

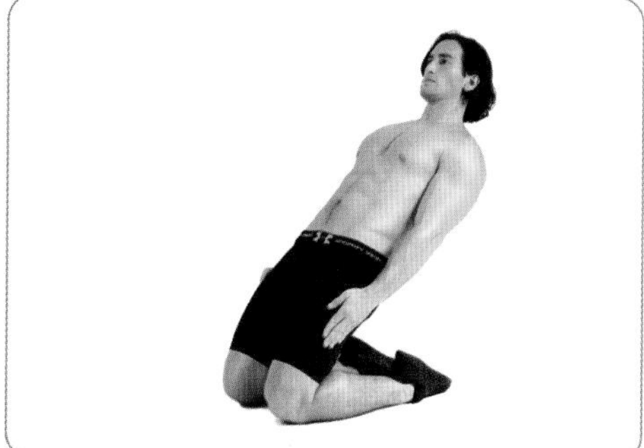
Thigh Rock-Back
pages 234-35

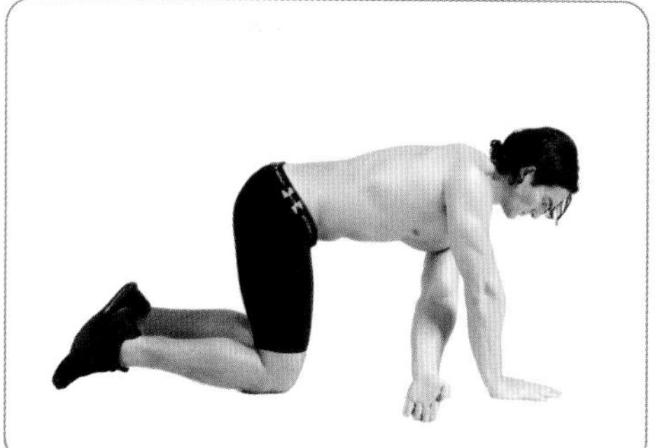
Thread the Needle
pages 154-55

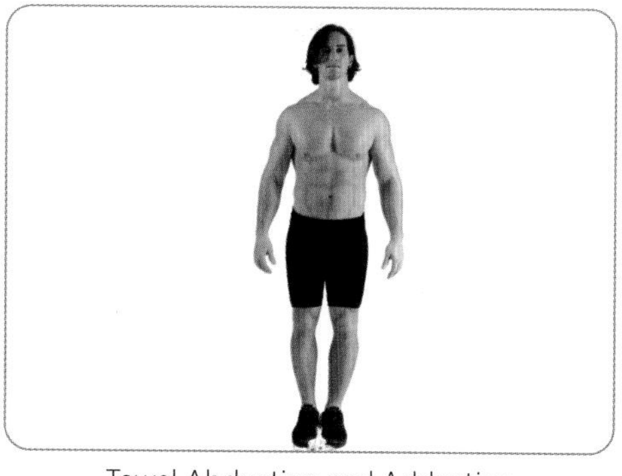
Towel Abduction and Adduction
page 275

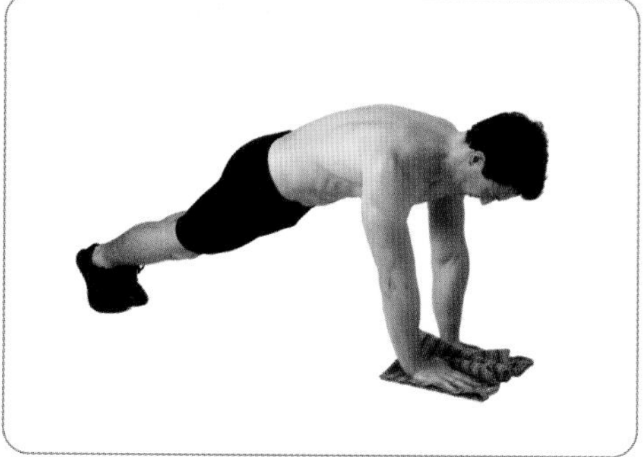
Towel Fly
pages 200-201

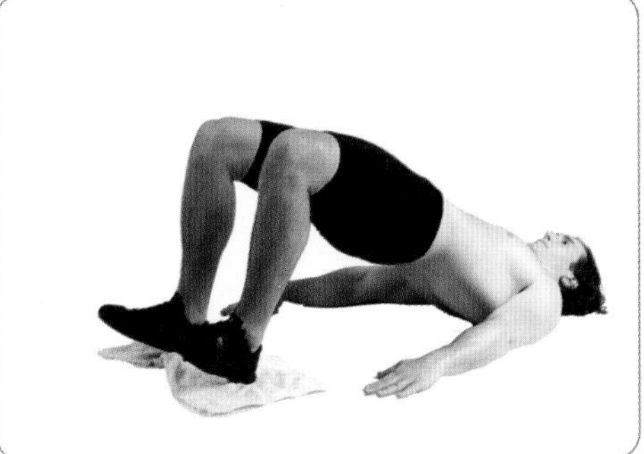

Towel Hamstrings Pull
page 274

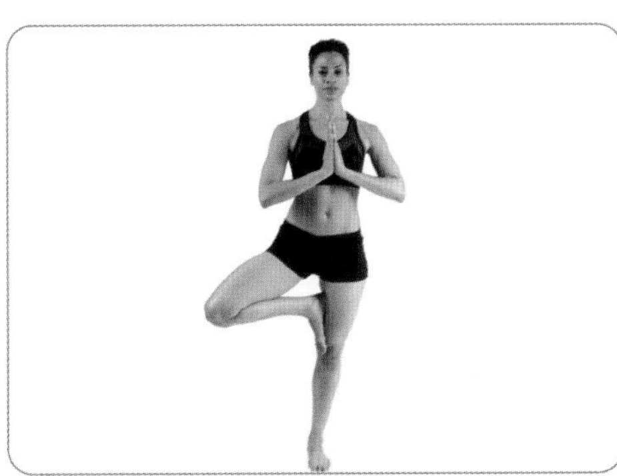

Tree Pose
pages 80-81

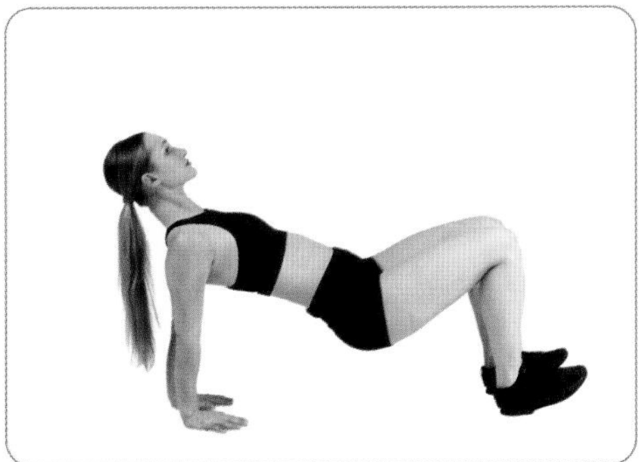

Triceps Dip
pages 188-89

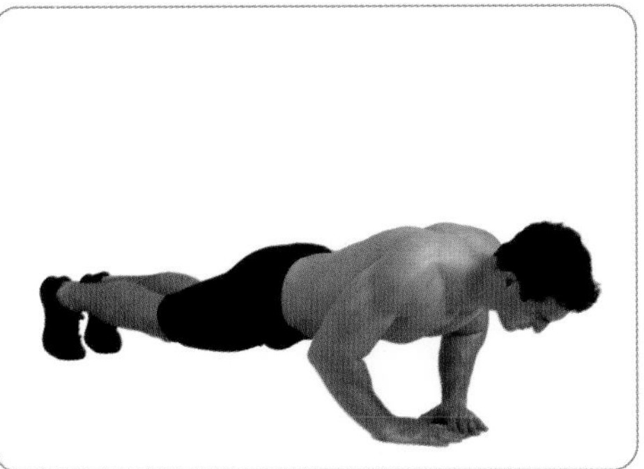

Triceps Push-Up
pages 178-79

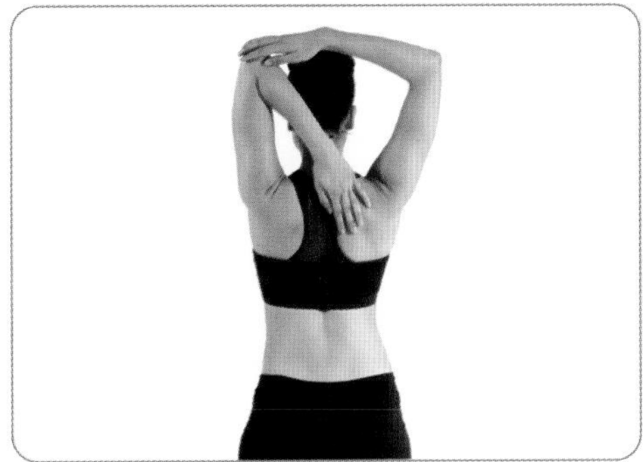

Triceps Stretch
page 36

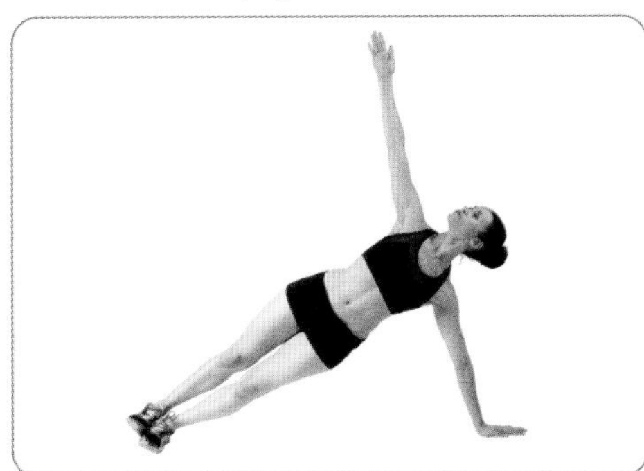

T-Stabilization
pages 310-11

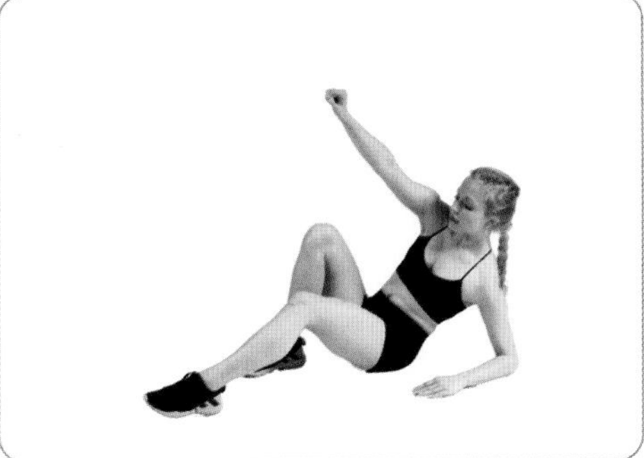

Turkish Get-Up
pages 304-5

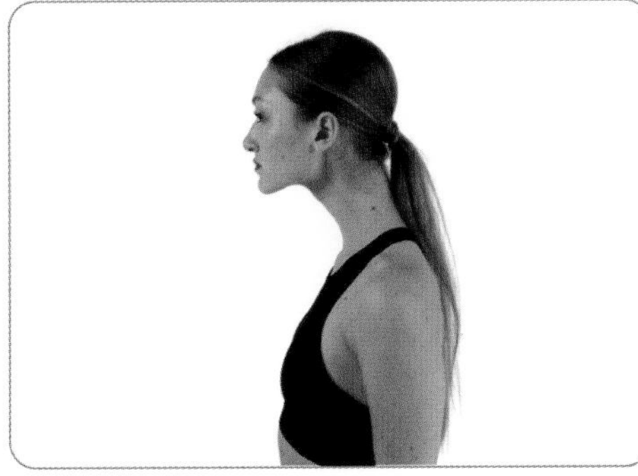

Turtle Neck
page 22

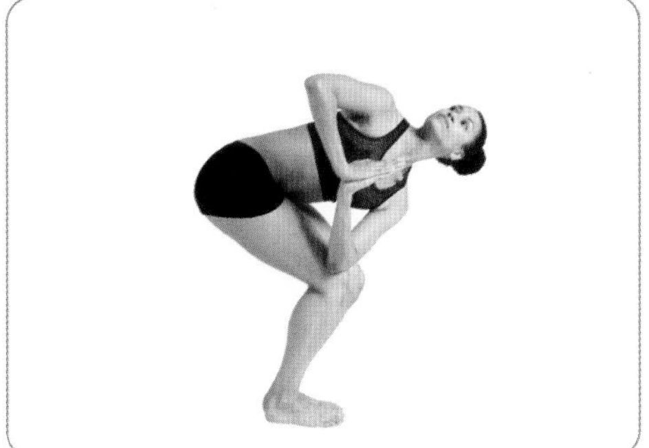

Twisting Chair Pose
pages 78-79

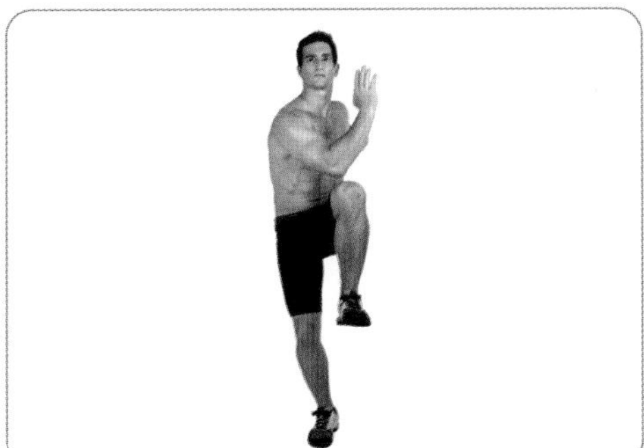

Twisting Knee Raise
pages 128-29

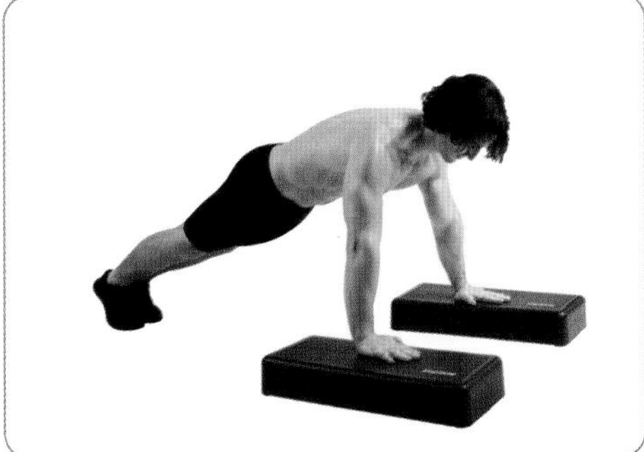

Two-Level Push-Up
pages 148-49

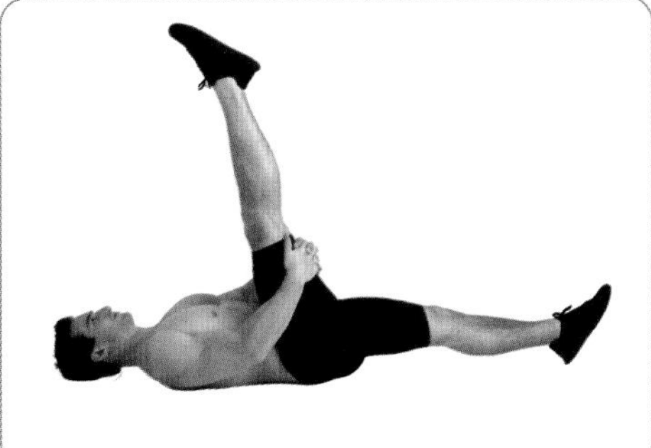

Unilateral Leg Raise
page 277

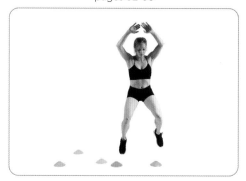

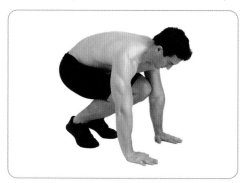

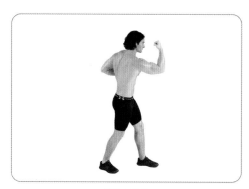

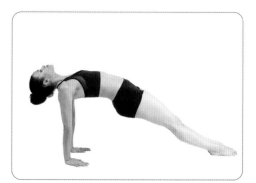

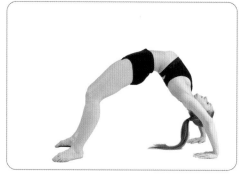

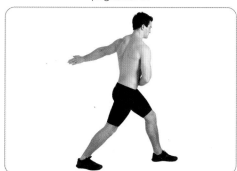

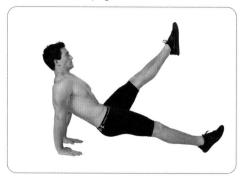

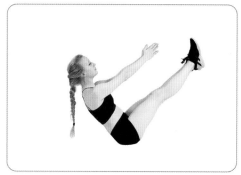

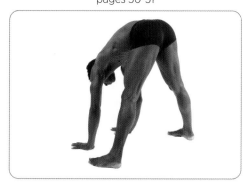

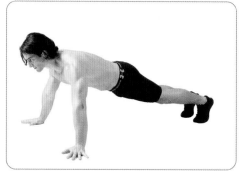

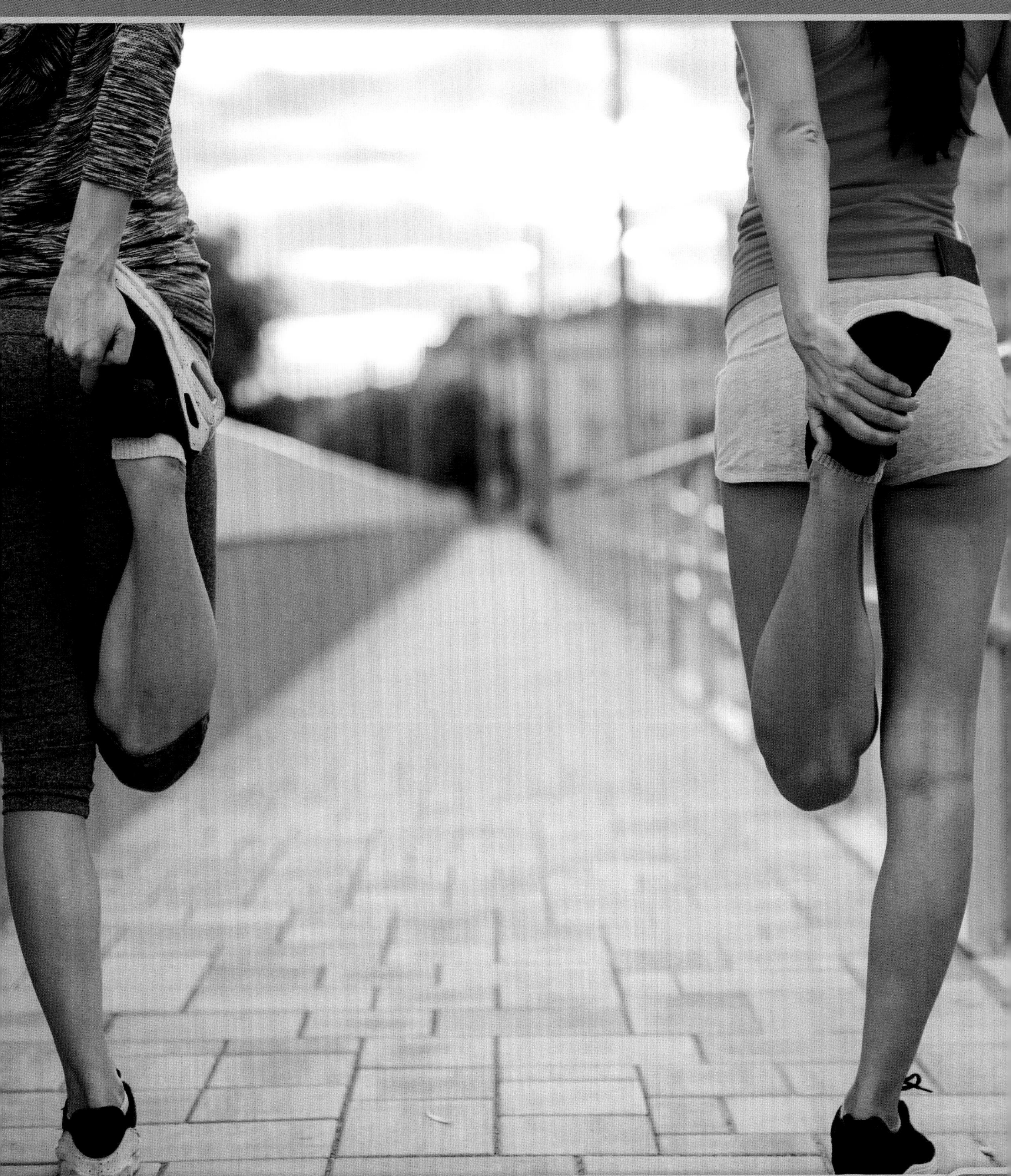

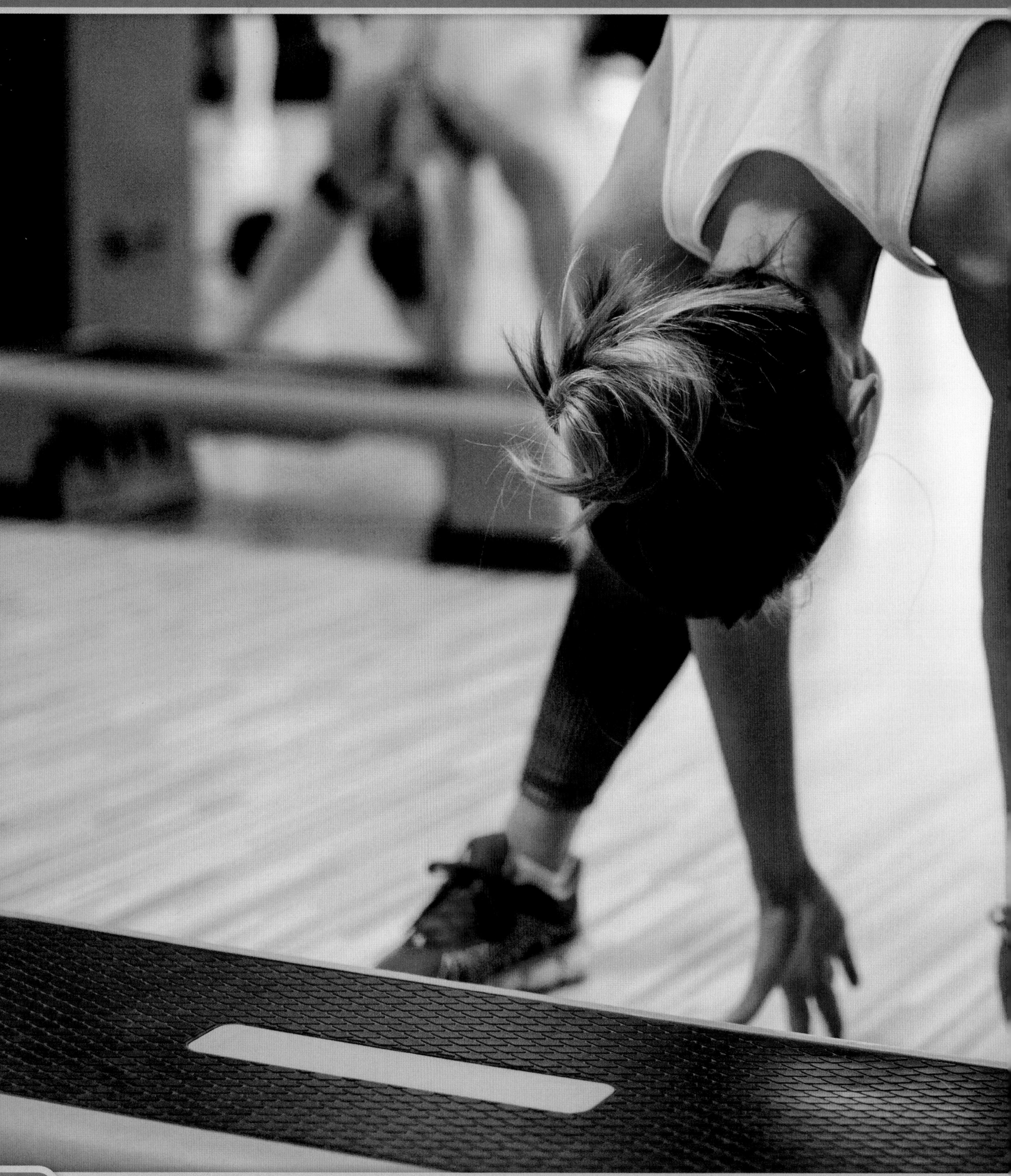

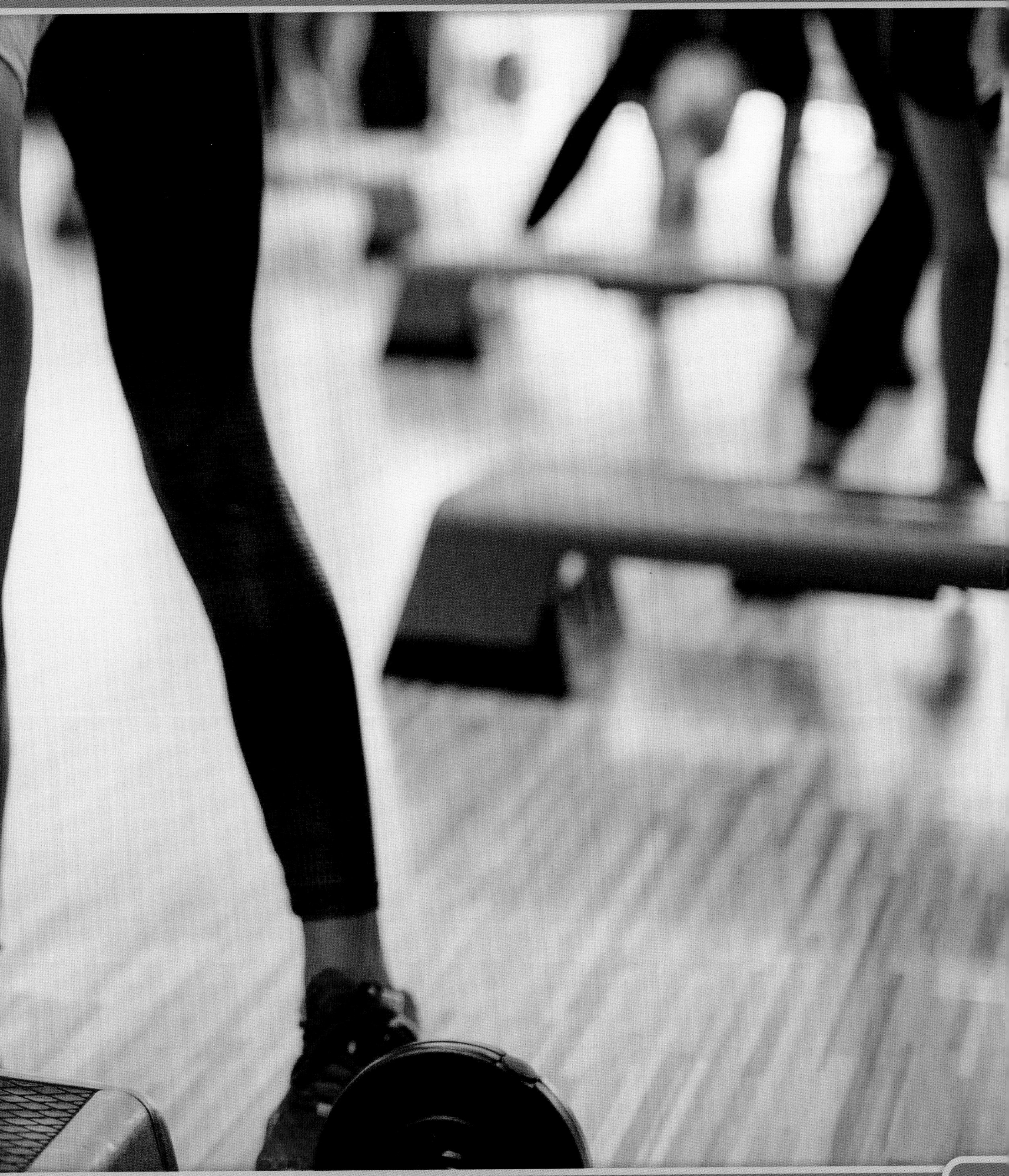

Index

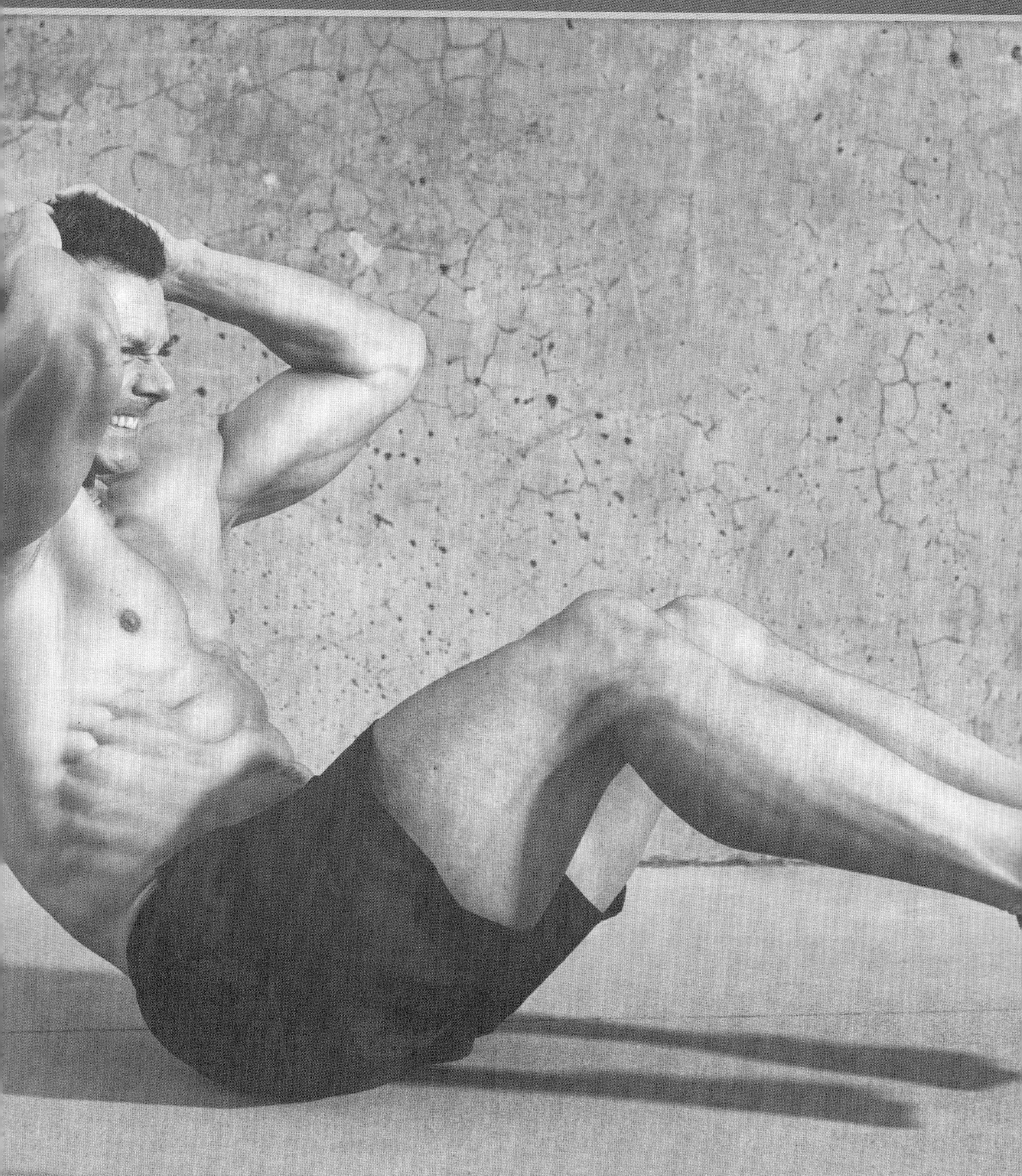

Index

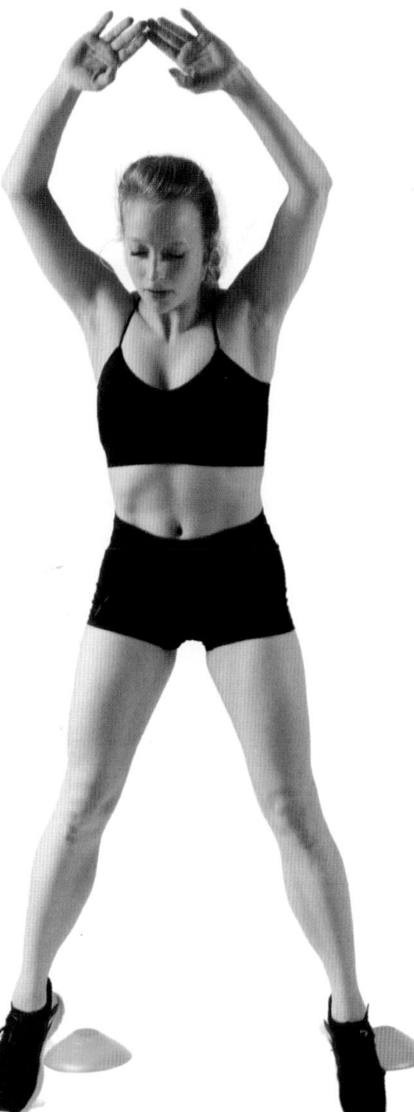

Index

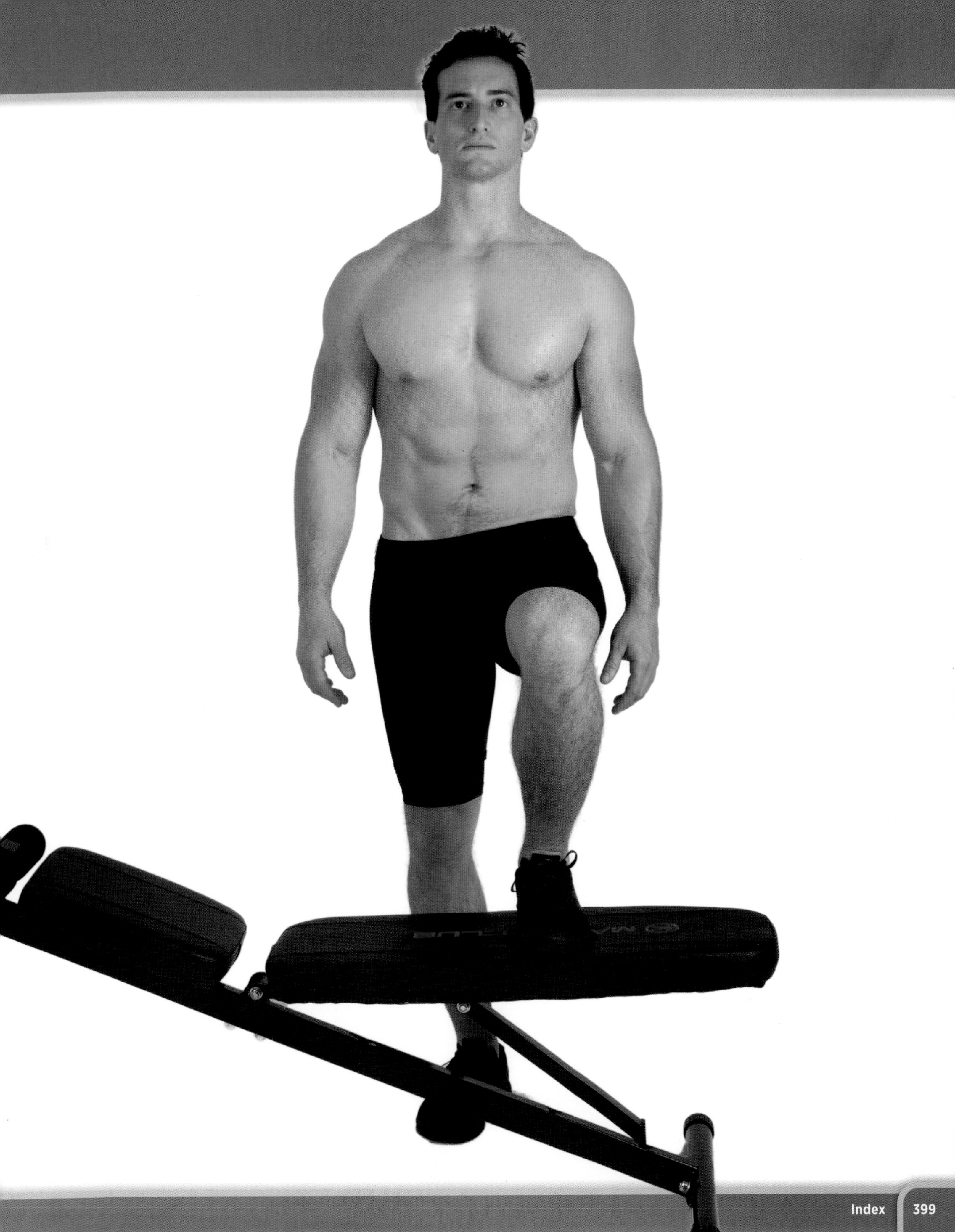

Image Credits

PHOTOGRAPHY

Naila Ruechel

MODELS

Philip Chan
Natasha Diamond-Walker
Jessica Gambellur
Alex Geissbuhler
Lloyd Knight
Larissa Terada

ADDITIONAL PHOTOGRAPHY

4 & 396 Volodymyr Tverdokhlib | Dreamstime.com
7 Andreadonetti | Dreamstime.com
8–9 Albertshakirov | Dreamstime.com
11 Albertshakirov | Dreamstime.com
13 Konstantin Yuganov | Dreamstime.com
16–17 mavo | Shutterstock.com
72–73 My Good Images | Shutterstock.com
120–21 Maridav | Shutterstock.com
152–53 GP PIXSTOCK | Shutterstock.com
174–75 Khwaneigq | Dreamstime.com
194–95 Antoniodiaz | Shutterstock.com
212–13 ESB Professional | Shutterstock.com
254–55 fizkes | Shutterstock.com
294–95 Roman Samborskyi | Shutterstock.com
315–16 engagestock | Shutterstock.com
374–75 fotoliza | Shutterstock.com
393 NDAB Creativity | Shutterstock.com
394–95 shevtsovy | Shutterstock.com

ILLUSTRATIONS

All anatomical illustrations by Adam Moore and Hector Diaz/
3DLabz Animation Limited. www.3dlabz.com
Full-body anatomy and insets by Linda Bucklin/Shutterstock.com